Neurologic Disorders of the Larynx

Second Edition

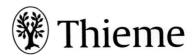

Neurologic Disorders of the Larynx

Second Edition

Andrew Blitzer, MD, DDS, FACS
Professor
Department of Otolaryngology–Head and Neck Surgery
College of Physicians and Surgeons
Columbia University
Director
New York Center for Voice and Swallowing Disorders
New York Head and Neck Institute
New York, New York

Mitchell F. Brin, MD
Clinical Professor
Department of Neurology
University of California–Irvine
Senior Vice President and Chief Scientific Officer
Allergan, LLC
Irvine, California

Lorraine O. Ramig, PhD, CCC-SLP
Professor
Department of Speech, Language, and Hearing Science
University of Colorado
Boulder, Colorado
Senior Scientist
National Center for Voice and Speech
Denver, Colorado

Thieme
New York • Stuttgart

Thieme Medical Publishers, Inc.
333 Seventh Ave.
New York, NY 10001

Executive Editor: Timothy Hiscock
Managing Editor: J. Owen Zurhellen IV
Editorial Assistant: Chad Hollingsworth
Editorial Director: Michael Wachinger
Vice President, Production and Electronic Publishing: Anne T. Vinnicombe
Production Editor: Print Matters, Inc.
Vice President, International Marketing: Cornelia Schulze
Chief Financial Officer: Peter Van Woerden
President: Brian D. Scanlan
Compositor: Thomson Digital Services
Printer: Sheridan Books, Inc.
Cover illustrations: Karl Wesker and Markus Voll

Library of Congress Cataloging-in-Publication Data

Neurologic disorders of the larynx / [edited by] Andrew Blitzer, Mitchell F. Brin, Lorraine O. Ramig. — 2nd ed.
  p. ; cm.
Includes bibliographical references and index.
ISBN 978-1-58890-498-0 (alk. paper)
  1. Larynx—Diseases. 2. Larynx—Innervation. I. Blitzer, Andrew. II. Brin, Mitchell F. III. Ramig, Lorraine O.
  [DNLM: 1. Laryngeal Diseases—physiopathology. 2. Laryngeal Nerves. 3. Larynx—physiology. WV 500 N4945 2009]
RF522 .N
616.2'2—dc22
                                           2009000788

Copyright ©2009 by Thieme Medical Publishers, Inc. This book, including all parts thereof, is legally protected by copyright. Any use, exploitation, or commercialization outside the narrow limits set by copyright legislation without the publisher's consent is illegal and liable to prosecution. This applies in particular to photostat reproduction, copying, mimeographing or duplication of any kind, translating, preparation of microfilms, and electronic data processing and storage.

Important note: Medical knowledge is ever-changing. As new research and clinical experience broaden our knowledge, changes in treatment and drug therapy may be required. The authors and editors of the material herein have consulted sources believed to be reliable in their efforts to provide information that is complete and in accord with the standards accepted at the time of publication. However, in view of the possibility of human error by the authors, editors, or publisher of the work herein or changes in medical knowledge, neither the authors, editors, or publisher, nor any other party who has been involved in the preparation of this work, warrants that the information contained herein is in every respect accurate or complete, and they are not responsible for any errors or omissions or for the results obtained from use of such information. Readers are encouraged to confirm the information contained herein with other sources. For example, readers are advised to check the product information sheet included in the package of each drug they plan to administer to be certain that the information contained in this publication is accurate and that changes have not been made in the recommended dose or in the contraindications for administration. This recommendation is of particular importance in connection with new or infrequently used drugs.

Some of the product names, patents, and registered designs referred to in this book are in fact registered trademarks or proprietary names even though specific reference to this fact is not always made in the text. Therefore, the appearance of a name without designation as proprietary is not to be construed as a representation by the publisher that it is in the public domain.

Printed in the United States

5 4 3 2 1

ISBN 978-1-58890-498-0

This second edition is dedicated to our patients, who constantly challenge us, teach us, and inspire us.

Contents

Foreword ix

Preface xi

Contributors xiii

I Physiology

1. **Anatomy of the Larynx** 3
   Margaret H. Cooper

2. **Laryngeal Sensory Receptors** 10
   Magalie Nelson, David M. Cooper, and William Lawson

3. **Central Laryngeal Motor Innervation** 21
   Leslie T. Malmgren Jr. and Richard R. Gacek

4. **Peripheral Laryngeal Motor Innervation** 32
   Phillip Song, Jerome S. Schwartz, Richard R. Gacek, Leslie T. Malmgren Jr., and Andrew Blitzer

II Clinical Evaluation

5. **Electromyography of Laryngeal and Pharyngeal Muscles** 41
   Tanya K. Meyer, Allen D. Hillel, and Andrew Blitzer

6. **Physical Examination of the Larynx and Videolaryngoscopy** 54
   Marshall E. Smith and Eiji Yanagisawa

7. **Pulmonary Function Evaluation** 59
   Christine M. Sapienza, Karen M. Wheeler-Hegland, and Anuja Chhabra

8. **Laryngeal Dysfunction in Sleep** 69
   Joan Santamaria and Alex Iranzo

9. **Acoustic Assessment of Vocal Function** 74
   Eugene H. Buder and Michael P. Cannito

10. **Stroboscopic Examination of the Normal Larynx** 85
    Minoru Hirano

11. **Flexible Endoscopic Evaluation of Swallowing with Sensory Testing (FEESST)** 89
    Jonathan E. Aviv and Thomas Murry

III Diseases and Treatment

12 Speech Treatment for Neurologic Disorders 95
Shimon Sapir, Lorraine O. Ramig, and Cynthia M. Fox

13 Diagnosis and Evaluation of Laryngeal Paralysis and Paresis 107
Alexander T. Hillel, Robin A. Samlan, and Paul W. Flint

14 Management of Vocal Fold Incompetence with Vocal Fold Injectable Fillers 117
Charles N. Ford and Karen A. Cooper

15 Vocal Fold Medialization, Arytenoid Adduction, and Reinnervation 127
Andrew Blitzer, Steven M. Zeitels, James L. Netterville, Tanya K. Meyer, and Marshall E. Smith

16 Diagnostic-Based Treatment Approaches 149
JoAnne Robbins, Stephanie K. Daniels, and Soly Baredes

17 Movement Disorders of the Larynx 160
Mitchell F. Brin, Andrew Blitzer, and Miodrag Velickovic

18 Botulinum Toxin Treatment of Spasmodic Dysphonia and Other Laryngeal Disorders 196
Lucian Sulica and Andrew Blitzer

19 Pyramidal Disease 204
Satish Mistry, Maxine Power, and Shaheen Hamdy

20 Neuromuscular Disorders of the Larynx 216
David S. Younger

Index 227

Foreword

Andrew Blitzer, Mitchell F. Brin, and Lorraine O. Ramig have provided a superb update to the well-received first edition of *Neurologic Disorders of the Larynx*, which was published by Thieme in 1992. The field of neurolaryngology has experienced unprecedented growth since then, and this edition's contents reflect the vitality of that growth.

Neurolaryngology is a relatively young subdiscipline of otolaryngology—head and neck surgery. The first meeting of the Neurolaryngology Study Group was held in 1989, and was attended by only 12 to 15 otolaryngologists (head and neck surgeons). All those in attendance practiced the subspecialty of laryngology as part of the larger specialty of otolaryngology. None of those in attendance had practices that consisted of only laryngology or neurolaryngology. Issues such as spasmodic dysphonia, laryngeal paralysis, laryngeal reinnervation, and laryngoplastic techniques were discussed at that first meeting of neurolaryngologists.

The ensuing years have seen a virtual explosion of technologies, knowledge, surgical techniques, and significant basic science research in this emerging field. Perhaps the best evidence of this newly focused interest on neurologic disorders of the larynx is the fact that through post-residency fellowship training in laryngology, a relatively large number of individuals on three or more continents are now practicing medicine and surgery exclusively in and of the larynx (laryngology). This has meshed nicely with the increasingly important concept of outcomes analysis, insofar as these focused laryngologists are now able to provide analysis of treatment of larger numbers of patients with laryngeal disorders. Accordingly this increased focus warrants such a superb comprehensive text as *Neurologic Disorders of the Larynx,* second edition.

In the years since the first edition was published, laryngologists and laryngeal scientists have provided profoundly significant advances in laryngeal videostroboscopy, laryngeal electromyography, laryngeal reinnervation, combinations of laryngoplastic surgical procedures, and electroglottographic analysis. There is indeed much new significant knowledge regarding neuroanatomy and the neurophysiology of the larynx. In addition, the return of high-speed laryngeal motion photography has provided scientists and surgeons with a better understanding of how the vocal folds produce sound, and how vocal fold disorders affect the emitted sound.

Of particular interest to many neurolaryngologists and laryngologists is the appropriate expansion of chapters regarding surgical procedures for laryngeal paralysis and paresis. Whereas in the first edition these issues were covered in two chapters (Chapters 17 and 18), in this new edition there are several excellent and more expansive chapters on evaluation of paralysis and paresis (Chapter 13), a full chapter on vocal fold injectable fillers (Chapter 14), and an expanded Chapter 15 discussing the techniques of medialization, arytenoid adduction, and reinnervation. This expansion reflects the evolution and progress of many of these newer surgical techniques in the treatment of laryngeal paresis and paralysis.

This book is indeed a timely summary of these most important changes in the field. It appears to have captured all of the excellence of the first edition as well as all of the important advances made in the last two decades. Neurolaryngologists, neurologists, speech pathologists and therapists, and indeed all physicians and scientists interested in voice, airway management, or the larynx will find much value in this excellent text. The authors have provided a distinct public and medical service by producing a book of this depth and breadth covering laryngeal research, science, medicine, and surgery.

Roger L. Crumley, MD
Professor and Chairman
Department of Otolaryngology–Head and Neck Surgery
University of California, Irvine
Chairman, Neurolaryngology Study Group
Irvine, California

Preface

The authors wrote the first edition of this book to fill the gap in the medical literature on the evaluation, diagnosis, and management of sensory and motor disorders of the larynx and associated structures. Since the first edition was published in 1992, the field of neurolaryngology has increased exponentially. Much more information is available for patients suffering with neuromuscular dysfunction of their larynx. This second edition provides an update for specialists who treat laryngeal dysfunction, as it addresses the information gained over the past two decades.

This edition continues to address the topics included in the first edition: physiology of the larynx, including anatomy, neural innervation, and electrophysiology; clinical evaluation, including electromyography, videolaryngoscopy, and stroboscopy; acoustic analysis and airflow studies; and treatment, including speech, medical, and surgical therapy for pyramidal, extrapyramidal, neuromuscular, cerebellar, and movement disorders. New to this second edition are chapters covering laryngeal dysfunction in sleep; flexible endoscopic evaluation of swallowing with sensory testing; evaluation of paresis and paralysis; vocal fold augmentation, medialization, arytenoids adduction, and reinnervation; and management of swallowing disorders and aspiration.

The book should be of value to all who provide care to patients with laryngeal disorders, including otolaryngologists, neurologists, speech scientists and pathologists, rehabilitationists, and pulmonologists. We believe the book presents not only the current knowledge, but also some of the perplexing questions that remain. It is hoped that this book will inspire others to seek the answers to these questions and thus provide better care for these patients.

Acknowledgments

We would like to thank all our contributors for sharing their expertise with the readers of this book. We also thank the editorial and production staff at Thieme Medical Publishers for their advice, effort, and encouragement throughout the writing of this book. A special thanks to Janice Pagoda for her editorial assistance.

Andrew Blitzer, MD, DDS, FACS
Mitchell F. Brin, MD
Lorraine O. Ramig, PhD, CCC-SLP

Contributors

Jonathan E. Aviv, MD, FACS
Professor
Department of Otolaryngology–Head and Neck Surgery
College of Physicians and Surgeons
Columbia University
New York-Presbyterian Hospital
New York, New York

Soly Baredes, MD
Professor and Chief
Department of Surgery
Division of Otolaryngology
New Jersey Medical School
University of Medicine and Dentistry of New Jersey
Newark, New Jersey

Andrew Blitzer, MD, DDS, FACS
Professor
Department of Otolaryngology–Head and Neck Surgery
College of Physicians and Surgeons
Columbia University
Director
New York Center for Voice and Swallowing Disorders
New York Head and Neck Institute
New York, New York

Mitchell F. Brin, MD
Clinical Professor
Department of Neurology
University of California-Irvine
Senior Vice President and Chief Scientific Officer
Allergan, LLC
Irvine, California

Eugene H. Buder, PhD
Associate Professor
School of Audiology and Speech-Language Pathology
University of Memphis
Memphis, Tennessee

Michael P. Cannito, PhD
Professor
School of Audiology and Speech-Language Pathology
University of Memphis
Memphis, Tennessee

Anuja Chhabra, MA
Department of Communication Sciences and Disorders
University of Florida
Gainesville, Florida

David M. Cooper, MD
Summit Medical Group
Berkeley Heights, New Jersey

Karen A. Cooper, MD
Clinical Assistant Professor
Department of Surgery
Division of Otolaryngology–Head and Neck Surgery
University of Wisconsin School of Medicine and Public Health
Madison, Wisconsin

Margaret H. Cooper, PhD
Professor
Department of Surgery
St. Louis University School of Medicine
St. Louis, Missouri

Stephanie K. Daniels, PhD
Assistant Professor
Department of Physical Medicine and Rehabilitation
Baylor College of Medicine
Michael E. DeBakey VA Medical Center
Houston, Texas

Paul W. Flint, MD
Professor and Chair
Department of Otolaryngology–Head and Neck Surgery
Oregon Health and Science University
Portland, Oregon

Charles N. Ford, MD
Professor
Department of Otolaryngology
Division of Otolaryngology–Head and Neck Surgery
University of Wisconsin School of Medicine and Public Health
Madison, Wisconsin

Cynthia M. Fox, PhD
Research Associate
National Center for Voice and Speech
Denver, Colorado

Richard R. Gacek, MD, FACS
Professor
Department of Otolaryngology
University of Massachusetts Medical School
UMass Memorial Medical Center
Worcester, Massachusetts

Shaheen Hamdy, MBChB, PhD, FRCP
Clinical Senior Lecturer and Associate Professor
School of Translational Medicine
Department of Gastrointestinal Sciences
Faculty of Medical and Human Sciences
University of Manchester
Salford, United Kingdom

Alexander T. Hillel, MD
Resident
Department of Otolaryngology–Head and Neck Surgery
Johns Hopkins University School of Medicine
Johns Hopkins Hospital
Baltimore, Maryland

Allen D. Hillel, MD
Associate Professor and Chief
Department of Otolaryngology–Head and Neck Surgery
University of Washington Medical Center
Seattle, Washington

Minoru Hirano, MD, PhD, FACS (Hon)
Retired
Kurume, Japan

Alex Iranzo, MD
Neurologist
Department of Neurology
University of Barcelona Medical School
Hospital Clinic of Barcelona
Barcelona, Spain

William Lawson, MD, DDS
Professor
Department of Otolaryngology
Mount Sinai School of Medicine
New York, New York

Leslie T. Malmgren Jr., PhD
Professor
Department of Otolaryngology and Communication Sciences
State University of New York Upstate Medical University
Syracuse, New York

Tanya K. Meyer, MD
Assistant Professor
Department of Otolaryngology
University of Maryland School of Medicine
Baltimore, Maryland

Satish Mistry, PhD
Post-Doctoral Research Associate
School of Translational Medicine
Department of Gastrointestinal Sciences
Faculty of Medical and Human Sciences
University of Manchester
Salford Royal NHS Foundation Trust–Hope Hospital
Salford, United Kingdom

Thomas Murry, PhD
Professor
Department of Otolaryngology–Head and Neck Surgery
College of Physicians and Surgeons
Columbia University
New York, New York

Magalie Nelson, MD
Trinitas Hospital
Elizabeth, New Jersey

James L. Netterville, MD
Professor
Department of Otolaryngology
Vanderbilt Medical Center
Vanderbilt-Ingram Cancer Center
Nashville, Tennessee

Maxine Power, PhD
Department of Stroke Medicine
Salford Royal NHS Foundation Trust–Hope Hospital
Salford, United Kingdom

Lorraine O. Ramig, PhD, CCC-SLP
Professor
Department of Speech, Language, and Hearing Science
University of Colorado
Boulder, Colorado
Senior Scientist
National Center for Voice and Speech
Denver, Colorado

JoAnne Robbins, PhD, CCC-SLP, BRS-S
Professor
Department of Medicine
University of Wisconsin School of Medicine and Public Health
University of Wisconsin Hospital and Clinics
Madison, Wisconsin

Robin A. Samlan, MS, CCC-SLP
Department of Speech, Language, and Hearing Sciences
University of Arizona
Tucson, Arizona

Joan Santamaria, MD
Assistant Professor
Department of Neurology
University of Barcelona Medical School
Barcelona, Spain

Christine M. Sapienza, PhD
Professor
Department of Communication Sciences and Disorders
University of Florida
Brain Rehabilitation Research Center
Malcolm Randall VA Medical Center
Gainesville, Florida

Shimon Sapir, PhD
Head
Department of Communication Disorders
University of Haifa
Haifa, Israel

Jerome S. Schwartz, MD
The Feldman ENT Group
Chevy Chase, Maryland

Marshall E. Smith, MD
Professor
Department of Surgery
Division of Otolaryngology–Head and Neck Surgery
University of Utah School of Medicine
University Hospital
Salt Lake City, Utah

Phillip Song, MD
Instructor
Department of Otology and Laryngology
Harvard Medical School
Massachusetts Eye and Ear Infirmary
Boston, Massachusetts

Lucian Sulica, MD
Assistant Professor
Department of Otorhinolaryngology
Weill Cornell Medical College
New York-Presbyterian Hospital
New York, New York

Miodrag Velickovic, MD
Assistant Clinical Professor
Department of Neurology
Mount Sinai School of Medicine
Movement Disorders Center
The Mount Sinai Medical Center
New York, New York

Karen M. Wheeler-Hegland, PhD
Department of Communication Sciences and Disorders
University of Florida
Gainesville, Florida

Eiji Yanagisawa, MD
Clinical Professor
Department of Surgery
Section of Otolaryngology
Yale School of Medicine
Southern New England Ear, Nose, Throat, and Facial
  Plastic Surgery Group, LLP
New Haven, Connecticut

David S. Younger, MD
Clinical Associate Professor and Chief
Department of Neurology
NYU School of Medicine
NYU Langone Medical Center
Lenox Hill Hospital
Saint Vincent Catholic Medical Centers
New York, New York

Steven M. Zeitels, MD, FACS
Professor
Department of Surgery
Harvard Medical School
Director
Center for Laryngeal Surgery
Massachusetts General Hospital
Boston, Massachusetts

Section I

Physiology

Chapter 1

Anatomy of the Larynx

Margaret H. Cooper

The larynx in the adult is located in the anterior neck and connects the hypopharynx and the trachea. It lies between the third and sixth cervical vertebrae anterior to the laryngopharynx, prevertebral muscles, and fascia. The upper poles of the thyroid gland are closely related to the inferolateral part of the larynx and the great vessels are located posterolaterally. Covering the larynx are the infrahyoid or strap muscles as well as superficial cervical fascia and skin.

The larynx develops from the endodermal lining and the mesoderm of the fourth to sixth branchial arches. At birth the tip of the epiglottis is at the level of the first cervical vertebra and may come in contact with the soft palate. Up to the age of 3 years the larynx descends in the neck and then little change occurs until puberty.[1] The larynx in the child is found between cervical vertebra three and five. At puberty the cricoid cartilage descends to the level of the sixth cervical vertebra, which results in part from growth of the thyroid cartilage. The latter cartilage increases in size and shape, especially in males. Growth of the thyroid prominence causes the angle between the thyroid laminae to become more acute in the male than in the female, hence the characteristic "Adam's apple." The adult male larynx is larger than that of the female.

The laryngeal framework comprises cartilages, muscles, membranes, and ligaments. It is lined with mucosa both within its cavity and on its pharyngeal surface. The mucosa of the cavity is continuous superiorly with the pharynx and inferiorly with that of the trachea. The mucosa of the outer surface of the larynx is the mucosa of the laryngopharynx. Contraction of the muscles will alter the positions of the cartilages and ligaments during respiration, phonation, and deglutition.

♦ Laryngeal Framework

The larynx comprises nine cartilages—three unpaired cartilages and three sets of paired cartilages. The unpaired cartilages are the thyroid, cricoid, and epiglottis. The paired cartilages, the arytenoids, are of more importance than the corniculates and cuneiforms.

Even though the hyoid bone is technically not part of the larynx, it is involved in movement of the larynx and therefore needs to be discussed with the larynx. The hyoid bone is a U-shaped bone consisting of a body and greater and lesser horns on each side. It derives from mesoderm of the second and third branchial arches and serves as attachment for numerous muscles of the tongue as well as some of the extrinsic muscles of the larynx. It is suspended from the tip of the styloid process of the temporal bone by the stylohyoid ligament and attached to the larynx by the thyrohyoid membrane. Because muscles of the tongue and larynx are attached to it, the hyoid bone plays an important role in movement of both structures.

♦ Cartilages

Thyroid Cartilage (Figs. 1.1 and 1.2)

The thyroid cartilage, the largest of the laryngeal cartilages, comprises two quadrilateral laminae fused in the midline as the laryngeal prominence. The angle formed at the prominence is more acute in the male adult (90 degrees) than the female (120 degrees). The superior border of the laminae meet in the midline in a V-shaped notch. Posteriorly, the laminae are incomplete and their edges become elongated as the inferior and superior horns. This configuration leaves the posterior aspect of the larynx open, with the laryngopharynx completed by the pharyngeal musculature. On the external surface of the laminae is the oblique line, a ridge that extends from the superior thyroid tubercle located inferior to the superior horn on its posterolateral edge. It extends inferomedially to the inferior thyroid tubercle. Three muscles attach to the oblique line (sternothyroid, thyrohyoid, and inferior constrictor). The superior border of the thyroid cartilage is concave and gives attachment to the thyrohyoid membrane. The superior horn is the lateral-most edge of attachment of the membrane, which is thickened in this area. This is the lateral thyroid ligament. The inferior border is concave posteriorly and convex anteriorly and gives attachment to the cricothyroid ligament. The inferior horn articulates with the cricoid cartilage at its lower end, forming the synovial cricothyroid joint. The thyroid cartilage comprises hyaline cartilage, which ossifies with age. Ossification usually begins at approximately 25 years of age.

I Physiology

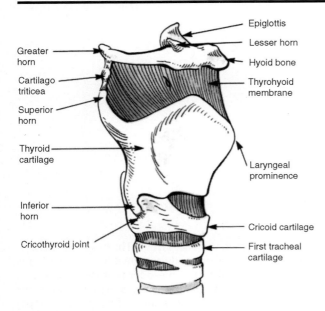

Fig. 1.1 Oblique view of the larynx.

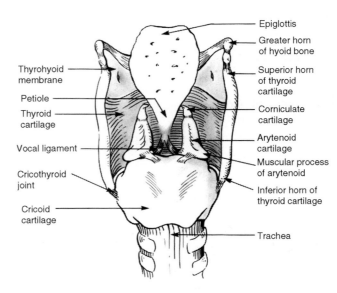

Fig. 1.2 Posterior view of the larynx.

Cricoid Cartilage (Figs. 1.1 and 1.2)

The cricoid cartilage lies between the thyroid cartilage and the trachea. In contrast to the thyroid cartilage, it is a complete ring, "signet" in shape. Posteriorly it has a large quadrate-shaped lamina that narrows into the arch anteriorly. The posterior lamina, which is 2 to 3 cm in vertical height, has a median vertical ridge with shallow depressions on each side. The posterior cricoarytenoid muscles originate in these depressions. The superior border of the lamina has two small oval convex facets that serve as the articular surfaces for the arytenoid cartilages. The cricoid's articular facet for the cricothyroid joint is at the point where the lamina narrows to become the arch. The cricoid cartilage is hyaline cartilage and with age undergoes various amounts of ossification.

Arytenoid Cartilage (Figs. 1.2, 1.3, and 1.4)

The arytenoid cartilages are paired pyramidal-shaped structures that sit on the superior border of the lamina of the

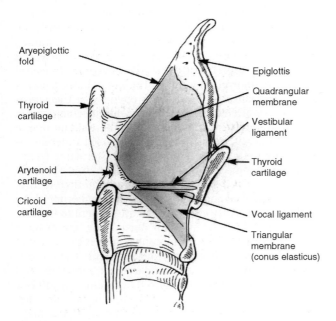

Fig. 1.3 Midsagittal cut of the larynx showing fibroelastic membrane attachments.

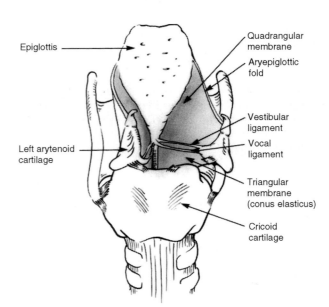

Fig. 1.4 Posterior view of the larynx showing fibroelastic membrane attachments. Arytenoid cartilage on right moved laterally to demonstrate membrane attachments to the ligaments.

cricoid cartilage. Each arytenoid cartilage has a base, three processes, and three surfaces. The base of the cartilage is concave and provides a smooth surface for articulation with the cricoid cartilage. Arising from the base are the vocal and muscular processes. The long vocal process projects anteriorly and gives attachment to the vocal ligament. The muscular process projects posterolaterally and gives attachment to the posterior cricoarytenoid muscle posteriorly and the lateral cricoarytenoid muscle anteriorly. The third process is the apex, which is directed superiorly, posteriorly, and medially. It articulates with the corniculate cartilage. The surfaces of the arytenoid are the posterior, medial, and anterolateral. The posterior surface is smooth, triangular, and concave; the medial surface is narrow, smooth, and flat; the anterolateral surface is rough and convex. On the lateral surface is a ridge that extends from the vocal process to the apex. This ridge separates two depressions. The superior depression gives attachment to the vestibular ligament, and the lower depression gives attachment to the vocal ligament and in part the lateral cricoarytenoid and the vocalis muscles, the latter being part of the thyroarytenoid muscle. Each cartilage comprises mainly hyaline cartilage with the apex being elastic cartilage.

Corniculate and Cuneiform Cartilages (Fig. 1.2)

The corniculate cartilages, comprising elastic cartilage, are paired and sit on the apex of the arytenoid cartilages. They extend the apex posteromedially. A synovial joint is usually formed with the arytenoid cartilage, but fusion can occur. The cuneiform cartilages are small, paired, elongated elastic cartilages that are located in the aryepiglottic fold. A small cartilage, the triticeal cartilage, also elastic in nature, is frequently found in each lateral thyrohyoid membrane.

Epiglottis (Figs. 1.2, 1.3, and 1.4)

The epiglottic cartilage is a single leaf-shaped structure. Its free superior portion is rounded and broad, whereas its inferior portion narrows to a stalklike structure, the petiole. The petiole is attached by the thyroepiglottic ligament to the inner surface of the thyroid cartilage in the midline just below the notch. The cartilage extends superiorly to the base of the tongue and its anterior surface faces it. The posterior surface is mainly concave, but there is some convexity at its superior border as well as at its inferior border. This elastic cartilage has numerous small pits into which mucous glands project.

◆ Membranes and Ligaments

The various portions of the larynx are held together by mucosal folds, ligaments, and membranes. The mucosal lining of the laryngeal cavity is continuous with that of the tongue and pharynx, and forms several folds. The median glossoepiglottic fold is in the midline between the tongue and epiglottis. On each side of it is a depression, vallecula. Extending laterally from the epiglottis to the pharyngeal wall are the paired lateral glossoepiglottic folds. The epiglottis and arytenoid cartilages are connected by the aryepiglottic folds, which contain the cuneiform cartilages and the upper part of the quadrangular membrane.

The ligaments and membranes can be divided into two groups: extrinsic and intrinsic.

Extrinsic

The thyrohyoid membrane is a broad fibroelastic membrane that extends from the lower border of the hyoid bone to the superior border of the thyroid cartilage. Laterally it is thickened as the lateral thyrohyoid ligament and in the midline becomes thickened as the median thyrohyoid ligament. Lateral to the latter ligament is the point where the superior laryngeal vessels and nerve enter the larynx (**Fig. 1.1**).

Intrinsic

The entire larynx is lined by mucosa overlying a sheet of fibroelastic tissue. This broad fibroelastic membrane forms the internal skeleton of the larynx and can be divided into two portions (**Figs. 1.3, 1.4, and 1.5**). The upper portion, the quadrangular membrane, extends between the arytenoid and epiglottic cartilages. Anteriorly the quadrangular membrane extends along the entire lateral border of the epiglottis and down to the thyroid cartilage near the attachment of the petiole of the epiglottis. Posteriorly it extends from the corniculate cartilage to the vocal process of the arytenoid cartilages. The superior border of the quadrangular membrane is free within the aryepiglottic folds, and the inferior border is the vestibular ligament, which is located in the false vocal cord (**Figs. 1.3, 1.4, and 1.5**).

The lower portion of the fibroelastic membrane is the triangular membrane, or conus elasticus. Inferiorly it is attached to the upper border of the arch of the cricoid cartilage and as it projects superiorly it attaches anteriorly to the midline of the inner surface of the angle of the thyroid cartilage and posteriorly to the vocal process of the arytenoids. The thick anterior part of the membrane is the cricothyroid ligament. It is situated in a position where an emergency cricothyroidotomy may be performed. As the triangular membrane extends superiorly to its free border, it becomes thin and is concave medially, forming a modified cone, thus the name conus elasticus. The superior end of the membrane is thickened and extends from the thyroid cartilage to the inferior depression of the arytenoid cartilage. This is the vocal ligament, and is located in the true vocal cord (**Figs. 1.3, 1.4, and 1.5**). The point at which the vocal ligaments attach to the thyroid cartilage is Broyles' ligament. The ligaments of both sides with the epithelium covering form the anterior commissure.[2]

◆ Muscles

The musculature of the larynx is divided into an extrinsic and intrinsic group (**Fig. 1.6**). The extrinsic muscles elevate or depress the larynx as a whole or effect the movement of

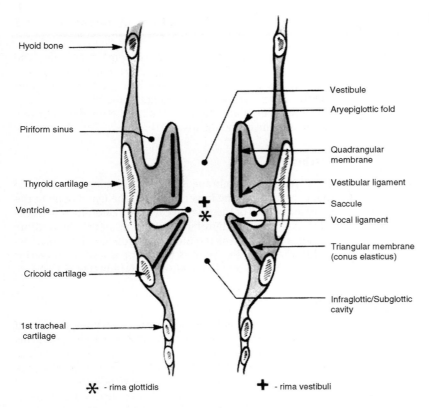

Fig. 1.5 Coronal section of the larynx.

∗ - rima glottidis + - rima vestibuli

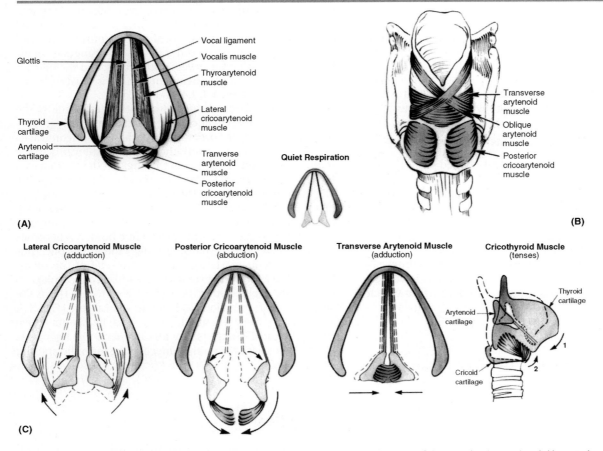

Fig. 1.6 Intrinsic muscles of the larynx **(A,B)** and the movement of the vocal cords caused by their contraction **(C)**. Dashed lines indicate position of vocal cords and arytenoid cartilages before movement caused by contraction of the muscles (arrows). Solid lines indicate position of vocal cords and arytenoid cartilage after contraction. Under cricothyroid muscle, 1 and 2 indicate possible movements of cartilages.

an individual cartilage. The intrinsic musculature changes the position and tension of the vocal cords, thus altering the shape of the glottis. Most intrinsic muscles have an attachment to an arytenoid cartilage.

Extrinsic

The extrinsic muscles include the infrahyoid or strap muscles, which lie anterior to the larynx. These are the sternohyoid, sternothyroid, thyrohyoid, and omohyoid muscles. Other muscles that also effect movement of the larynx include the stylohyoid, digastric, mylohyoid, stylopharyngeus, palatopharyngeus, and middle and inferior pharyngeal constrictors.[2]

Intrinsic

Cricothyroid Muscle

The cricothyroid muscle originates from the cricoid cartilage lateral to the attachment of the median cricothyroid ligament. The anterior portion arises from the superior border of the cricoid cartilage, whereas the posterolateral portion originates from the lateral surface. The anterior fibers insert on the posterolateral border of the thyroid cartilage and posterolateral or oblique fibers insert onto the inferior border of the thyroid cartilage posterior to the anterior fibers as well as the entire anterior aspect of the inferior horn.

Action Contraction of the muscle causes either the thyroid cartilage to be tilted anteriorly and inferiorly toward the cricoid cartilage or the arch of the cricoid to be drawn superiorly and the lamina inferiorly (**Fig. 1.6C**). The actual action is controversial.[2-5] The muscle, however, increases the distance between the arytenoid and thyroid cartilages, causing the vocal cord to be stretched and therefore tensed.

Nerve Supply External branch of the superior laryngeal nerve.

Posterior Cricoarytenoid Muscle

The posterior cricoarytenoid muscle arises from the depression on the posterior aspect of the cricoid lamina. The fibers are directed laterally and superiorly to insert onto the posterior aspect of the ipsilateral muscular process of the arytenoid. The upper fibers are almost horizontal, the middle fibers oblique, and the lower fibers almost vertical.

Action Contraction of this muscle causes the muscular process to be pulled posteriorly and toward the opposite arytenoid. The vocal process in turn is pulled laterally, thus causing the abduction of the vocal cord.

Nerve Supply Recurrent laryngeal nerve.

Lateral Cricoarytenoid Muscle

The lateral cricoarytenoid muscle arises from the superior border of the lateral cricoid cartilage. The fibers insert onto the anterior surface of the muscular process of the arytenoid cartilage.

Action Contraction of the muscle causes the muscular process to be pulled anteriorly and the arytenoid to rotate with the vocal process turning medially. This action causes adduction of the vocal cords.

Nerve Supply Recurrent laryngeal nerve.

Interarytenoid Muscle

The interarytenoid muscle is the only unpaired intrinsic muscle. It comprises two portions. The transverse arytenoid muscle arises from the posterior surface of both arytenoid cartilages, thus crossing in the midline. The oblique portion of the muscles originates on the posterior aspect of the muscular process, crosses the midline, and inserts on the apex of the contralateral arytenoid cartilage. Some of the fibers continue within the aryepiglottic fold as the aryepiglottic muscle.

Action Contraction of the interarytenoid muscle pulls the arytenoid cartilages toward one another, thus causing adduction of the vocal cords.

Nerve Supply Recurrent laryngeal nerve.

Thyroarytenoid Muscle

The thyroarytenoid muscle arises from the inner surface of the angle of thyroid cartilage and cricothyroid ligament. This thin broad muscle passes posteriorly, laterally, and superiorly to insert on the anterolateral surface of the arytenoid cartilage. The fibers that are most medial and inferior and partially within the vocal fold constitute the vocalis muscle. It lies just lateral and is attached to the vocal ligament.

Action Contraction of the thyroarytenoid muscle alters the height of the vocal cord surfaces. It causes the vocal cord to relax as well as adduct.

Nerve Supply Recurrent laryngeal nerve.

♦ Cavity of the Larynx

The cavity of the larynx (**Fig. 1.5**) communicates with the pharynx at the superior laryngeal aperture. The aperture is bounded by the epiglottis anteriorly, the aryepiglottic folds laterally, and the interarytenoid notch posteriorly. The cavity of the larynx is completely lined by mucosa and is divided into different regions: vestibule, rima vestibulis, rima glottidis, ventricle, and infraglottic or subglottic space.

The vestibule is the part of the cavity between the aperture and the vestibular or false vocal cords and is bounded by the quadrangular membrane deep to the mucosa of the aryepiglottic fold. The actual space between the folds is the vestibular slit or rima vestibulis. The vestibular folds are thick pads of mucosa covering the vestibular ligament and are attached to the thyroid cartilage just inferior to the petiole attachment of the epiglottis.

The space between the false and true vocal cords is the ventricle (**Figs. 1.5** and **1.7**). On the lateral edges of the larynx the mucous membrane evaginates as a diverticulum extending superiorly from the ventricle as the laryngeal saccule. It normally extends superiorly under the false vocal cord, but can extend as far as the superior border of the thyroid cartilage.

The vocal folds or cords and the space between them is the glottis. The rima glottidis, the space between the vocal cords and vocal processes of the arytenoids, is divided into the longer intermembranous space (between the former) and intercartilaginous space (between the latter). It is the narrowest part of the laryngeal cavity and its shape and width change with movement of the cartilages and vocal cords during respiration and phonation. The vestibular slit between the false vocal cords is wider than the glottis, enabling the true vocal cords to be visualized easily during laryngoscopy. Below the vocal cords and extending inferiorly to the inferior border of the cricoid cartilage is the subglottic or infraglottic space. It is continuous with the lumen of the trachea.

Other true spaces that are related to the larynx include the valleculae, which are between the epiglottis and base of the tongue and the piriform sinus (fossa), which is on each side of the larynx within the laryngopharynx and is bounded by the aryepiglottic fold (**Fig. 1.5**). Potential spaces of the larynx are the pre-epiglottic space, which lies between the epiglottis and the superior portion of the thyroid cartilage and thyrohyoid membrane and the paraglottic space, a potential space bounded by the thyroid cartilage and conus elasticus.

The mucosal lining of the larynx is continuous with that of the pharynx and the trachea. The epithelium of the mucosa of the cavity of the larynx is pseudostratified columnar with the exception of the epithelium of the epiglottis and true vocal cord, which is stratified squamous. The space deep to the epithelium and superficial to the fibroelastic membrane is Reinke's space. The epithelium of the posterior surface of the larynx is stratified squamous because it is actually part of the laryngopharynx. The glands within the mucosa are mainly mucous with some scattered serous cells.[6] There are numerous glands within the saccule that secrete mucous to lubricate the true vocal cord.

♦ Innervation

The larynx is innervated by the vagus nerve, which contains motor, sensory, and secretory (parasympathetic) fibers. At the level of the inferior ganglion of the vagus nerve, the superior laryngeal nerve originates and descends toward the larynx medial to the carotid arteries. The nerve divides into internal and external branches. The internal branch pierces the thyrohyoid membrane along with the superior laryngeal artery to supply the mucosa of the epiglottis, the aryepiglottic folds, and the cavity of the larynx as far inferior as the vocal cords. It contains sensory and secretory fibers. The external branch remains outside the larynx lying on the inferior constrictor muscle in close relationship to the superior thyroid artery and ends in the cricothyroid muscle, which it innervates (**Fig. 1.8**). It is solely a motor nerve. The rest of the cavity of the larynx as well as the remaining muscles are supplied by the recurrent laryngeal nerve (inferior laryngeal nerve). On the right side of the body it arises from the vagus nerve anterior to the subclavian artery, winds posteromedially around the artery in close relationship to the inferior thyroid artery, and ascends in or adjacent to the tracheoesophageal groove posterior to the thyroid gland.

It enters the larynx posterior to the cricothyroid joint just inferior to the attachment of the inferior constrictor muscle, the cricopharyngeus (**Fig. 1.8**). On the left side the nerve arises to the left of the aorta arch and winds posteromedially around the ligamentum arteriosum. It ascends to the larynx in a similar fashion to the right recurrent nerve. The nerve on both sides divides into an anterior and posterior branch either outside or inside the larynx.[7] The anterior branch supplies the lateral cricoarytenoid, thyroarytenoid, and vocalis muscles. The posterior branch supplies the posterior cricoarytenoid and the interarytenoid muscles. The mucosa of the infraglottic space receives both sensory and secretory innervation via the recurrent laryngeal nerve.

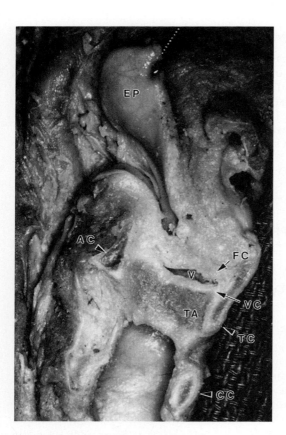

Fig. 1.7 Larynx cut just lateral to the midline showing the relationship of the vestibular and vocal cords (FC [false cord] and VC), thyroarytenoid muscle (TA), ventricle (V), and thyroid, arytenoid, and cricoid cartilages (TC, AC, and CC). EP, epiglottis.

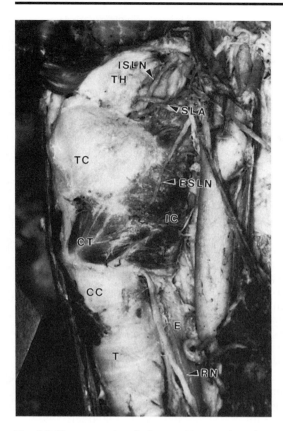

Fig. 1.8 Nerves entering the larynx. CC, cricoid cartilage; CT, cricothyroid muscle; E, esophagus; ESLN, external branch of the superior laryngeal nerve; IC, inferior constrictor muscle; ISLN, internal branch of the superior laryngeal nerve; RN, recurrent laryngeal nerve; SLA, superior laryngeal artery; T, trachea; TC, thyroid cartilage; TH, thyrohyoid membrane.

♦ Blood Supply

The blood supply of the larynx arises from both the carotid and the subclavian arteries. The superior thyroid artery, a branch of the external carotid artery, gives rise to the superior laryngeal artery, which enters the larynx through the thyrohyoid membrane with the internal branch of the superior laryngeal nerve (**Fig. 1.1**). It is always inferior to the nerve and may pass through a foramen in the thyroid cartilage. The inferior thyroid artery, a branch of the thyrocervical trunk of the subclavian artery, enters the larynx with the recurrent laryngeal nerve at the inferior border of the inferior constrictor muscle. The two arteries anastomose. The laryngeal veins parallel the arteries.

♦ Lymphatics

The lymphatics drainage of the larynx is either superior or inferior in nature from the true vocal cords. In the area superior to the cord, the supraglottic region, the drainage follows the superior laryngeal vessels to the superior group of deep cervical lymph nodes. Inferiorly the subglottic region is drained anteriorly and laterally. The anterior drainage channel pierces the cricothyroid membrane to terminate in the prelaryngeal or Delphian node. The lateral channels pass through the cricotracheal membrane to drain into the paratracheal nodes. Both sets of channels eventually drain into the inferior deep cervical lymph nodes. The true vocal cord appears to be almost devoid of lymphatic channels.[8,9]

References

1. Westhorpe RN. The position of the larynx in children and its relationship to the ease of intubation. Anaesth Intensive Care 1987;15:384–388
2. Hollinshead WH. Anatomy for Surgeons: Vol. I, The Head and Neck. 3rd ed. Philadelphia: Harper & Row; 1982:411–439
3. Williams PL, Warwick R, Dyson M, Bannister LH, eds. Gray's Anatomy. 37th ed. London: Churchill Livingstone; 1989
4. Negus VE. Certain anatomical and physiological considerations in paralysis of the larynx. Proc R Soc Med 1947;40:849–853
5. O'Rahilly R. Anatomy: A Regional Study of Human Structure. 5th ed. Philadelphia: WB Saunders; 1986
6. Fawett DW. A Textbook of Histology. 11th ed. Philadelphia: WB Saunders; 1986
7. Steinberg JL, Khane GJ, Fernandes CMC, Nel JP. Anatomy of the recurrent laryngeal nerve: a redescription. J Laryngol Otol 1986;100:919–927
8. Pressman J, Dowdy A, Libby R, Fields M. Further studies upon the submucosal compartments and lymphatics of the larynx by the injection of dyes and radioisotopes. Ann Otol Rhinol Laryngol 1956;65:963–980
9. Welsh LW. The normal human laryngeal lymphatics. Ann Otol Rhinol Laryngol 1964;73:569–582

Chapter 2

Laryngeal Sensory Receptors

Magalie Nelson, David M. Cooper, and William Lawson

The larynx subserves several important functions including airway protection, respiration, and phonation, which are derived from a complex interrelationship of diverse reflexive and involuntary actions. The laryngeal reflexes are initiated when chemical or mechanical stimuli contact receptors in the laryngeal mucosa, which trigger afferent neural activity. The reflexes include apnea, swallowing, coughing, bradycardia, hypertension, and changes in peripheral vascular resistance. The laryngeal chemoreflexes have clinical significance and can have fatal consequences as is seen by their association with sudden infant death syndrome.[1] The structure, function, and physiologic reflexes produced by these sensory receptors will be discussed.

♦ Morphology of Laryngeal Sensory Receptors

It is well established that the sensory innervation to the supraglottic larynx is derived from the internal branch of the superior laryngeal nerve; below the true vocal folds, sensation is mediated by the recurrent laryngeal nerve.[2] Afferent impulses are delivered through the nodose ganglion to the brainstem tractus solitarius. The laryngeal mucosa is the source of afferent neural activity and has been the focus of countless research efforts to better understand the laryngeal sensory system. The most commonly described sensory structures in the laryngeal mucosa include free nerve endings, taste buds, muscle spindles, and glomerular and corpuscular receptors. Investigations are still underway to better define the morphologic and topographic characteristics of these sensory structures and to correlate with specific reflexes. Morphologic descriptions of the different receptor types present in the larynx widely vary because of the study of many different species, ranging from mouse to humans. In addition, it has been difficult to correlate which receptor causes a specific recorded afferent nerve discharge and reflex. Historically, Konig[3] in 1881, Simanowsky[4] in 1883, Retzius[5] in 1892, and Ploschko[6] in 1897, all described the sensory innervation of the laryngeal mucosa. Konig, using serial section and light microscopy, identified a fine network of neurofibrils in the subepithelium, approximately 150 to 250 μm for the epithelium, which disappeared when the stratified squamous epithelium of the glottis changed to columnar respiratory epithelium. He described sensory nerve corpuscles resembling retiform and fungiform as well as efferent neurofibrils that project toward the epithelial surfaces. These neural structures were predominantly present in the posterior portions of the larynx. In the anterior glottic region, only isolated neurofibrils and scant free epithelial nerve endings were documented. Some of the fibers become myelinated after they leave the epithelium and others remain unmyelinated. These findings matched those of Jabonero,[7] who in 1958, noted subepithelial plexuses, intraepithelial nerve endings, and sensory corpuscles in the mucous membrane of the epiglottis.

More recently, using modern techniques including immunohistochemistry and immunoelectron microscopy, several authors have further clarified the morphology of various sensory structures in the laryngeal mucosa. In 1986 Shin et al[8] performed morphologic investigations of sensory nerve endings in human and canine larynges with silver impregnation, immunohistochemistry, and electron microscopy. They discovered intraepithelial free nerve endings with simple and complex branching patterns, corpuscles endings with glomerular patterns, and taste bud-like structures. In the equine laryngeal mucosa, Yamamoto et al[9] found the highest density of intraepithelial free nerve endings in the corniculate process of the arytenoid region and lowest in the vocal cord mucosa. Lima-Rodrigues et al[10] described intraepithelial nerve fiber endings that protrude into the laryngeal lumen among the cilia of the apical epithelial cells, which may explain the mechanism of airborne airway irritants.

In summary, free nerve endings are found throughout the laryngeal mucosa, from the epiglottis to the subglottis, including in the vocal folds, and they have a wide array of morphology. Although they are located in the subepithelial plexuses, they send projections into the intercellular space of the epithelium, and new evidence points to intralumen projections. These nerve endings are often surrounded by polygonal stratified epithelial cells in the supraglottic region, and by ciliated cells in the subglottic region. Immunologic studies have identified substance P (SP), calcitonin gene-related peptide (CGRP), choline acetyltransferase (CHAT), and nitric oxide in some fibers.

Taste Buds

Taste buds are found mainly in the mucosa of the epiglottis, arytenoid cartilages, aryepiglottic fold, and the posterior glottic region. Morphologically, they resemble the taste buds present at the base of the tongue, although they are not contained in papillae and are not believed to play a role in gustation. Studies of various animals have shown abundant taste buds in the laryngeal surface of the epiglottis, whereas a variable number have been found in human epiglottis. The ultrastructure of the laryngeal taste buds was described by Idé and Munger in 1980.[11] They found three cell types in the taste buds of monkeys: basal cells or stem cells; sustentacular cells, which are characterized by the presence of microvilli and dark granules near apices; and chemosensory cells, which project synaptic specializations and microvillar extensions into the surface. Sweazey et al[12] compared the ultrastructural details of epiglottal taste buds with those in the oral cavity and concluded that epiglottal taste buds share many of the same structural characteristics as oral taste buds, having basal cells, which did not extend a process into the taste pore, as well as type I (dark) and type II (light) cells, which have synaptic connections with primary afferent fibers. Taste buds contain small clear and large dense-cored vesicles containing neurotransmitters such as SP, CGRP, 5-hydroxytryptamine (5-HT), galanin, and enkephalin (ENK). In some cases, the taste buds were arranged around the opening of the duct of the epiglottic glands. The taste buds function as chemoreceptors and their reflex actions include swallowing and associated apnea, which protect the airway against aspiration.

Other Sensory Receptors

The remaining sensory receptors are less well defined. Glomerular, corpuscular, and lamellar receptors are complex structures with surrounding sheaths, which have been frequently described in the laryngeal mucosa. Their sizes vary and some are found inside the squamous cell epithelium. Their functions have not been well established, but by analogy to the skin, it is likely that they respond to pressure, touch, and cold.[13] Sbarbati et al[14] in 2004 discovered a new type of chemoreceptor organ organized in plates of a modified, highly permeable mucosa that they coined specific laryngeal sensory epithelium (SLSE). The SLSE contains arrays of solitary chemoreceptor cells (SCCs), which are single epithelial cells contacted by nerves, and are located primarily in highly reflexogenic regions such as the posterior commissure. These chemoreceptor cells had previously been described only in aquatic vertebrates, and their recent discovery in rat laryngeal epithelium encourages further investigations as to their role in the human larynx.

♦ Chemoreceptors

Neurophysiology

As early as 1876, Schofield[15] discovered the presence of taste bud-like structures in the laryngeal of the dog and cat. In the first quantitative investigation of epiglottal taste bud-like structures, Lalonde and Eglitis[16] counted approximately 1000 receptors in a human newborn. Whether or not these receptors functioned for taste or other stimuli was debated. Bradley et al,[17] studying sheep of different ages, noted six stages in the development of epiglottal taste buds identifiable by their changing cellular morphology. The buds of all six morphologic stages were never present in a single epiglottis at any of the ages examined. As the animals matured, the morphologic features of the buds changed until a single population of similar structure was noted, indicating that the stages are distinct landmarks in the development of these sensory structures.

The maturational changes noted early on by Bradley et al,[17] along with the large number of these sensory structures, seem to imply an important physiologic role. Wilson,[18] reviewing the early literature in 1905, thought the epiglottal taste bud-like structures to be either a phylogenetic residue with no functional role, or to serve as chemoreceptors. He used a laryngeal mirror to apply chemical stimuli to his larynx and noted the ability to discern the four primary tastes, although quantitatively inferior to the tongue. It was postulated that the sensory buds were important multichemical receptors and part of the reflex mechanism protecting the airway. Supporting such a role is the fact that the buds maintain a constant density throughout the life span of an organism. Storey,[19] using cat larynges in an electrophysiologic study, demonstrated the response patterns of chemosensitive fibers in the nerve supply of the epiglottis, including specificity. He dissected free the superior laryngeal nerve and severed it near the nodose ganglion. Action potentials were recorded and photographed from single-sensory units consisting of a receptor and afferent fiber using a cathode ray oscilloscope. Receptor units were found by systematically applying a range of chemical stimuli to the exposed laryngeal mucosa. Test solutions included various concentrations of sodium chloride, sodium acetate, calcium chloride in water, sucrose in water, sucrose in Ringer's solution, as well as acid and alkaline solutions. By dripping these test solutions onto the larynx, together with puffs of air and tactile stimulation, he was able to demonstrate proprioceptive, pressure, tactile, water-sensitive, and hybrid-receptive units responding to multiple chemicals. No receptor was specifically responsive to sodium chloride, sucrose, or acid. He noted that only stimulation of tactile and water-sensitive units were adequate to induce swallowing and coughing, concluding that these were the receptors initiating such reflexes. These receptor units were also noted to have the shortest response latencies and were sensitive to topical anesthetics, indicating their proximity to the mucosal surface. The chemoreceptor discharge patterns associated with reflex swallowing and coughing were noted to be different from those recorded from lingual taste buds. Free nerve endings were therefore thought to be the primary receptors of these two laryngeal chemoreflexes.

Boushey et al[20] described the site, method of excitation, and the resulting reflexes produced by chemical irritation of the larynx in cats. By stroking the laryngeal epithelium with a single linen thread containing an applied chemical stimulus, they were able to detect the exact site from which a reflex reaction was initiated. They concluded that the receptors involved were of a hybrid nature, being sensitive to both mechanical stimulation as well as chemical irritants. Two groups of such receptors were established based on their spontaneous electrical discharges: group 1 fibers had little or no spontaneous activity, and group 2 fibers had regular spontaneous discharges. Group 1 units were stimulated by cigarette smoke, NH3, SO2, CO2, and distilled water. The adaptation time was variable, and the units were mechanosensitive. Group 2 units were stimulated by NH3 and distilled water, but inhibited by cigarette smoke, CO2, and had slow adaptation times. This study also confirmed data showing that the superior laryngeal nerve fibers have receptive fields in the supraglottic larynx.

By 1975, the chemoreflexes reported to be associated with chemical stimulation of the larynx included coughing, apnea, bronchoconstriction, laryngeal constriction, increased blood pressure, and swallowing.[19-22] However, the specific chemoreceptor units could not yet be matched to the various known reflexes produced. Prolonged and sometimes fatal apnea could be initiated reflexively in newborn lambs breathing via a tracheotomy by the introduction into the larynx of water but not isotonic saline. Preliminary investigation of afferent units in superior laryngeal nerve fibers by Storey and Johnson[23] revealed the presence of water-sensitive receptors with short response latencies, slow rates of adaptation, and insensitivity to isotonic saline. They considered these to be the chemoreceptor units responsible for the apnea reflex in lambs. Harding et al[24] extended the work of Storey and Johnson by recording the action potentials generated in single afferent units of the superior laryngeal nerve with various chemical stimuli in neonatal and adult sheep, cats, and monkeys. Two types of receptors sensitive to water were detected to be present in each species from birth. The most common unit responded after a latency period of less than 1 second, discharged maximally in the first 1 to 3 seconds, and became inactive when the stimulus was withdrawn. The other receptor responded after only several seconds, with the discharge frequency gradually increasing and continuing after removal of the stimulus. Reproducible responses were elicited by tactile stimuli to the laryngeal mucosa over the receptive field of each of the long latency units. The short latency units responded to milk, gastric contents, saliva, and isotonic solutions of sugar. Harding et al believed that the water-sensitive chemoreceptors represented the unspecified epithelial endings previously described by Koizumi.[25] It is apparent from these electrophysiologic data that distinct groups of chemoreceptors exist that initiate various chemoreflexes in response to the same or different stimuli.

Bradley et al[26] used various concentrations of KCl, NH4Cl, NaCl LiCl, HCl, citric acid, and distilled water to stimulate sheep larynges to better define the chemical specificity of laryngeal chemoreceptors. All the chemicals were dissolved in a solution of NaCl of very low concentration, which elicited minimal activity. The responses recorded in the superior laryngeal nerve fibers varied among fibers and within a single fiber depending on the chemical stimulus. In lambs and ewes, KCl was the most effective chemical stimulus followed by NH4Cl, with NaCl and LiCl being much less effective. HCl was a more effective acidic stimulant than citric acid. The difference in response frequency between each chemical and a solution of 0.5 molar KCl (used as a standard) was calculated for the entire stimulation period. It was evident that plotting the peripheral neural response pattern over time enabled discrimination among salts, between some salts and acids, and between some salts and water during stimulation of the epiglottis. This demonstrated that various chemicals produced characteristic discharge patterns, when decoded by central nervous system processing centers, and initiated an appropriate laryngeal chemoreceptor reflex. Sucrose, glucose, HCl, quinine, and water all initiated reflex apnea and swallowing. Shingai and Shimada[27] elicited similar results in rabbits.

Kovar et al[28] in 1978 compared the swallowing and apnea reflexes in response to 194 chemical stimuli in lambs. They found that the reflexes did not follow an all-or-none principle but showed a graded relationship between the strength of the stimulus and the respiratory response. They also noted that salts and acids produced different respiratory responses for various stimuli. Data using sugars as stimuli supported the belief that laryngeal taste bud–like structures function as chemoreflex receptors. Lambs reacted with increasing apnea to progressively more concentrated glucose solutions. Potassium gymnetate, known to suppress taste sensitivity to sweet substances by binding to the sweet receptor site of lingual taste buds, markedly reduced this response to glucose. However, the response to saline or water was not altered. Accordingly, there appears to be some contribution by laryngeal taste bud–like structures to specific stimuli-induced chemoreflexes.

The question now arose as to what common features did the various stimulating substances possess that induced excitation of the chemoreceptors. Harding et al[24] noted that hypotonicity was not a requirement because receptors were excited by isotonic solutions of sugars, milk, saliva, and gastric juice. They concluded that it was a lack of Na$^+$ or Cl$^-$ ions that was responsible for the excitatory effect of the many isotonic solutions tested. Boggs and Bartlett[29] used puppies to elucidate further the common features of chemoreceptor stimulants initiating reflex apnea. The laryngeal lumen was perfused with various substances while ventilation through a tracheal cannula was recorded. Water consistently elicited apnea, which could be terminated by a NaCl solution. Sucrose and urea solutions also consistently produced apnea, supporting data indicating that osmolarity is not a critical factor. Phosphate buffer solutions of various concentrations and pH did not produce apnea. Cation substitutions in chloride salts also did not elicit apnea with the exception of potassium. Large anion salts, sucrose, urea, and milk ceased to be effective stimulants in the presence of chloride ion in concentrations of 80 mEq/L or more.

This clearly indicated that the common characteristic of apnea-inducing substances is a chloride concentration below that which is normally present in extracellular fluid. This suggests the existence of a receptor normally held in a low ionic conductance state by the presence of chloride ions in the extracellular fluid. The receptor membrane may have specific chloride or other small anion binding sites. Removal of chloride must somehow increase the conductance of nerve membranes to other ions, notably Na^+, resulting in depolarization.

It is now widely accepted that the taste buds of the larynx respond to several chemical stimuli and to water. They tend to be stimulated by the pH and the tonicity of the solution, and do not respond to NaCl solutions close to physiologic concentrations (0.154 M), but do respond at both lower and higher concentrations. In addition, stimulation of the larynx with taste stimuli does not give rise to taste sensation. These results reveal a fundamental difference between the chemoreceptors of the oral cavity and the larynx, and lead to the conclusion that chemoreceptors of the larynx do not play a role in gestation but are adapted to detect nonsaline chemicals.

There appear to be species and age-dependent differences in laryngeal chemoreflexes. When adult dogs were tested with known apnea-inducing solutions, little or no effect on breathing was noted, but reflex swallowing or coughing did occur.[29] A clear decrease in the magnitude of the chemoreflex-induced apnea occurs after 2 weeks of life, which gradually decreased to an inconsequential level when the puppies reached 7 weeks of age. The maturational component of laryngeal chemoreflex-induced apnea observed in puppies has also been noted in piglets[30] and kittens.[31,32] It was suggested that the absence of the apneic reflex in mature animals was the result of a maturation of central respiratory control mechanisms.

Age-related laryngeal neural dysfunction is evident by the high incidence of dysphonia and dysphagia encountered in the elderly. Mortelliti et al[33] reported an age-related loss of small myelinated nerve fibers in the human superior laryngeal nerve. Rosenberg et al[34] also noted age-related changes in the cytoplasm of Schwann cells from the superior laryngeal nerve of Wistar rats, although the number of axons was preserved with age. This suggested that the changes began at the terminal portion of the neurons. In an attempt to correlate changes in laryngeal neural structures with laryngeal dysfunction in elderly cats, Yamamoto et al[35] compared the density, distribution, and morphology of various types of sensory nerve endings in laryngeal neurons tissue of rats of different ages. They discovered a significant decrease in the number of taste buds as well as degeneration of nerve endings with age. A variable amount of taste buds were found in postmortem human adult epiglottis, but no comparison was made to that of children.

Chemoreceptors and Reflexes

The initiation and magnitude of chemoreceptors response require significant central nervous system input as well as a modulation from the peripheral system. Although apnea is the chemoreflex most commonly measured in the study of laryngeal receptor function, major cardiovascular reflexes may be initiated by laryngeal chemostimulation. These cardiovascular reflexes may also be duplicated by electrical stimulation of the superior laryngeal nerves and can be abolished by their sectioning, indicating their relationship to the laryngeal chemoreceptors.[36,37] The receptors respond to substances that are chemically different from the normal secretions present in the larynx, and therefore have a protective function to prevent aspiration of foreign substance into the airway.

Lee et al[38] studied the cardiorespiratory responses to chemoreceptor stimulation in piglets varying in age from 1 to 79 days. The introduction of water or milk into the piglet larynx previously was noted to produce persistent apnea and asphyxial death in a high proportion of animals. Upon the introduction of saline, only transient alterations of blood pressure and respiration were noted. Replacement of saline with water or KCl solutions resulted in reflex apnea and gasping. Accompanying this respiratory response was a rise in arterial blood pressure and fall in heart rate. Electrical stimulation of the superior laryngeal nerves in animals older than 1 month, as compared with younger piglets, did not produce an apneic reflex, with only a mild reduction in respiratory rate and depth noted. No significant hypertension or bradycardia was recorded either. These findings support the concept that important changes in the respiratory control system occur as the organism matures. This has important clinical implications in the pathophysiology of sudden infant death syndrome (SIDS), which will be discussed later.

Grogaard et al[39] studied the cardiovascular reflexes produced by chemoreceptor stimulation in unanesthetized lambs to examine the influence of central mechanisms on them. Marked bradycardia, hypertension, increased systemic vascular resistance, and blood flow redistribution were noted with water infusion into the larynx. The associated apneic reflex was known to be associated with hypoxia and a decreased arterial oxygen tension, which should stimulate arterial chemoreceptors primarily in the carotid body. A decrease in the reflex cardiovascular response to laryngeal chemoreceptor stimulation during hyperoxia was demonstrated. This suggested that carotid body receptors operating through a central mechanism were modulators of the laryngeal chemoreflex response. Other workers demonstrated in newborn lambs a postnatal maturation effect on the carotid body–mediated hypoxic ventilatory response during the first 10 days after birth.[40,41] It appears that the age-dependent magnitude of the chemoreflex response is related to the maturation of the modulating carotid bodies, which initiate the secondary central nervous system reflexes. The carotid bodies were shown to modify the respiratory and cardiovascular responses to laryngeal chemostimulation in 2- to 4-week-old lambs. Postnatal maturation of the carotid-body central respiratory reflex is required, as the reduced hypoxic ventilatory response noted in the first postnatal week of life was associated with an increased apneic reflex response. This observation was not altered by carotid body denervation.

Clinically, the laryngeal chemoreceptor reflexes discussed evolved as a protective mechanism to preserve vital functions when the organism was not breathing. The laryngeal chemoreflex has been implicated in the apnea associated with gastroesophageal reflux in infants[42,43] and SIDS.[30] As discussed, a striking feature of laryngeal chemoreflex apnea is its disappearance with age. In no species has a fatal or sustained apneic response been elicited in an adult animal or even an immature animal after a certain developmental period.[30,44] It is the difference in the central respiratory drive mechanism, modulated by the carotid body receptor response to hypoxia that accounts for these observations. It is probable that carotid body maturation is necessary for optimal central control of the chemoreflex response.

Sasaki[45] noted a period of laryngeal hyperexcitability in the postnatal period that is probably critical in fatal cases of chemoreflex-induced apnea associated with SIDS. SIDS victims usually die at night, presumably because of an inadequate arousal response to apnea. Quiet and rapid eye movement (REM) sleep have both been noted to be vulnerable activity states for prolonged apnea in the newborn period.[46,47] Marchal et al[1] studied unanesthetized premature newborn lambs to evaluate the effect of activity on chemoreflex responses. Apnea, hypertension, and bradycardia were more pronounced during quiet and REM sleep, particularly when no arousal occurred. These observations were attributed to a decreased response to hypoxia due to immaturity of the central respiratory control centers or the modulating carotid body chemoreceptors in newborns. Therefore, it becomes apparent how laryngeal chemoreceptor stimulation, producing reflex apnea in a newborn with immature respiratory control mechanisms, could result in a fatal outcome as is seen in SIDS. Immature, abnormal, or malfunctioning carotid bodies are a critical factor in the lack of arousal associated with SIDS.[48]

Nishino et al[49] found that stimulation of human laryngeal mucosa with a small amount of distilled water during wakefulness elicited the expiration, cough, and swallowing reflexes. By contrast, the same stimulation causes more variable, prolonged, and exaggerated responses during light anesthesia. Deepening the anesthesia abolishes the cough and expiration reflexes, whereas the laryngeal closure and apneic reflexes persist. It was also noted that the site of stimulation affects the respiratory reflex responses to airway stimulants. Bronchial stimulation caused little or no respiratory response, whereas both laryngeal and tracheal stimulation caused vigorous respiratory responses. In effect, the site of stimulation is crucial in determining the pattern of respiratory responses elicited by human airway stimulants.

In summary, we have presented some of the past studies describing the laryngeal chemoreceptors and the reflexes their stimulation produce. Free intraepithelial nerve endings, taste bud–like structures, as well as solitary chemoreceptor cells function as laryngeal chemoreceptors. The receptors themselves appear to depolarize when a relative decrease in the chloride ion concentration around their membranes occurs. The receptor units have their afferent fibers in the superior laryngeal nerves. Various chemical stimuli can result in specific discharge patterns produced by different receptors. This electrophysiologic information is then decoded by the central nervous system through the nodose ganglion and appropriate secondary reflexes elicited.

Maturation of the organism's central respiratory drive system and the modulating carotid body receptors will determine the magnitude and ultimate physiologic outcome of the cardiorespiratory reflexes.

♦ Mechanoreceptors

The larynx also contains a variety of mechanoreceptors in its muscles and joints responding to and influencing laryngeal function. These mechanoreceptors include muscle spindles, articular receptors, and other proprioceptive nerve endings that have significant input into respiratory reflexes and control mechanisms.

Muscle Spindles and Related Encapsulated Endings

Since the late 1880s, physiologists have spent considerable time studying the presence and nature of spindle-like receptors in groups of nonskeletal muscles in the face, tongue, eye, and larynx. Studies by Hines,[50] Hinsey,[51] Barker,[52] Tiegs,[53] and Cooper et al[21] provide conflicting evidence of their existence even in the same animal species. Fernand and Young[54] studied nerve fibers innervating muscles in the rabbit and attempted to relate nerve fiber size to the presence of muscle spindles. They suggested that groups of muscles such as those found in the larynx and face, which are simple in action and non–weight bearing, would have small proprioceptive requirements and therefore lack muscle spindles. They also proposed that spindle receptors were associated with muscle groups having large-caliber nerve fibers. Cooper et al,[21] using electrophysiologic techniques in cats, reported recording afferent impulses from extrinsic ocular muscles in which no spindle receptors were identified. This suggested that non–weight-bearing muscles contained other forms of low threshold stretch receptors. Fulton[55] also proposed that non–weight-bearing muscles, such as the laryngeal muscle groups, lacked spindle receptor units.

However, continued work has refuted this notion. Bowden and Mahran[56] using rabbits, and Kadanoff[57] in humans, demonstrated spindle receptors in facial muscles. Goerttler,[58] in 1950, demonstrated muscle spindle receptors in the vocalis muscle in man, and Paulsen,[59] in 1958, described their presence in small numbers only in the posterior cricoarytenoid and cricothyroid muscles in humans. In contrast to Paulsen, Keene[60] demonstrated large numbers of neuromuscular spindles in all the intrinsic muscles of the larynx. He also recorded other types of muscle endings described as claw and spiral, but could not establish any pattern of fiber size related to muscle spindle presence. The spindles were noted to be of the classic form and pattern described by Sherrington[61] in 1894.

Ibrahim et al[62] used dogs to study the presence and structure of proprioceptors in the cricothyroid muscle. They noted three types of spindle units in all muscles examined. In spindle type I, annulospiral nerve endings were seen enwrapping the intrafusal fibers together with other branched sensory fibers. Spindle types II and III showed the presence of juxtaequatorial motor axons in addition to the polar ones. Spiral and atypical forms of sensory endings were also identified. In the latter forms, axons were noted to encircle one or two extrafusal fibers and give twigs to them. Classical spindles were noted infrequently. Capsulated ganglia containing multipolar neurons were detected at the site of entry of the external laryngeal nerve into the cricothyroid muscle. Smaller ganglia were found between the bundles of muscle fibers. However, it should be noted that Geacheva[63] and Martensson[64] failed to find muscles spindles in the laryngeal muscles of dogs. These contradictory data are probably explainable by the lack of serial sectioning as a uniform protocol in such work. The fiber diameters in the external branch of the superior laryngeal nerve were noted to be from 2 to 16 μm. Fibers above 12 μm in diameter were believed to represent spindle afferents, which have a known range of 12 to 20 μm. However, Ibrahim et al concluded that spindle receptor afferents from the cricothyroid muscle travel in the external branch of the laryngeal nerve of the dog after finding degenerated spindles after neurectomy.

There is also experimental support for sensory innervation of laryngeal muscles by proprioceptors other than spindle receptor units. Such innervation has been described as consisting of terminal ramifications of nerve fibers and sensory end organs in the intermuscular connective tissue.[63] Their functional significance is not entirely clear. Electron microscopic studies by Nagai[65] provided further insight into the sensory receptors of the human vocal cords and their encapsulated nerve structures. These proprioceptors are located in the intermuscular connective tissue and the subepithelium of the vocal cord. Encapsulated nerve structures in the vocalis muscle are found near the vocal ligament where bundles of muscle fibers cross and terminate. The nerve fibers were noted to run a tortuous course within the capsule, often sending out branches from the side of the nerve trunk. A distinctive identifying feature of these structures is the presence of a striated muscle fiber, which is seen to narrow and finally end within the capsular space. This peculiar striated muscle fiber arrangement within the capsule, with respect to both its termination and the absence of sensory innervation, resembles the Golgi tendon organ.[66] The relation of axon terminals and collagen fibers within the capsule of these proprioceptors also resembles the fine structure of the Ruffini corpuscle. Nagai believes the similarities between the encapsulated nerve structures and known proprioceptive organs implicate them as mechanoreceptors. The location of these proprioceptors suggests that they may monitor the degree of rigidity of the vocal cord during phonation. These encapsulated structures may detect tension within the vocalis muscle where it terminates in the vocal ligament and provide sensory input to centers controlling the shape of the vocal cord in phonation. Their location in the submucosa beneath stratified squamous epithelium is a region of frequent mechanical stimuli by adducting vocal cords.

By 1962, muscle spindles as well as nonspindle forms of proprioceptors had been identified in laryngeal muscles, mostly by histologic examination. However, there was no experimental evidence of spindle receptor neuroactivity analogous to laryngeal chemoreceptors. Bianconi and Molinari,[67] in an early electrophysiologic study of few fiber and single-fiber recurrent laryngeal nerve preparations, recorded activity from spindle receptor units of the thyroarytenoid muscle in cats. These workers had previously identified proprioceptive fibers in the recurrent laryngeal nerve that ended in the intrinsic laryngeal muscles and demonstrated their association with muscle spindle receptors.

Granit[68] identified spindle receptor units by showing interruption of stretch discharge during contraction of the same muscle with direct electrical stimulation. He noted a slowly adapting discharge to be elicited by passive traction of the vocal cord that was interrupted by contraction of the thyroarytenoid muscle initiated by electrical stimulation. Direct pressure with a probe on the intrinsic muscle's spindle unit made the nerve endings discharge as long as the pressure was maintained. When the ending was already firing, probing increased the discharge frequency, and upon releasing the pressure, a sudden temporary arrest occurred.

Bianconi and Molinari[67] were also able to identify nerve endings other than the spindle units described in thyroarytenoid and posterior cricoarytenoid muscles, which showed different patterns of activity. In contrast to the spindle units, the nonspindle receptors fired steadily during stretching of the vocal cord. These nonspindle receptors were also made to fire by the contraction of the thyroarytenoid muscle itself, as well as the antagonistic posterior cricoarytenoid muscle. Direct electrical stimulation of the thyroarytenoid muscle was not always followed by a discharge of these receptor endings. Receptors with a similar pattern of activity were also found in the posterior cricoarytenoid muscle with spontaneous discharge increasing in frequency occurring with strong adduction. This response was interrupted by the abduction of the vocal cord. The significance of this work is that it provided direct functional evidence of muscle spindle activity by nerve endings in parallel with the muscular fibers. Intrinsic laryngeal muscles are therefore equipped with a stretch-receptor mechanism providing myotatic control, contributing to the integration of respiratory and phonatory innervation.

The presence and role of muscle spindles in the larynx is still controversial. Sanders et al[69] examined the distribution of muscle spindles throughout the human thyroarytenoid muscle using histologic cross sections. They found an average of 6.1 muscle spindles from each region. Brandon et al,[70] however, did not find muscle spindles in the human thyroarytenoid. In 2003, Tellis's group[71] evaluated the interarytenoid (IA) muscle immunohistochemically and found evidence of muscle spindles in five patients. Given the conflicting results in various studies of laryngeal muscle spindles, further research is warranted.

Touch Receptors

Touch receptors comprise another group of mechanoreceptors. Sampson and Eyzaguirre[72] studied such receptors in cat larynges and identified two types based on the types of discharge recorded from the cut ends of superior laryngeal nerve fibers. The touch receptive fields of single nerve fibers were quite discrete and had distinct patterns both at rest and during stimulation. The first type was elicited after either gentle touch of the mucosal surface or application of an air jet, with gentle touch being the most effective. Stimulating the vocal cord mucosa with puffs of air elicited short high-frequency bursts of receptor discharge followed by a period of no discharge before a return to baseline discharge occurred. Such data indicated that the touch receptors were a slowly adapting type, with the pause that followed increased activity probably the result of hyperpolarization. These receptors were noted to behave similarly to skin touch receptors. Touch receptors were also noted to have variable patterns of discharge. Some touch mechanoreceptor units were silent at rest, others discharged spontaneously without stimulation, and still others showed an intermittent background discharge that became more regular with stimulation.

The second type did not respond to light touch but was readily activated either by displacement of the vocal cords or by compression or displacement of the outer laryngeal walls. These receptors were termed "deep touch mechanoreceptors" because of their embedded location. They consisted of touch receptors located superficially in the mucosa and mechanoreceptors located deep within laryngeal structures. Sampson and Eyzaguirre[72] found the former to be activated by light touch and low-amplitude vibratory stimuli. The deep receptors were activated primarily by displacement of the vocal cords or extrinsic displacement of laryngeal segments.

Unlike the superficial touch mechanoreceptors, the deep mechanoreceptors have not been studied thoroughly and their nature is less clear. They could only be located in or near the vocal cords. At rest, most receptor units were noted to have a high-frequency background discharge, although some were silent. As with the superficial touch receptors, baseline discharge was synchronous with expiration and inspiration. Their discharge activity was modified by displacement of either the vocal cords or laryngeal segments. All rhythmic patterns of receptor function disappeared after section of the homolateral recurrent laryngeal nerve. These mechanoreceptors appeared most numerous rostral to the base of the vocal cords and possibly function as detectors of foreign bodies in the airway. It has also been suggested that the sensitivity of deep mechanoreceptors to vocal cord movement and vibratory stimuli gives them a role in modulating phonation.[73]

Articular Receptors

Articular receptors form another distinct group of laryngeal mechanoreceptors. Andrew[73] identified Golgi-type endings in the thyroepiglottic joints of the rat whose function was unclear. Kirchner and Wyke[74] described afferent nerve endings supplying the laryngeal joints. They demonstrated electromyographically that stimulation of the afferent nerves innervating these corpuscular receptors resulted in the contraction or relaxation of laryngeal muscles. Passive movements of laryngeal joints can induce reflexively coordinated changes in the tone of laryngeal muscles. Kirchner and Wyke,[75] using oscillographic analysis, were further able to show that the identified mechanoreceptor discharges produced by passive laryngeal joint movement elicited reflex laryngeal muscular responses. They demonstrated that medial and anteromedial movement of the cricothyroid joint produced bursts of rapidly adapting potentials recorded from articular afferent nerves. Release of a displaced joint gave rise to a brief burst of rapidly adapting potentials in the articular afferent nerves. These responses were eliminated by infiltrating the cricothyroid joint capsule with local anesthetic. Recurrent laryngeal nerve recordings during joint movement produced transient rapidly adapting potentials that after a short interval were followed by a more prolonged episode of irregular asynchronous potentials that were accompanied by a twitch of the laryngeal adductor muscles. Section of the recurrent laryngeal nerve abolished this delayed asynchronous discharge and muscle twitch, but not the initial rapidly adapting response. These experiments confirmed the presence of articular mechanoreceptors whose stimulation by specific passive movements of laryngeal joints resulted in recurrent nerve afferent impulses that alter laryngeal muscle tone.[74,75] Therefore, the rapidly adapting mechanoreceptors of the laryngeal joint capsule contributed to coordinated reflex adjustments of intrinsic laryngeal muscle tone.

Kirchner and Wyke further noted that the above-described articular mechanoreceptor reflex system was phasic, with no sustained influence on the tone of the laryngeal muscles. However, precise continuous reflex laryngeal muscle adjustment also occurred during both respiration and phonation. Kirchner and Wyke then postulated that a tonic proprioceptive reflex system must exist, although they had only noted rapidly adapting mechanoreceptors present within laryngeal joints. Abo-el-Enein[76] believed that such a system would require very slow adapting mechanoreceptors located in the laryngeal muscles themselves, rather than joints. Histologic and physiologic studies of the laryngeal muscles of cats provided evidence of the presence of mechanoreceptors producing sustained adjustments of laryngeal muscular tone. Investigators had previously identified mechanoreceptors in laryngeal muscles that could possibly function as the slowly adapting mechanoreceptors sought in this study. Abo-el-Enein demonstrated laryngeal myotatic reflexes distinct from the phasic articular reflexes previously described by Kirchner and Wyke.

Abo-el-Enein's[76] study found two types of myotatic reflexes that originated in laryngeal muscles undergoing passive stretch. One was facilatory and the other inhibitory. The facilatory reflex was evidenced by a sustained increase in the amplitude and frequency of motor unit discharges from the muscle recorded as soon as the stretch was applied. This discharge activity persisted throughout the period of stimulation and disappeared at its termination. As the stretch stimulus was incrementally increased from 5 g to beyond 15 g, the discharge recorded was noted to convert from a facilatory to an inhibitory response. An additional facilatory reflex effect was usually observed with application of stretch to the thyroarytenoid muscle. At the moment the stretch stimulus was applied, a brief burst of high-amplitude motor unit potentials was recorded from the stretched muscle and also in the ipsilateral cricothyroid muscle. These bursts of discharge were noted only at the beginning and end of each sustained stretch reflex response and increased with increasing stimulus. This characteristic "on-off" transient response was also noted in the previously described articular mechanoreceptor reflex response.[77] The author concluded that the phasic articular mechanoreceptor reflex response was superimposed on the slowly adapting muscle mechanoreceptors. Facilatory reflex responses were noted to disappear with active contraction of the muscle tested, in contrast to the inhibitory myotatic reflex response. This inhibitory response continued during contraction of the stretched muscle, which suggests that the mechanoreceptors differ for the two myotatic reflex responses described. Finally, it was observed that most of the reflex afferent impulses passed through the recurrent laryngeal nerve, with the internal laryngeal nerve providing a small contribution.

Flow, Pressure, Pharyngeal Muscle, and Tracheal Motion Receptors

The last group of mechanoreceptors to be discussed include those responsive to air flow, transmural pressure change, and pharyngeal receptors. With each respiratory cycle the larynx experiences significant changes in pressure, airflow, and intrinsic muscle tone, and responds to the effects of contraction of the associated oropharyngeal muscles. The afferent stimuli generated by such activity must have receptor units, which probably plays a significant role in the reflex control of breathing. Sant'Ambrogio et al[78] studied dog laryngeal single-fiber preparations searching for such mechanoreceptors recording activity from one internal branch of the superior laryngeal nerve during (1) normal upper airway breathing; (2) tracheostomy breathing with the larynx subjected only to the action of the upper airway muscles; (3) occlusion of the upper airway; and (4) occlusion of the trachea, which subjected the larynx to the action of only the upper airway muscles. Each condition eliminated one or two of the three stimuli being tested: transmural pressure, airflow, and laryngeal movement. The authors noted that breathing through the tracheostomy eliminated airflow and transmural pressure changes from the larynx and therefore mechanoreceptor discharges could be attributed to contraction of the upper airway muscles.

Drive was the term coined to define upper airway (pharyngeal) muscle activity affecting laryngeal receptor discharge. Using this approach Sant'Ambrogio et al[78] identified flow, pressure, and drive mechanoreceptors. Flow receptors were those discharging only during airflow across the larynx and represented approximately 15% of the samples tested. Most of these receptors responded to inspiratory flow. Pressure mechanoreceptors were those discharging during both the inspiratory and expiratory phases of upper airway breathing, with marked stimulation noted during airway occlusion. These receptors were not recruited during tracheotomy or tracheal occlusion situations and represented 64% of the total sample. The collapsing pressure generated at end expiration was the most significant stimulus. The so-called drive receptors discharged in response to laryngeal and pharyngeal muscle contraction changes. These drive receptors had a baseline output in all respiratory situations tested. A marked decrease in drive receptor output was noted with laryngeal nerve block. These receptors comprised 22% of the sample and included some hybrid receptors. Several investigators concluded that receptors previously described as touch and deep mucosal,[72] joint capsule,[75] and muscle spindle and atypical endings[65] may function as the pressure, flow, or drive endings. The distending and collapsing forces generated during respiration probably stimulated mechanoreceptors located at different depths from submucosal to deep joint receptors. Several other investigators have demonstrated the larynx to be a source of reflex responses that affect respiratory rate and pattern and that are elicited by pressure or airflow stimuli.[79-81] The reflex responses elicited by the receptors described by Sant'Ambrogio et al[78,82,83] were found to be abolished by the topical application of local anesthetics to the laryngeal mucosa by Mathew et al.[80,84-87] This finding makes deep muscle and joint capsule mechanoreceptors less likely to be the primary mediators of the respiratory-modulating laryngeal reflexes. Mathew et al also demonstrated that collapsing pressure of the upper airway produced a reflex that augmented laryngeal muscle tone and enhanced airway patency. Such a reflex would have obvious benefit for avoiding oropharyngeal obstruction. Felman et al[88] showed that elimination of airflow and pressure in the larynx resulted in a marked reduction in upper airway muscle activity, as occurs in sleep apnea.

Mathew et al observed upper airway pressure changes to affect the activity of the upper airway dilating muscles. They noted that topical anesthesia, or section of both superior laryngeal nerves, reduced the response to upper airway pressure changes. Mathew et al used dogs to quantitate the reflex effect of stimulation of the pressure mechanoreceptors on breathing pattern and airway patency. Stepwise changes of negative and positive pressure were both applied to the upper airway for intervals of at least 3 seconds, and the discharge frequency of the pressure receptors was recorded. Most of the pressure mechanoreceptors responded to either positive or negative transmural pressure, with only a small percentage responding to both. Pressure receptors showed characteristics of rapidly adapting receptors.

Sant'Ambrogio et al[83] realized that the coexistence of both rapidly and slowly adapting discharge patterns in one group of receptors was unique among airway mechanoreceptors. They noted that the response of the pressure receptors under conditions of normal breathing, tracheotomy breathing, and airway occlusion indicated two populations of such mechanoreceptors. One group altered its discharge pattern with transmural pressure change during eupnea, and the other group functioned with a high threshold necessitating airway obstruction to alter the discharge pattern. Most receptors functioned at low thresholds. It would follow that when the airway is subjected to a large collapsing pressure, the low-threshold pressure receptors that are already firing increase their discharge and are joined by high-threshold receptors being recruited. The exact location of these high threshold receptors remains unclear.

Investigators have demonstrated mechanoreceptors that generate afferent impulses phasically during breathing in the absence of airflow and pressure—the so-called drive receptors.[2,87] They recognized the role of intrinsic laryngeal muscle activity in stimulating these receptors and identified persistent activity even after laryngeal paralysis indicating that the receptors also responded to oropharyngeal muscle activity or passive tracheal motion. Sant'Ambrogio et al[78] studied the specific role of muscle contraction and tracheal motion on the function of laryngeal mechanoreceptors. Action potentials were counted during both inspiration and expiration, and the receptors were designated accordingly. Laryngeal receptors were sensitive to laryngeal muscle activity and unaffected, or affected less than 10%, by tracheal motion. The tracheal motion receptors were unaffected by laryngeal muscle activity. Single-fiber recordings of the superior laryngeal nerve indicated that the intrinsic laryngeal muscles and transmitted tracheal motion modulating inspiration have a baseline input for respiratory control. The majority of this group of receptors represents a special contribution to the mechanical coupling of respiration. Although most laryngeal mechanoreceptors play a role in upper airway patency, breathing pattern, and probably vocalization, head movements alter resistance to tracheal flow and therefore influence the modulating effect of tracheal motion receptors.

Impulses from the laryngeal mechanoreceptors initiate reflexes that make a significant contribution to the regulation of respiration, including upper airway patency. Sant'Ambrogio et al[82] indicated that the pressure mechanoreceptors sensitive to collapsing pressure played the greatest role. In tracheotomized and anesthetized dogs, diversion of the airflow above and below the larynx as well as airway occlusion showed that flow receptors did not appear to alter significantly the pattern of breathing. Drive receptors have been shown to be responsive to intrinsic laryngeal muscle activity. These studies suggest a role of these receptors in respiratory regulation and airway patency. The contribution of the pressure receptors was assessed by comparing their responses to upper airway and tracheal occlusion. The negative pressure present in the larynx during airway occlusion accompanied by the increased posterior cricoarytenoid activity was interpreted by Sant'Ambrogio et al as indicating a role of these receptors in maintaining airway patency. These negative pressure responses were abolished by sectioning the superior laryngeal nerves.[89]

These reflexes assume clinical importance in tracheotomized patients and those with obstructive sleep apnea. Sasaki et al[90] noted a significant decrease in posterior cricoarytenoid activity immediately after tracheotomy and a total lack of activity within 1 week. Abu-Osba et al[91] demonstrated that such a decrease in intrinsic laryngeal muscle function resulted in oropharyngeal collapse in rabbits. Remmers et al[92] reported obstructive sleep apnea to occur at the level of the oropharynx. The resulting intense negative pressure in the larynx triggers a reflex to maintain airway patency through excitation of the negative-pressure receptors. This reflex mechanism is what prevents obstructive apnea from being a uniformly fatal affliction.

Paraganglia

Small discrete bodies comprising clusters of epithelium-like cells in a richly vascular connective tissue stroma that are chromaffin-negative histologically make up a system of nonchromaffin paraganglia.[93] These bodies are generally noted along branches of the cranial parasympathetic nerves, often juxtavascularly. These cells generally have a sensory innervation, produce only small quantities of biogenic amines resulting in a negative chromaffin response, and probably function as chemoreceptor organs.[94] The carotid body is the best known member of this system and its function as a chemosensory organ is well established. However, there exist clusters of nonchromaffin cells in the temporal bone, nodose ganglion of the vagus nerve, larynx,[93] and mediastinum, whose functions are not clearly elucidated. More than 70 cases of laryngeal paraganglioma have been reported to date that correlate with the naturally occurring paraganglia in the area.[95,96]

In a study of serially sectioned larynges, Watzka,[97] in 1963, recorded the first observation of nonchromaffin paraganglia in the larynx. Kleinsasser[98] and the group of Lawson and Zak then independently discovered subglottic paraganglia using this method. Paraganglia have been described in the human larynx at two main sites. The upper collection, known as the superior laryngeal glomus, measures 0.1 to 0.3 mm in diameter. The inferior laryngeal glomus body occurs bilaterally between the inferior horn of the thyroid cartilage and measures 0.3 to 0.4 mm in diameter. A variable midline body was reported anterior to the cricothyroid membrane by Kleinsasser, which he labeled an anterior laryngeal glomus. Scattered ectopic foci have also been noted in laryngeal tissue other than at the above sites.[93]

The laryngeal glomus bodies are related to the autonomic system via the cranial nerves IX and X, with clusters of cells present within their branches and ganglia. Although the laryngeal bodies are structurally identical to the carotid bodies, the question as to whether they have chemoreceptor activity is not undisputed. There is increasing data indicating that they function as chemoreceptors. These cells have been reported to contain several neuropeptides such as substance P, dopamine, 5-hydroxytryptamine, and neuropeptide Y.[94] Schonberger[22] and Kleinsasser believed the close association between laryngeal paraganglia (glomus bodies) and nervous elements indicated a chemoreceptor function. Lack[99] noted hyperplastic changes in the vagal bodies of patients with chronic hypoxia and considered this to represent morphologic evidence of their chemoreceptor function. O'Leary et al[100] demonstrated that hypoxia triggered firing of rat superior laryngeal nerve fibers as well as chemoreceptor response to small volumes of the chemostimulant sodium cyanide. The physiologic role of the laryngeal paraganglia is unclear, and further investigation is needed.

References

1. Marchal F, Corke B, Sundell H. Reflex apnea from laryngeal chemo-stimulation in the sleeping premature newborn lamb. Pediatr Res 1982;16:621–627
2. Sanders I, Mu L. Anatomy of the human internal superior laryngeal nerve. Anat Rec 1998;252:646–656
3. Konig WF. Histologische untersuchungen uber die sensiblen nervosen endigungen im stimmband des menschen. Arch Miker Anat 1881;19:53
4. Simanowsky N. Der taschenband muskel die nervenendigangen in den wahlem stimmbandem des menschen und der saugetiere. Arch Mikr Anat 1883;22:698–707
5. Retzius G. Uber die sensib1en nervenendigangen in den epithe1ien bei den wirbelthieren. Biol Untersuch 1982;4:42–44
6. Ploschko A. Die nervenendigangen und pathogischehistologie der innervation des kehlkopfes. Z Mikrosk Anat Forsch 1958;64:364–416
7. Jabonero V. Uber die normale und pathogischehistologie der innervation des kehlkopfes. Z Mikrosk Anat Forsch 1958;64:364–416
8. Shin T, Watanabe S, Wada S, Maeyama T. Sensory nerve endings in the mucosa of the epiglottis-morphologic investigations with silver impregnation, immunohistochemistry, and electron microscopy. Otolaryngol Head Neck Surg 1987;96:55–62
9. Yamamoto Y, Atoji Y, Hobo S, et al. Morphology of the nerve endings in laryngeal mucosa of the horse. Equine Vet J 2001;33:150–158
10. Lima-Rodrigues M, Nunes R, Almeida A. Intraepithelial nerve fibers project into the lumen of the larynx. Laryngoscope 2004;114:1074–1077
11. Idé C, Munger BL. The cytologic composition of primate laryngeal chemosensory corpuscles. Am J Anat 1980;158:193–209
12. Sweazey RD, Edwards CA, Kapp BM. Fine structure of taste buds located on the lamb epiglottis. Anat Rec 1994;238:517–527
13. Bradley RM. Sensory receptors of the larynx. Am J Med 2000;108(Suppl 4a):47S–50S
14. Sbarbati A, Merigo F, Benati D, et al. Identification and characterization of a specific sensory epithelium in the rat larynx. J Comp Neurol 2004;475:188–220
15. Schofield RH. Observation of taste goblets in the epiglottis of the dog and cat. J Anat Physiol. 1876;10:475–477
16. Lalonde ER, Eglittis JE. Number and distribution of taste buds on the epiglottis, pharynx, larynx, softpalate and uvula in a human newborn. Anat Rec 1961;140:91–95
17. Bradley RM, Cheal ML, Kim YH. Quantitative analysis of developing epiglottal taste buds in sheep. J Anat 1980;130:25–32
18. Wilson JG. The structure and function of taste buds on the larynx. Brain 1905;28:339–351
19. Storey AT. A functional analysis of sensory units innervating epiglottis and larynx. Exp Neurol 1968;20:366–383
20. Boushey HA, Richardson PS, Widdicombe JG, Wise JC. The response of laryngeal afferent fibres to mechanical and chemical stimuli. J Physiol 1974;240:153–175
21. Cooper S, Daniel PM, Whitteridge D. Muscle spindles and other sensory endings in the extrinsic eye muscles; the physiology and anatomy of these receptors and of their connexions with the brainstem. Brain 1955;78:564–583
22. Schonberger W. On paraganglia in plica ventricularis of newborn infants. Anat Anz 1966;119:296–304
23. Storey AT, Johnson P. Laryngeal water receptors initiating apnea in the lamb. Exp Neurol 1975;47:42–55
24. Harding R, Johnson P, McClelland ME. Liquid-sensitive laryngeal receptors in the developing sheep, cat and monkey. J Physiol 1978;277:409–422
25. Koizumi H. On sensory innervation of larynx in dog. Tohoku J Exp Med 1953;58:199–210
26. Bradley RM, Stedman HM, Mistretta CM. Superior laryngeal nerve response patterns to chemical stimulation of sheep epiglottis. Brain Res 1983;276:81–93
27. Shingai T, Shimada K. Reflex swallowing elicited by water and chemical substances applied in the oral cavity, pharynx, and larynx of the rabbit. Jpn J Physiol 1976;26:455–469
28. Kovar I, Selstam U, Catterton WZ, Stahlman MT, Sundell HW. Laryngeal chemoreflex in newborn lambs: respiratory and swallowing response to salts, acids, and sugars. Pediatr Res 1979;13:1144–1149
29. Boggs DF, Bartlett D Jr. Chemical specificity of a laryngeal apneic reflex in puppies. J Appl Physiol 1982;53:455–462
30. Downing SE, Lee JC. Laryngeal chemosensitivity: a possible mechanism for sudden infant death. Pediatrics 1975;55:640–649
31. Long WA, Lawson EE. Maturation of the superior laryngeal nerve inhibitory effect. Am Rev Respir Dis 1981;123:166
32. GE, Storey AT, Sessle BJ. Effects of upper respiratory tract stimuli on neonatal respiration: reflex and single neuron analyses in the kitten. Biol Neonate 1979;35:82–89
33. Mortelliti AJ, Malmgren LT, Gacek RR. Ultrastructural changes with age in the human superior laryngeal nerve. Arch Otolaryngol Head Neck Surg 1990;116:1062–1069
34. Rosenberg SI, Malmgren LT, Woo P. Age-related changes in the internal branch of the rat superior laryngeal nerve. Arch Otolaryngol Head Neck Surg 1989;115:78–86
35. Yamamoto Y, Tanaka S, Tsubone H, et al. Age-related changes in sensory and secretomotor nerve endings in the larynx of F344/N rat. Arch Gerontol Geriatr 2003;36:173–183
36. Angell-James JE, Daly MB. Some aspects of upper respiratory tract reflexes. Acta Otolaryngol 1975;79:242–252
37. Iriuchijima J, Kumada M. On the cardioinhibitory reflex originating from the superior laryngeal nerve. Jpn J Physiol 1968;18:453–461
38. Lee JC, Stoll BJ, Downing SE. Properties of the laryngeal chemoreflex in neonatal piglets. Am J Physiol 1977;233:R30–R36
39. Grogaard J, Lindstrom DP, Stahlman MT, Marchal F, Sundell H. The cardiovascular response to laryngeal water administration in young lambs. J Dev Physiol 1982;4:353–370
40. Belenky DA, Standaert TA, Woodrum DE. Maturation of hypoxic ventilatory response of the newborn lamb. J Appl Physiol 1979;47:927–930
41. Bureau MA, Zinman R, Foulon P, Begin R. Diphasic ventilatory response to hypoxia in newborn lambs. J Appl Physiol 1984;56:84–90
42. Herbst JJ, Minton SD, Book LS. Gastroesophageal reflux causing respiratory distress and apnea in newborn infants. J Pediatr 1979;95(5 Pt 1):763–768
43. Leape LL, Holder TM, Franklin JD, Amoury RA, Ashcraft KW. Respiratory arrest in infants secondary to gastroesophageal reflux. Pediatrics 1977;60:924–928
44. Sutton D, Taylor EM, Lindeman RC. Prolonged apnea in infant monkeys resulting from stimulation of superior laryngeal nerve. Pediatrics 1978;61:519–527
45. Sasaki CT. Development of laryngeal function: etiologic significance in the sudden infant death syndrome. Laryngoscope 1979;89:1964–1982
46. Baker TL, McGinty DJ. Reversal of cardiopulmonary failure during active sleep in hypoxic kittens: implications for sudden infant death. Science 1977;198:419–421
47. Gabriel M, Albani M, Schulte FJ. Apneic spells and sleep states in preterm infants. Pediatrics 1976;57:142–147
48. Naeye RL, Fisher R, Ryser M, Whalen P. Carotid body in the sudden infant death syndrome. Science 1976;191:567–569

49. Nishino T, Tagaito Y, Isono S. Cough and other reflexes on irritation of airway mucosa in man. Pulm Pharmacol 1996;9:285–292
50. Hines M. Nerve and muscle. Q Rev Biol 1927;2:149–180
51. Hinsey JE. The innervation of skeletal muscle. Physiol Rev 1934;14: 514–585
52. Barker D. The innervation of the muscle spindle. Q J Microsc Sci 1948;89:143–186
53. Tiegs OW. Innervation of voluntary muscle. Physiol Rev 1953;33: 90–144
54. Fernand VS, Young JZ. The sizes of the nerve fibres of muscle nerves. Proc R Soc Lond B Biol Sci 1951;139:38–58
55. Fulton JF. Howell's Textbook of Physiology. 15th ed. Philadelphia: WB Saunders; 1946:190
56. Bowden RE, Mahran ZY. The functional significance of the pattern of innervation of the muscle quadratus labii superioris of the rabbit, cat and rat. J Anat 1956;90:217–227
57. Kadanoff D. Sensitive nerve endings in human mimic muscles. Z Mikrosk Anat Forsch 1956;62:1–15
58. Goerttler K. Die anordnung histologie und histogenese der quergestreifen muskulator im menschlichen stimmband. Z Anat Entwicklungsgesch 1950;115:352–401
59. Paulsen K. Occurrence and number of muscle spindles in intermallaryngeal muscles of humans (m. cricoarytenoideus & m. cricothyreoideus). Z Zellforsch Mikrosk Anat 1958;48:349–355
60. Keene MF. Muscle spindles in human laryngeal muscles. J Anat 1961;95:25–29
61. Sherrington CS. On the anatomical constitution of nerves of skeletal muscles; with remarks on recurrent fibres in the ventral spinal nerve root. J Physiol 1894;17:210–258
62. Ibrahim MK, Abd EI, Rahman S, Mahran ZY. Experimental studies on the afferent innervation of the cricothyroid muscle in dogs. Acta Anat (Basel) 1980;106:171–179
63. Gracheva MS. On sensory innervation of the framework of the motor apparatus of the larynx. Arkh Anat Gistol Embriol 1963;44:77–83
64. Martenson A. Communication. Acta Physiol Scand 1964;62:176
65. Nagai T. Encapsulated nerve structures in the human vocal cord. An electron microscopic study. Acta Otolaryngol 1987;104:363–369
66. Schoultz TW, Swett JE. The fine structure of the Golgi tendon organ. J Neurocytol 1972;1:1–26
67. Bianconi R, Molinari G. Electroneurographic evidence of muscle spindles and other sensory endings in the intrinsic laryngeal muscles of the cat. Acta Otolaryngol 1962;55:253–259
68. Granit R. Receptors and Sensory Perception, XL. New Haven: Yale University Press; 1955
69. Sanders I, Han Y, Wang J, Biller H. Muscle spindles are concentrated in the superior vocalis subcompartment of the human thyroarytenoid muscle. J Voice 1998;12:7–16
70. Brandon CA, Rosen C, Georgelis G, Horton MJ, Mooney MP, Sciote JJ. Staining of human thyroarytenoid muscle with myosin antibodies reveals some unique extrafusal fibers, but no muscle spindles. J Voice 2003;17:245–254
71. Rosen C, Tellis CM, Thekdi A, Sciote JL. Anatomy and fiber type composition of human interarytenoid muscle. Ann Otol Rhinol Laryngol 2004;113:97–107
72. Sampson S, Eyzaguirre C. Some functional characteristics of mechanoreceptors in the larynx of the cat. J Neurophysiol 1964;27: 464–480
73. Andrew BL. The respiratory displacement of the larynx: a study of the innervation of accessory respiratory muscles. J Physiol 1955;130: 474–487
74. Kirchner JA, Wyke BD. Articular reflex mechanisms of the larynx. Ann Otol Rhinol Laryngol 1965;74:749–767
75. Kirchner JA, Wyke BD. Innervation of laryngeal joints, and laryngeal reflexes. Nature 1964;201:506
76. Abo-el-Enein MA. Laryngeal myotatic reflexes. Nature 1966;209: 682–686
77. Lawson W. Glomus bodies and tumors. N Y State J Med 1980;80: 1567–1575
78. Sant'Ambrogio G, Mathew OP, Sant'Ambrogio FB. Role of intrinsic muscles and tracheal motion in modulating laryngeal receptors. Respir Physiol 1985;61:289–300
79. Al-Shway SF, Mortola JP. Respiratory effects of airflow through the upper airways in newborn kittens and puppies. J Appl Physiol 1982;53:805–814
80. Mathew OP, Sant'Ambrogio G, Fisher JT, Sant'Ambrogio FB. Laryngeal pressure receptors. Respir Physiol 1984;57:113–122
81. McBride B, Whitelaw WA. A physiological stimulus to upper airway receptors in humans. J Appl Physiol 1981;51:1189–1197
82. Sant'Ambrogio FB, Mathew OP, Clark WD, Sant'Ambrogio G. Laryngeal influences on breathing pattern and posterior cricoarytenoid muscle activity. J Appl Physiol 1985;58:1298–1304
83. Sant'Ambrogio G. Role of the larynx in cough. Pulm Pharmacol 1996;9:379–382
84. Mathew OP, Abu-Osba YK, Thach BT. Influence of upper airway pressure changes on genioglossus muscle respiratory activity. J Appl Physiol 1982;52:438–444
85. Mathew OP, Abu-Osba YK, Thach BT. Genioglossus muscle responses to upper airway pressure changes: afferent pathways. J Appl Physiol 1982;52:445–450
86. Mathew OP, Abu-Osba YK, Thach BT. Influence of upper airway pressure changes on respiratory frequency. Respir Physiol 1982;49: 223–233
87. Mathew OP. Upper airway negative-pressure effects on respiratory activity of upper airway muscles. J Appl Physiol 1984;56:500–505
88. Felman AH, Loughlin GM, Leftridge CA Jr, Cassisi NJ. Upper airway obstruction during sleep in children. AJR Am J Roentgenol 1979; 133:213–216
89. Van Lunteren E, Van de Graaff WB, Parker DM, et al. Nasal and laryngeal reflex responses to negative upper airway pressure. J Appl Physiol 1984;56:746–752
90. Sasaki CT, Fukuda H, Kirchner JA. Laryngeal abductor activity in response to varying ventilatory resistance. Trans Am Acad Ophthalmol Otolaryngol 1973;77:ORL403–ORL10
91. Abu-Osba YK, Mathew OP, Thach BT. An animal model for airway sensory deprivation producing obstructive apnea with postmortem findings of sudden infant death syndrome. Pediatrics 1981;68: 796–801
92. Remmers JE, deGroot WJ, Sauerland EK, Anch AM. Pathogenesis of upper airway occlusion during sleep. J Appl Physiol 1978;44: 931–938
93. Lawson W, Zak FG. The glomus bodies ("paraganglia") of the human larynx. Laryngoscope 1974;84:98–111
94. Lawson W. The neuroendocrine nature of the glomus cells: an experimental, ultrastructural, and histochemical tissue culture study. Laryngoscope 1980;90:120–144
95. Pellitteri PK, Rinaldo A, Myssiorek D, et al. Paragangliomas of the head and neck. Oral Oncol 2004;40:563–575
96. Peterson KL, Fu YS, Calcaterra T. Subglottic paraganglioma. Head Neck 1997;19:54–56
97. Watzka M. On the paraganglia in the plica ventricularis of the human larynx. Acta Anat (Basel) 1966;63:300–308
98. Kleinsasser O. The inferior laryngeal glomus: a nonchromaffin paraganglion, unknown so far, of the structure of the so-called carotid gland in human larynx. Arch Ohren Nasen Kehlkopfheilkd 1964;184: 214–224
99. Lack EE. Hyperplasia of vagal and carotid body paraganglia in patients with chronic hypoxemia. Am J Pathol 1978;91:497–516
100. O'Leary DM, Murphy A, Pickering M, Jones JF. Arterial chemoreceptors in the superior laryngeal nerve of the rat. Respir Physiol Neurobiol 2004;141:137–144

Chapter 3

Central Laryngeal Motor Innervation

Leslie T. Malmgren Jr. and Richard R. Gacek

Control of laryngeal function has evolved from a simple respiratory reflex (sphincteric and dilation) protecting the pulmonary system in lung fish, into midbrain and subcortical pathways in higher species serving phonatory capabilities associated with warning, mating, and anger as well as with more complex respiratory reflexes. Ultimately, the acquisition of voluntary phonation (speech) in humans was paralleled by direct connections between the laryngeal motoneurons and the cerebral cortex. The central nuclei and pathways providing these roles are reviewed in this chapter (**Fig. 3.1**).

◆ Functional Organization of the Laryngeal Motoneurons in the Nucleus Ambiguus

The functional and topographical organization of the laryngeal motoneurons (LMNs) in the nucleus ambiguus (NA) reflects the evolutionary origin of the larynx from accessory respiratory muscles as well as more recent adaptations to vocalization and speech. Phylogenetically, the NA is first seen in reptiles with the differentiation of the visceral efferent vagus into distinct dorsal and ventrolateral motor nuclei,[1] possibly to support the evolution of the orienting reflex, which is characterized by focusing of exteroreceptors, freezing of movement, and neurogenic bradycardia.[2] With the evolution of mammals, the additional capacity for voluntary attention, emotions, and communication in the form of facial expressions and vocalizations was added to this orienting behavior as well as adaptations to the greatly increased oxidative metabolism of mammals.[2] As such, the mammalian NA projects to supradiaphragmatic structures including the larynx, pharynx, soft palate, esophagus, bronchi, and heart (primary cardioinhibitory motoneurons) with only minor projections to subdiaphragmatic structures restricted to rostral NA. The major innervation to these subdiaphragmatic structures is provided by projections from the dorsal motor nucleus of the vagus.[3] The most rostral NA neurons are separated from the main (caudal) division of the NA at birth and are known as the retrofacial nucleus (RFN), which merges with the NA neurons during development.[4]

Early lesion studies[5,6] and horseradish peroxidase (HRP) retrograde labeling investigations in a variety of species[4,7–13] have shown that the most rostral LMN group projects to the cricothyroid (CT) muscle and that they extend to or overlap the caudal margin of the facial nerve nucleus. In the caudal two thirds of the NA, the adductor LMNs are located in the dorsolateral division of the NA, running within the recurrent laryngeal nerve. These include, from rostral to caudal, the LMN for the thyroarytenoid (TA), lateral cricoarytenoid (LCA), and interarytenoid (IA) muscles. Although concentrated pools of these LMNs can be distinguished, there is considerable overlap. The LMN pool for the posterior cricoarytenoid (PCA) is located in the middle one third of the NA. The adductor neurons have a diffuse arrangement in the dorsolateral portion of the NA, whereas the PCA abductor neurons are more compactly grouped ventromedially to the adductor neurons.[4,7–11,14]

Although the topographical representation of the groups of LMNs innervating the individual laryngeal muscles is established, less is known about the functional organization within the motoneuron pools of the laryngeal muscles. In nonlaryngeal muscles the diversity of motoneuron size, synaptic input, and neuromodulator content are integral to the mechanisms underlying motor control, but the extent to which similar relationships extend to the laryngeal muscles is unclear. Increases in muscle force are generally achieved by the progressive recruitment of individual motor units, which consist of a motoneuron and the set of muscle fibers that it innervates (muscle unit).[15,16] Because the characteristics of the muscle unit are primarily controlled by the motoneuron, the physiologic and histochemical profiles of all muscle fibers within each muscle unit are uniform.[17,18] Furthermore, motor unit characteristics cluster into categories based on their fatigability and their twitch contraction time. In adult human limb muscles, these include type 1 (slow twitch, fatigue resistant), type 2A (fast twitch, fatigue resistant), and type 2X (previously called 2B; fast twitch, fatigable).[19] In most nonlaryngeal muscles, motor units are recruited in an orderly size-ordered sequence in which the smallest force and slowest contracting type 1 motor units are recruited first, progressing to the larger force and faster type 2A motor units, and finally to the largest force, 2B motor units.[17] This stereotypic recruitment of increasingly larger motor units with greater conduction velocities and

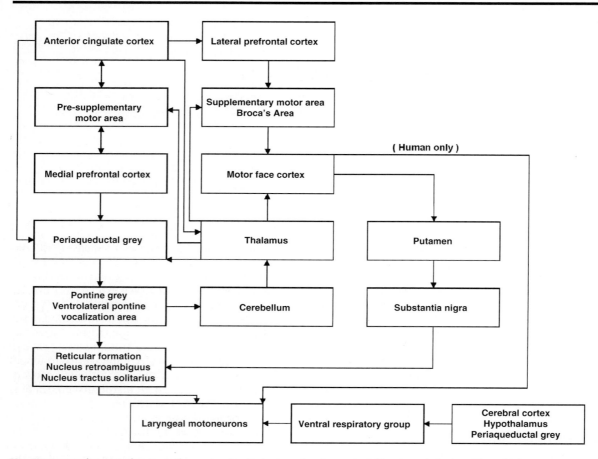

Fig. 3.1 Circuit diagram of major pathways involved in laryngeal motor control. Structures in boxes with multiple structures are directly connected with each other.

larger soma size is known as the "size principle."[16] However, there is evidence that this stereotypic recruitment sequence is modified for the laryngeal motor units as an adaptation to the coordination of their diverse roles in phonation, deglutition, Valsalva maneuver, coughing, and respiration, and possibly also to corresponding functional topographic gradients (compartments or fiber bundles) that have been described in some of the laryngeal muscles. Possibly consistent with these diverse adaptations, some laryngeal motor unit types express unusual myosin heavy chain isoforms such as extraocular myosin or mixtures of myosin heavy chain isoforms.[18,20–22]

There is evidence for such functional and topographic diversity within the TA muscles and their innervation. Studies in the awake monkey have demonstrated subsets of motoneurons in the NA that are recruited during multiple behaviors for control of generalized laryngeal functions, and other subsets that are recruited during specific behaviors such as vocalization, swallowing, or respiration.[23,24] Consistent with these findings, retrograde tracer studies using cholera toxin B have demonstrated distinct muscle fiber bundles in feline TA muscles that are likely to play different roles in laryngeal function.[25] Motoneurons innervating muscle fiber bundles in the vocalis were located more medially than the motoneurons of other TA motor units, but there was no apparent rostral to caudal functional diversity among TA motoneurons.[25] The motoneuron size did not differ among these TA muscle fiber bundles.[25] Although motor unit pools have generally been considered to be equivalent to motor nuclei, reports that some animal limb muscles, such as the cat anterior sartorius, are innervated by two functionally distinct motor unit pools are consistent with this finding.[17,26]

Cholera toxin tracer studies have also suggested functional diversity within the feline PCA motoneuron pool in that motoneurons projecting to the vertical component of the PCA are located dorsomedially to motoneurons projecting to the oblique subdivision.[25] However, there was no significant difference in the soma diameter of these two groups.[25] Studies concerning the synaptology of PCA motoneurons provide further support for a diversity of motoneuron pools and recruitment mechanisms. Retrograde transport of cholera toxin subunit B-conjugated HRP was used to label PCA motoneurons in the rat for the determination of their ultrastructure and synaptic organization.[27] Two types of neurons were identified in the PCA. One type (PCA-A) was significantly smaller than the other (PCA-B) in frontal sections at the level of the nucleolus. The mean number of axosomatic synapses per section also differed significantly between these motoneuron populations with the largest input to the PCA-B motoneurons (57) followed by the PCA-A motoneurons (36).[27] In the PCA-A motoneurons, the majority (65%) of axosomatic terminals were excitatory (Gray's type II), whereas in the PCA-B motoneurons the majority (61%) were inhibitory (Gray's type I).[27] The ratios of excitatory to inhibitory axodendritic terminals were similar to the data for axosomatic terminals in the respective motoneuron type.[27] Based on these findings, it was suggested that PCA-A neurons receive inhibitory inputs containing γ-aminobutyric acid (GABA) from the nucleus tractus solitarius (NTS). This is consistent with GABA-containing neurons in the lateral part of the NTS,[28] GABAergic fibers in the caudal part of the NA,[28] and physiologic data showing many GABA receptors in the same area.[29] It was hypothesized that this inhibitory input to the PCA-A motoneurons is used to relax the PCA, causing the closing of the glottis during swallowing, while the excitatory input to the PCA-B motoneurons would open the glottis during inspiration.[27] Possibly consistent with this finding, the human PCA muscle has two divisions: a vertically oriented component, which inserts on the body of the arytenoid cartilage, and a more obliquely directed muscle component, which inserts on the posterior surface of the muscular process of the arytenoid. It has been proposed that the action of the former would be to stabilize the arytenoid in the phonatory action of the cricothyroid (CT), thus lengthening the vocal ligament. In contrast, the oblique portion of the PCA is reported to abduct the vocal ligament during inspiration. In contrast, it has been reported that the dog PCA includes transverse, oblique, and lateral divisions.[30] However, muscle stimulation studies indicate that the vertical and oblique divisions are both related to inspiratory abduction, whereas the transverse division regulates the position of the vocal process during phonation.[31]

It has also been demonstrated that motoneurons projecting to the vertical component of the CT are located ventromedially to those of the oblique part, suggesting a functional diversity within the CT motoneuron pool.[25] However, there is no difference between the soma size of these two groups, although they are both smaller than other laryngeal motoneurons.[25] Also, cholera toxin tracer studies concerning the ultrastructural synaptology of CT motoneurons report a single type of neuron in the CT with the majority (70%) of axosomatic terminals being excitatory (Gray's type II).[27] It was suggested that the recruitment of the CT motoneurons during swallowing and respiration is achieved primarily by excitatory input.[27] The CT exhibits peripheral subdivisions, suggesting different effects on the vocal cord and voice. The ventral portion of the CT, by closing the cricothyroid gap, would stretch the vocal ligament in apposition to the PCA. The oblique division of the CT could assist in enlarging the glottic aperture during inspiration. Such varied actions of muscle subunits would require separate neural inputs to appropriate motoneurons in the NA.

♦ Laryngeal Respiratory Motor Innervation

Ventral Respiratory Group

The respiratory patterns of laryngeal motoneurons during eupnea are mainly generated by inhibitory and excitatory inputs from neurons in the ventral respiratory group (VRG).[32–36] The VRGs in the rat, cat, and rabbit are basically similar, consisting of three divisions. An expiratory division (Botzinger complex) is ventral to the rostral NA, and a second expiratory group extends from the caudal NA though the retroambiguus.[35,37] Expiratory neurons in the Botzinger complex project to inspiratory neurons in the rostral VRG.[38] The inspiratory division is between the two groups of expiratory neurons.[35,37] The respiratory activity patterns originate within the VRG in a neuronal network known as the respiratory central pattern generator (RCPG).[39] Augmenting inspiratory neurons in the VRG drive the respiratory spinal motoneurons and interneurons.[40] Accessory respiratory muscles are driven by collateral branches of these neurons, which innervate the retrofacial nucleus, the hypoglossal nucleus, and laryngeal motoneurons in the NA.[40,41] Neuroanatomic studies based on the retrograde transport of double fluorescent dyes after injection into the cervical spinal cord and the laryngeal muscles have demonstrated that the locations of some bulbospinal interneurons overlap with the NA in both rats and cats.[42] Furthermore, in both species they are consistently distributed within the spread of the LMN's dendritic trees.[42] Because there were no double-labeled neurons, none of these laryngeal neurons projected to the spinal cord.[42] Although this overlap of bulbospinal interneurons with laryngeal neurons is present throughout the NA in both species, there are rostrocaudal and interspecies variations in the predominant localizations of bulbospinal neurons.[42] In both species they were mainly ventrolateral to the LMN in the rostral NA, but at more caudal levels they were predominantly ventromedial and ventrolateral in cats and more concentrated within the NA in rats.[42] Physiologic studies have also noted this overlap between the VRG and the NA, and that respiration-related neurons modify their discharge rates during vocalization and swallowing. Most cells have a higher discharge rate during vocalization than during quiet respiration.[43]

Nucleus Tractus Solitarius

The nucleus tractus solitarius (NTS) plays a major role in the coordination of alimentary and respiratory functions (see also Chapter 2).[44,45] However, the neuroanatomic pathways involved in input from this nucleus to the LMN remain unclear in spite of the vital role of these neuronal networks in preventing aspiration. Based on synaptic delay, it has been concluded that the glottic closure reflex in humans following stimulation of the internal branch of the ipsilateral internal branch of the superior laryngeal nerve (SLN) involves at least two synapses, one in the ipsilateral NTS and one in the NA.[45] However, the contralateral reflex response has a greater latency, suggesting two or three additional interneurons within the reticular formation.[45] It was further proposed that the increased synaptic complexity of the contralateral pathway accounts for the observed greater vulnerability of the crossed adductor reflex to anesthesia due to an increased effect of central facilitation.[45] Neuroanatomic tracer studies demonstrating projections from the NTS to the NA and reticular formation are consistent with these findings.[46–48]

Cortical Respiratory Centers

Although the respiratory patterns of LMN are initiated by the RCPG within the VRG during eupnea, the cerebral cortex plays an essential role in the initiation of volitional respiration such as during breath holding or voluntary inspiratory or expiratory efforts. In humans, premotor cerebral potentials can be recorded in the area of the motor cortex prior to voluntary inspiratory or expiratory efforts, but not during spontaneous quiet breathing.[49] Positron emission tomography (PET) has been used to determine the three-dimensional distribution of neuronal activation in the human cerebral cortex during volitional inspiration and expiration.[50] During voluntary inspiration, increased blood flow was detected in the right and left primary cortices dorsolateral to the vertex, in the supplementary motor area, the right lateral pre-motor cortex, and the left ventrolateral thalamus.[50] The localization of neuronal activity associated with volitional expiration was similar, but more extensive with the inclusion of the ventrolateral thalamus bilaterally and the cerebellum.[50] Recently, PET demonstrated increased activity in the ventral rolandic cortex that increased during both voiced and whispered speech.[51] It was suggested that the greater activity seen with whispered speech may reflect the greater cortical control of the chest wall and diaphragm during the rapid air loss that occurs during whispering.[51] In addition, the observation that this increased activity was left lateralized was suggested to reflect the dominance of the left hemisphere in praxis, because the temporal coordination of the respiratory and laryngeal muscles as well as the rapid and precise recruitment of the laryngeal muscles during pitch adjustments in voiced speech may constitute a praxic demand.[51,52]

Laryngeal Motor Innervation for Vocalization and Speech

Premotor Neurons

Medullary Reticular Formation

The medullary reticular formation plays a key role in vocal motor coordination. Studies using the anterograde tracer biotin dextran amine have demonstrated numerous efferent projections from the laryngeal motor cortex to the parvicellular, intermediate, and dorsal reticular nuclei,[53] but retrograde tracer studies with wheat germ agglutinin HRP indicate that there are no reciprocal projections from these nuclei to the laryngeal cortex.[54] Because these reticular nuclei also project to the nucleus ambiguus,[55] it has been suggested that they function as a cortico-ambigual relay for motor coordination of learned vocal patterns.[53] In addition, these nuclei also receive inputs from the periaqueductal gray for the coordination of innate vocal patterns. Single-unit recordings in the monkey have shown that the parvocellular reticular formation has a greater number of cells with vocalization-related activity changes than other reticular nuclei.[56] Because these cells are not active during quiet inspiration, their primary role is not respiratory.[56] Conversely, the parvocellular reticular formation contained the greatest number of cells that were active immediately before, but not during, vocalization, indicating that they are more likely involved in the initiation of vocalization or pre-phonatory processes.[56] In this respect, they resemble cells with similar activity in the periaqueductal gray (PAG). However, the parvocellular and dorsal reticular nuclei contain neurons with a discharge rate that correlates with changes in the fundamental frequency and intensity,[56] whereas the PAG does not contain pattern generating neurons.[57]

Nucleus Retroambiguus

Anterograde tracer studies with wheat germ agglutinin have demonstrated projections from the nucleus retroambiguus (NRA) to the dendrites of LMNs in the monkey and cat.[58,59] These projections are bilateral with a contralateral predominance.[59] In both species, the dendrites of cholera toxin–labeled CT motoneurons receive asymmetrical synaptic contacts, containing spherical vesicles, suggesting that they are excitatory.[58,59] Physiologic evidence,[60,61] neuroanatomic studies,[62] and 2-deoxyglucose uptake techniques show that the NRA plays a role in vocalization.[63] However, the laryngeal adductor response, following a single stimulus to the internal branch of the superior laryngeal nerve, does not involve neuronal activation of the NRA.[64] It has been suggested that this pathway is involved in control of the LMN during vocalization and straining activities.[59]

Midbrain Centers

Periaqueductal Gray and Laterally Bordering Reticular Formation

Electrical stimulation of the PAG produces vocalizations similar to species-specific calls such as laughing in humans,[65] trilling in the squirrel monkey,[66] meowing in the cat,[67] and ultrasonic vocalizations in the rat.[52,68] Ablation of the PAG or its outflow tract in the later tegmental field abolishes all vocalization (mutism).[69] However, partial destruction of the PAG generally results in the loss of certain call types with no change in the acoustic structure of the remaining calls, as occurs with lower brainstem lesions.[69-71] The observation that these vocalizations can be elicited not only by electrical stimulation but also by glutamate agonists and GABA antagonists demonstrates that they are due to activation of PAG neurons rather than fibers of passage.[70,71] Furthermore, single-unit recordings in the PAG have demonstrated vocalization-correlated activity, demonstrating that the PAG is involved in the coordination of brainstem nuclei during vocalization.[72] More recent telemetric single-unit studies in the squirrel monkey studies have shown that vocalization-correlated activity with the same reaction profiles extends into the reticular formation bordering the PAG.[57]

The PAG receives inputs from several limbic structures,[69,73] and activities in vocalization-correlated neurons in the PAG correspond to different motivational states.[74]

Furthermore, all vocalizations elicited from the limbic forebrain require an intact PAG.[69,75-77] Recent stereologic studies have demonstrated some regions in the PAG that produce call types differing in the degree of "aversiveness" when pharmacologically stimulated to receive inputs from the same structures, but with quantitative differences in the number of retrogradely labeled cells from certain regions.[78] For example, the cell count from the posterior hypothalamus correlated positively with aversiveness, whereas the preoptic area and the nucleus striae terminalis showed a negative correlation.[78] Because vocalization-correlated neurons in the PAG do not reflect frequency modulation and have only scarce projections to laryngeal motoneurons, it has been suggested that they do not function in pattern generation but rather to code vocal responses to different motivational states (species-specific calls). However, a recent PET study has demonstrated highly correlated activity in the PAG during voiced speech but not in whispered speech in humans,[51] although part of this activation may be related to sensory feedback to the PAG during phonation.[79]

◆ Ventrolateral Pontine Vocalization Area

Because direct connections between the PAG and the NA are scarce, it is likely that additional areas contribute to vocal motor coordination.[55,80-82] Stereotaxic injections of a nonspecific glutamate antagonist into the ventrolateral pons directly dorsal to the superior olivary complex blocks ipsilateral PAG-elicited vocalization in squirrel monkeys, demonstrating the role of synaptic integration in this pontine vocalization area (VOC).[83] However, only vocalizations having a characteristic frequency modulation (4 kHz/25 milliseconds) can be synaptically blocked, namely cackling, trilling, and clucking calls.[83] Moreover, vocalizations can be elicited from the VOC, independent of the PAG, following pharmacologic inactivation of the PAG or a transaction between the PAG and the pons.[84,85] Furthermore, it appears that the VOC is a descending branch of this vocalization-controlling pathway because only lesions caudal to the pons can block vocalizations elicited from this area.[84] Most importantly, the activities of some neurons in the VOC reflect frequency-modulated call types.[86] Because frequency modulation is lacking in PAG neurons,[57] the PVA is the highest center in this pathway serving as a vocal pattern generator. Recently, anterograde tracer studies using injections of biotin dextranamine (BDA) into the VOC demonstrated projections into all cranial motor and sensory nuclei involved in phonation, including the NA.[87,88] Projections into several auditory nuclei were also reported, including the nucleus cochlearis complex, superior olive, ventral and dorsal nuclei of the lateral lemniscus, and inferior colliculus.[88] In addition, tracer studies using wheat germ agglutinin-conjugated HRP into the VOC revealed retrograde labeling throughout the PAG,[88] and BDA injections into a vocalization-eliciting site in the PAG demonstrated projections into this ventral paralemniscal area.[88] These connections to all cranial nuclei involved in phonation make it possible for the PVA to control complex phonatory behaviors. Furthermore, the demonstrated projections to various auditory nuclei[88] have been shown to function in audio-vocal interactions.[89] Recently, a telemetric single-unit recording study in squirrel monkeys compared the activities of motoneurons in the trigeminal motor nucleus, facial nucleus, and NA to those in the VOC, and confirmed that the VOC is, in fact, able to control motoneurons in each of these nuclei during frequency-modulated vocalizations.[86]

◆ Cortical Representation

Medial Premotor Areas

Cortical neurons in the area of the interhemispheric fissure play a key role in the initiation of spontaneous vocalizations in both humans and animals. However, humans differ from other primates with respect to the organization of this area for the volitional control of learned motor patterns. When genetically determined calls are conditioned to occur at increased frequency in macaques, they require an intact anterior cingulate cortex (ACC).[90,91] However, these animals retain a normal response to unconditioned stimuli, such as grasping them.[92] The ACC is similarly essential for spontaneous long-distance contact calls in socially isolated squirrel monkeys, but not for the same calls when uttered in response to identical calls from other conspecifics.[93]

Penfield and colleagues[94,95] first demonstrated a role of the supplementary motor area (SMA) in speech production based on arrest and prolongation of vowel sounds in patients during stimulation of this region. This area is located in the medial aspect of Broca's area (BA) 6 and includes two subregions that differ in their cytoarchitecture, connectivity, and function: the SMA proper and the more caudally located pre-SMA.[96,97] Studies in monkeys demonstrate a key role of both of these areas in the control of movement sequences.[98] Recent studies have demonstrated that the macaque pre-SMA contains neurons that monitor behavior sequences using a binary code with different cells representing odd-numbered and even-numbered trials, similar to counting mechanisms used in computers.[99] It has been proposed that this binary code is employed to register the progress of events in behavioral sequences for use in the generation of signals to start and end sequential behaviors.[99] In contrast, neurons displaying this type of activity were very rare in the SMA.[99] The more extensive connections between the pre-SMA and the prefrontal cortex and between the pre-SMA and the anterior striatum have been interpreted as evidence for a planning function, whereas the SMA is thought to play a role in motor performance based on its stronger connection with the motor cortex and posterior striatum.[100-103] Consistent with these findings, a recent functional magnetic resonance imaging (MRI) study in humans demonstrated that activity in the pre-SMA increased with both the complexity of individual nonlexical syllables and the sequential complexity of the syllables.[100] In contrast, the SMA only increased activity with the initiation of speech production and not with increases in the demand for planning of speech production.[100] Based on these findings, it was suggested that the pre-SMA represents syllables to coordinate serial position/timing signals, which are processed in the SMA for transmission to the motor apparatus.[100]

Frontal Operculum

The frontal operculum includes Broca's area proper (BA44, BA45), which is a premotor area that is related to speech production in humans. It is homologous to area F5 in nonhuman primates, which contains "mirror neurons" that form a system for grasping objects by employing a common neural code for executed and observed manual actions.[104] It is hypothesized that this capacity was extended in the course of evolution to permit imitation of complex object-oriented sequences through much repeated exposures.[104] It is proposed that this capacity to generate and recognize a set of actions provided the substrate for the evolution of language, and that projections between mirror neurons and the parietal and temporal cortex were essential to this process.[104] Subsequent stages of language evolution are thought to involve a progression from hand movements from praxis to an open repertoire of manual voluntary gestures ("protosign") and then to the substitution of vocalizations ("protospeech") within the mechanisms evolved for this manual-based communication system.[104] In *Homo sapiens* language evolution is hypothesized to have progressed from action-object frames to verb-argument structures and ultimately to syntax and semantics.[104]

In humans, several techniques have demonstrated segregation of Broca's area proper into two structurally and functionally distinct areas (BA44, BA45). The cytoarchitecture of BA44 is characterized by conspicuously large pyramidal cells in deep layer III and layer V without a prominent dysgranular layer IV, whereas, in contrast, a clearly visible layer IV is present in BA45.[105] The volume of BA44 is significantly greater in the dominant (usually left) hemisphere, whereas that of BA45 is more symmetric.[105] It is also well established that the left 44/45 is dominant in language-related function. In the great apes, the volume of the corresponding area in the left hemisphere is also greater, and it has been suggested that this is consistent with the hypothesis that the neuroanatomic substrates for left hemisphere dominance progressed from a manual gestural system in apes to include the predominance of vocal language during late human evolution, possibly with a mutation in the *FOXP2* gene.[106-108] Area F5 in monkeys, which is possibly homologous to Broca's area in humans, is connected to the anterior intraparietal cortex, the superior temporal sulcus, the parietal cortex, the cerebellum, and Wernicke's area.[109] However, since Broca's area likely plays a key role in the human capacity for speech, extreme caution is essential in the interpretation of connectivity results in nonhuman primates. Similarities have been supported by primate electrophysiologic studies reporting both a dorsal and a ventral pathway between the monkey F5 and Wernicke's area[110] as well as diffusion tensor imaging and tractography data showing the same parallel pathways between Broca's area and Wernicke's area in humans.[111] It has been hypothesized that the anatomic and functional topology demonstrated between the anterior (pars triangularis and BA45) and posterior (pars opercularis and BA44) divisions of Broca's area is integral with parallel anterior and posterior channels within the basal ganglia/thalamocortical circuits subserving, respectively, the anterior/ventral cortical regions and posterior/dorsal cortical regions.[112] It has been further suggested that this anterior channel subserves the retrieval of lexical and conceptual-semantic knowledge stored in declarative memory. The posterior channel is thought to subserve procedural memory for the acquisition and real-time expression of primarily sequential motor and cognitive skills.[112] Consistent with this hypothesis, human functional MRI studies indicate that BA44 plays a key role in syntactic processing, whereas BA45 is more active during lexically based processes.[113] Recent functional MRI studies of nonlexical syllable utterances demonstrate a left-lateralized activation of BA44 with an increase in the number of syllables ("sequence complexity") independent of semantic effects.[100] Although the dominance of the left hemisphere BA44/BA45 in language function is established, the function of the right Broca's area is less clear.[113]

Speech-related activity has also been reported in areas of the frontal operculum outside of Broca's area proper (BA44, BA45). Recent PET studies have demonstrated that the highest activation in the operculum during vocalization is in the ventral pars orbitalis, BA47.[51] Furthermore, covariance analyses indicate that BA47 activity is coupled to that of the PAG during vocalization.[51] Based on these findings, it has been suggested that BA47 may play a key role in voluntary regulation of visceromotor systems during human speech.[51] More recently, diffusion-weighted MRI studies have used probabilistic tractographic methods to parcellate BA47 from BA44 and BA45.[114] The studies also report the parcellation of a third region cortical band that extends as a cortical band from the crown of the opercular part of Broca's area to the anterior insula.[114] The studies refer to this area as the "deep frontal operculum."[114] As is the case with BA47,[51] probabilistic tractograms indicate that the deep frontal operculum projects to structures of the limbic system, in contrast to BA44 and BA45.[114] Furthermore, event-related functional MRI also indicates that this area differs from BA44 and BA45 in that the activity of the left deep frontal operculum is greatest during the processing of sentences having syntactic violations.[115]

Subcortical Pathways and Cerebellum

Broca's area is connected to both subcortical and cortical structures via basal ganglia thalamocortical pathways.[112] These pathways are organized into two anatomically and functionally segregated but parallel channels, also called circuits or loops.[112,116-118] It has been hypothesized that an anterior channel connects anterior/ventral cortical areas to the pars triangularis and BA45, and subserves the retrieval of lexical and semantic memory.[112] A second, posterior channel encompasses posterior/dorsal cortical regions with connections to the pars opercularis and BA44.[112] It is suggested that this posterior channel supports procedural memory, especially for the acquisition of sequential and grammatical knowledge.[112] Overt production of nonlexical syllables results in increased bilateral activation of the putamen, which coincides with increased cortical activation.[100] With additional sequence complexity there is activation of the caudate nucleus or anterior thalamus.[100] There was an interaction between increased sequential complexity and syllabic complexity in both of these areas.[100] Because the activation of the anterior thalamus lacked a significant main effect for increased complexity of the individual syllables, it was suggested that this activation corresponded to the complexity of the overall speech plan.[100] Because stimulation of either the dominant head of the caudate nucleus or the anterior thalamic nuclei evoke compulsory speech,[119,120] it is thought that both of these regions play a role in release of the speech/language plan, although the activation focus may vary with the syllable type.[100]

Functional MRI studies have reported increasing, moderately right lateralized activity of the superior and inferior cerebellum with increasing sequence complexity of nonlexical syllables.[100] Activation of the right inferior cerebellum differed from areas of the brain activated during syllable production in that it increased activation with increasing number of syllables but with no statistical interaction with the complexity of the individual syllables.[100] It has been suggested that this area processes abstract "chunks" of verbal working memory transmitted from the inferior parietal lobe (BA40) without regard for syllable complexity.[100,121] The activity in the superior cerebellum extended more laterally with an interaction between the sequence complexity and the syllable complexity in lateral regions of the right hemisphere,[100] consistent with reports indicating higher order processes in more lateral portions.[122] It was hypothesized that this area interacts with frontal regions for mental rehearsal.[100]

Motor Cortex

The motor cortex exerts control over the acoustic nature of vocalizations via pyramidal and extrapyramidal pathways. An intact forebrain is responsible for the initiation and suppression of these vocalizations. Early macrostimulation studies by Penfield and Rasmussen[123] demonstrated a cortical representation for human speech located near the area for control of the facial muscles, but current spread to adjacent areas of cortex limited their accuracy. Subsequent microstimulation studies by Hast et al,[124] Jurgens,[125] and Zealear et al[126] demonstrated a similar representation of the laryngeal muscles in the lower lateral face region of the motor cortex in monkeys (**Fig. 3.2**). This area is bordered by the arcuate sulcus, the central sulcus, and the sylvian fissure, and overlaps the motor area for facial muscle control. Microstimulation studies in the macaque laryngeal motor cortex report bilateral excitation of multiple but not single laryngeal muscles, typically recruiting one or more adductor muscles with inhibition of the laryngeal abductor muscle (the PCA).[127] This indicates that these cortical neurons project to motoneurons in multiple areas of the NA. Cortical laryngeal motoneurons responsible for PCA inhibition are spread over a larger area than the neurons activating adductor muscles. A somatotopic organization for laryngeal muscles in the motor cortex was not seen in these

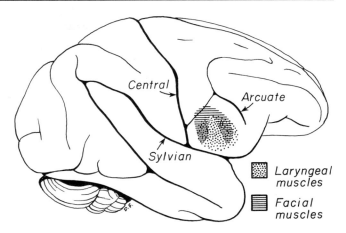

Fig. 3.2 The location of motor units for laryngeal and facial muscles in the cerebral cortex of the monkey.

stimulation studies. Stimulation of this area in the human led to the production of various phonemes or vowel-like sounds and may be considered the locus for speech (verbal phonation).[123] Lesions involving this cortical area produce aphasia or apraxia but not total loss of phonation.

It might be expected that the evolution of the human capacity for speech would require major neuroanatomic adaptations. Evidence that cortical motor projections differ between humans and other primates is found in the fact that the production or arrest of vocalization by electrical or transcranial magnetic stimulation appears to be unique to humans.[123,124,126,128] A latency of approximately 40 to 60 milliseconds for laryngeal muscle response from cortical stimulation in the macaque indicates that the pathway is a polysynaptic rather than a direct projection from the cortex to the laryngeal motoneurons in the NA. However, postmortem anatomic studies in humans, based on the distribution of degenerating fibers resulting from cerebral vascular accidents, have reported direct corticobulbar projections to the NA as well as other brainstem nuclei.[129,130] In addition, human studies using transcranial magnetic stimulation have reported approximately 12-millisecond latencies, which provide further support for the possibility of monosynaptic corticomotoneuronal projections to the human NA.[131-133]

The functional significance of monosynaptic corticomotoneuronal projections to the human NA is suggested by the selective occurrence of direct corticomotoneuronal input in certain other motor pathways. In monkeys, monosynaptic corticomotoneuronal projections to the distal limb muscles are present only in species that are capable of independent (fractionated) finger movements,[134] and in humans, it has been suggested that there is a positive correlation between the strength of monosynaptic corticomotoneuronal projections to finger muscles and differences in the maximum rate of voluntary contraction between fingers.[135] In human arm muscles, these fast, monosynaptic corticomotoneuronal pathways contribute mainly to tonic voluntary contractions, but less to rhythmic arm movement.[136] Transcranial magnetic stimulation studies have also recently demonstrated that human masseter motoneurons receive corticobulbar monosynaptic input, primarily from the contralateral hemisphere.[137] It has been proposed that this input pattern may contribute to independent (fractionated) activation of the masseter muscles at low bite forces on one side when food is held between the teeth.[137] It also is likely that direct corticomotoneuronal input is involved in reflexive compensatory adjustments of the upper lip during speech articulation.[138] Taken together, these studies suggest that monosynaptic corticomotoneuronal projections are adaptations for rapid, voluntary, and fractionated control of muscles, and it would seem that there would have been strong selection for direct corticomotoneuronal projections during the evolution of the human capacity for speech.

It remains to be determined how direct corticomotoneuronal input would be integrated with noncortical projections to the laryngeal motoneurons. However, recent studies on monosynaptic corticomotoneuronal input to human extensor carpi radialis longus muscles have suggested what may be a general mechanism for dynamic modulation of α-motoneurons by cognitive demands.[139] It was reported that the efficacy of direct corticomotoneuronal inputs may be modulated not only by the mean rate of the action potential but also by the strength of gamma-band (40–60 Hz) coherence between the motor cortex and the α-motoneuron.[139] This mechanism could be dynamically modulated by cognitive demands to provide highly selective regulation of the efficiency of input as a function of the phase-lock status of the target motoneuron.[140]

References

1. Barbas-Henry HA, Lohman AH. The motor nuclei and sensory neurons of the IIIrd, IVth, and VIth cranial nerves in the monitor lizard, Varanus exanthematicus. J Comp Neurol 1988;267:370–386
2. Porges SW. Orienting in a defensive world: mammalian modifications of our evolutionary heritage. A polyvagal theory. Psychophysiology 1995;32:301–318
3. Kalia M, Mesulam MM. Brain stem projections of sensory and motor components of the vagus complex in the cat: II. Laryngeal, tracheobronchial, pulmonary, cardiac, and gastrointestinal branches. J Comp Neurol 1980;193:467–508
4. Davis PJ, Nail BS. On the location and size of laryngeal motoneurons in the cat and rabbit. J Comp Neurol 1984;230:13–32
5. Szentagothai J. Die lokalisation der kehlkoph muskulatur in der vagus kernen. Z Anat Entwicklungsgesch 1943;112:704–710
6. Lawn AM. The localization, in the nucleus ambiguus of the rabbit, of the cells of origin of motor nerve fibers in the glossopharyngeal nerve and various branches of the vagus nerve by means of retrograde degeneration. J Comp Neurol 1966;127:293–306
7. Hinrichsen CF, Ryan AT. Localization of laryngeal motoneurons in the rat: morphologic evidence for dual innervation? Exp Neurol 1981;74:341–355
8. Yoshida Y, Miyazaki T, Hirano M, Shin T, Kanaseki T. Arrangement of motoneurons innervating the intrinsic laryngeal muscles of cats as demonstrated by horseradish peroxidase. Acta Otolaryngol 1982;94:329–334
9. Yoshida Y, Mitsumasu T, Hirano M, Kanaseki T. Somatotopic representation of the laryngeal motoneurons in the medulla of monkeys. Acta Otolaryngol 1985;100:299–303
10. Hisa Y, Sato F, Fukui K, Ibata Y, Mizuokoshi O. Nucleus ambiguus motoneurons innervating the canine intrinsic laryngeal muscles by the fluorescent labeling technique. Exp Neurol 1984;84:441–449
11. Hisa Y, Matsui T, Sato F, et al. The localization of the motor neurons innervating the cricothyroid muscle in the adult dog by the fluorescent retrograde axonal labeling technique. Arch Otorhinolaryngol 1982;234:33–36
12. Basterra J, Chumbley C, Dilly PN. Topographic distribution of laryngeal motor neurons in the nucleus ambiguus of the guinea pig studied by horseradish peroxidase (HRP) technique. Acta Otolaryngol 1987;103:105–110
13. Okubo J, Kitamura S, Ogata K, Sakai A. Localization of rabbit laryngeal motoneurons in the nucleus ambiguus. Exp Neurol 1987;96:528–539
14. Gacek RR. Localization of laryngeal motor neurons in the kitten. Laryngoscope 1975;85:1841–1861
15. Liddell EGT, Sherrington CS. Recruitment and some other factors of reflex inhibition. Proc R Soc Lond B Biol Sci 1925;97:488–518
16. Burke RE. Motor units: anatomy, physiology, and functional organization. In: Brooks VB, ed. Motor Control. American Physiological Society; 1981:345–422
17. Burke RE. The structure and function of motor units. In: Engel A, Franzini-Armstrong C, eds. Myology. 3rd ed. Palatino: McGraw-Hill; 2004:104–118
18. Rhee HS, Lucas CA, Hoh JF. Fiber types in rat laryngeal muscles and their transformations after denervation and reinnervation. J Histochem Cytochem 2004;52:581–590
19. Bottinelli R, Reggiani C. Human skeletal muscle fibres: molecular and functional diversity. [Review] [370 refs] Prog Biophys Mol Biol 2000;73:195–262
20. D'Antona G, Megighian A, Bortolotto S, et al. Contractile properties and myosin heavy chain isoform composition in single fibre of human laryngeal muscles. J Muscle Res Cell Motil 2002;23:187–195
21. Sciote JJ, Morris TJ, Brandon CA, Horton MJ, Rosen C. Unloaded shortening velocity and myosin heavy chain variations in human laryngeal muscle fibers. Ann Otol Rhinol Laryngol 2002;111:120–127
22. Perie S, Agbulut O, St Guily JL, Butler-Browne GS. Myosin heavy chain expression in human laryngeal muscle fibers. A biochemical study. Ann Otol Rhinol Laryngol 2000;109:216–220
23. Zealear DL, Larson CR. A microelectrode study of laryngeal motoneurons in the nucleus ambiguus of the awake vocalizing monkey. In: Fujimura O, ed. Vocal Physiology: Voice Production, Mechanisms, and Functions. New York: Raven Press; 1988:29–37
24. Yajima Y, Larson CR. Multifunctional properties of ambiguous neurons identified electrophysiologically during vocalization in the awake monkey. J Neurophysiol 1993;70:529–540
25. Yoshida Y, Yatake K, Tanaka Y, et al. Morphological observation of laryngeal motoneurons by means of cholera toxin B subunit tracing technique. Acta Otolaryngol Suppl 1998;539:98–105
26. Hoffer JA, Loeb GE, Sugano N, Marks WB, O'Donovan MJ, Pratt CA. Cat hindlimb motoneurons during locomotion. III. Functional segregation in sartorius. J Neurophysiol 1987;57:554–562
27. Hayakawa T, Zheng JQ, Maeda S, Ito H, Seki M, Yajima Y. Synaptology and ultrastructural characteristics of laryngeal cricothyroid and posterior cricoarytenoid motoneurons in the nucleus ambiguus of the rat. Anat Embryol (Berl) 1999;200:301–311
28. Mugnaini E, Oertel WH. An atlas of the distribution of GABAergic neurons and terminal. In: Bjorklund A, Hokfelt T, eds. Handbook of Chemical Neuroanatomy. GABA and Neuropeptides in. 13313 ed. New York: Elsevier; 1985:436–608

29. Yajima Y, Hayashi Y. GABA(A) receptor-mediated inhibition in the nucleus ambiguus motoneuron. Neuroscience 1997;79:1079–1088

30. Sanders I, Jacobs I, Wu BL, Biller HF. The three bellies of the canine posterior cricoarytenoid muscle: implications for understanding laryngeal function. Laryngoscope 1993;103:171–177

31. Sanders I, Rao F, Biller HF. Arytenoid motion evoked by regional electrical stimulation of the canine posterior cricoarytenoid muscle. Laryngoscope 1994;104:456–462

32. Barillot JC, Grelot L, Reddad S, Bianchi AL. Discharge patterns of laryngeal motoneurones in the cat: an intracellular study. Brain Res 1990;509:99–106

33. Richter DW, Camerer H, Meesmann M, Rohrig N. Studies on the synaptic interconnection between bulbar respiratory neurones of cats. Pflugers Arch 1979;380:245–257

34. Ezure K. Synaptic connections between medullary respiratory neurons and considerations on the genesis of respiratory rhythm. Prog Neurobiol 1990;35:429–450

35. Ezure K, Manabe M, Yamada H. Distribution of medullary respiratory neurons in the rat. Brain Res 1988;455:262–270

36. Richter DW, Ballanyi K, Ramirez JM. Respiratory rhythm generation. In: Miller AD, Bianchi AL, Bishop BP, eds. Neural Control of the Respiratory Muscles. Boca Raton, FL: CRC Press; 1997:119–130

37. Jiang C, Shen E. Respiratory neurons in the medulla of the rabbit: distribution, discharge patterns and spinal projections. Brain Res 1991;541:284–292

38. Bryant TH, Yoshida S, de Castro D, Lipski J. Expiratory neurons of the Botzinger complex in the rat: a morphological study following intracellular labeling with biocytin. J Comp Neurol 1993;335:267–282

39. Grelot L, Bianchi AL. Multifunctional medullary respiratory neurons. In: Miller AD, Bianchi AL, Bishop BP, eds. Neural Control of the Respiratory Muscles. Boca Raton, FL: CRC Press; 1997:297–304

40. Sasaki H, Otake K, Mannen H, Ezure K, Manabe M. Morphology of augmenting inspiratory neurons of the ventral respiratory group in the cat. J Comp Neurol 1989;282:157–168

41. Ezure K, Manabe M. Monosynaptic excitation of medullary inspiratory neurons by bulbospinal inspiratory neurons of the ventral respiratory group in the cat. Exp Brain Res 1989;74:501–511

42. Portillo F, Pasaro R. Location of bulbospinal neurons and of laryngeal motoneurons within the nucleus ambiguus of the rat and cat by means of retrograde fluorescent labelling. J Anat 1988;159:11–18

43. Larson CR, Yajima Y, Ko P. Modification in activity of medullary respiratory-related neurons for vocalization and swallowing. J Neurophysiol 1994;71:2294–2304

44. Sasaki CT, Hundal JS, Kim YH. Protective glottic closure: biomechanical effects of selective laryngeal denervation. Ann Otol Rhinol Laryngol 2005;114:271–275

45. Sasaki CT, Jassin B, Kim YH, Hundal J, Rosenblatt W, Ross DA. Central facilitation of the glottic closure reflex in humans. Ann Otol Rhinol Laryngol 2003;112:293–297

46. Beckstead RM, Morse JR, Norgren R. The nucleus of the solitary tract in the monkey: projections to the thalamus and brain stem nuclei. J Comp Neurol 1980;190:259–282

47. Zec N, Kinney HC. Anatomic relationships of the human nucleus of the solitary tract in the medulla oblongata: a DiI labeling study. Auton Neurosci 2003;105:131–144

48. Waldbaum S, Hadziefendic S, Erokwu B, Zaidi SI, Haxhiu MA. CNS innervation of posterior cricoarytenoid muscles: a transneuronal labeling study. Respir Physiol 2001;126:113–125

49. Macefield G, Gandevia SC. The cortical drive to human respiratory muscles in the awake state assessed by premotor cerebral potentials. J Physiol 1991;439:545–558

50. Ramsay SC, Adams L, Murphy K, et al. Regional cerebral blood flow during volitional expiration in man: a comparison with volitional inspiration. J Physiol 1993;461:85–101

51. Schulz GM, Varga M, Jeffires K, Ludlow CL, Braun AR. Functional neuroanatomy of human vocalization: an H2150 PET study. Cereb Cortex 2005;15:1835–1847

52. Kimura D, Archibald Y. Motor functions of the left hemisphere. Brain 1974;97:337–350

53. Simonyan K, Jurgens U. Efferent subcortical projections of the laryngeal motorcortex in the rhesus monkey. Brain Res 2003;974:43–59

54. Simonyan K, Jurgens U. Afferent subcortical connections into the motor cortical larynx area in the rhesus monkey. Neuroscience 2005;130:119–131

55. Thoms G, Jurgens U. Common input of the cranial motor nuclei involved in phonation in squirrel monkey. Exp Neurol 1987;95:85–99

56. Luthe L, Hausler U, Jurgens U. Neuronal activity in the medulla oblongata during vocalization. A single-unit recording study in the squirrel monkey. Behav Brain Res 2000;116:197–210

57. Dusterhoft F, Hausler U, Jurgens U. Neuronal activity in the periaqueductal gray and bordering structures during vocal communication in the squirrel monkey. Neuroscience 2004;123:53–60

58. Boers J, Klop EM, Hulshoff AC, de Weerd H, Holstege G. Direct projections from the nucleus retroambiguus to cricothyroid motoneurons in the cat. Neurosci Lett 2002;319:5–8

59. VanderHorst VG, Terasawa E, Ralston HJ III. Monosynaptic projections from the nucleus retroambiguus region to laryngeal motoneurons in the rhesus monkey. Neuroscience 2001;107:117–125

60. Zhang SP, Bandler R, Davis PJ. Brain stem integration of vocalization: role of the nucleus retroambigualis. J Neurophysiol 1995;74:2500–2512

61. Zhang SP, Davis PJ, Carrive P, Bandler R. Vocalization and marked pressor effect evoked from the region of the nucleus retroambigualis in the caudal ventrolateral medulla of the cat. Neurosci Lett 1992;140:103–107

62. Holstege G. Anatomical study of the final common pathway for vocalization in the cat. J Comp Neurol 1989;284:242–252

63. Jurgens U, Ehrenreich L, De Lanerolle NC. 2-Deoxyglucose uptake during vocalization in the squirrel monkey brain. Behav Brain Res 2002;136:605–610

64. Ambalavanar R, Tanaka Y, Selbie WS, Ludlow CL. Neuronal activation in the medulla oblongata during selective elicitation of the laryngeal adductor response. J Neurophysiol 2004;92:2920–2932

65. Sem-Jacobsen C, Torkildsen A. Depth recording and electrical stimulation in the human brain. In: Ramey ER, O'Doherty DS, eds. Electrical Studies on the Unanesthetized Brain. New York: Paul B. Hoeber; 1960:275–287

66. Jurgens U, Ploog D. Cerebral representation of vocalization in the squirrel monkey. Exp Brain Res 1970;10:532–554

67. Magoun HW, Atlas D, Ingersoll EH, Ranson SW. Associated facial, vocal and respiratory components of emotional expression: an experimental study. J Neurol Psychopathol 1937;17:241–255

68. Yajima Y, Hayashi Y, Yoshii N. The midbrain central gray substance as a highly sensitive neural structure for the production of ultrasonic vocalization in the rat. Brain Res 1980;198:446–452

69. Jurgens U, Pratt R. Role of the periaqueductal grey in vocal expression of emotion. Brain Res 1979;167:367–378

70. Bandler R, Depaulis A. Elicitation of intraspecific defence reactions in the rat from midbrain periaqueductal grey by microinjection of kainic acid, without neurotoxic effects. Neurosci Lett 1988;88:291–296

71. Lu CL, Jurgens U. Effects of chemical stimulation in the periaqueductal gray on vocalization in the squirrel monkey. Brain Res Bull 1993;32:143–151

72. Larson CR, Kistler MK. The relationship of periaqueductal gray neurons to vocalization and laryngeal EMG in the behaving monkey. Exp Brain Res 1986;63:596–606

73. Beitz AJ. The organization of afferent projections to the midbrain periaqueductal gray of the rat. Neuroscience 1982;7:133–159

74. Jurgens U. Reinforcing concomitants of electrically elicited vocalizations. Exp Brain Res 1976;26:203–214

75. Jurgens U. Amygdalar vocalization pathways in the squirrel monkey. Brain Res 1982;241:189–196
76. Jurgens U, Pratt R. The cingular vocalization pathway in the squirrel monkey. Exp Brain Res 1979;34:499–510
77. Jurgens U, Lu CL. The effects of periaqueductally injected transmitter antagonists on forebrain-elicited vocalization in the squirrel monkey. Eur J Neurosci 1993;5:735–741
78. Dujardin E, Jurgens U, Dujardin E, Jurgens U. Call type-specific differences in vocalization-related afferents to the periaqueductal gray of squirrel monkeys (Saimiri sciureus). Behav Brain Res 2006;168:23–36
79. Ambalavanar R, Tanaka Y, Damirjian M, Ludlow CL. Laryngeal afferent stimulation enhances Fos immunoreactivity in periaqueductal gray in the cat. J Comp Neurol 1999;409:411–423
80. Carrive P. The periaqueductal gray and defensive behavior: functional representation and neuronal organization. Behav Brain Res 1993;58:27–47
81. Ennis M, Xu SJ, Rizvi TA. Discrete subregions of the rat midbrain periaqueductal gray project to nucleus ambiguus and the periambigual region. Neuroscience 1997;80:829–845
82. VanderHorst VG, Terasawa E, Ralston HJ III, Holstege G. Monosynaptic projections from the lateral periaqueductal gray to the nucleus retroambiguus in the rhesus monkey: implications for vocalization and reproductive behavior. J Comp Neurol 2000;424:251–268
83. Jurgens U. Localization of a pontine vocalization-controlling area. J Acoust Soc Am 2000;108:1393–1396
84. Kanai T, Wang SC. Localization of the central vocalization mechanism in the brain stem of the cat. Exp Neurol 1962;6:426–434
85. Siebert S, Jurgens U. Vocalization after periaqueductal grey inactivation with the GABA agonist muscimol in the squirrel monkey. Neurosci Lett 2003;340:111–114
86. Hage SR, Jurgens U, Hage SR, Jurgens U. On the role of the pontine brainstem in vocal pattern generation: a telemetric single-unit recording study in the squirrel monkey. J Neurosci 2006;26:7105–7115
87. Cameron AA, Khan IA, Westlund KN, Cliffer KD, Willis WD. The efferent projections of the periaqueductal gray in the rat: a phaseolus vulgaris-leucoagglutinin study. I. Ascending projections. J Comp Neurol 1995;351:568–584
88. Hannig S, Jurgens U, Hannig S, Jurgens U. Projections of the ventrolateral pontine vocalization area in the squirrel monkey. Exp Brain Res 2006;169:92–105
89. Hage SR, Jurgens U, Ehret G, Hage SR, Jurgens U, Ehret G. Audio-vocal interaction in the pontine brainstem during self-initiated vocalization in the squirrel monkey. Eur J Neurosci 2006;23:3297–3308
90. Sutton D, Trachy RE, Lindeman RC. Primate phonation: unilateral and bilateral cingulate lesion effects. Behav Brain Res 1981;3:99–114
91. Aitken PG. Cortical control of conditioned and spontaneous vocal behavior in rhesus monkeys. Brain Lang 1981;13:171–184
92. Sutton D, Larson C, Lindeman RC. Neocortical and limbic lesion effects on primate phonation. Brain Res 1974;71:61–75
93. MacLean PD, Newman JD. Role of midline frontolimbic cortex in production of the isolation call of squirrel monkeys. Brain Res 1988;450:111–123
94. Penfield W, Welch K. The supplementary motor area of the cerebral cortex; a clinical and experimental study. AMA Arch Neurol Psychiatry 1951;66:289–317
95. Penfield W, Roberts L. Speech and Brain Mechanisms. Princeton, NJ: Princeton University Press; 1959
96. Picard N, Strick PL. Motor areas of the medial wall: a review of their location and functional activation. Cereb Cortex 1996;6:342–353
97. Hoshi E, Tanji J. Differential roles of neuronal activity in the supplementary and presupplementary motor areas: from information retrieval to motor planning and execution. J Neurophysiol 2004;92:3482–3499
98. Tanji J. Sequential organization of multiple movements: involvement of cortical motor areas. [Review] Annu Rev Neurosci 2001;24:631–651
99. Shima K, Tanji J. Binary-coded monitoring of a behavioral sequence by cells in the pre-supplementary motor area. J Neurosci 2006;26:2579–2582
100. Bohland JW, Guenther FH. An fMRI investigation of syllable sequence production. Neuroimage 2006;32:821–841
101. Jurgens U. The efferent and afferent connections of the supplementary motor area. Brain Res 1984;300:63–81
102. Johansen-Berg H, Behrens TE, Robson MD, et al. Changes in connectivity profiles define functionally distinct regions in human medial frontal cortex. Proc Natl Acad Sci U S A 2004;101:13335–13340
103. Lehericy S, Ducros M, Krainik A, et al. 3-D diffusion tensor axonal tracking shows distinct SMA and pre-SMA projections to the human striatum. Cereb Cortex 2004;14:1302–1309
104. Arbib MA. From monkey-like action recognition to human language: an evolutionary framework for neurolinguistics. Behav Brain Sci 2005;28:105–124
105. Amunts K, Schleicher A, Burgel U, Mohlberg H, Uylings HB, Zilles K. Broca's region revisited: cytoarchitecture and intersubject variability. J Comp Neurol 1999;412:319–341
106. Corballis MC. From mouth to hand: gesture, speech, and the evolution of right-handedness. Behav Brain Sci 2003;26:199–208
107. Corballis MC. FOXP2 and the mirror system. [see comment] Trends Cogn Sci 2004;8:95–96
108. Gentilucci M, Corballis MC. From manual gesture to speech: a gradual transition. [Review] Neurosci Biobehav Rev 2006;30:949–960
109. Arbib M, Bota M. Language evolution: neural homologies and neuroinformatics. Neural Netw 2003;16:1237–1260
110. Kaas JH, Hackett TA. "What" and "where" processing in auditory cortex. Nat Neurosci 1999;2:1045–1047
111. Romanski LM, Tian B, Fritz JB, Mishkin M, Goldman-Rakic PS, Rauschecker JP. Reply to "What," "where" and "how" in auditory cortex. Nat Neurosci 2000;3:966
112. Ullman MT. Is Broca's area part of a basal ganglia thalamocortical circuit? [Review] Cortex 2006;42:480–485
113. Bookheimer S. Functional MRI of language: new approaches to understanding the cortical organization of semantic processing. [Review] Annu Rev Neurosci 2002;25:151–188
114. Anwander A, Tittgemeyer M, von Cramon DY, Friederici AD, Knosche TR. Connectivity-based parcellation of Broca's area. Cereb Cortex 2007;17:816–825
115. Friederici AD, Fiebach CJ, Schlesewsky M, Bornkessel ID, von Cramon DY. Processing linguistic complexity and grammaticality in the left frontal cortex. Cereb Cortex 2006;16:1709–1717
116. Alexander GE, DeLong MR, Strick PL. Parallel organization of functionally segregated circuits linking basal ganglia and cortex. Annu Rev Neurosci 1986;9:357–381
117. Middleton FA, Strick PL. Basal ganglia and cerebellar loops: motor and cognitive circuits. Brain Res Brain Res Rev 2000;31:236–250
118. Middleton FA, Strick PL. Basal ganglia output and cognition: evidence from anatomical, behavioral, and clinical studies. Brain Cogn 2000;42:183–200
119. Schaltenbrand G. The effects on speech and language of stereotactical stimulation in thalamus and corpus callosum. Brain Lang 1975;2:70–77
120. Vanburen JM. Confusion and disturbance of speech from stimulation in vicinity of the head of the caudate nucleus. J Neurosurg 1963;20:148–157
121. Chen SH, Desmond JE. Cerebrocerebellar networks during articulatory rehearsal and verbal working memory tasks. Neuroimage 2005;24:332–338
122. Leiner HC, Leiner AL, Dow RS. Cognitive and language functions of the human cerebellum. Trends Neurosci 1993;16:444–447
123. Penfield W, Rasmussen T. Vocalization and arrest of speech. Arch Neurol Psychiatry 1949;61:21–27

124. Hast MH, Fischer JM, Wetzel AB, Thompson VE. Cortical motor representation of the laryngeal muscles in Macaca mulatta. Brain Res 1974;73:229–240
125. Jurgens U. Projections from the cortical larynx area in the squirrel monkey. Exp Brain Res 1976;25:401–411
126. Zealear DL, Hast MH, Kurago Z. Functional organization of the primary motor cortex controlling the face, tongue, jaw, and larynx in the monkey. In: Titze IR, Scherer RC, eds. Vocal Fold Physiology: Biomechanics, Acoustics, and Phonatory Control. Denver: Denver Center for the Performing Arts; 1983:57–73
127. Zealear DL. The brainstem connections with the laryngeal region of the motor cortex in the monkey. In: Baer T, Sasaki C, Harris K, eds. Laryngeal Function in Phonation and Respiration. Boston: Little, Brown; 1987:168–177
128. Pascual-Leone A, Gates JR, Dhuna A. Induction of speech arrest and counting errors with rapid-rate transcranial magnetic stimulation. Neurology 1991;41:697–702
129. Kuypers HG. Corticobular connexions to the pons and lower brainstem in man: an anatomical study. Brain 1958;81:364–388
130. Iwatsubo T, Kuzuhara S, Kanemitsu A, Shimada H, Toyokura Y. Corticofugal projections to the motor nuclei of the brainstem and spinal cord in humans. Neurology 1990;40:309–312
131. Maccabee PJ, Amassian VE, Cracco RQ, Cracco JB, Eberle L, Rudell A. Stimulation of the human nervous system using the magnetic coil. [Review] Clin Neurophysiol 1991;8:38–55
132. Cracco JB, Amassian VE, Cracco RQ, Maccabee PJ. Brain stimulation revisited. J Clin Neurophysiol 1990;7:3–15
133. Ludlow CL, Lou G. Observations on human laryngeal muscle control. In: Fletcher N, Davis P, eds. Vocal Fold Physiology: Controlling Complexity and Chaos. 9th ed. San Diego: Singular; 1996:201–218
134. Bortoff GA, Strick PL. Corticospinal terminations in two new-world primates: further evidence that corticomotoneuronal connections provide part of the neural substrate for manual dexterity. J Neurosci 1993;13:5105–5118
135. Ziemann U, Ilic TV, Alle H, Meintzschel F. Cortico-motoneuronal excitation of three hand muscles determined by a novel penta-stimulation technique. Brain 2004;127(Pt 8):1887–1898
136. Carroll TJ, Baldwin ER, Collins DF, Zehr EP. Corticospinal excitability is lower during rhythmic arm movement than during tonic contraction. J Neurophysiol 2006;95:914–921
137. Pearce SL, Miles TS, Thompson PD, Nordstrom MA. Responses of single motor units in human masseter to transcranial magnetic stimulation of either hemisphere. J Physiol 2003;549(Pt 2):583–596
138. Ito T, Kimura T, Gomi H. The motor cortex is involved in reflexive compensatory adjustment of speech articulation. Neuroreport 2005;16:1791–1794
139. Schoffelen JM, Oostenveld R, Fries P. Neuronal coherence as a mechanism of effective corticospinal interaction. Science 2005;308:111–113
140. Schreiber S, Fellous JM, Tiesinga P, Sejnowski TJ. Influence of ionic conductances on spike timing reliability of cortical neurons for suprathreshold rhythmic inputs. J Neurophysiol 2004;91:194–205

Chapter 4

Peripheral Laryngeal Motor Innervation

Phillip Song, Jerome S. Schwartz, Richard R. Gacek, Leslie T. Malmgren Jr., and Andrew Blitzer

The laryngeal peripheral motor innervation system has evolved to reflect the constant dynamic function of the larynx. Unlike many muscle groups, the laryngeal muscles are constantly active and in motion—a fact very well known to those who study laryngeal electromyography. This dynamic homeostasis is a function of our constant need to breathe, swallow, cough, and speak. Vocal behavior and the laryngeal innervation system are adapted to meet these requirements.

The laryngeal functions of respiration involve baseline, unconscious input from the brainstem, as well as rapid, reflexive responses to sensory receptors from the pulmonary system. Deglutination and airway protection similarly require highly reliable responses from the brainstem and sensory system. Phonation requires rapid adduction and abduction as well as fine control of cord tension for pitch adjustments.[1] In addition, high tensile strength is needed to resist the forces produced at the vibratory margin of the vocal fold. The laryngeal muscles and nerves are adapted to be rapid, reliable, and highly resistant to fatigue. Anatomic dissection and histologic analysis have revealed several specialized features of the motor innervation system in the intrinsic larynx that differ markedly from other skeletal muscles groups.

◆ Nerve Anatomy

Recurrent Laryngeal Nerve Anatomy

The recurrent or inferior laryngeal nerve (RLN) and the superior laryngeal nerve (SLN) are responsible for the motor function of the larynx. These nerves carry a mixture of motor and sensory fibers from the brainstem. The vagus nerve is supplied by four nuclei within the medulla: the nucleus ambiguus, the nucleus of the tractus solitarius, the dorsal nucleus of the vagus, and the sensory nucleus of the trigeminal nerve.

The nucleus ambiguus is the source of motor innervation carried to the RLN via the vagus nerve to the larynx. Within the vagus, the laryngeal motor axons are located in the anterior aspect of the trunk superiorly. It rotates medially as the vagus nerve trunk descends the neck. The vagus leaves the jugular foramen anterior to the jugular vein, but as it descends within the carotid sheath, it assumes a posterior position. The left RLN loops under the aorta before beginning its ascent along the tracheoesophageal groove to enter the larynx at the cricothyroid membrane. The right RLN has a shorter course and loops underneath the right subclavian artery. The right RLN is approximately 5 to 6 cm in length, whereas the left RLN is approximately 12 cm. As the RLN enters the larynx, it divides into motor and sensory branches to innervate the laryngeal muscles and carry sensory information from the subglottis.[2]

Superior Laryngeal Nerve

The anatomic course of the SLN is more variable than that of the RLN. The SLN originates from the nodose ganglion and then travels with the vagus nerve. The external branch of the SLN (EBSLN), which carries the motor fibers to the cricothyroid (CT) muscle, separates from the vagus nerve via the superior laryngeal nerve approximately 4 cm above the bifurcation of the common carotid. The larger internal branch of the SLN carries primarily sensory fibers from the ipsilateral hemilarynx. The EBSLN then descends along the larynx crossing dorsal to the superior thyroid artery. In approximately 42 to 62% of cases, the EBSLN crosses behind the superior thyroid artery 2 cm or greater in the cranial direction from the superior pole of the thyroid gland. In 11 to 27% of patients, the distance is less than 2 cm. In 13 to 14% of cases, the EBSLN passes behind the superior lobe of the thyroid gland. In 13% of cases, the EBSLN does not cross the thyroid artery at the trunk, but runs dorsal to the artery until it has ramified.[3] The variability in relationship to the thyroid gland is important for prevention of inadvertent injury during thyroidectomy.

The EBSLN lies lateral to the inferior constrictor when it reaches the CT muscle. It then divides into two main branches to supply the two bellies of the CT muscle.[4] The action of the CT is to reduce the anterior angle between the cricoid and thyroid cartilages. The result of this action is to increase the distance between the anterior thyroid lamina and the arytenoids, which are anchored to the posterior cricoid. This tenses and thins the vocal cords, resulting in higher pitch.

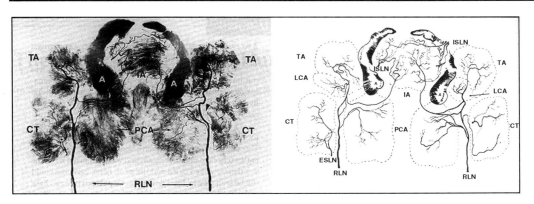
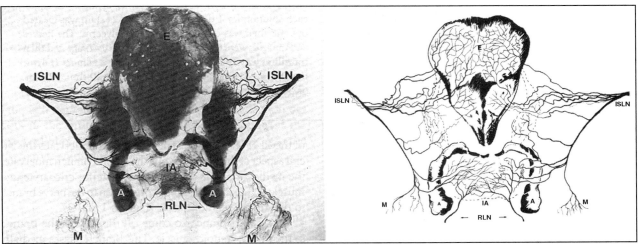

Fig. 4.1 Innervation of the recurrent laryngeal nerve and superior laryngeal nerves in the intrinsic muscles of the larynx. CT, cricothyroid; IA, interarytenoid; PCA, posterior cricoarytenoid; RLN, recurrent laryngeal nerve; TA, thyroarytenoid. (From Sanders I, Wu B, Mu L, Li Y, Biller H. The innervation of the human larynx. Arch Otolaryngol Head Neck Surg 1993;119:934–939. Reprinted with permission.)

Intralaryngeal Anatomy

A modification of Sihler's staining, a technique that stains nerves and in the process renders nonneural tissue opaque, has been used successfully to trace the small nerve branches to the individual laryngeal muscles. Sanders et al[4] published a series of papers utilizing this technique, uncovering more complexity and variability of the intralaryngeal nerve distribution than previously recognized. After the RLN enters the larynx, the first branch innervates the posterior cricoarytenoid (PCA) muscle. The PCA was innervated by two branches in 50% of the specimens studied. It is estimated that the PCA may receive 25% of all motor axons carried by the RLN, underscoring its importance as the primary abductor of the glottis. The next branch to come off the RLN goes to the interarytenoid muscle. This branch passes medially around the cricoarytenoid joint and underneath the PCA. The interarytenoid receives bilateral innervation, and the right and left sides of the nerve anastomose with each other and with branches from the SLN. The terminal branches of the RLN innervate the lateral cricoarytenoid (LCA) and thyroarytenoid (TA) muscles. The LCA is innervated by a single nerve branch. The RLN terminates in the thyroarytenoid muscle, forming multiple dense anastomotic networks throughout the muscle (**Fig. 4.1**).

Intralaryngeal connections between the RLN and SLN have been studied. The anastomosis of Galen (a connection between the inferior division of the SLN and RLN) has been found with variable frequency and is thought to be primarily sensory.[5] The existence of an anastomosis between the branches of the SLN with RLN fibers between the interarytenoid and thyroarytenoid muscles has also been described.[6,7] Human anatomic studies have revealed another connection between the EBSLN and RLN in the paraglottic space that is thought to be sensory for the subglottis.[8] As of yet, a motor anastomosis between the SLN and RLN has not been confirmed.

Based on Sanders et al's examination of individual laryngeal muscles and nerve branches, they hypothesized that the laryngeal muscles may be partitioned into subcompartments that can undergo individualized activity and perform far more complex actions than previously known. Sanders et al have shown two to three compartments for the PCA, TA, and CT muscles. The CT muscle has two muscle bellies that are innervated by two branches of the external branch of the SLN. One branch enters the oblique belly, whereas the second supplies the rectus. The PCA was found to have multiple neuromuscular compartments divided by fascial planes. The human vocalis muscle appears to contain two subcompartments — a superiorly based compartment composed of multiple small fascicles, and an inferiorly based compartment made of a single large muscle fascicle.[9]

The composition of slow and fast twitch muscle fibers as well as the arrangement of the muscle fascicles and neural innervation suggest an ability to individually stimulate different subcompartments of the muscle.[10] Within the larynx, individual muscles have different composition of fast and slow muscle fibers that display multiple innervation.[11,12] In the TA muscle, type I (slow) muscle fibers had multiple innervations in 67% of fibers. In type II (fast) muscle fibers, 28% had multiple innervations. This feature may reflect the highly elastic and tremendous vocal range of the human larynx.

◆ Nerve Physiology

The RLN and SLN carry both motor and sensory fibers. Early histologic examination of the RLN and SLN showed a mixture of myelinated and unmyelinated fibers. Myelin is the component of the nerve sheath, the Schwann cell, that provides many support functions for the nerve including increasing transmission velocity for neural signal. Motor signals are generally carried via the large and intermediate myelinated nerves, whereas sensory signals are carried by small myelinated fibers. Autonomic parasympathetic fibers are also carried by myelinated fibers. The unmyelinated fibers are thought to be branches of cervical sympathetic fibers and postganglionic parasympathetic fibers.[13]

Differentiation of the neural components of the RLN and SLN can be made by immunohistochemical techniques. Staining for myelin, acetylcholinesterase, as well as the use of both anterograde and retrograde tracers such as biotin and horseradish peroxidase have increased our understanding of the composition of the peripheral nerves. Animal experiments involving disruption of different segments of nerve with examination of peripheral nerve degeneration has been instrumental for the understanding of composition as it relates to function. Experimental sectioning of the RLN from the motor signal origin (nucleus ambiguus) results primarily in the degeneration of intermediate and large myelinated nerve fibers. These laryngeal motor fibers are myelinated and 4 to 12 μm in diameter.[14] Similar studies of denervation of the SLN by vagoaccessory root destruction shows degeneration of 23% of the myelinated nerve fibers within the SLN. Almost all are motor and all go to the external branch of the SLN.[15]

The left RLN has a larger diameter than the right and may reflect adaptation to synchronize nerve signals. Conduction time recordings have shown that large diameter fibers have higher conduction velocities. Because the left RLN is approximately twice as long as the right, the larger diameter of the nerve is believed to compensate for this additional distance.

Peytz et al[16] compared conduction times between the right and left RLN and discovered that impulses from the right side arrives 3 milliseconds before those from the left.[17] This difference is not felt to be important physiologically.

◆ Nerve Topography

In the brainstem, topographic localization of adductor and abductor neurons is feasible; however, this separation is lost in the peripheral nervous system. Using retrograde axoplasmic tracers such as horseradish peroxidase, abductor and adductor motor groups were found to be preferentially located within the nucleus ambiguus. Abductor motor neurons are located in the ventral division of the nucleus ambiguus, whereas the adductor neurons are located in the dorsal division.[18,19] The separation between abductor and adductor motor neurons is not apparent in the peripheral nerve system. Using retrograde tracers, abductor and adductor motor neurons were found to be scattered within the fascicle of the RLN and not partitioned.[20]

Immunohistologic examination of RLN shows that the nerve fiber content is divided into two primary fascicles separating the laryngeal and nonlaryngeal components. The nonlaryngeal fascicles carry smaller myelinated nerves supplying trachea and esophagus. In animal studies, the nonlaryngeal component is composed of smaller nerve fibers and segregated into discrete units.[21-24] In human studies using immunohistochemical techniques and fiber diameter, the RLN also shows differential segregation between laryngeal and nonlaryngeal nerve groups.[25] The largest fascicle is usually the laryngeal motor axons.[26]

The intraneural distribution of fibers to different muscle groups has been a source of study in developing reinnervation procedures and nerve reanastomosis. Based on the observation by Semon[27] that partial injuries result in greater loss of abductor function, it was theorized that there was a superficial circumferential distribution of abductor fibers.[28] Sunderland and Swaney[29] constructed a three-dimensional topographic map of the RLN that displayed the relationship among various fascicles. They found that fascicles to different muscle groups formed a plexus along the length of the nerve, and that the fibers supplying a particular muscle became redistributed to various fascicles. In addition, retrograde tracer injection studies in the cat showed that axons innervating the abductor muscle, such as those of the TA, were diffusely distributed in the RLN.[30] Based on the diffused distribution of different fascicles throughout the nerve peripherally, it is unlikely that partial mechanical damage to the RLN would consistently result in selective loss of abductor or adductor function.[31] Distally, as the RLN divides into anterior and posterior branches, the fascicles become aligned to stimulate the individual muscles. These findings correlate with clinical observations of the difficulty encountered during nerve anastomosis in the peripheral nervous system. This feature has helped explain why anastomosis to nerve stumps results in mixed adductor/abductor responses. Correct alignment of individual abductor and adductor fascicles requires microsurgical and histologic techniques that have not been developed.

◆ Neuromuscular Junctions

The neuromuscular innervation of the larynx differs from other skeletal muscle groups because the laryngeal muscle fibers receive input from multiple motor end plates.[32,33] In the mammalian skeletal muscle system, multiple neuromuscular junctions (NMJ) are found in middle ear muscles[34,35] and extrinsic eye muscles.[36] Based on anatomic and immunohistologic studies of acetylcholinesterase, distances between end plates were found to vary greatly, with a range of 50 to 1000 μm. The number of end plates per muscle also varies from two to five.

Comparison of adult and perinatal larynges show that the motor end plates are not static entities but grow and develop with age. Innervation of multiple motor end plates in the adult are generally unineuronal; a single neuron stimulates multiple end plates. In contrast, embryonic motor end plates often have multiple neuronal inputs with apoptosis of motor neurons during development.[37] During the perinatal and early neonatal period, laryngeal muscles often have polyneuronal innervation. Synaptic elimination may occur as a normal process of development, a feature seen in the central nervous system. During aging, the end plate of the muscles mature from early fetal plate-like NMJs to complex NMJs. This may represent NMJ splintering or segmental growth.[38]

Three-dimensional reconstruction of the distribution of motor end plates have been performed that details the distribution of neuromuscular junctions throughout each of the muscles. Each laryngeal muscle appears to have different patterns of distribution. The end plates are diffused throughout the thyroarytenoid,[39] whereas in the posterior cricoarytenoid the motor end plates are distributed in an arc-like pattern with few end plates at the superior and inferior poles.[40] In the CT muscles, the external branch of the SLN distribute themselves primarily to the medial two thirds of the muscle belly.[41] The motor end plates adopt an inverted Y configuration in the interarytenoid muscle with a central broad band at the midpoint. In the inferior border of the muscle, the end plates diverge laterally.[42] The lateral cricoarytenoid end plates form a distinct band at the midlength of the muscle.[43] Knowledge of these end plate locations has utility in neurolaryngology, especially during electromyography and botulinum toxin injections (**Fig. 4.2**).

There are several theories describing the reason for multiple innervations in the larynx. Bendiksen et al[44] noted that in eye muscles, multiple innervations result in muscles that are less compliant than singly innervated fibers. This feature may be adaptive for the thyroarytenoid because it makes it highly resistant to vibration. Multiple neuromuscular junctions may also create more reliable transmissions that are adaptive to perform high-frequency repetitive stimulation.[45,46] Simultaneous activation may increase the rate of tension increase and reflect the rapid response needed for airway protection.[47]

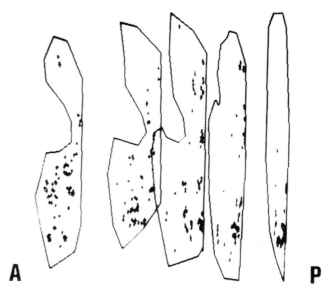

Fig. 4.2 Three-dimensional computer reconstruction of the motor end plates of the thyroarytenoid muscle. A, anterior; P, posterior. (From Rosen M, Malmgren LT, Gacek RR. Three-dimensional computer reconstruction of the distribution of neuromuscular junctions in the thyroarytenoid muscle. Ann Otol Rhinol Laryngol 1983;92(5 Pt 1): 424–429. Reprinted with permission.)

◆ Denervation and Regeneration

The PCA denervated by transection of the RLN undergoes rapid degeneration over the first 2 to 3 weeks. However, the muscle reorganizes and achieves near baseline size over the next several months. This regrowth may reflect the observation that vacated neuromuscular junctions are reoccupied by autonomic neurons. With motor end plate degeneration, the postsynaptic site secretes neurotrophic factors (theory) that may attract autonomic neuron ingrowth. These features suggest that opportunities for reinnervation should be taken early after nerve injury to capitalize on the release of neurotrophic factors and to prevent ingrowth of local autonomic neurons into the neuromuscular junction.[48]

◆ Conclusion

The peripheral motor innervation system of the larynx reflects the specialized functions required for respiration, phonation, and deglutination. The realization that the muscles of the larynx have multiple muscular subcompartments, numerous neuromuscular junctions, and neural innervations reveal new levels of plasticity and complexity. Fundamental knowledge of the laryngeal innervation system continues to expand and evolve our understanding of laryngeal function.

References

1. Hirose H, Ushijima T, Kobayashi T, Sawashima M. An experimental study of the contraction properties of the laryngeal muscles in the cat. Ann Otol Rhinol Laryngol 1969;78:297–306
2. Myssiorek D. Recurrent laryngeal nerve paralysis: anatomy and etiology. Otolaryngol Clin North Am 2004;37:25–44
3. Kierner AC, Aigner M, Burium M. The external branch of the superior laryngeal nerve. Arch Otolaryngol Head Neck Surg 1998;124:301–303
4. Sanders I, Wu B, Mu L, Li Y, Biller HF. The innervation of the human larynx. Arch Otolaryngol Head Neck Surg 1993;119:934–939
5. Wu BL, Sanders I, Mu L, Biller HF. The human communicating nerve: an extension of the external superior laryngeal nerve that innervates the vocal fold. Arch Otolaryngol Head Neck Surg 1994;120:1321–1328
6. Mu L, Sanders I, Wu BL, Biller HF. The intramuscular innervation of the human interarytenoid muscle. Laryngoscope 1994;104:33–39
7. Nasri S, Beizae P, Ye M, Sercarz JA, Kim YO, Berke GS. Cross-innervation of the thyroarytenoid muscle by a branch from the external division of the superior laryngeal nerve. Ann Otol Rhinol Laryngol 1997;106:594–598
8. Maranillo E, Leon X, Quer M, Orus C, Sanudo JR. Is the external laryngeal nerve an exclusively motor nerve? The cricothyroid connection branch. Laryngoscope 2003;113:525–529
9. Sanders I, Rai S, Han Y, Biller HF. Human vocalis contains distinct superior and inferior subcompartments: possible candidates for the two masses of vocal fold vibration. Ann Otol Rhinol Laryngol 1998;107(10 pt 1):826–833
10. Sanders I, Jacobs I, Wu BL, Biller HF. The three bellies of the canine posterior cricoarytenoid muscle: implications for understanding laryngeal function. Laryngoscope 1993;103:171–177
11. Bach-y-Rita P, Ito F. In vivo studies on fast and slow muscle fibers in cat extraocular muscles. J Gen Physiol 1966;49:1177–1198
12. Lennerstrand G. Electrical activity and isometric tension in motor units of the cat's inferior oblique muscles. Acta Physiol Scand 1974;91:438–478
13. Gacek RR, Lyon MJ. Fiber components of the recurrent laryngeal nerve in cats. Ann Otol Rhinol Laryngol 1976;85:460–472
14. Malmgren LT, Gacek RR. Acetylcholinesterase staining of fiber components in feline and human recurrent laryngeal nerve. Topography of laryngeal motor fiber regions. Acta Otolaryngol 1981;91:337–352
15. Dubois FS, Foley JO. Experimental studies on the vagus and spinal accessory nerves in the cat. Anat Rec 1936;64:285–307
16. Peytz F, Rasmussen H, Buchthal F. Conduction time and velocity in the human recurrent laryngeal nerve. Dan Med Bull 1965;12:125–127
17. Atkins JP. An electromyographic study of recurrent laryngeal nerve conduction and its clinical applications. Laryngoscope 1973;83:796–807
18. Gacek RR. Localization of laryngeal motor neurons in the kitten. Laryngoscope 1975;85:1841–1861
19. Yoshida Y, Mitsumasu T, Hirano M, Morimoto M, Kanaseki T. Afferent connections to the nucleus ambiguous in the brainstem of the cat—an HRP study. In: Baer T, Sasaki C, Harris K, eds. Laryngeal Function in Phonation and Respiration. Boston: Little, Brown; 1987:45–61
20. Gacek RR, Malmgren LT, Lyon MJ. Localization of adductor and abductor motor nerve fibers to the larynx. Ann Otol Rhinol Laryngol 1977;86:771–776
21. Dubois FS, Foley JO. Experimental studies on the vagus and spinal accessory nerves in the cat. Anat Rec 1936;64:285–307
22. Brocklehurst RJ, Edgeworth FH. The fibers components of the laryngeal nerves of the Macaca mulatta. J Anat 1940;74:386–389
23. Evans DHL, Murray JG. Histological and functional studies on the fiber composition of the vagus nerve of the rabbit. J Anat 1954;88:320–337
24. Malmgren LT, Lyons MJ, Gacek RR. Localization of abductor fibers in the kitten recurrent laryngeal nerve: use of a variation of the horseradish peroxidase tracer technique. Exp Neurol 1977;55:187–198
25. Dahlqvist A, Carlsoo B, Hellstrom S. Fiber components of the recurrent laryngeal nerve of the rat: a study by light and electron microscopy. Anat Rec 1982;204:365–370
26. Malmgren LT, Gacek RR. Acetylcholinesterase staining of fiber components in feline and human recurrent laryngeal nerve. Topography of laryngeal motor fiber regions. Acta Otolaryngol 1981;91:337–352
27. Semon F. Clinical remarks on the proclivity of the abductor fibres of the recurrent laryngeal nerve to become affected sooner than the adductor fibres; or even exclusively in cases of undoubted central or peripheral injury or disease of the roots or trunks of the pneumogastric, spinal accessory or recurrent nerves. Arch Laryngol. 1881;2:197–222
28. MacKenzie M. A Manual of Disease of the Throat and Nose, Vol. 1: Diseases of the Pharynx, Larynx and Trachea. New York: William Wood; 1880:321
29. Sunderland S, Swaney WE. The intraneural topography of the recurrent laryngeal nerve in man. Anat Rec 1952;114:411–426
30. Malmgren LT, Lyons J, Gacek RR. Localization of abductor fibers in the kitten recurrent laryngeal nerve: use of a variation of the horseradish peroxidase tracer technique. Exp Neurol 1977;55:187–198
31. Dyer KR, Duncan ID. The intraneural distribution of myelinated fibres in the equine recurrent laryngeal nerve. Brain 1987;110:1531–1543
32. Rossi G, Cortesina G. Morphological study of the laryngeal muscles in man. Acta Otolaryngol 1965;59:575–592
33. Bendiksen FS, Dahl HA, Teig E. Innervation pattern of different types of muscle fibers in the human thyroarytenoid muscle. Acta Otolaryngol 1981;91:391–397
34. Erulkar SD, Shelanski ML, Whitsel BL, Ogle P. Studies of muscle fibers of the tensor tympani of the cat. Anat Rec 1964;149:279–298
35. Fernand VSV, Hess A. The occurrence, structure and innervation of slow and twitch muscles fibers in the tensor tympani and stapedius of the cat. J Physiol 1969;200:547–555
36. Hess A, Pilar G. Slow fibers in the extraocular muscles of the cat. J Physiol 1963;169:780–798
37. Van Essen DC, Gordon H, Soha JM, Fraser SE. Synaptic dynamics at the neuromuscular junction: mechanisms and models. J Neurobiol 1990;21:223–249
38. Perie S, St Guily JL, Sebille A. Comparison of prenatal and adult multi-innervation in human laryngeal muscle fibers. Ann Otol Rhinol Laryngol 1999;108:683–688
39. Rosen M, Malmgren LT, Gacek RR. Three dimensional computer reconstruction of the distribution of neuromuscular junctions in the thyroarytenoid muscle. Ann Otol Rhinol Laryngol 1983;92:424–429
40. Gambino DR, Malmgren LT, Gacek RR. Three dimensional computer reconstruction of the neuromuscular junction distribution in the human posterior cricoarytenoid muscle. Laryngoscope 1985;95:556–560
41. De Vito MA, Malmgren LT, Gacek RR. Three dimensional distribution of neuromuscular junctions in human cricothyroid. Arch Otolaryngol 1985;111:110–113
42. Freije J, Malmgren LT, Gacek RR. Motor endplate distribution in the human interarytenoid muscle. Arch Otolaryngol Head Neck Surg 1987;113:63–68
43. Freije J, Malmgren LT, Gacek RR. Motor endplate distribution in the human lateral cricoarytenoid muscle. Arch Otolaryngol Head Neck Surg 1986;112:176–179
44. Bendiksen FS, Dahl HA, Teig E. Innervation pattern of different types of muscle fibers in the human thyroarytenoid muscle. Acta Otolaryngol 1981;91:391–397

45. Pilar G. Further study of the electrical and mechanical responses of slow fibers in cat extraocular muscles. J Gen Physiol 1967;50:2289–2300

46. Lennerstrand G. Motor units in eye muscles. In: Lennerstrand G, Bach-y-Rita P, eds. Basic Mechanisms of Ocular Motility and Their Clinical Implications. Oxford: Pergamon Press; 1975:119–142

47. Kupfer C. Motor innervation of extraocular muscle. J Physiol 1960;153:522–526

48. Nomoto M, Yoshihara T, Kanda T, Kaneko T. Synapse formation by autonomic nerves in the previously denervated neuromuscular junctions of the feline intrinsic laryngeal muscles. Brain Res 1991;539:276–286

Section II

Clinical Evaluation

Chapter 5

Electromyography of Laryngeal and Pharyngeal Muscles

Tanya K. Meyer, Allen D. Hillel, and Andrew Blitzer

Electromyography (EMG) samples the electrical activity of muscle, thereby reflecting the neural signal delivered to that muscle. EMG can give valuable information regarding the pertinent muscle and also the function of the innervating nervous system, particularly the lower motor neuron. Most commonly a needle electrode is used as the active/recording electrode, and surface electrodes are used as the reference and ground electrodes. The patterns of electrical activity, evaluated both at rest and during contraction, have been characterized. Normal patterns of activity are well defined, and abnormal findings, taken in context within the clinical scenario, can aid in diagnosis, prognosis, and influence timing and choice of therapeutic intervention.

Although laryngeal EMG (LEMG) can provide valuable diagnostic information in conditions in which there is suspicion of neuromuscular injury, it is also used for other purposes, most commonly therapeutic injection of the intrinsic laryngeal musculature (**Table 5.1**).

◆ History

Laryngeal electromyography was first described in 1944 by Weddell et al[1] even before the technique was standard in the evaluation of truncal and limb neurologic disorders.

Table 5.1 Common Clinical Uses of Laryngeal Electromyography

- Estimating the degree and prognosis of paralysis
- Differentiating laryngeal paralysis from mechanical fixation of the cricoarytenoid joint
- Determining a neurologic diagnosis: myasthenia gravis, amyotrophic lateral sclerosis, myopathy
- Determining the site of neurologic lesion (SLN, RLN, high vagal)
- Evaluating laryngeal synkinesis or dysfunctional reinnervation
- Intraoperative nerve monitoring
- Therapeutic injection of laryngeal muscles (botulinum toxin)
- Biofeedback in speech and swallowing disorders

It was one year later when the first EMG machine designed specifically for clinical use was made by Golseth.[2,3] Over the course of the next 30 years, electromyography gradually became accepted as the clinical standard for diagnostic and prognostic evaluation of the neuromuscular system.

The field of LEMG was greatly advanced in the late 1950s by Faaborg-Anderson,[4] who published a detailed treatise describing the activity of the laryngeal muscles during both phonatory and nonphonatory tasks. Buchthal[5] and Hirano[6] were also early pioneers in the field, applying newer findings of motor unit morphology to EMG studies of the larynx. The success of EMG-guided botulinum toxin injections for the treatment of laryngeal dystonia, as reported by Blitzer,[7] stimulated more widespread incorporation of LEMG into clinical practice. The utility of LEMG in the evaluation of suspected laryngeal neurologic disorders has been described by many investigators, and it is rapidly becoming accepted as the standard of care in the diagnosis and treatment of the injured and neurologically impaired larynx.[8–23]

◆ Electromyography Recording and Techniques

For the most part, LEMG is performed using a needle recording electrode and surface reference and ground electrodes. The electrical activity at the recording electrode is compared with that of the reference electrode, which has been designated as zero. The difference between these two points is determined and displayed on the oscilloscope or computer screen and via loudspeaker, enabling visual and audio interpretation.

The electrical charges are represented as either positive or negative. By convention electrical positivity is represented by a downward deflection, whereas electrical negativity is represented by an upward deflection of the tracing. It is important to note that the acoustic signal is essential to the proper performance of the EMG exam, and experienced electromyographers can identify the abnormal patterns more efficiently by ear than by visualization.

In brief, a needle electrode (the active or sampling electrode) is inserted through the skin and into the muscle of interest. Reference and ground electrodes are placed over the skin of the neck or upper chest. Proper insertion is verified by asking the patient to perform appropriate verification tasks (such as vocalization for the vocalis muscle or sniffing for the posterior cricoarytenoid muscle). EMG evaluation consists of sampling three types of electrical activity—insertional, spontaneous, and volitional muscle activity.

When a needle is inserted into a relaxed muscle there is a short burst of normal electrical activity that occurs due to disruption of the muscle membrane, which is termed insertional activity. If the test muscle is completely at rest, after the dissipation of the insertional activity, there should be almost complete electrical silence in a normal muscle. Any electrical activity present is termed spontaneous activity and is abnormal. Volitional activity is evaluated by asking the individual to contract the test muscle. During volitional contraction, the morphology of individual motor unit potentials (MUPs) is evaluated. The individual is then asked to perform a sustained contraction and the recruitment pattern of the muscle is sampled.

Although the basic principles are similar, laryngeal and pharyngeal EMG has some differences as compared with the EMG of limb musculature. Because the intrinsic laryngeal musculature is phasically activated to a low degree with respiration, it can be challenging to evaluate insertional and spontaneous activity, which relies on evaluation of electrical activity at rest. In addition, it can be difficult to evaluate interference patterns in selected muscles because individuals may not be able to reliably perform a sustained contraction of the test muscle (sniffing and swallowing are by nature intermittent processes). Finally, correct electrode placement may be difficult due to the fact that each target muscle is small, close to other muscles, and nonpalpable. In cases of paralysis or synkinesis, absent or misleading electrical activity may make electrode placement even more challenging. Thus, extensive familiarity with anatomy is mandatory for accurate electrode placement.

The spectrum of abnormal EMG findings is broad; none are pathognomonic for a specific disease entity, and in themselves cannot provide a definitive diagnosis. The significance of any finding depends on the frequency of its occurrence, pattern of occurrence among various muscles, time course in relation to the original injury, and clinical context; for this reason there are few lists of strict diagnostic criteria for specific diseases in the EMG literature.

Laryngeal Electromyography Techniques

There are six basic components of the technique of laryngeal EMG **(Table 5.2)**, which are discussed in the following subsections.

Table 5.2 Technique of Laryngeal Electromyography

1. Electrode placement with attention to insertional activity
2. Verification of correct electrode placement by appropriate verification gestures
3. Evaluation of electrical activity of the muscle at rest (absence/presence of spontaneous activity)
4. Examination of individual motor unit potentials for phase, amplitude, and duration
5. Examination of the recruitment pattern
6. Evaluation for synkinetic reinnervation

Patient Positioning and Preparation

Consent is obtained. Patients are counseled that the major risks are bleeding and infection, with a diminutive risk of airway compromise. They may have a transient change in their voice due to needle manipulation. Testing is deferred if there is overlying skin infection or an acute laryngitis. We do not routinely request patients to stop anticoagulants, including aspirin, nonsteroidal antiinflammatory drugs (NSAIDs), and Coumadin, and we have not encountered airway complications in over 20 years of testing. Although the pacemaker spike is seen on the oscilloscope, the EMG tracing can be recorded and the pacemaker artifact ignored. Routine diagnostic EMG does not affect electrical cardiac pacing. Deep brain stimulation and vagal nerve stimulation create an extensive artifact that precludes meaningful testing, and must be temporarily turned off to allow for diagnostic LEMG.

We prefer to position the patient reclining in a chair with the neck extended using a modest shoulder roll. Although some examiners prefer to sit at the head of the patient, we prefer to stand at the patient's side. A local anesthetic can be used at the cutaneous insertion site, although this may affect the signal given by the cricothyroid muscle if the anesthetic diffuses to this area. If the patient reacts strongly with coughing, anesthetic can be dribbled into the airway via the cricothyroid membrane, although this can also blunt the EMG reading.[24] For most individuals we do not find it necessary to use an anesthetic.

Electrode Placement and Verification (Fig. 5.1)

- *Cricothyroid:* The needle is inserted 5 mm lateral to the midline at the level of the lower edge of the cricoid cartilage and directed toward the inferior tuberculum of the thyroid cartilage.

    Verification gesture:

    Activity with glissando (slide pitch of voice from low to high)

    No activity with raising head (straps)

- *Thyroarytenoid:* The needle is inserted at or just lateral to midline at the level of the cricothyroid membrane and

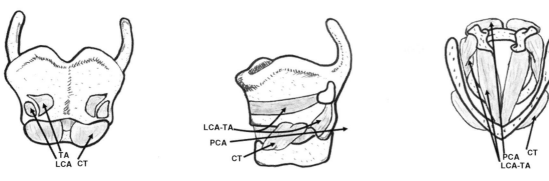

Fig. 5.1 Needle electrode placement for the thyroarytenoid (TA), cricothyroid (CT), lateral cricoarytenoid (LCA), and posterior cricoarytenoid (PCA).

directed superolaterally toward the superior tuberculum of the thyroid cartilage.

Verification gesture:

Activity with phonation of /e/

No activity with sniffing (posterior cricoarytenoid, PCA) or with raising head (straps)

- *Lateral cricoarytenoid:* The needle is inserted 7 to 8 mm lateral to midline at the level of the cricothyroid membrane and directed superolaterally toward the superior tuberculum of the thyroid cartilage.

Verification gesture:

Activity with phonation of /e/

No activity with sniffing (PCA) or with raising head (straps)

- *Posterior cricoarytenoid:* The PCA muscle can be sampled transcutaneously by two methods. If the patient is sufficiently relaxed, the examiner can rotate the larynx by catching the thumb of the noninjecting hand behind the posterior edge of the thyroid lamina. The anterior aspect of the cricoid ring is palpated with the index finger. The needle is inserted just superior and lateral to the index finger, traversing the inferior constrictor until it stops against the rostrum of the cricoid cartilage. Alternatively, the needle may be inserted through the cricothyroid membrane in the midline, traversing the subglottic space (there will be the characteristic airway "buzz" from the amplifier) and piercing the posterior lamina of the cricoid cartilage just to one side of the midline. The needle will often harbor a cartilage plug requiring moderate force to inject the medication. This approach is most successful in younger patients before extensive cartilage ossification has occurred.

Verification gesture:

Activity with sniffing

No activity during phonation

- *Interarytenoideus:* With endoscopic guidance, the needle is inserted transglottically, piercing the interarytenoideus muscle in the midline between the arytenoids towers.

Verification gesture:

Activity with phonation

- *Cricopharyngeus:* The cricoid cartilage is palpated, and if possible, the larynx is rotated for injection of the PCA. The insertion site is just at the inferior border of the cricoid cartilage, hugging the trachea. The patient should be asked to sniff, and if there is muscular activity with this gesture the needle should be repositioned more inferiorly. The cricopharyngeus is tonically constricted, but relaxes with swallowing; thus there will be a tonic EMG signal that temporarily abates with each swallow.

Verification gesture:

There will be tonic activity that silences during swallow

No activity with sniffing (PCA) or with raising head (straps)

- *Many intrinsic laryngeal muscles* can also be sampled transorally using curved instruments and hook-wire electrodes, with the exception of the cricothyroideus (**Table 5.3**).

Table 5.3 Other Craniocervical Muscles Amenable to Electromyography

Muscle	Nerve	Verification Gesture
Levator palatine	X	/s/
Palatoglossus/ palatopharyngeus	X	Swallow
Genioglossus/hyoglossus	XII	Protrude tongue
Sternocleidomastoid/trapezius	XI	Turn head/raise shoulder
Anterior belly digastric	V	Open mouth
Masseter/temporalis/internal pterygoid	V	Clench jaw
External pterygoid	V	Move jaw from side to side
Facial musculature	VII	Facial expression

Electromyography Patterns

Electromyography activity can be classified into three types: insertional, spontaneous, and volitional. Upon insertion into a relaxed muscle, irritation by the needle itself causes sporadic individual fibers to depolarize. This activity is normal and should not persist 400 milliseconds beyond the time of any needle movement. Prolonged insertional activity is considered a sign of pathologic muscle membrane instability. Alternatively, a needle placed into a muscle in which there is only a very small burst of electrical activity may indicate atrophy, as occurs with long-standing paralysis. There is nothing specifically diagnostic about insertional activity; it is simply an evaluation of the irritability of the muscle membrane. It is difficult to evaluate for insertional activity during LEMG because laryngeal muscles are never truly at rest.

After correct needle position is confirmed with performance of appropriate verification gestures, the patient is asked to relax all muscles to evaluate spontaneous activity. In general, with complete relaxation of a healthy striated muscle, there will be no EMG activity. Muscles that have suffered neurologic damage with denervation develop abnormal spontaneous activity such as fibrillation potentials and positive sharp waves (**Figs. 5.2** and **5.3**). In the intrinsic

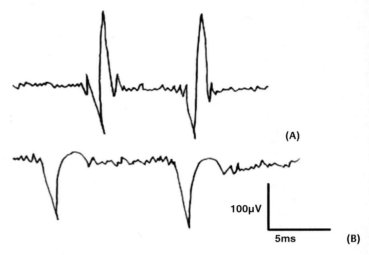

Fig. 5.2 Diagrams of abnormal spontaneous activity suggestive of denervation. **(A)** Fibrillation potential. **(B)** Positive sharp wave.

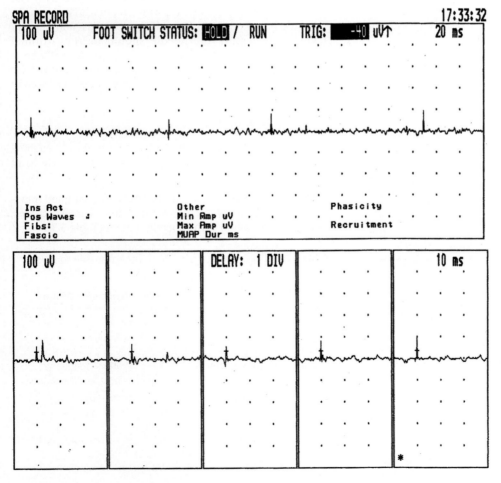

Fig. 5.3 Fibrillation potentials. Note that the duration of this waveform is approximately 1 millisecond.

laryngeal musculature, complete relaxation is rarely achieved due to continuous activation during the respiratory cycle. Thus the presence of pathologic spontaneous activity may be detected through a background of voluntary motor unit potentials in instances where there has been an incomplete denervation injury.

Pathologic spontaneous activity usually represents muscle membrane instability that develops with denervation and loss of appropriate neurotrophic input. Over time, the resting potential of a muscle cell that has lost neural input will fall to near the depolarization threshold. At regular intervals, it will cross the threshold, spontaneously depolarize, and then repolarize to repeat the cycle. This somewhat random activity represents the abnormal spontaneous activity termed positive sharp waves (PSWs) and fibrillation potentials (fibs). In the absence of neural regeneration, spontaneous activity persists until the muscle atrophies. PSWs and fibs usually indicate recent or ongoing denervation.

Many believe that fibrillation potentials and positive sharp waves represent the same electrical activity seen from different distances. They have been referred to as denervation potentials, but this is technically incorrect. Although denervation is the most common reason for their existence, they can also been seen in myopathic conditions.

Fibrillation potentials are described as sounding like light rain on a tin roof. They have an initially positive deflection (down), an amplitude of 50 to 300 microvolts, a duration of 1 to 2 milliseconds, and occur at a frequency of 20 to 200 Hz. Positive waves have a characteristic shape with a predominately positive component, as the name implies. The values for amplitude, duration, and frequency are similar to that for fibrillation potientials. There are other less common forms of spontaneous activity including fasciculations (pop-thud), complex repetitive discharges (motor boats), myotonic discharges (dive bombers), myokymia (marching soldiers), and neuromyotonia (continuous spikes).

Volitional activity is measured by asking the patient to contract the muscle of interest. In the larynx this usually consists of appropriate vocal tasks, which results in the appearance of MUPs on the oscilloscope (**Figs. 5.4** and **5.5**). The MUP is characterized by the number of phases, duration, and amplitude.

The MUP from each motor unit has its own reproducible characteristics. Usually the signal from multiple motor units can be identified at any given insertional location. A normal MUP is bi- or triphasic (phases are counted by noting the number of times the potential crosses the baseline). Greater than four phases is abnormal and termed polyphasic. Polyphasia occurs when the single muscle fibers are not well synchronized. Although this may occur for many different reasons, it most often occurs with muscle reinnervation (there can be up to 15% polyphasia in certain muscles in normal individuals, and this increases with patient age).

Duration and amplitude are proportional to the number of muscle fibers in each motor unit, and each muscle has its own normal values. For instance, the number of muscle fibers per motor unit in the laryngeal muscles ranges from five to 10, but is in the hundreds for the soleus. Normals

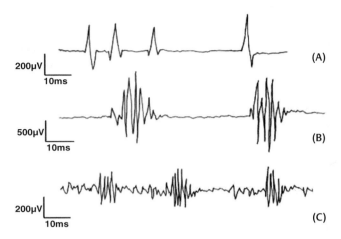

Fig. 5.4 Examples of motor unit potentials. **(A)** Normal units. **(B)** Neuropathic units. **(C)** Myopathic units.

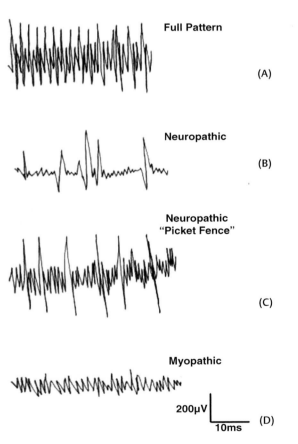

Fig. 5.5 Examples of recruitment patterns. **(A)** Normal pattern with a full interference pattern obliterating the baseline. **(B)** Reduced recruitment seen with a neuropathic process. Note that the baseline is not obliterated. **(C)** "Picket fence" pattern characteristic of a neuropathic process. **(D)** Early recruitment pattern seen with a myopathic process. The baseline is obliterated quickly with an overall lower amplitude.

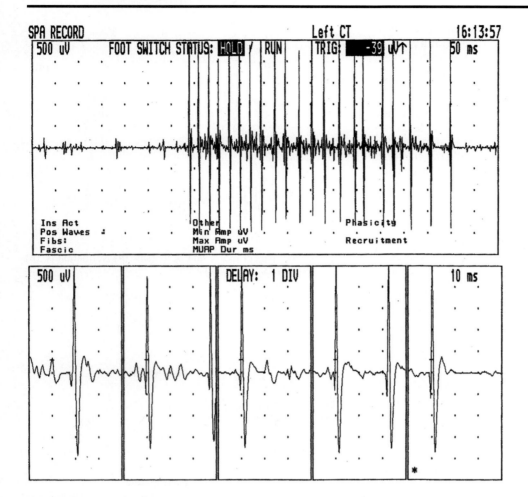

Fig. 5.6 Large amplitude motor unit depicting an old but stable peripheral nerve injury. The amplitude is approximately 4 mV (500 μV/division) with under 2 mV being the normal range. Note that the waveform is triphasic and that the duration of the waveform is approximately 7 milliseconds.

are also dependent on the type of needle used. For concentric needles, laryngeal MUPs generally have amplitudes ranging from 220 to 360 microvolts with a mean duration of 3.5 to 5.5 milliseconds.[4,5] For monopolar needles, the mean amplitude can be up to 500 microvolts, with a similar duration.

In neuropathic conditions with reinnervation, a given nerve makes connections to additional muscle fibers and the amplitude of the associated MUP increases. Because the new nerve sprouts have a slower conduction than the older, mature nerves, there is some disynchrony during firing between the original motor fibers and the newly reinnervated fibers. Therefore, the MUPs are polyphasic and increased in duration. These are termed polyphasic potentials, or "polys." In mature neuropathic lesions, the synchrony of a motor unit improves over time, decreasing the polyphasia and duration, although the amplitude increases, producing a giant wave (**Fig. 5.6**). This "mature" polyphasic potential reflects the discharge of more muscle fibers than a normal motor unit, and although it has the normal triphasic appearance, it is much larger in amplitude. These large amplitude motor units indicate an old but stable peripheral nerve injury.

In myopathic conditions, the number of functioning muscle fibers in a motor unit decreases, and the amplitude of the associated MUP also decreases. Therefore, the MUPs are polyphasic but have decreased amplitude and duration (brief small-amplitude polyphasic potentials [BSAPs]).

After the individual motor unit potentials have been examined for phase, amplitude, and duration, and the presence or absence of pathologic spontaneous activity has been determined, the patient is instructed to perform a sustained contraction of the muscle to evaluate the recruitment or interference pattern (**Figs. 5.7** and **5.8**). When a muscle is contracted lightly, motor units begin to fire. As the force of contraction increases, the frequency of motor unit firing increases, and additional motor units are "recruited" to start

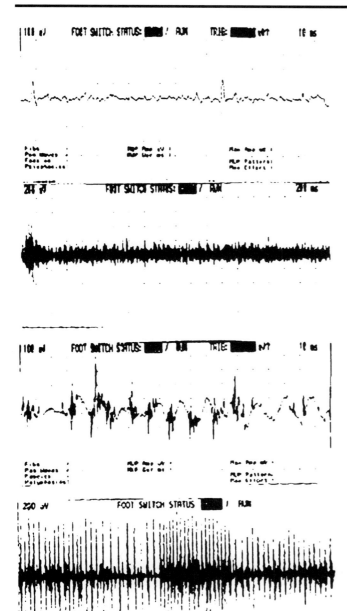

Fig. 5.7 Laryngeal electromyography sequence of a patient with a left vocal fold paralysis due to injury of the recurrent laryngeal nerve. **(A)** Tracing of the electrical activity of the right thyroarytenoid muscle taken during quiet respiration showing isolated firing of motor unit potentials of normal morphology. **(B)** The normal, full interference pattern for the right thyroarytenoid, obliterating the baseline. **(C)** Tracing of the electrical activity of the left thyroarytenoid muscle taken during phonatory effort shows multiple polyphasic giant waves indicative of reinnervation. **(D)** A decreased interference pattern for the left thyroarytenoid demonstrating the picket-fence pattern characteristic of neuropathy.

firing. At full contraction, the display screen is filled with MUPs such that individual patterns are not discernible and the baseline is obliterated. With a neuropathic process, there are fewer functioning motor units available, and even firing rapidly they are unable to obliterate the baseline. This is a decreased recruitment pattern, and it sounds like a stick being dragged along a picket fence (**Fig. 5.9**).

With a myopathic process, there is a loss of functioning muscle fibers within a motor unit; the muscle is therefore weak and all available motor units are recruited quickly—termed early full recruitment. This produces an interference pattern that is reduced in amplitude but still able to obliterate the baseline.

Laryngeal synkinesis is a common sequela of a neuropathic lesion to the vagus nerve. Synkinesis occurs when there is cross-reinnervation between adductor and abductor muscle groups after an injury. After evaluating the interference pattern of an adductor muscle such as the thyroarytenoid using a typical gesture such as vowel vocalization, the patient is then asked to perform an abductor task such as sniffing. If cross-innervation has occurred, there will be electrical signal with both tasks (**Fig. 5.10**).

Repetitive Stimulation

Repetitive stimulation testing records the simultaneous muscle contraction (compound muscle potential) when the recurrent nerve is stimulated. The EMG machine must have a setting that allows repetitive recording and analysis of the waveform. This examination is most useful when a diagnosis of myasthenia gravis is suspected. The test looks for degradation of the response with rapid repetitive stimulation. Because it is critical to have accurate comparisons of each waveform, a hook wire electrode is used, as it will not move during the testing. An example would be placing a hooked wire electrode in the thyroarytenoid (TA) muscle. The recurrent nerve is then stimulated transcutaneously in the area of the tracheoesophageal groove as low in the neck as possible. The distance from the TA is very short, so the latencies of response that are often measured in nerve conduction testing are not useful in laryngeal evaluation. The threshold of stimulation that provides a good response is determined, and then a train of five rapid stimulations is performed at a rate of 3 Hz. The fifth response is compared with the first response. The test is considered abnormal if there is a degradation of 10% or more.

The laryngeal muscles are then activated by asking the patient to vocalize for 30 seconds. This exercise activates the release of acetylcholine, and for a short time there is a postexercise facilitation of acetylcholine release. The patient is then asked to remain quiet for 2 to 4 minutes. At this point, there will be a postexercise exhaustion, and another train of five rapid stimulations at 3 Hz is performed. Degradation of the response is again measured, and if there is a degradation of 10% when comparing the fifth response to the first response, a likely diagnosis of myasthenia is considered. This can be confirmed with antiacetylcholine antibody studies. An example of a degradation of response is seen in **Fig. 5.9**.

48 II Clinical Evaluation

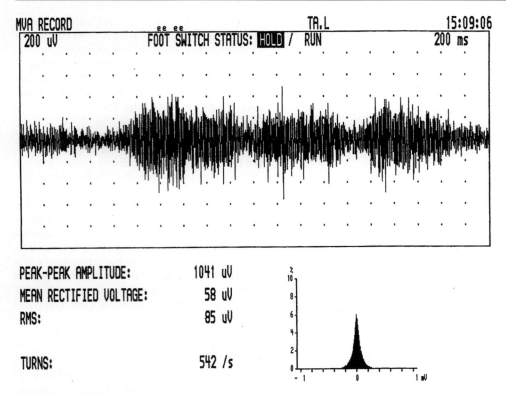

Fig. 5.8 Normal recruitment pattern during the phonation task of "eee,eee,eee"(/i/i/i). Note the dense recruitment representing the firing of many motor units.

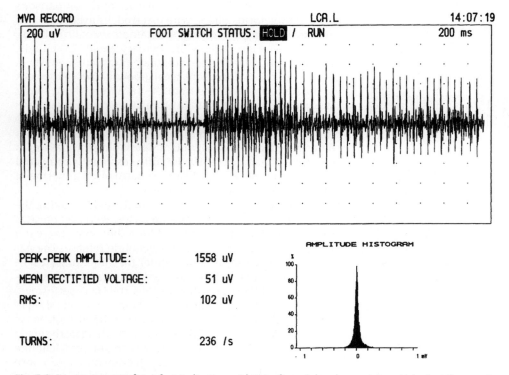

Fig. 5.9 Few motor units firing fast, indicating evidence of a peripheral nerve injury. Note that the recruitment pattern is less dense than in **Fig. 5.8**. Also note that in contrast to **Fig. 5.8**, individual motor units can be seen and are repetitive at a rate indicating fast firing.

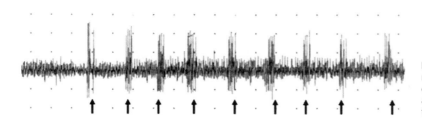

Fig. 5.10 Synkinesis. A recording from the thyroarytenoid muscle of a patient with long-standing vocal fold immobility demonstrating inappropriate activation when the patient is asked to sniff (*arrows*), an abductory task during which the thyroarytenoid muscle is normally not active.

Multiple Fine-Wire Electromyography

This test is the only test that can provide real-time recordings of many muscles of the larynx simultaneously. These recordings show the timing of muscle activation, and, to a degree, the relative activity of the muscles during specific tasks. Fine-wire EMG has been useful in defining some of the cases of laryngeal dystonia and in understanding some of the cases of laryngeal synkinesis.

The technique of fine-wire EMG is valuable whenever stable electrodes are needed. The technique of repetitive stimulation is an example of a situation in which a single stable fine-wire electrode is necessary. Multiple fine-wire EMG allows for comparative testing of many muscles. The EMG machine must have a program that allows multiple free-run EMG recordings. The placement of the fine wires is similar to the placement of other needle electrodes, but searching that can be done with a simple needle electrode is not possible with a fine wire. If the needle needs to be relocated, it must be removed and a new wire inserted.

The multiple fine-wire EMGs can be used to study patients with suspected synkinesis and for testing in patients with laryngeal dystonia. For synkinesis, the fine-wire electrodes are placed in the TA and posterior cricoarytenoid (PCA) muscles. The patient is asked to sniff, and a normal burst of potentials is seen in the PCA. The patient is then asked to vocalize, and a normal burst of potentials is noted in the TA and not in the PCA. In cases of synkinesis, mixed signals may be seen in both muscles.

For adductor laryngeal dystonia, fine wires are placed in the TA, LCA, and interarytenoid (IA) muscles. For abductor or mixed dystonia, a wire is also placed in the PCA muscles. Recordings are taken during quiet and voice tasks. The timing and participation of the muscles is examined for normal and abnormal responses. In many of the cases, this technique has proven valuable to tailor the treatment to the specific dystonic patterns. An example of multiple fine-wire EMG in a normal subject and dystonic subject is seen in **Figs. 5.11** and **5.12**.

◆ Common Clinical Uses of Laryngeal Electromyography

Prognosis of Paralysis

Investigators have reported highly variable success in regard to prognosticating return of vocal fold function in cases of identified immobility. This is due to a wide variation in the EMG criteria used, the time period of study, and differences in neural injury patterns among the study populations.

Min et al[25] studied 14 patients with unilateral vocal fold paralysis and describe a correct prognosis rate of 89% if the following criteria were satisfied: normal MUP morphology, overall EMG activity characterized by a root-mean-square value greater than 40 microvolts in any one task, and no electrical silence during voluntary tasks. They also suggest that patients should be studied within the time period of 6 weeks to 6 months.

Sittel et al[26] studied 98 patients with 111 paralyzed vocal folds of various etiology (53 due to thyroid surgery and 18 idiopathic). LEMG was performed at least 14 days after the onset of paralysis and classified as neuropraxia, axontotmesis, or neurotmesis with vocal fold mobility at 6 months as the outcome parameter. Partial recovery was correctly predicted in 94.4% of cases, but complete recovery was only accurately predicted in 12.8% of cases.

Munin et al[27] studied 31 consecutive cases of vocal fold paralysis with LEMG at 3 weeks to 6 months after onset of symptoms using vocal fold motion at 6 months from onset of symptoms as the outcome measure. Prognostic criteria used were presence or absence of spontaneous activity and recruitment, which enabled the accurate prediction of 44.4% of recovered cases.

Mostafa et al[28] compared 35 patients with unilateral vocal fold immobility to 10 normal controls and found a specificity of 100% and sensitivity of 65.7% in detecting vocal fold immobility. Clinical evaluation at 6 months of the patients with immobility showed recovery in 10 of 25 cases. None of the recovered patients showed abnormal EMG data at presentation, whereas 13 out of 15 cases of nonrecovered patients showed abnormal EMG data; that is, the specificity of EMG was 100%, whereas the sensitivity was 86.6% in predicting recovery in patients with vocal fold immobility. These authors feel that quantitative analysis of the interference pattern is a more sensitive indicator for predicting recovery after injury.

Despite the wide variation in reports, some generalizations regarding prognosis can be made. Preservation of normal MUPs with brisk recruitment implies an excellent prognosis, whereas the presence of spontaneous activity, aberrant MUP morphology, decreased recruitment, or electrical silence is an ominous indicator. Although 6 months is the time period used in many studies, it is the experience of the authors that mobility rarely returns in the absence of voluntary MUPs at 3 months. In the instance of an initial ambiguous EMG result, a second study

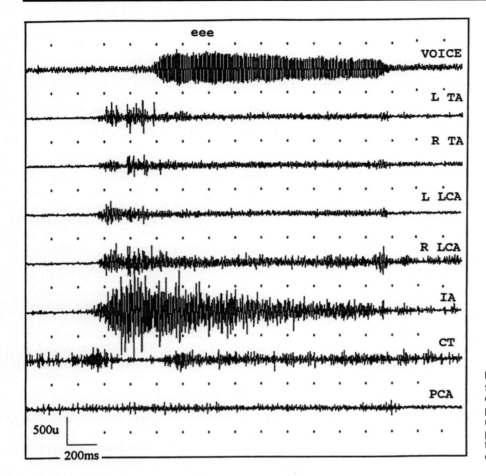

Fig. 5.11 Fine-wire EMG tracing in a normal subject with seven wires in place. The upper channel is the voice recorded with a microphone. Note the latency between onset of the muscle activity and the voice production is approximately 400 milliseconds. Note also that the TA and LCA muscles diminish in activity once phonation begins.

can be performed at a 6-week interval. If there has been interval improvement, then a favorable prognosis can be entertained; conversely, if the study is unchanged or deteriorates, then return of motion is unlikely and the patient can be counseled accordingly.

Determining Paralysis from Fixation

Laryngeal EMG can differentiate mechanical from neurogenic causes of vocal fold immobility and help the patient avoid the need for operative laryngoscopy with arytenoid palpation. In isolated cases of cricoarytenoid arthritis, dislocation, or posterior glottic scarring, the LEMG pattern should be normal. Unfortunately, it is possible that some etiologies, such as prolonged intubation, may yield both a mechanical and neurologic component, which may cause some diagnostic confusion. This may account for the observation by Yin[29] that some abnormal patterns may occur in long-standing dislocation.

Site of Lesion Testing Along the Vagal Nerve

Although EMG tests only striated muscle, because the superior and recurrent division of the vagus innervate discrete muscles, a high vagal or an isolated peripheral lesion can be determined. Comparison of findings between the cricothyroid and the thyroarytenoid indicates the site of the lesion. If there are neuropathic findings in both muscles, a high injury is suspected, and imaging of the skull base and central nervous system is warranted. If there are abnormalities in only the thyroarytenoid, the recurrent nerve is implicated, directing attention to the lower neck and mediastinum. Rarely, an isolated superior nerve palsy can cause laryngeal sensory abnormalities and vague vocal symptoms, confirmation of which can be reassuring to both the frustrated patient and physician.

Synkinetic and Dysfunctional Reinnervation (Fig. 5.10)

The recurrent branch of the vagus contains both adductor and abductor fibers. After nerve injury, recovery can occur along a spectrum from fully appropriate to partial to synkinetic. Likely there is some component of each type of reinnervation in many cases of neuropathic injury, and the end result depends on the final predominant pattern. Evaluation of synkinetic reinnervation was discussed earlier.

5 Electromyography of Laryngeal and Pharyngeal Muscles   51

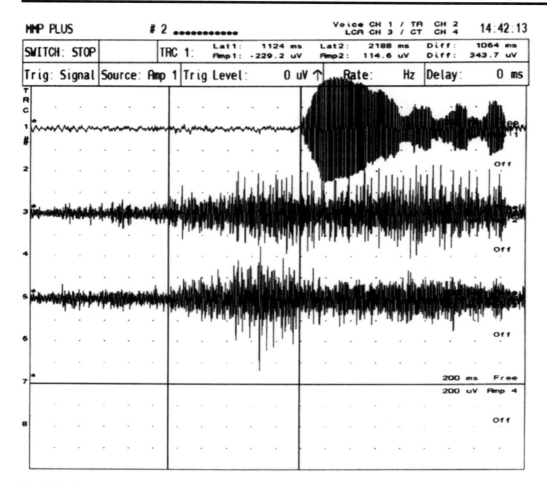

Fig. 5.12 Fine-wire EMG tracing in a patient with adductor laryngeal dystonia. Note the abnormally long latency between onset of muscle activity and voice production of over 1000 milliseconds also note the continued activity of the TA, and LCA muscles during voice production.

Upper Motor Neuron Injury

In the first 3 to 6 weeks after an upper motor neuron (UMN) injury there may be abnormal spontaneous activity seen in the muscles affected by the UMN lesion. After that time, examination should show electrical silence at rest with no abnormal spontaneous activity. With incomplete UMN lesions, individual motor units appear normal in morphology but may fire in clumps and have a "ratchety" recruitment pattern. However, EMG is neither sensitive nor specific in the diagnosis of UMN dysfunction.

Other Neurologic Disorders[30–32]

Myasthenia gravis is an autoimmune disorder characterized by fatigue with repetitive movement that is restored after rest. The condition is caused by immunoglobulin G (IgG) antibodies directed against the postsynaptic acetylcholine receptor. If disease is localized to the throat, patients may have difficulty speaking, breathing, or swallowing, and examination of the larynx and palate reveals fatigue with repetitive movements. EMG shows decreased amplitude and number of MUPs with repetitive use[8] (**Fig. 5.13**), which

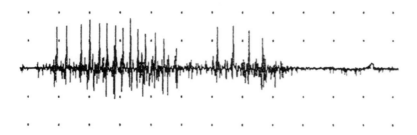

Fig. 5.13 Laryngeal EMG recording of the thyroarytenoid muscle showing decreasing amplitude and number of potentials with continued function characteristic of myasthenia gravis.

normalizes with the administration of edrophonium. Most patients are positive for antibody against the acetylcholine receptor, and early detection is invaluable because medical treatment is effective and potentially lifesaving.

Although the diagnosis of spasmodic dysphonia is usually made by history, vocal characteristics, and fiberoptic laryngeal exam across multiple speech tasks, in ambiguous cases, the diagnosis can be confirmed by EMG studies[33] (**Fig. 5.12**). In general, inappropriate, dystonic muscular activity is noted, with onset of electrical activity significantly before onset of voice, and persistent electrical activity despite voice breaks.

Electromyography-Guided Laryngeal Injections

Electromyography guidance is the standard of care in the therapeutic injection of botulinum toxin for spasmodic dysphonia and also for other hyperfuncional craniocervical muscular disorders such as hemifacial spasm, torticollis, and temporal mandibular joint syndrome. EMG enables the physician to confirm delivery of toxin into the correct muscle and also placement within the most active portion of that muscle.[7]

♦ Conclusion

Laryngeal electromyography provides the clinician with the best diagnostic information to evaluate the neurophysiology of vocal fold and pharyngeal function. It can provide valuable information to guide treatment planning and evaluate therapeutic results. We recommend that all laryngologists become familiar with LEMG to promote advancement of our field through refinement of diagnostic skills and correlation of therapeutic outcome to specific diagnoses.

References

1. Weddell G, Feinstein B, Paattle R. The electrical activity of voluntary muscle in man under normal and pathological conditions. Brain 1944;67:178–242
2. Golseth JG. Diagnostic contributions of the electromyogram. Calif Med 1950;73:355–357
3. Golseth JG. Electromyographic examination in the office. Calif Med 1957;87:298–300
4. Faaborg-Anderson K. Electromyographic investigation of intrinsic laryngeal muscles in humans. Acta Physiol Scand 1957;41(Suppl 140):1–149
5. Buchthal F. Electromyography of intrinsic laryngeal muscles. Q J Exp Physiol Cogn Med Sci 1959;44:137–148
6. Blitzer A, Brin MF, Fahn S, Lange D, Lovelace RE. Botulinum toxin (Botox) for the treatment of "spastic dysphonia" as part of a trial of toxin injections for the treatment of other cranial dystonias. Laryngoscope 1986;96:1300–1301
7. Mao VH, Abaza M, Spiegel JR, et al. Laryngeal myasthenia gravis: report of 40 cases. J Voice 2001;15:122–130
8. Maronian N, Waugh P, Robinson L, Hillel A. Electromyographic findings in recurrent laryngeal nerve reinnervation. Ann Otol Rhinol Laryngol 2003;112:314–323
9. Maronian NC, Robinson L, Waugh P, Hillel AD. A new electromyographic definition of laryngeal synkinesis. Ann Otol Rhinol Laryngol 2004;113:877–886
10. Maronian NC, Waugh PF, Robinson L, Hillel AD. Tremor laryngeal dystonia: treatment of the lateral cricoarytenoid muscle. Ann Otol Rhinol Laryngol 2004;113:349–355
11. Hillel AD. The study of laryngeal muscle activity in normal human subjects and in patients with laryngeal dystonia using multiple fine-wire electromyography. Laryngoscope 2001;111(Suppl.97):1–47
12. Hillel AD, Benninger M, Blitzer A, et al. Evaluation and management of bilateral vocal cord immobility. Otolaryngol Head Neck Surg 1999;121:760–765
13. Hillel AD, Robinson LR, Waugh P. Laryngeal electromyography for the diagnosis and management of swallowing disorders. Otolaryngol Head Neck Surg 1997;116:344–348
14. Dray TG, Robinson LR, Hillel AD. Idiopathic bilateral vocal fold weakness. Laryngoscope 1999;109:995–1002
15. Benninger MS, Crumley RL, Ford CN, et al. Evaluation and treatment of the unilateral paralyzed vocal fold. Otolaryngol Head Neck Surg 1994;111:497–508
16. Heman-Ackah YD, Batory M. Determining the etiology of mild vocal fold hypomobility. J Voice 2003;17:579–588
17. Koufman JA, Postma GN, Whang CS, et al. Diagnostic laryngeal electromyography: The Wake Forest experience 1995–1999. Otolaryngol Head Neck Surg 2001;124:603–606
18. Koufman JA, Postma GN, Cummins MM, Blalock PD. Vocal fold paresis. Otolaryngol Head Neck Surg 2000;122:537–541
19. Mostafa BE, Gadallah NA, Nassar NM, Al Ibiary HM, Fahmy HA, Fouda NM. The role of laryngeal electromyography in vocal fold immobility. ORL J Otorhinolaryngol Relat Spec 2004;66:5–10
20. Sulica L, Blitzer A. Electromyography and the immobile vocal fold. Otolaryngol Clin North Am 2004;37:59–74
21. Sulica L. Vocal fold paralysis and electromyography. Arch Phys Med Rehabil 2003;84:1906
22. Jacobs IN, Finkel RS. Laryngeal electromyography in the management of vocal cord mobility problems in children. Laryngoscope 2002;112:1243–1248
23. Dray TG, Robinson LR, Hillel AD. Laryngeal electromyographic findings in Charcot-Marie-Tooth disease type II. Arch Neurol 1999;56:863–865
24. Chitkara A, Meyer TK, Cultrara A, Blitzer A. Dose response of topical anesthetic on laryngeal neuromuscular transmission. Ann Otol Rhinol Laryngol 2005;114:819–821
25. Min YB, et al. A preliminary study of the prognostic role of electromyography in laryngeal paralysis. Otolaryngol Head Neck Surg 1994;111(6):770–775
26. Sittel C, et al. Prognostic value of laryngeal electromyography in vocal fold paralysis. Arch Otolaryngol Head Neck Surg 2001;127(2):155–160
27. Munin MC, Rosen CA, Zullo T. Utility of laryngeal electromyography in predicting recovery after vocal fold paralysis. Arch Phys Med Rehabil 2003;84(8):1150–1153
28. Mostafa BE, et al. The role of laryngeal electromyography in vocal fold immobility. ORL J Otorhinolaryngol Relat Spec 2004;66(1):5–10

29. Yin SS, Qiu WW, Stucker F J. Value of electromyography in differential diagnosis of laryngeal joint injuries after intubation. Ann Otol Rhinol Laryngol 1996;105(6)446–451

30. Sulica L, Blitzer A, Lovelace RE, Kaufmann P. Vocal fold paresis of Charcot-Marie-Tooth disease. Ann Otol Rhinol Laryngol 2001;110:1072–1076

31. Dumitru D, Zworts MJ, Amato AA. Electrodiagnostic Medicine. 2nd ed. Amsterdam: Elsevier; 2001

32. Woo P. Laryngeal electromyography is a cost-effective clinically useful tool in the evaluation of vocal fold function. Arch Otolaryngol Head Neck Surg 1998;124:472–475

33. Klotz DA, Maronian NC, Waugh PF, Shahinfar A, Robinson L, Hillel AD. Findings of multiple muscle involvement in a study of 214 patients with laryngeal dystonia using fine-wire electromyography. Ann Otol Rhinol Laryngol 2004;113:602–612

34. Hillel AD, Maronian NC, Waugh PF, Robinson L, Klotz DA. Treatment of the interaytenoid muscle with botulinum toxin for laryngeal dystonia. Ann Otol Rhinol Laryngol 2004;113:341–348

Chapter 6

Physical Examination of the Larynx and Videolaryngoscopy

Marshall E. Smith and Eiji Yanagisawa

It has been suggested that the laryngeal system can be regarded as a microcosm of the entire speech mechanism,[1] and therefore the larynx may reflect neurologic impairments before other speech components. Neurologic voice disorders can be isolated problems or occur in the context of extensive systemic disease. Because voice disorders have been reported as initial symptoms of various neurologic disorders, such as Parkinson disease[2] and myasthenia gravis,[3–6] phonatory evaluation should be considered for its contribution to neurologic assessment.[7] The laryngologist, speech pathologist, and neurologist caring for these patients recognize several clinically important issues. They are aware of (1) disorders for which voice problems and complaints may initially present to the laryngologist or voice clinician; and (2) disorders for which medical, surgical, or behavioral intervention may improve laryngeal function, in the context of the individual's general physical condition. These key considerations should not be minimized because voice characteristics may contribute to neurologic differential diagnosis, and various intervention procedures may significantly improve quality of life, even in a patient otherwise suffering from a terminal illness. An example that applies particularly to these issues is the patient with early symptoms of bulbar amyotrophic lateral sclerosis (ALS), presented in detail in an excellent review by Hillel et al.[8]

◆ Physical Examination (Neurolaryngologic and Voice Evaluation)

The neurolaryngologic examination involves several components. These include medical history, phonation assessment, general otolaryngology–head and neck examination, laryngeal imaging examination, directed neurologic examination, and, when appropriate, special diagnostic testing. Aspects of the laryngeal imaging examination are discussed in further detail later in the chapter.

The physical examination of the larynx of a patient begins when the clinician observes the patient walk into the room. The examination proceeds while listening to the patient relate his or her complaints and details of medical history. While physicians are trained in observational skills, those caring for laryngeal disorders require use of the ears as well as the eyes. A careful history of both medical and neurologic symptoms provides the basis for evaluation of the patient with a neurologic voice disorder. The voice history includes the nature of the vocal complaint. In general, voice complaint symptoms may be described as hoarseness, vocal fatigue, breathiness, reduced phonation range, aphonia, pitch breaks or inappropriately high pitch, strain/strangle voice, and tremor.[9] One or (frequently) several of these complaints may be given by a patient with a neurologic voice disorder. Voice problems in conjunction with other speech production difficulties such as unclear speech, slurring, or unintelligible speech suggest an underlying neurologic disease. The same applies to the presence of concomitant symptoms of dysphagia. The onset and progression of symptoms is elicited, as well as what improves and worsens the voice. Voice and speech problems that are intermittent do not suggest a neurologic disease. When underlying organic neuromotor disease is present, though symptoms may vary to some degree, the speech or the voice is usually not totally normal.[10] Stress worsens most neurologic voice disorders, so this should not be taken as an indication of purely functional etiology of symptoms. Other symptoms of laryngeal dysfunction, for example, swallowing or respiratory complaints, are reviewed; if these also occur, a neurologic disease may be suspected. The patient's complete medication history is discussed. A review of systems pays particular attention to respiratory, gastrointestinal, endocrine, and neurologic areas. Questions about fatigue, balance, gait disturbance, tremor, changes in handwriting, sensation, and weakness all pertain to the neurologic system review.

The next portion of the examination comprises the phonation assessment. Ideally, it should be conducted jointly by a voice/speech pathologist and a laryngologist. Separately or together, they assess the quality of the patient's voice, speech, resonance, articulation, prosody, and breath support. Such examination begins while listening as the patient relates his or her medical history. In addition, sustained vowel phonation allows evaluation of phonatory stability, tremor, and movement of laryngeal supporting structures. If the patient is a singer and has complaints related to singing, then observation of the patient while singing is mandatory so that the problem may be demonstrated. Professional vocalists may develop neurologic voice disorders; problems during the vocally demanding tasks of singing may be an initial symptom.[11] Testing of the articulators (tongue, lip, jaw) can be done by having the patient rapidly repeat /pa/,/ta/,/ka/. Lack of precision or crispness suggests lower motor neuron or muscular compromise. Testing for velopharyngeal incompetence is done by asking the patient to sustain phonation of the vowels "ah" and "ee" while alternately pinching and releasing the nares together. The patient is also asked to read sentences with high pressure and nasal sounds such as "Suzy stayed all summer" or counting aloud from 60 to 70. Increased nasal resonance or nasal air emission during these tasks suggests lack of adequate velopharyngeal closure. Comprehensive assessment of the laryngeal mechanism in the context of motor speech control is summarized by Yorkston and Beukelman,[12] and in the textbook by Duffy.[13]

The general otolaryngologic–head and neck examination should be conducted, including assessment of ears, nasal passages, facial structures, oral cavity and oropharynx, nasopharynx, and neck inspection and palpation.

The patient with a neurologic voice disorder may have other neurologic examination findings that aid the physician in diagnosis. These have been reviewed in an excellent summary by Rosenfield et al.[10] Although this neurologic assessment may not replace a complete evaluation by a neurologist, it helps the laryngologist to understand the nature of the illness of which the voice may be only a part. It also facilitates communication with the neurologist about the patient's problem. Components include a cranial nerve examination, assessment of muscle strength and tone (motor and extrapyramidal), and coordination (cerebellar). Though cranial nerve testing is familiar to the otolaryngologist, other aspects of neurologic examination are not. However, these should be routinely performed in cases of suspected neurologic voice disorders. In the elderly patient, a screening examination for tone (resistance to passive movement) may be more revealing than an assessment of muscle strength.[14] Increased tone on passive movement of the limbs may be an upper motor neuron sign, and rigidity of wrist or elbow movement may be an early sign of Parkinson disease. Coordination and cerebellar function are assessed by observation of gait and by the Romberg sign. Following the Romberg test, the coordination of the upper extremities is evaluated by finger-nose testing. Observation of the outstretched limbs allows evaluation of postural (cerebellar) tremor. Resting tremor that improves with movement is seen in Parkinson disease. During the examination the patient is observed for adventitious (unintended or involuntary) movements (e.g., tremor of head or limbs, circumoral twitches, blepharospasm, dyskinesias, or dystonias). Observation of the patient's handwriting may be helpful in identifying ataxia or tremor.

Special diagnostic tests are indicated in selected cases. Laryngeal electromyography has been found to be helpful in the diagnostic assessment of vocal fold paralysis, differentiating paralysis from fixation, and in determining prognosis for recovery.[15–19] It can provide helpful information in determining etiology and treatment of a variety of neurolaryngologic disorders.[20] The workup of vocal fold paralysis, in the absence of identifiable etiology, involves imaging studies along the entire course of the nerve on the affected side.[21] Regarding spasmodic dysphonia, in the absence of secondary causes for dystonia,[22,23] Rosenfield et al[24] recommended additional medical evaluation with a thyroid-stimulating hormone (TSH) level to identify concomitant hypothyroidism, and Swenson et al[23] suggested a complete blood count and sedimentation rate to rule out systemic vasculitis. In the patient with suspected myasthenia gravis an acetylcholine receptor antibody assay or edrophonium (Tensilon) test should be performed. Those with presumed underlying central neurologic lesions are evaluated with magnetic resonance imaging (MRI).

◆ Laryngeal Imaging Examination and Videolaryngoscopy

Since Manuel Garcia, a Spanish-born voice teacher observed the motion of the vocal cords with a dental mirror in 1854 and presented his technique at the Royal Society of London in 1855, indirect mirror laryngoscopy of the awake patient eventually was popularized. It became a basic skill upon which the specialty of laryngology was founded. It is a fundamental tool of otolaryngologists and part of the core examination of the ears, nose, throat, head, and neck. Visualization of the laryngopharynx has greatly expanded our diagnostic capabilities. Many voice disorders can be diagnosed with mirror laryngoscopy. Technologic advances have yielded improved methods for observing the structure and function of the laryngopharynx. These have expanded upon the basic procedure of indirect mirror laryngoscopy. They include fiberoptic laryngoscopy, telescopic laryngoscopy, and stroboscopic laryngoscopy. For the patient with a neurologic disorder affecting the larynx, these tools are very useful. They provide the ability to examine the larynx under a variety of conditions and tasks. They allow for observation of fine details of laryngeal movement not always seen with the mirror. The examination can be video recorded for study, review with the patient, and teaching and research purposes. All the capabilities create a great advantage so that they are now considered necessary tools of those who care for patients with voice disorders.

The topic of visual examination of the laryngopharynx requires discussion in the context of neurolaryngologic assessment. There are several ways to examine the laryngopharynx. The way the examination is conducted, the endoscope used, and the type of disorder all affect the interpretation of the findings.

An example of this is the use of mirror laryngoscopy. It is a basic component of the general ear, nose, and throat (ENT) physical examination. The examination is conducted with the patient leaning forward, with the neck extended in the so-called sniffing position. The tongue is extended and the mirror placed above the base of the tongue with its back end at the soft palate. The appearance of the tissues in the hypopharynx and larynx is observed, and movement of the larynx observed during respiration. The patient is then instructed to say /i/. Often a high-pitch falsetto production of /i/ is required to elevate the larynx and tip the epiglottis forward to view the vocal folds. A cough may be elicited to view brisk vocal fold adduction and abduction.

Mirror laryngoscopy can identify gross visual structural abnormalities in tissue or gross asymmetries in vocal fold movement such as seen in vocal fold paralysis. It may allow observation of a tremor of the larynx. But, because of the task the patient is asked to do (sustained-vowel high-pitch phonation with the tongue extended), the clinician's ability is limited to identify abnormalities during the tasks (speech, swallow) in which the symptoms are present. For example, mirror laryngoscopy does not identify breaks in phonation of spasmodic dysphonia. Indeed, a characteristic finding of spasmodic dysphonia is that sustained-vowel or high-pitch phonation is generally normal. Subtle or task-dependent movement abnormalities present during connected speech cannot be observed. Although mirror laryngoscopy is a basic component of the general ENT examination, it is insufficient for many if not most patients with a suspected neurologic disorder of the larynx.

There are two endoscopes in laryngology practice that are now routinely used in addition to the laryngeal mirror. They are the flexible laryngoscope and rod-lens indirect laryngeal telescope. The instrument of choice for examination of the laryngopharynx in a patient with neurologic voice disorder is flexible transnasal laryngoscopy.[25] The flexible fiberoptic laryngoscope was introduced in 1968, was applied to examine otolaryngologic patients in the 1970s, and by the 1980s and 1990s became a standard routine procedure in ENT office practice. It is particularly useful in the examination of children and patients with a hypersensitive gag reflex or an overhanging or "omega-shaped" epiglottis.

The rod-lens laryngeal telescope is an excellent instrument to obtain a magnified well-illuminated view of the pharynx and larynx that can be photographed or video-recorded.[26,27] But it has all the task-limitations described above for mirror laryngoscopy.

Videolaryngoscopy, a videographic documentation of the laryngeal examination, is a most useful office procedure for the clinical practice of laryngology. It can be done with either a flexible fiberoptic laryngoscope or a rigid rod-lens telescope.[28] It allows excellent visualization and documentation of the physiologic function and pathologic conditions of the larynx. It is of significant value for the assessment of neurologic disorders of the larynx. It has been described in several reports, including use of a low-cost home color video camera by Yanagisawa et al[29] in 1981. Twenty-five years later there are now a variety of office systems available for this purpose. The examination is recorded on a videotape recorder or a digital video recorder. It is a routine component of most ENT physician practices. Because of video technology, the procedure itself has changed. The examiner often watches the video monitor instead of looking through the endoscope.

Videolaryngoscopy allows for the documentation of dynamic physiologic functions of respiration, swallowing, cough, and phonation. The capability for immediate feedback is of great value in communicating with the patient. Video printers or color ink-jet computer printers permit the creation of hardcopy still images that can be given to the patient or placed in the patient's chart. It provides an effective means of patient education, communication with other practitioners, teaching, and publication.[30]

Both fiberoptic and telescopic videolaryngoscopy have advantages and disadvantages. One of the most significant advantages of flexible transnasal laryngoscopy is the ease of the examination. It can be used in examination of children and for adults with a hypersensitive gag reflex who cannot be examined by either a mirror or a telescope. It is of great value for voice analysis of functional and organic disorders and for evaluation of the physiologic functions of the larynx. Respiration, phonation, glottal effort closure (Valsalva maneuver), connected speech, whistling, and swallowing and velopharyngeal function can be studied effectively with a flexible laryngoscope. It can be useful for singers who wish to study and improve their methods of singing. It also allows observation and documentation of disorders of the upper airway structures such as the nasal cavity, nasopharynx, and nasal surface of the soft palate.

In the past, telescopic laryngoscopy provided a clearer, sharper, brighter, more magnified image of the larynx than fiberoptic laryngoscopy. This advantage has been substantially minimized with the development of flexible endoscopes that have the video and lens apparatus at the tip of the endoscope, or "tip-chip" technology.[31,32] The images acquired from the endoscopes are much less distorted, bright, and not subject to the moiré effect. Examples of tip-chip flexible laryngoscopes currently available include the Olympus ENF-V (3.9 mm), Olympus ENF-V2 (3.2 mm), Pentax VNL 1170K (4.1 mm), and Pentax VNL 1130 (3.8 mm). A comparison of images of the larynx in the same subject obtained with a telescopic laryngoscope, a flexible laryngoscope, and a tip-chip flexible laryngoscope are shown in **Fig. 6.1**.

Stroboscopic videolaryngoscopy is commonly used in evaluation of voice disorders,[33] but it has limitations in the assessment of neurolaryngologic voice disorders. The great utility of stroboscopy is in the visualization of the illusion of mucosal wave movement in the steady or quasi-steady state of sustained vowel production. This can be done at a constant vocal pitch or varying pitch. Stroboscopic laryngoscopy is most helpful for the evaluation of subtle mass lesions of the vocal fold that affect vibration such as nodules, polyps, cysts, or mucosal diseases of dysplasia or early carcinoma. However, most neurologic disorders of the larynx do not need stroboscopic examination of the vocal folds to make the diagnosis or influence treatment decisions. Observation of the mucosal wave and glottic configuration may be helpful in some forms of neurologic impairment. These may include subtle stiffness

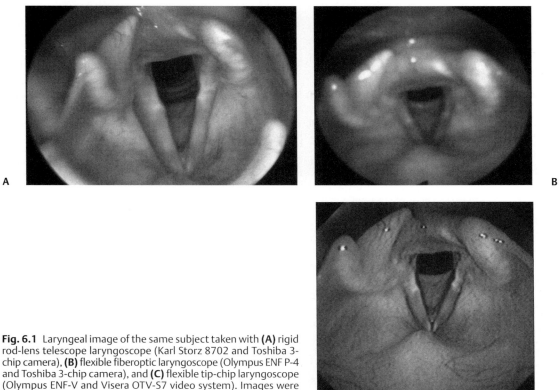

Fig. 6.1 Laryngeal image of the same subject taken with **(A)** rigid rod-lens telescope laryngoscope (Karl Storz 8702 and Toshiba 3-chip camera), **(B)** flexible fiberoptic laryngoscope (Olympus ENF P-4 and Toshiba 3-chip camera), and **(C)** flexible tip-chip laryngoscope (Olympus ENF-V and Visera OTV-S7 video system). Images were captured with the Kay Elemetrics digital workstation.

or movement asymmetries of vocal fold paresis, or the increased open phase of glottal incompetence in Parkinson disease. Interesting asymmetric vibratory phase patterns can be seen in unilateral vocal fold paralysis if glottal incompetence is not too great and the dysphonia is not diplophonic or aphonic (in which case the strobe light will not trigger).

Table 6.1 summarizes the various instruments for laryngeal examination in patients with neurologic disorders of the larynx. Recognition of these instruments helps the clinician to use them effectively in accurate diagnosis. An accurate diagnosis, which is obtained through the intellectual synthesis of data from history, physical examination findings, and medical knowledge, is essential to the appropriate care of each patient.

Table 6.1 Common Endoscopes Used in Laryngeal Examination

	Advantages	Disadvantages
Flexible fiberoptic laryngoscopy	Tolerated by nearly all patients	View mildly distorted, less magnified, less well illuminated
	Dynamic observation of laryngeal and velopharyngeal function	
Rigid telescopic laryngoscopy	Magnified, bright view of laryngopharynx	Task limitations
		Gag reflex
Laryngostroboscopy (flexible or rigid)	Observe vocal fold mucosa structural abnormalities and mucosal wave movement	Not needed for most neurologically based voice disorders

References

1. Barlow S, Netsell R, Hunker CJ. Phonatory disorders associated with CNS lesions. In: Cummings CW, et al, eds. Otolaryngology–Head and Neck Surgery. St. Louis: CV Mosby; 1986:2087–2093
2. Ramig LO, Scherer RC, Klasner ER, et al. Acoustic analysis of voice in amyotrophic lateral sclerosis: a longitudinal case study. J Speech Hear Disord 1990;55:2–14
3. Younger D, Lange DJ, Lovelace RE, et al. Neuromuscular disorders of the larynx. In: Blitzer A, et al, eds. Neurologic Disorders of the Larynx. New York: Thieme; 1992:246
4. Mastaglia F. Genetic myopathies. In: Swash M, Oxbury J, eds. Clinical Neurology. New York: Churchill Livingstone; 1991:1286
5. Ramig LO, Scherer RC, Titze IR, et al. Acoustic analysis of voices of patients with neurological disease: rationale and preliminary data. Ann Otol Rhinol Laryngol 1988;97:164–172
6. Salomonson J, Kawamoto H, Wilson L. Velopharyngeal incompetence as the presenting symptom of myotonic dystrophy. Cleft Palate J 1988;25:296–300
7. Darley FL, Aronson A, Brown J. Differential diagnostic patterns of dysarthria. J Speech Hear Res 1969;12:246–269
8. Hillel A, Dray T, Miller R, et al. Presentation of ALS to the otolaryngologist/head and neck surgeon: getting to the neurologist. Neurology 1999;53(8, Suppl 5):S22–S25; discussion S35–36
9. Colton RH, Casper J, Leonard R. Understanding Voice Problems: A Physiological Perspective for Diagnosis and Treatment. Philadelphia: Lippincott Williams & Wilkins; 2005:464.
10. Rosenfield DB. Neurolaryngology. Ear Nose Throat J 1987;66:323–326
11. Sataloff RT. The physical examination. In: Sataloff RT, ed. Professional Voice: The Science and Art of Clinical Care. San Diego: Plural; 2005
12. Yorkston K, Beukelman DR, Bell KR. Laryngeal Function: Clinical Management of Dysarthric Speakers. Boston: College Hill Press; Little, Brown; 1988:241–267
13. Duffy J. Motor Speech Disorders. St. Louis: Mosby; 1995
14. Glick T. Neurologic Skills: Examination and Diagnosis. Boston: Blackwell Scientific; 1993
15. Hirano M, Nozoe I, Shin T, Maeyama T. Electromyography for laryngeal paralysis. In: Hirano M, Kirchner JA, Bless DM, eds. Neurolaryngology: Recent Advances. Boston: College-Hill; 1987:232–248
16. Miller RH, Rosenfield DB. The role of electromyography in clinical laryngology. Otolaryngol Head Neck Surg 1984;92:287–291
17. Parnes SM, Satya-Murti S. Predictive value of laryngeal electromyography in patients with vocal cord paralysis of neurogenic origin. Laryngoscope 1985;95:1323–1326
18. Munin MC, Murry T, Rosen CA. Laryngeal electromyography: diagnostic and prognostic applications. Otolaryngol Clin North Am 2000;33:759–770
19. Sataloff RT, Mandel S, Mañon-Espaillat R, Heman-Ackah YD, Abaza M. Laryngeal Electromyography. San Diego: Plural; 2005
20. Yin S, Qiu WW, Stucker FJ, Batchelor BM. Critical evaluation of neurolaryngological disorders. Ann Otol Rhinol Laryngol 2000;109:832–838
21. Terris DJ, Arnstein DP, Nguyen HH. Contemporary evaluation of unilateral vocal cord paralysis. Otolaryngol Head Neck Surg 1992;107:84–90
22. Brin MF, Fahn S, Blitzer A, Ramig LO. Movement disorders of the larynx. In: Blitzer A, Brin MF, Sasaki CT, Fahn S, Harris KS, eds. Neurologic Disorders of the Larynx. New York: Thieme; 1992:248–278
23. Swenson M, Zwirner P, Murry T, et al. Medical evaluation of patients with spasmodic dysphonia. J Voice 1992;6:320–324
24. Rosenfield DB, Donovan DT, Sulek M, et al. Neurologic aspects of spasmodic dysphonia. J Otolaryngol 1990;19:231–236
25. Koufman JA. Approach to the patient with a voice disorder. Otolaryngol Clin North Am 1991;24:989–998
26. Bless DM. Measurement of vocal function. Otolaryngol Clin North Am 1991;24:1023–1033
27. Ward P, Berci G, Calcaterra TC. Advances in endoscopic examination of the respiratory system. Ann Otol Rhinol Laryngol 1974;83:754–760
28. Yanagisawa E, Owens T, Strothers G, Honda K. Videolaryngoscopy—a comparison of fiberscopic and telescopic documentation. Ann Otol Rhinol Laryngol 1983;92:430–436
29. Yanagisawa E, Casuccio J, Suzuki M. Video laryngoscopy using a rigid telescope and video home system color camera. A useful office procedure. Ann Otol Rhinol Laryngol 1981;90:346–350
30. Yanagisawa E, Carlson R. Videophotolaryngography using a new low cost video printer. Ann Otol Rhinol Laryngol 1985;94:584–587
31. Sato K, Umeno H, Nakashima T. Stroboscopic observation of vocal fold vibration with the videoendoscope. Ann Otol Rhinol Laryngol 2003;112:965–970
32. Kawaida M, Fukuda H, Kohno N. Observations of laryngeal lesions with a rhinolarynx electronic videoendoscope system and digital image processing. Ann Otol Rhinol Laryngol 1998;107:855–859
33. Hirano M, Bless DM. Videostroboscopic Examination of the Larynx. San Diego: Singular; 1993:167–169

Chapter 7

Pulmonary Function Evaluation

Christine M. Sapienza, Karen M. Wheeler-Hegland, and Anuja Chhabra

Respiratory function testing is common practice in the medical setting as it helps to identify disease and disability and may clinically indicate why a patient is complaining of shortness of breath or having difficulty ventilating. Typically, a combination of pulmonary function tests is used to help differentially diagnose a patient's respiratory problem. And although appropriate referral to a pulmonologist is necessary to diagnose a pulmonary disease, there are general principles every clinician should be familiar with regarding pulmonary function, pulmonary function screening procedures, and interpretation of pulmonary function outcome variables. Individual pulmonary function tests give information regarding specific lung functions. Disruptions of lung function can look similar across distinct pathologic conditions. Subsequently, there are times when more detailed pulmonary function tests must be pursued to manage the patient effectively. This chapter provides an overview of ventilation, and reviews the pulmonary function tests and screening procedures.

♦ Ventilation

Overview

The primary biologic purpose of ventilation is gas exchange between the body and the atmosphere. Oxygen (O_2) is transported from the atmosphere into the lungs and ultimately to body tissues. Carbon dioxide (CO_2) needs to be carried from the tissues, to the lungs, and expelled from the body.

Gas exchange begins with inspiration. Air flows into the mouth, through the upper airway, larynx, and into the trachea. The trachea divides into two main stem bronchi at the carina, which in turn continue dividing into smaller bronchi, bronchioles, and the terminal bronchioles. The terminal bronchioles then divide into respiratory bronchioles, alveolar ducts, and alveolar sacs.[1–5] The trachea, bronchi, and bronchioles comprise the conducting airways, and are sometimes termed "anatomic dead space," because no gas exchange occurs in those structures. The primary role of the conducting airways is to warm, clean, and humidify atmospheric air before it reaches the alveoli. Respiratory bronchioles, alveolar ducts, and alveolar sacs comprise the alveolar air space, and this is where gas exchange of O_2 and CO_2 takes place.[2,3,6]

Because gas exchange occurs within the alveolar air space, the volume of air that moves into the alveoli (alveolar ventilation; V_A) from the atmosphere is very important. On average, approximately 500 mL of air enters the airway with each breath (tidal volume; TV). Of this, 150 mL remains in the conducting airways and 350 mL reach the alveoli. Tidal volume multiplied by the number of breaths per minute (on average, 12) is equal to the minute ventilation (mL/min). Minute volume ventilation refers to the amount of air that is moved in and out of the lungs in a minute[2,5,7,8] and can be altered by either changing the number of breaths per minute or by changing the TV. Either one of these parameters is relatively easy to manipulate, and both are important, for example, when considering ventilator settings for ventilator-dependent patients. If ventilator settings are such that there is asynchrony between respiratory muscle contraction and the respiratory cycle timing imposed by the ventilator, gas trapping, or failure to move O_2 and CO_2 in and out of the lungs, may occur.[9–12]

To calculate alveolar ventilation (V_A), or the amount of air reaching the alveoli, simply subtract the volume of air in the conducting airways (150 mL) from the TV (500 mL), and then multiply by the number of breaths per minute. Thus, for an average healthy adult male breathing at a rate of 12 breaths per minute, the V_A is 4200 mL/minute [12 breaths/min × (500 mL − 150 mL)]. That is, 4200 mL of air reaches the alveoli per minute of tidal breathing. This is an important value when considering a person's ability to adequately oxygenate the body tissues. Decreased alveolar ventilation may result from several pathologies, including airway obstruction (i.e., asthma, chronic obstructive pulmonary disease [COPD], laryngeal cancer) or decreased inspiratory drive (weakness in the muscles of inspiration). Alveolar ventilation can be increased by either increasing the respiratory rate (minute ventilation) or by increasing TV. Because increasing respiratory rate can lead to hypoxemia (discussed later), TV is typically thought of as the more important factor in determining how well the alveoli are ventilated.[3,5–7]

Changes of Partial Pressures of Atmospheric Gases During Ventilation

Atmospheric air is composed of a mixture of gases, including O_2, CO_2, nitrogen (N_2), and trace amounts of water vapor. Dalton's law of gases indicates that the total pressure exerted by a mixture of gases is equal to the total of partial pressures exerted by each gas in the mixture.[2,5,6,8] The partial pressure of an individual gas is dependent on the percentage concentration of that gas in the mixture. At sea level, atmospheric pressure, or barometric pressure (P_B) of atmospheric air, is 760 mm Hg. Oxygen makes up approximately 20.8% of atmospheric air, and therefore the partial pressure of oxygen (P_{O_2}) at sea level is 158 mm Hg (20.8% × 760 mm Hg). See **Table 7.1** for partial pressures of gases comprising atmospheric air.[2,7]

As air flows from the atmosphere to the alveoli, the composition of the gas mixture changes. Inspired air is warmed and humidified; as this occurs approximately 47 mm Hg of water vapor is added to the mixture. Thus, the adjusted P_{O_2} of inspired air ($P_{I}O_2$) is 150 mm Hg [(760 − 47) × 20.8%]. Subsequent mixing of inspired air with air already in the lungs also changes the partial pressures. An estimate of the partial pressure of oxygen in the alveoli (P_AO_2) is given by the alveolar gas equation:

$$P_AO_2 = P_{IO_2} − (P_ACO_2/R), \text{ where R is a constant equal to 0.8.}$$

Thus, the P_{AO2} at sea level is 100 mm Hg [150 − (40/0.8)]. It is the P_{AO2} that is important in examining the oxygenating capacity of the lungs.[2,5,7] P_{AO2} is an indirect measure of arterial P_{O_2} (Pa_{O_2}), which gives information about gas exchange between the alveoli and alveolar capillaries. A decreased P_AO_2 will lead to a decreased Pa_{O_2}, which leads to decreased oxygen delivery to the tissues. In the case of normal P_{AO2} (100 mm Hg) and decreased Pa_{O_2}, the problem likely exists at the level of the actual gas exchange across the alveolar and capillary membranes, as is the case in intrinsic pulmonary diseases, such as emphysema.[8,13]

The partial pressures change in the blood after gas exchange takes place across the alveolar and capillary membranes, in the tissues, and in the venous return blood after cellular respiration has occurred. A summary of partial pressures of O_2 and CO_2 from atmosphere to lungs, blood, tissue, and back to the lungs is given in **Fig. 7.1**. Keep in mind that as the P_B changes, so does the partial pressure of each gas.[5,7,13–16] For example, at an altitude of 10,000 feet P_B is 523 mm Hg. The percentage composition of oxygen remains the same, and the P_{O_2} is 110 mm Hg (20.8% × 523 mm Hg) as compared with 158 mm Hg at sea level. Pulmonologists, respiratory physiologists, and clinicians involved in respiratory monitoring must attend to this important information. Normal values undergo a change at altitude, which must be considered when planning therapeutic intervention. Partial pressures in the alveoli and arterial blood are lower at higher altitudes. This is problematic for some patients, especially those with already compromised respiratory function. In these cases, giving oxygen can increase the partial pressures and subsequently improve the oxygenating capacity of the lungs and oxygen delivery to the tissues.[17]

Gas Exchange

Once inspired air has reached the alveolus, the airflow has slowed and the predominant means of air movement is diffusion. The rate of diffusion is governed by Fick's law of diffusion. Fick's law of diffusion states that the rate of diffusion of a gas across a membrane is directly proportional to the differences in partial pressure (partial pressure gradient), and to the area of the membrane, and inversely proportional to the thickness of the membrane. In more general terms, the rate of diffusion increases with increases in partial pressure gradients and increasing area of the membrane. The rate of diffusion decreases with increasing membrane thickness. Fick's law is given by the following equation:

$$J = DA\alpha(\Delta P/X)$$

where J is the rate of molecular movement, D is the permeability constant of the membrane, A is the area of the membrane, α is the solubility of the gas, P is the concentration gradient (partial pressure gradient), and X is the thickness of the membrane.[4,5,18–20] In terms of respiratory physiology, the rate of diffusion, J, for gas consumption is the consumption rate of oxygen (V_{O2}) or the release rate of CO_2, (V_{CO2}).

The blood entering the capillaries from the tissues, or venous return blood, contains O_2 and CO_2 with partial pressures of 40 mm Hg and 46 mm Hg, respectively. In the alveoli, the P_{AO2} is 100 mm Hg, and the P_{ACO2} is 40. Thus, partial pressure gradients are set up between alveolar and venous oxygen and CO_2, resulting in a net diffusion of oxygen into the blood and CO_2 into the lungs. The membrane separating the alveolus and the blood is very thin, approximately 0.5 mm. In the lung, A, D, and X are typically constant, and they can be combined into a term D_L, which is called the diffusing capacity. Thus, the rate of diffusion for respiratory gases can be expressed as:

$$V_{gas} = D_L(\Delta P_{gas})$$

Because many diseases result in diffusion impairment by their effects on membrane thickness (pulmonary edema) or surface area (such as emphysema), determining the D_L is a useful tool to diagnose diffusion impairment that can result in low arterial oxygen and high arterial CO_2.[4,5,18–20] For

Table 7.1 Partial Pressures of Gases that Comprise Atmospheric Air (Sea Level)

	Percentage Concentration	Partial Pressure (mm Hg)
Nitrogen (N_2)	79%	600.40
Oxygen (O_2)	20.8%	158.08
Carbon dioxide (CO_2)	Trace	0.30
Water (H_2O)	Trace	0.00
Total atmospheric		760.00

example, with pulmonary edema, Fick's law indicates that the rate of diffusion is decreased secondary to increased membrane thickness, resulting in decreased oxygen delivery to the tissues and decreased CO_2 extracted from venous return blood.

Once this gas exchange between the alveoli and pulmonary capillaries occurs, the freshly oxygenated blood is routed back through the left heart and subsequently pumped to body tissues where cellular respiration takes place. As a result of cellular respiration, O_2 is consumed by the tissue in the production of adenosine triphosphate (ATP), and CO_2 is created as a waste product. Carbon dioxide then plays a role in blood buffering and keeping an appropriate acid–base balance in the body.[2,3,5,7,21,22]

Ventilation/Perfusion Matching

Pulmonary circulation sends the total cardiac output through the pulmonary vasculature, where the gas exchange takes place. Blood accumulates in the right heart after returning from systemic circulation, where it has accumulated CO_2 and released O_2 in the distal tissues. The right heart provides the energy, or pump, to drive blood flow into pulmonary capillaries. Blood flows through the pulmonary capillary typically at a rate that results in a 0.75-second transit time past the alveoli. Fortunately, blood reaches an equilibrium with the alveolar gas levels (exchange of O_2 and CO_2) in approximately 0.25 seconds, so there is a built-in safety buffer in the transit time that helps ensure equilibrium will occur even if the flow rate should change.[2,7,8,23–25]

Pulmonary blood flow is measured by perfusion, denoted "Q." That is, Q is a measure of how much blood is flowing to the lungs. The ratio of ventilation to perfusion is called the V_A/Q ratio. The V_A/Q ratio provides an estimate of the match between blood perfusion of a pulmonary capillary around an alveolus and the ventilation of the alveolus. In healthy individuals the V_A/Q should be approximately 1.0, indicating a match between ventilation and perfusion. A high V_A/Q is indicative of good ventilation but poor perfusion. Conversely, a low V_A/Q indicates poor ventilation and good perfusion. High and low V_A/Q both result in inadequate gas exchange.[1,23,25–30] Many clinical symptoms, including shortness of breath, wheezing, coughing, nausea, and dizziness, can be manifestations of V_A/Q mismatch. Respiratory, cardiac, or metabolic disorders are all suspects in a patient with these symptoms, and appropriate referrals should be made.[21]

◆ Hypoxemia

Matching O_2 and CO_2 levels in the alveoli with levels in the blood is paramount for adequate removal of CO_2 and oxygenation. This means there must be an appropriate match between ventilation and perfusion (e.g., $V_A/Q = 1.0$). A mismatch results in hypoxemia, which is a decrease in Pa_{O2}.[1,5,8,23,25,29]

Hypoxemia can be considered in four main categories, which are discussed in the following subsections.

Hypoxic Hypoxemia

Hypoxic hypoxemia is due to a decrease in P_{IO2} and can result from decreased P_B, as occurs at high altitudes. This results in decreased P_{O2} and subsequent decreased P_{IO2}. Additionally, decreased P_{IO2} may occur at normal P_B, but in cases where the gas has decreased oxygen content (i.e., <20.8%) due to dilution by other gases. In either scenario, P_{IO2} is reduced, leading to decreased P_{AO2} and low Pa_{O2}. This may be helped by increasing the P_{O2} of inspired air.[5,19,21,25,27,30]

Alveolar Hypoventilation

Alveolar hypoventilation can also lead to hypoxemia and results from decreased ventilation where alveolar gas is not sufficiently refreshed to maintain normal levels of P_{AO2}. Some causes of this include a physical obstruction of the airway, such as asthma or COPD, or weakness of the respiratory muscles secondary to some neuromuscular diseases, such as Parkinson disease. Additionally, decreased respiratory drive from the central nervous system (CNS) can result in alveolar hypoventilation. Alveolar hypoventilation results in low P_{AO2}, low Pa_{O2}, and high Pa_{CO2}.[1,2,15,18,21,22,28,31]

Diffusion Limitation

Conditions that limit the diffusing capacity of O_2 and CO_2 between the alveoli and capillary membranes may result in hypoxemia. A decrease in Pa_{O2} would likely result, and this may be remedied by increasing the oxygen content of inspired air (i.e., instead of 20.8%, increase to 50.0%), which should increase the rate of oxygen transfer by increasing the partial pressure gradient (remember Fick's law of diffusion). Some examples include emphysema, which decreases the surface area of the alveoli, and pulmonary edema, which increases the membrane thickness. Decreasing surface area and increasing membrane thickness both lead to decreased rate of diffusion, and subsequent limitation of O_2 and CO_2 exchange.[5,7,8,18,21,25]

V_A/Q Imbalance

Under normal conditions, the V_A/Q should be approximately equal to 1.0, indicating a ventilation-perfusion match and, subsequently, adequate gas exchange. With a ventilation-perfusion imbalance, the V_A/Q is not equal to 1.0. When ventilation and perfusion do not match, Pa_{O2} and Pa_{CO2} are affected (see normal values of P_{O2} and P_{CO2} in **Fig. 7.1**). With a normal V_A/Q, Pa_{O2} should approximate the P_{AO2}. A low V_A/Q is caused by decreased ventilation with normal perfusion, as with airway obstruction such as mucous plugs. In the poorly ventilated lung, P_{AO2} is decreased. This leads to decreased reoxygenation of the returning venous blood going to the alveoli of that affected lung.[5,6,8,14,15,24] For example, if the P_{AO2} is decreased to 50 mm Hg due to decreased V_A, the P_{VO2} of 40 mm Hg, which is typically increased to a Pa_{O2} of 100 mm Hg, might only increase to $Pa_{O2} = 50$ mm Hg with the underventilated lung.

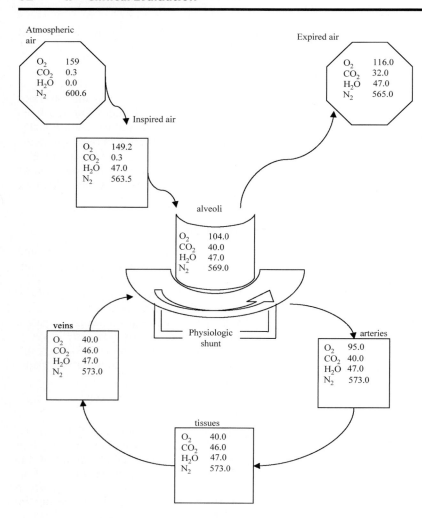

Fig. 7.1 Partial pressures in the alveoli, in the blood entering and leaving the alveolar capillaries, and in the body tissues (sea level).

A high V_A/Q is indicative of normal ventilation and poor perfusion. When one lung unit is receiving normal perfusion and the other is decreased or not perfused, the ventilation of the nonperfused lung is wasted and essentially acts as additional anatomic dead space. The P_{AO_2} and P_{ACO_2} of the nonperfused lung approaches the P_{IO_2} and P_{ICO_2} because of this lack of gas exchange.[5,6,8,15,19,24,25] The body may compensate by increasing the volume of blood flow (and, subsequently, rate of flow) to this region, which may increase the rate of diffusion. However, if the flow rate is sufficiently high to pass the blood through the gas exchange region before equilibrium is reached, the Pa_{O_2} will decrease. In this case, increasing the P_{AO_2} may help by increasing the pressure gradient (increasing the rate of diffusion).[8,18]

It is important to note that some of the above-mentioned causes of hypoxemia may overlap. For example, asthma, which results in swelling in the conducting airways, can be grouped under "alveolar hypoventilation" or "V_A/Q imbalance." Both are correct, and, in this case, alveolar hypoventilation leads to the V_A/Q imbalance. Of importance are the observable signs and symptoms, such as shortness of breath, coughing, and wheezing, which may be indicative of underlying respiratory, cardiac, or metabolic pathology. Knowledge of diseases that affect respiration and subsequent gas exchange capacity is valuable when considering the appropriateness of therapeutic interventions. For example, respiratory muscle strength training may be helpful in improving alveolar ventilation in a patient with respiratory muscle strength weakness secondary to Parkinson disease. However, for a patient with V_A/Q mismatch secondary to right-to-left pulmonary shunt, respiratory muscle strength training would not be an appropriate or helpful intervention.

♦ Alveolar Pressure

The driving force for the respiratory system is the pressure gradient between the alveoli and the atmosphere. Boyle's law tells us that air flows from areas of higher pressure to areas of low pressure. Thus, for air to flow into and out of the lungs, pressure gradients must be present. To inflate the lung the alveolar pressure must be less than atmospheric pressure, creating a negative pressure gradient and allowing air to flow into the lung. This is called inspiration. In order

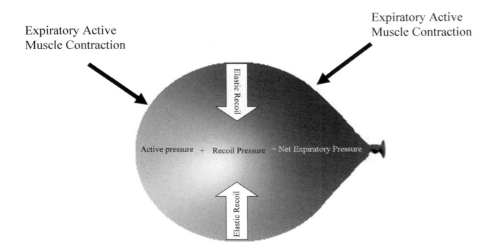

Fig. 7.2 Schematic of a balloon depicting active and passive mechanisms during expiration. The arrows squeezing the balloon illustrate the addition of an active expiratory force.

for expiration to occur, the alveolar pressure must be greater than atmospheric pressure generating a positive pressure gradient and allowing air to flow out of the lung.

The alveolar pressure is changed by two forces: (1) the passive, elastic properties of the respiratory system; and (2) active contraction of the respiratory muscles (**Fig. 7.2**). Inspiration is normally active, requiring the contraction of the diaphragm primarily and the external intercostals muscles that lift the ribs during inspiration. Accessory muscles of inspiration may aid in more effortful tasks and include such muscles as the sternocleidomastoids, scalene muscles, and others. Conversely, the principal action of expiration is passive. The elastic recoil properties of the lungs and thorax unit generate enough force to increase alveolar pressure adequately for air to flow out of the body. However, when the pressures produced by the passive recoil of the lung thorax unit cannot meet the pressure demand for a task, active expiratory muscle contraction must occur. The principal muscles of expiration include the abdominal muscles (transversus abdominis, external and internal obliques, and rectus abdominis) as well as the internal intercostals muscles, which act to pull the ribs downward and inward.

The best example of the passive and active properties of the respiratory system is a balloon (**Fig. 7.2**). To overcome the balloon's stiffness, active muscle force is required, forcing air into the balloon. With the balloon inflated and the opening closed, there is a pressure inside the balloon that is produced by the balloon retracting toward its rest position, compressing the air inside the balloon. This is an elastic force that is a property inherent to the balloon. The strength of the elastic force is a passive property of the balloon and directly proportional to the stretch of the balloon. The greater the balloon volume, the greater the stretch of the balloon wall, the greater the elastic recoil of the balloon, and the greater the pressure inside the balloon. The pressure inside the balloon can be further increased if the outside of the balloon is squeezed. This squeeze is the result of an active contraction of muscles and is an *active* pressure. The total pressure within the balloon is the sum of the passive elastic pressure and the active squeeze pressure (i.e., muscle contraction).

The elastic behavior of the total results from a combination of both the lung and thoracic elastic forces. When the respiratory system is at rest, the lung is partially inflated to approximately 40% of the total lung capacity (TLC). This rest position is referred to as the functional residual capacity (FRC). At FRC, neither the lung nor the thorax is at their respective rest positions. In other words, FRC is the lung volume at which the chest wall's tendency to spring outward is balanced by the lungs tendency to recoil inward. The elastic neutral position for the lung (without the influence of the chest wall) is a volume actually much smaller than FRC, so that the lung has a natural affinity to collapse at FRC. The thoracic elastic neutral position (without the influence of the lungs) is a volume much greater that FRC, approximately 75% of TLC, which means the thorax has a natural affinity to expand at FRC.

With the lungs in their natural position in the thorax, the outer surface of the lung is apposed to the inner surface of the thorax by hydrostatic forces. The lung is covered by a membrane called the visceral pleura. The thorax is covered by a similar membrane called the parietal pleura. The pleural fluid between the visceral and parietal pleurae holds the lung against the thoracic wall while allowing the lung to slide freely during volume changes. However, mechanically linking the lung and chest wall means that the combined system elastic behavior is a result of the interaction of the lung and thoracic elastic forces. The lung is at a volume above its elastic neutral position and has a collapsing force. The thorax is at a volume smaller than its elastic neutral position and has an expanding force. Application of pressures to the combined system results in a system pressure-volume curve (**Fig. 7.3**). Recall, that the FRC is the system elastic neutral position and is a volume of approximately 40% of the TLC. If the system volume is increased above FRC, there is a net collapsing force for the respiratory system. The greater the volume, the greater the collapsing force. Similarly, the volume below FRC will result in an expanding force. The lower the volume below FRC, the greater the expanding force.

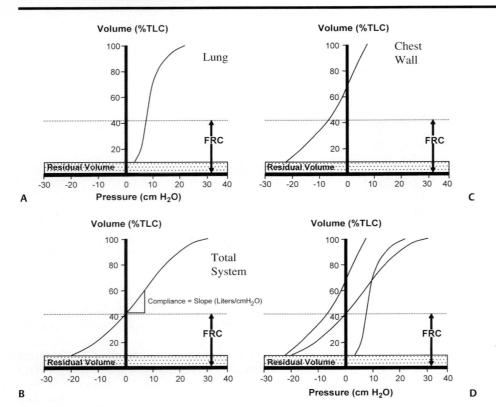

Fig. 7.3 Pressure-volume curves for **(A)** the lung, **(B)** chest wall, and **(C)** total system. **(D)** The relationship of all three pressure-volume curves for the lung, chest wall, and total system; note that the passive relaxation point for the total system, functional residual capacity (FRC), is the volume point where the lung and chest-wall pressures are equal.

♦ Measurement of Respiratory-related Pressures

Most pressure measurements of respiratory-related events use a pressure transducer fit with connecting tubes or adaptors coupled to the mouth. The frequency response of these transducers should be flat up to 10 to 15 Hz and this response should be tested when coupled to the tubing/adaptors. Resolution should be on the order of 0.5 cm H_2O with a range anywhere from 0 to 200++ cm H_2O depending on the pressure of interest. There are several pressures of interest, but only a few are discussed here.

Maximum Respiratory Pressures

Measures of maximum respiratory pressure are used as an index of respiratory muscle function. These measures provide an indirect measure of respiratory muscle strength. Depending on whether the individual exhales or inhales air with maximal effort, maximum expiratory and inspiratory pressures are measured. The maximal pressures that are generated during these maximal respiratory maneuvers (i.e., maximum expiratory pressure [MEP] and maximum inspiratory pressure [MIP]) have been linked to the strength of the respective muscles of expiration and inspiration.

Maximum Inspiratory Pressure

Maximum inspiratory pressure is an indirect measure of inspiratory muscle strength.[32,33] Digital manometers are typically used to measure MIP. They consist of a pressure transducer with an attached mouthpiece. Patients are asked to exhale maximally, and then to place the mouthpiece in the mouth and suck in with maximal force (**Fig. 7.4**). The manometer provides a measurement of the maximal pressure generated during the task.

Maximum Expiratory Pressure

Maximum expiratory pressure is defined as the pressure generated following a maximal expiration and is indicative of expiratory muscle strength.[32,33] MEP measurements are obtained using the same equipment as for MIP, with the difference being that patients are asked to inhale maximally and then place the mouthpiece between their lips and exhale maximally through their mouth (**Fig. 7.4**).

The MIP and MEP measures are of enormous value in the evaluation of respiratory muscle strength and can be useful when monitoring interventions, such as respiratory muscle strength training. Respiratory muscle strength training is a technique that can be used with several different populations, including healthy young and elderly individuals, sedentary elderly individuals, individuals with neuromuscular disorders not characterized by muscle fatigue, and individuals with spinal cord injuries. In the clinical context, indices of respiratory muscle strength can be helpful in determining an individual's ability to maintain adequate ventilation and achieve airway clearance. Respiratory muscle strength may be compromised in several patient populations, including those with progressive neuromotor disease affecting respiratory muscles and COPD.[34–36] To draw

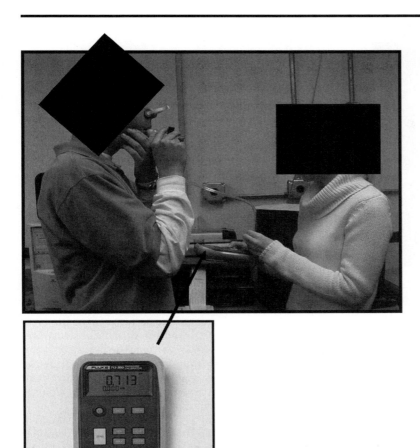

Fig. 7.4 Fluke 713 30G pressure gauge (Cole-Parmer, Montreal, Canada) used to measure maximum respiratory pressures.

comparisons between healthy individuals and those with reduced respiratory strength, it is essential to have a current, valid, and reliable normative respiratory pressure database for use in both clinical and research settings.

One of the most commonly referenced databases was created by Black and Hyatt[32] in 1969. This database was developed using information from 120 subjects, 60 males and 60 females, with an age range of 20 to 70 years. Subjects were grouped by age according to 10-year periods. Each group consisted of 10 males and 10 females. The oldest age group consisted of 10 males and 10 females over age 70. To date, only a few studies have used sample sizes that are comparable to Black and Hyatt's; however, these studies have not provided specific data on changes in MIP/MEP values longitudinally across the life span.[37,38] Other databases have been developed in Brazil, Canada, China, Germany, and Italy.[33,39–43] There are additional studies that have examined more limited age ranges (typically either young or old).[43–46] These studies have not gained much popularity as they are not felt to meet the need for a comprehensive, well-documented respiratory pressure database.

Intraoral Air Pressure

The intraoral air pressure (P_{io}) is measured as the air pressure generated behind a point of constriction in the oral cavity. This measure may be helpful in determining the adequacy of lip closure during articulation or the integrity of the velopharyngeal port during oral productions. Normative data abounds for this measure for children and adults for speech sounds produced with constriction of the oral cavity.[47–50] The peak pressure averages around 5 cm H_2O for most consonants (p,b,t,d, k,g,s,z,) produced at a comfortable effort level.

Pulmonary Function Testing

Long-established measurements of respiratory function like volumes, flows, and indices of gas exchange are nonspecific with regard to diagnosis but give useful information about respiratory muscle functioning.

Static Lung Volumes

These measures are independent of airflow velocity. The sum of two or more lung volume subdivisions makes a

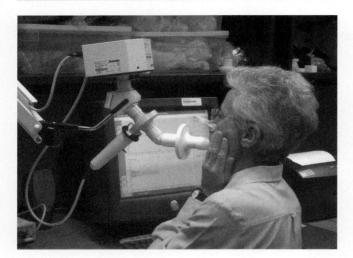

Fig. 7.5 Digital spirometric measuring device using a Jaeger Master Screen Pulmonary Function Testing and Impulse Oscillometry unit (Viasys Health Care, Conshohocken, PA).

capacity. Typically these capacities are expressed in liters, accounting for body temperature and pressure saturated with water vapor (BTPS).

Spirometry

Spirometry is the technique used to gather data on lung volume (**Fig. 7.5**). A spirometer is a device that assesses lung function. It is one of the simplest and most common pulmonary function tests and may be necessary for any of the following reasons:

- To determine how well the lungs receive, hold, and utilize air
- To monitor a lung disease
- To monitor the effectiveness of treatment
- To determine the severity of a lung disease
- To determine whether the lung disease is restrictive (decreased airflow) or obstructive (disruption of airflow)

Some common spirometric measures are discussed in the following subsections.

Forced Vital Capacity

Simply put, this is the amount of air in a full breath. More specifically, it is the volume change of the lung between a full inspiration to total lung capacity and a maximal expiration to residual volume. The measurement is performed during forceful exhalation; the preceding maximal inhalation need not be performed forcefully. The maneuver is almost invariably performed in conjunction with the assessment of the forced expiratory volume in 1 second (FEV_1) and of maximal expiratory flow-volume curves. At least three successful forced vital capacity (FVC) maneuvers should be performed, with the largest value of the three being reported. If FVC is 85% or below the predicted value for age, gender, and body type, it is likely indicative of pulmonary disease.[51]

Functional Residual Capacity

Functional residual capacity (FRC) is the volume of air remaining in the lungs at the end of a normal, quiet expiration. It is the sum of the residual volume and the expiratory reserve volume. The residual volume is the amount of air that cannot be blown out after forceful exhalation. In obstructive diseases, as emphysema and asthma, this value may increase due to air trapped in the lung behind blocked airways. The expiratory reserve volume is the largest amount of air that can be forced out of the lungs after a normal breath has already been breathed out.

Flow-Volume Loops

The flow volume relationships in particular diagnoses may indicate the presence and assess the effect of large (central) airway obstruction. Characteristic patterns of the flow volume loop also distinguish fixed from variable obstructions, and extra- from intrathoracic location. The overall shape of the flow volume loop is important when interpreting the results of this spirometric test. The speed of air movement in and out of the lungs is assessed by the flow rate. Volume measures the amount of air moved.

The major landmarks of a flow volume loop are shown in **Fig. 7.6**. They include the following: The *peak expiratory flow rate* (PEFR) is the first peak of air exhaled from the patient. Peak flow rate judges if the patient is giving maximal effort, and tests the overall strength of the expiratory muscles and the general condition of the large airways, such as the trachea and main bronchi. The *forced expiratory flow at 25% of FVC* (FEF_{25}) is the flow rate at the 25% point of the total volume (FVC) exhaled. Assuming maximal effort, this

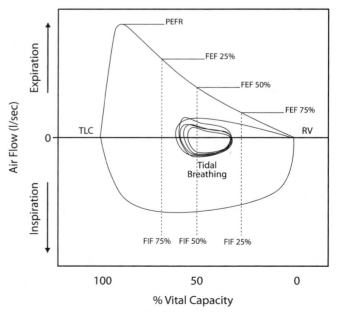

Fig. 7.6 Flow-volume loop indicating major flow and volumetric landmarks during expiratory and inspiratory cycle.

flow rate is still indicative of the condition of fairly large to medium-size bronchi. The *forced expiratory flow at 50% of FVC* (FEF_{50}) is the flow rate at the 50% point of the total volume (FVC) exhaled. This landmark is at the midpoint of the FVC and indicates the status of medium to small airways. The *forced expiratory flow at 75% of FVC* (FEF_{75}) is the flow rate at the 75% point of the total volume (FVC) exhaled. This landmark indicates the status of small airways. The *forced inspiratory flow at 25% of FVC* (FIF_{25}) is the flow rate at the 25% point on the total volume inhaled. Abnormalities here are indicators of upper airway obstructions. Areas of the mouth, upper and lower pharynx (back of the throat), and vocal folds impact the inspiratory flow rates. The *peak inspiratory flow rate* is the fastest flow rate achieved during inspiration. The *forced inspiratory flow at 50% of FVC* (FIF_{50}) is the flow rate at the 50% point on the total volume inhaled. The *forced inspiratory flow at 75% of FVC* (FIF_{75}) is the flow rate at the 75% point on the total volume inhaled.[51]

Spirometric values stated in clinical reports are typically presented in absolute numbers as well as percent predicted based on normative values. The normative values are race-, gender-, and age-dependent, and the standards may vary across clinical laboratories. If the spirometric data rules out lower airway disease, or the flow volume loop data indicate upper airway obstruction, then appropriate care can focus on the remediation of a laryngeal condition and with that intervention the sensation of dyspnea should diminish.

♦ Devices for Pulmonary-function Testing

Chest Pneumographs

There are several devices that are common to pulmonary function testing. Spirometry was discussed earlier. Chest pneumographs are strain gauges that measure thoracic circumference, thus enabling evaluation of thoracic contribution during breathing tasks, such as breathing during speech. Pneumographs are relatively inexpensive and are good for indicating gross respiratory movement patterns, but are not as specific for disorders that result in less stereotypical movement patterns.

Magnetometers

Magnetometers have been used routinely in the past for quantification of anteroposterior chest-wall displacements. Magnetometers use a small pair of electromagnetic coils fixed to the skin.[52] This device is precise with appropriate calibration, repeatable, and valid for documenting chest-wall distortions with disease. However, magnetometry that is used only for measuring anteroposterior movement may not be able to account for respiratory movements characterized by complex elliptical movements. In these cases, magnetometers are advised only for making transverse measurement. Unfortunately, the availability of these devices is limited.

Additionally, there are optical devices available that provide detailed information about kinematics of the chest wall related to lung volume. The advantages of these devices are often outweighed by their expense and time-consuming data analysis.

♦ Terminology for Breath Patterns and Breath Control

There are many terms that may be used to describe a patient's breathing pattern or breath control during speech. These terms include *support, diaphragmatic breathing, clavicular breathing, circular breathing, breathing exercises,* and others. The term *support* is vague and does not indicate the physiological status of the respiratory pump. The term *diaphragmatic breathing* is a play on words, given that the diaphragm is a muscle of inspiration and so it does not make much physiologic sense to use this term when directing instruction of expiration to the patient. If the term is used to indicate the piston-like mechanism of the abdominal wall, then the term should be changed to *abdominal force* and the terminology would make more physiologic sense with regard to the mechanics of breathing. *Clavicular breathing* commonly refers to the type of breathing used by raising the pectoral area of the chest wall and shoulders. It is, in fact, commonly used to classify the way women breathe. However, this usage of the term is also inaccurate, as those who have normal respiratory structure and function of the chest wall would not use a less efficient system voluntarily or reflexively. For those with solely laryngeal conditions and intact respiratory muscle tone, clavicular breathing is unlikely.

♦ Conclusion

Adequate ventilation is critical for gas exchange. Pulmonary function for speech is critical for developing the respiratory pressures to initiate vocal fold vibration and maximal pressures are indices of respiratory strength. Awareness of measures and terms are important for enhancing the clinical understanding of pulmonary-related disease.

References

1. Chapman RF. Ventilatory influences on arterial saturation maintenance during exercise in normoxia and mild hypoxia. Ph.D. dissertation, Indiana University, 1996
2. Martin DE. Respiratory Anatomy and Physiology. St. Louis: Mosby; 1988.
3. Wasserman K, Whipp BJ, Davis JA. Respiratory physiology of exercise: metabolism, gas exchange, and ventilatory control. Int Rev Physiol 1981;23:149–211
4. Workman JM, Penman RW, Bromberger-Barnea B, Permutt S, Riley RL. Alveolar dead space, alveolar shunt, and transpulmonary pressure. J Appl Physiol 1965;20:816–824

5. West JB. Respiratory Physiology—The Essentials. 5th ed. Baltimore: Williams & Wilkins; 1995

6. Wasserman K. Exercise gas exchange, breath-by-breath. Am J Respir Crit Care Med 2002;165:325–326

7. Spence AP, Mason EB. Human Anatomy and Physiology. 4th ed. St. Paul: West; 1992

8. West JB, Wagner PD. Pulmonary gas exchange. Am J Respir Crit Care Med 1998;157(4 Pt 2):S82–S87

9. Fernandez R, Mendez M, Younes M. Effect of ventilator flow rate on respiratory timing in normal humans. Am J Respir Crit Care Med 1999; 159:710–719

10. Laghi F, Karamchandani K, Tobin MJ. Influence of ventilator settings in determining respiratory frequency during mechanical ventilation. Am J Respir Crit Care Med 1999;160(5 Pt 1):1766–1770

11. Puddy A, Younes M. Effect of inspiratory flow rate on respiratory output in normal subjects. Am Rev Respir Dis 1992;146:787–789

12. West JB. Effects of ventilation-perfusion inequality on over-all gas exchange studied in computer models of the lung. J Physiol 1969; 202:116P

13. Clark FJ, von Euler C. On the regulation of depth and rate of breathing. J Physiol 1972;222:267–295

14. Johnson C. Clinical evaluation of pulmonary function. 1. Normal respiration. Postgrad Med 1966;39:357–361

15. Kim BM, Refsum HE. Changes in alveolar-arterial oxygen tension difference (A-aDO2) during variations in alveolar ventilation. Acta Physiol Scand 1968;73:36–41

16. Wasserman K, Whipp BJ, Koyl SN, Beaver WL. Anaerobic threshold and respiratory gas exchange during exercise. J Appl Physiol 1973;35: 236–243

17. Marks D, Milzman D, Jay B, Regan Z, Yoo P. Changes in hemodynamics and oxygenation in healthy normals during acute ascent to high altitude (14,500 ft): therapeutic considerations. Acad Emerg Med 2000;7:505

18. Ayers LN, Ginsberg ML, Fein J, Wasserman K. Diffusing capacity, specific diffusing capacity and interpretation of diffusion defects. West J Med 1975;123:255–264

19. Sue DY, Oren A, Hansen JE, Wasserman K. Diffusing capacity for carbon monoxide as a predictor of gas exchange during exercise. N Engl J Med 1987;316:1301–1306

20. West JB. Analysis of pulmonary gas exchange using a time-sharing computer. J Physiol 1969;202:9P

21. http://www.nhlbi.nih.gov

22. Howard P, Penman RW. The effect of breathing 30 per cent oxygen on pulmonary ventilation-perfusion inequality in normal subjects and patients with chronic lung disease. Clin Sci 1967;32:127–137

23. Johnson C. Clinical evaluation of pulmonary function. 3. Uneven ventilation. Postgrad Med 1966;39:601–606

24. Lenfant C, Okubo T. Distribution function of pulmonary blood flow and ventilation-perfusion ratio in man. J Appl Physiol 1968;24:668–677

25. Peters RM. Coordination of ventilation and perfusion. Ann Thorac Surg 1968;6:570–590

26. Daly WJ. Pulmonary diffusing capacity for carbon monoxide and topography of perfusion during changes in alveolar pressure in man. Am Rev Respir Dis 1969;99:548–553

27. Haab P, Held DR, Ernst H, Farhi LE. Ventilation-perfusion relationships during high-altitude adaptation. J Appl Physiol 1969;26:77–81

28. Haas F, Bergofsky EH. Effect of pulmonary vasoconstriction on balance between alveolar ventilation and perfusion. J Appl Physiol 1968;24: 491–497

29. Wasserman DH, Whipp BJ. Coupling of ventilation to pulmonary gas exchange during nonsteady-state work in men. J Appl Physiol 1983;54: 587–593

30. West JB. Ventilation-perfusion inequality and overall gas exchange in computer models of the lung. Respir Physiol 1969;7:88–110

31. Daly ID, Michel CC, Ramsay DJ, Waaler BA. Conditions governing the pulmonary vascular response to ventilation hypoxia and hypoxaemia in the dog. J Physiol 1968;196:351–379

32. Black LF, Hyatt RE. Maximal respiratory pressures: normal values and relationship to age and sex. Am Rev Respir Dis 1969;99:696–702

33. McElvaney G, Blackie S, Morrison NJ, Wilcox PG, Fairbarn MS, Pardy RL. Maximal static respiratory pressures in the normal elderly. Am Rev Respir Dis 1989;139:277–281

34. Saleem A, Sapienza CM, Okun M. Response to respiratory muscle strength training and its treatment duration in a patient with early idiopathic Parkinson's disease. NeuroRehabilitation, 2005;20(4); 323–333

35. Weiner P, Magadle R, Beckerman M, Weiner M, Berar-Yanay N. Comparison of specific expiratory, inspiratory, and combined muscle training programs in COPD. Chest 2003;124:1357–1364

36. Gosselink R, Kovacs L, Ketelaer P, Carton H, Decramer M. Respiratory muscle weakness and respiratory muscle training in severely disabled multiple sclerosis patients. Arch Phys Med Rehabil 2000;81: 747–751

37. Scott GC, Burki NK. The relationship of resting ventilation to mouth occlusion pressure. An index of resting respiratory function. Chest 1990;98:900–906

38. Berry JK, Vitalo CA, Larson JL, Patel M, Kim MJ. Respiratory muscle strength in older adults. Nurs Res 1996;45:154–159

39. Bruschi C, Cerveri I, Zoia MC, et al. Reference values of maximal respiratory mouth pressures: a population-based study. Am Rev Respir Dis 1992;146:790–793

40. Chen HI, Kuo CS. Relationship between respiratory muscle function and age, sex, and other factors. J Appl Physiol 1989;66:943–948

41. Hautmann H, Hefele S, Schotten K, Huber RM. Maximal inspiratory mouth pressures (PIMAX) in healthy subjects—what is the lower limit of normal? Respir Med 2000;94:689–693

42. Neder JA, Andreoni S, Castelo-Filho A, Nery LE. Reference values for lung function tests. I. Static volumes. Braz J Med Biol Res 1999;32:703–717

43. Szeinberg A, Marcotte JE, Roizin H, et al. Normal values of maximal inspiratory and expiratory pressures with a portable apparatus in -children, adolescents, and young adults. Pediatr Pulmonol 1987;3: 255–258

44. Enright PL, Adams AB, Boyle PJ, Sherrill DL. Spirometry and maximal respiratory pressure references from healthy Minnesota 65- to 85-year-old women and men. Chest 1995;108:663–669

45. Ng GY, Stokes MJ. Maximal inspiratory and expiratory mouth pressures in sitting and half-lying positions in normal subjects. Respir Med 1991;85:209–211

46. Wagener JS, Hibbert ME, Landau LI. Maximal respiratory pressures in children. Am Rev Respir Dis 1984;129:873–875

47. Arkebauer HJ, Hixon TJ, Hardy JC. Peak intraoral air pressures during speech. J Speech Hear Res 1967;10:196–208

48. Baken RJ. Clinical Measurement of Speech and Voice. Boston: College-Hill Press; 1987

49. Stathopoulos ET. Relationship between intraoral air pressure and vocal intensity in children and adults. J Speech Hear Res 1986;29: 71–74

50. Williams WN, Brown WS Jr, Payne A, Turner GE, Wharton PW. Intraoral air pressure discrimination under conditions of partial and complete resistance. Folia Phoniatr Logop 2001;53:99–109

51. American Thoracic Society/European Respiratory Society. ATS/ERS Statement of Respiratory Muscle testing. Am J Respir Crit Care Med 2002;166:518–624

52. Hixon TJ. Respiratory Function in Speech and Song. San Diego: Singular; 1991

Chapter 8

Laryngeal Dysfunction in Sleep

Joan Santamaria and Alex Iranzo

Sleep is an essential behavior in humans and many other species. Although it may look externally very simple, sleep is in fact an elaborate state resulting from a complex interplay of different central nervous system areas. There are two types of sleep: rapid eye movement (REM) and non–rapid eye movement (NREM) sleep, which are differentiated mainly by the presence or absence of rapid eye movements, muscle atonia, and characteristic electroencephalogram (EEG) activity. There are many changes in physiologic function during sleep that result in significant modifications in respiration, blood pressure, heart rate, muscle tone, and brain metabolism. Respiration, for example, is significantly altered, and the clinical relevance of this is illustrated in obstructive sleep apnea/hypopnea syndrome in which patients breathe normally while awake but experience repeated upper airway occlusions during sleep, most likely precipitated by relaxation of the upper airway muscles. The larynx also modifies its function during sleep. In a normal subject, the vocal cords abduct on inspiration, increasing the glottic area and reducing airway resistance, and adduct on expiration, both during wakefulness and sleep. Animal experiments have shown that during all stages of sleep, and particularly during REM sleep, there is a marked reduction in activity of the intrinsic muscles of the larynx, including the posterior cricoarytenoid muscle, the lone vocal cord abductor. As a result, the glottic caliber is narrowed and upper airway resistance increases, resulting in a more negative laryngeal pressure.[1,2] If this physiologic change occurs in combination with any underlying abnormality in the laryngeal function (e.g., vocal cord abductor paralysis) or anatomy (e.g., laryngomalacia) that reduces the glottic area, further increases in airway resistance may reach the critical level for significant glottic obstruction during sleep. This explains why some patients with laryngeal obstruction only show clinical signs of dysfunction (such as nocturnal stridor or obstructive sleep apnea) during sleep. Laryngeal dysfunction during sleep occurs in several neurologic diseases that affect supranuclear structures, the nucleus ambiguus, or the recurrent laryngeal nerves, and it has been described, for example, in several neurodegenerative diseases, sporadic or inherited, such as multiple system atrophy, spinocerebellar ataxia, and Parkinson disease. In some of these conditions, laryngeal dysfunction during sleep may be the presenting symptom of the disease and may be associated with sudden death often during sleep.

Laryngeal function during sleep may be evaluated by different methods. Fiberoptic laryngoscopy enables visualizing the vocal cord movements during fully inspiration, expiration, and phonation. This procedure is usually performed in the awake patient, but it can be achieved under drug-induced sleep with intravenous diazepam.[3] This is particularly interesting because laryngeal narrowing is exacerbated by sleep, and therefore some subjects with normal vocal cord movements during wakefulness may present vocal cord abductor restriction or paradoxical movements of the vocal cords only during sleep, both leading to nocturnal stridor. On the other hand, nocturnal polysomnography with synchronized audiovisual recording (videopolysomnography [VPSG]) allows for identification of the presence and severity of stridor, apneas, and oxyhemoglobin desaturations. Although laryngoscopy during natural sleep is the ideal procedure to define the mechanism, characteristics, and severity of laryngeal dysfunction during sleep, it is bothersome and difficult to tolerate. Because nocturnal stridor may be mistaken for soft-palate snoring or other respiratory noises, a tape recording while the patient sleeps at home may be useful in distinguishing these sounds. Laryngeal electromyography, although technically very difficult, may help to evaluate the presence of denervation or dystonia. This chapter briefly reviews the characteristics of the laryngeal dysfunction in sleep that occurs in the setting of several conditions, using multiple system atrophy as the prototypical disorder.

♦ Multiple System Atrophy

Multiple system atrophy (MSA) is a sporadic neurodegenerative disease characterized by parkinsonism, cerebellar syndrome, and autonomic failure in any combination. Mean life expectancy is less than 10 years, and the most frequent causes of death are bronchopneumonia and sudden death.[4] There are two different causes of sleep-disordered breathing (SDB) in MSA. One is central alveolar hypoventilation leading to central sleep apnea (CSA) due to degeneration of the pontomedullary respiratory centers. The other is obstructive sleep apnea/hypopnea (OSAH) and nocturnal stridor, which result from upper airway obstruction at the pharyngeal and laryngeal levels.[5]

Importance and Characteristics of Upper Airway Obstruction and Stridor

Detection of stridor in MSA is very important because it is associated with life-threatening episodes of respiratory failure, nocturnal choking episodes, sudden death during sleep, and short survival.[5,6] Nocturnal stridor occurs in all clinical stages of MSA, and it may be the initial symptom of the disease. Patients with stridor have similar age, gender, body mass index, duration and severity of the disease, and MSA subtype (cerebellar or parkinsonian) than those without stridor, but have a higher number of apneas and hypopneas during sleep, oxyhemoglobin desaturations, and vocal cord abnormalities on laryngoscopy. Severity of nocturnal stridor gradually worsens with disease progression. Patients are usually unaware themselves of their nocturnal stridor, and unexpected stridor may be found in routine VPSG studies. Stridor during wakefulness appears in patients who already have nocturnal stridor and reflects a marked laryngeal obstruction that may herald respiratory failure.[7]

Fiberoptic Laryngoscopy Findings[3,6,7]

In patients without stridor, laryngoscopy may show asymptomatic partial vocal cord abduction restriction. In patients with stridor, laryngoscopy during wakefulness usually detects normal adduction of the vocal cords in phonation, and partial or complete abduction restriction of the vocal cords during inspiration. In addition, peculiar twisting-like dystonic movements may also be observed in vocal cords with impaired abduction. Abduction restriction may be unilateral or bilateral. Subjects with complete unilateral vocal cord abduction restriction do not present severe dyspnea because the glottic space is relatively wide during inspiration. Subjects with complete bilateral abduction restriction usually have diurnal and nocturnal stridor. These subjects may not experience dyspnea because their vital capacity is so low and their activity is so limited that the narrowed airway is sufficient, although they are at a high risk of developing episodes of respiratory insufficiency. Normal movements of the vocal cords during wakefulness, however, may be seen in a few subjects with mild nocturnal stridor. In these subjects, laryngoscopy during diazepam-induced sleep discloses either paradoxical movements of the vocal cords or partial vocal cord abduction.[3] Vocal abductor restriction is exacerbated during sleep, and partial abduction limitation during wakefulness may become total during sleep. Isozaki et al[3] classified vocal cord abnormalities in MSA as follows: stage 1, normal movement during wakefulness and paradoxical movements during sleep; stage 2, abduction restriction during wakefulness and paradoxical movements during sleep; stage 3, almost midline position during both wakefulness and sleep.

Polysomnography with Video Recording Findings

In most subjects with stridor, VPSG reveals OSAH with associated oxyhemoglobin desaturations. Alternatively, a few subjects with stridor do not show OSAH, probably because the laryngeal narrowing during sleep is not severe enough to cause critical upper airway obstruction.[7] Conversely, in some subjects with partial vocal cord abduction dysfunction without stridor, the presence of OSAH at VPSG may suggest airway obstruction at the pharynx level.[5,6]

Pathophysiology of Laryngeal Obstruction

The origin of laryngeal obstruction in MSA is unclear, but it is thought to be related to the vocal cord abductors, or overactivation of the vocal cord adductors, or a combination of the two. MSA patients with stridor and vocal cord abductor restriction have neuronal loss of the nucleus ambiguus, axonal loss of the recurrent laryngeal nerve, and prominent or selective neurogenic atrophy of the posterior cricoarytenoid muscle.[3,8-10] On the other hand, other studies have reported preservation of the nucleus ambiguus, and abnormal tonic and phasic activity of the vocal cord adductors during inspiration,[11-13] suggesting that dystonia rather than paralysis might be the cause of stridor. The most likely mechanism of stridor in MSA is an unbalanced coactivation of the adductors and abductors of the larynx in response to increased upper airway resistance.[12]

Management of Upper Airway Obstruction in Multiple System Atrophy

Laryngeal Surgery

Several surgical techniques such as vocal cord lateralization, cordectomy, and arytenoidectomy have been proposed to increase glottic aperture. These surgical procedures are associated with an increased risk of aspiration and hoarseness, and experience is limited to a few cases.[14] MSA patients with autonomic failure are at increased risk during anesthesia as they may develop hypotension, respiratory depression, and acute laryngospasm.

Botulinum Toxin

Experience with botulinum toxin is limited to one study.[13] In two subjects with stridor, unilateral injection into the thyroarytenoid muscle resulted 1 month later in improvement of stridor, increased vocal cord mobility, and decreased tonic electromyographic activity. In a third patient there was no improvement. Botulinum toxin therapy may increase the risk of bronchial aspiration, and aggravate dysphonia and dysphagia, and it requires electromyographic guidance and repeated injections.

Tracheostomy

Tracheostomy is required as an emergency procedure in subjects with bilateral vocal cord abduction restriction presenting with an acute or subacute episode of respiratory failure. In the past, MSA patients with stridor were treated solely with elective tracheostomy.[5] Tracheostomy completely eliminates diurnal and nocturnal stridor because it bypasses the vocal cord obstruction and increases survival in MSA.[6] Tracheostomy is limited by local complications such as infection and tracheal stenosis, and is frequently not accepted by patients.

Continuous Positive Airway Pressure[7,15]

In MSA, continuous positive airway pressure (CPAP) is a long-term effective treatment for eliminating stridor and OSAH. The best CPAP compliance is achieved in patients at earlier stages of disease. Optimal CPAP pressures needed to abolish stridor and obstructive sleep apneas are similar to those used in subjects with typical sleep apnea syndrome (range, 5–11 cm H20). CPAP abolishes stridor because by opening the airway it eliminates the overactivity of the vocal cord adductors, thereby reducing the laryngeal resistance and increasing the glottic aperture.[12] However, in a few patients with immobile vocal cords fixed at midline, CPAP may sometimes not completely abolish stridor and apneas. Although untreated stridor is associated with short survival,[6] median survival is no different in subjects without stridor and in those with stridor treated only with CPAP.[7] Successful long-term CPAP therapy is associated with patients' subjective improvement in sleep quality and daytime alertness, although this improvement may not be reflected in polysomnography (PSG) studies,[15] probably because other problems that interfere with sleep, such as rigidity, urinary incontinence, and coexisting depression may still be present. Bed partners also have a more restorative sleep after the elimination of the patient's stridor. It is important to note, though, that some patients with SDB and stridor may refuse to be treated with CPAP, or any other therapy, because their sleep complaints are not felt as problematic or because of their advanced disease stage.

The available data allow the following practical recommendations to be made for the difficult management of SDB in patients with MSA: (1) Early diagnosis and treatment is advised to reduce morbidity and mortality. Treatment strategies need to be highly individualized. (2) At the earliest stages of disease and during routine visits, patients and their bed partners should be questioned about stridor, snoring, witnessed apneas, and excessive daytime somnolence. (3) If SDB is suspected, VPSG and laryngoscopy should be performed. Laryngoscopy, if possible, should be performed with the patient awake and asleep. (4) If SDB is detected, patients and their relatives should be informed about its importance, prognostic implications, and available therapeutic options. (5) CPAP therapy is recommended in patients at early and moderate stages with nocturnal stridor but no daytime stridor. Patients, family members, and caregivers must receive intensive education and support about CPAP use. CPAP compliance must be assessed and encouraged in routine follow-up visits. (6) In advanced MSA, with nocturnal but no daytime stridor, the decision to treat must be made after careful evaluation of the state of the patient. If treatment is recommended, CPAP should be considered first because it is noninvasive. If CPAP is not tolerated despite intensive support, tracheostomy should be then considered. (7) In patients with daytime stridor, elective tracheostomy should be advised because this condition leads to subacute episodes of dramatic respiratory failure.

◆ Autosomal Dominant Spinocerebellar Ataxias

Autosomal dominant spinocerebellar ataxias (ADSCAs) are inherited neurodegenerative disorders of the adult characterized by cerebellar syndrome, ophthalmoplegia, peripheral neuropathy, and parkinsonism. Vocal cord abductor restriction during inspiration has been described in ADSCA types 1 and 3 (Machado-Joseph disease) but it is less frequent than in MSA. Partial vocal cord abductor restriction is asymptomatic but complete bilateral vocal cord abduction restriction is associated with nocturnal stridor and subacute episodes of diurnal stridor and respiratory failure that may require tracheostomy. Vocal cord dysfunction in ADSCA types 1 and 3 is thought to result from neuropathy of the nucleus ambiguus, impairing the recurrent laryngeal nerve function.[9,16] Unlike MSA, in ADSCA there is neurogenic atrophy of all intrinsic laryngeal muscles.[17]

◆ Parkinson Disease

Parkinson disease (PD) is caused by neuronal loss in the substantia nigra and is characterized by tremor, bradykinesia, rigidity, postural instability, and responsiveness to dopaminergic agents. Voice disorders due to abnormal laryngeal muscle activity are also common. In advanced PD, laryngoscopy during wakefulness frequently shows vocal fold bowing and paradoxical movements of the vocal cords, leading to partial obstruction of the glottis.[18] It has been reported that advanced PD patients may occasionally exhibit episodes of acute dyspnea and inspiratory stridor during wakefulness requiring emergency tracheostomy. These episodes are thought to be related to overactivity of the laryngeal adductors and tensors occurring in patients with severe dysphagia. In these cases, stridor, unlike MSA, is not worsened during sleep, and laryngeal muscles show no abnormalities on autopsy.[10,17]

◆ Syringomyelia and Syringobulbia[19]

Syringomyelia (SM) is a central cavitation of the cervical spinal cord of undetermined origin that may extend into the medulla (syringobulbia [SB]). Some subjects with SM and SB may have cranial nerve IX and X impairment, OSAH, and sudden death during sleep. Others may exhibit bilateral vocal cord abductor paralysis and acute respiratory failure during wakefulness. PSG studies in most patients with SM and SB show central as well as obstructive sleep apnea despite the lack of respiratory or sleep symptoms. These abnormalities are associated with dysphagia and dysphonia and are attributable to damage by the syrinx of the nucleus ambiguus, the respiratory center in the medulla, and the phrenic neurons in the cervical spinal cord, in various combinations.

Sleep breathing disorders are rare in subjects with SM not involving the medulla, but bilateral vocal cord abductor paresis, stridor, and OSAH have been described in subjects with SM associated with Arnold-Chiari malformation.

♦ Amyotrophic Lateral Sclerosis

Amyotrophic lateral sclerosis (ALS) is characterized by progressive loss of the motor neurons in the cortex, medulla, and spinal cord. Death usually occurs less than 5 years after disease onset and is usually due to respiratory failure. In subjects with bulbar symptoms, laryngoscopy shows weakness of the vocal cords, adduction during phonation is incomplete causing dysphonia, and abduction during inspiration is impaired leading to glottic narrowing.[20] PSG studies may show OSAH due to obstruction of the upper airway in subjects with the bulbar form of ALS, with preserved diaphragm strength, but only a few require tracheostomy or other treatments because of SDB.[21] Pathologic studies show neurogenic atrophy of all intrinsic muscles of the larynx.[17] Central alveolar hypoventilation associated with nocturnal hypercapnia and oxygen desaturations is more frequent than OSAH, and is mainly related to the common occurrence in ALS of muscle weakness of the diaphragm and the accessory respiratory muscles.[21] In ALS, respiratory muscle strength has a prognostic value, and therapy with noninvasive positive pressure ventilation during sleep can prolong survival.

♦ Charcot-Marie-Tooth Disease[22,23]

Charcot-Marie-Tooth (CMT) disease is a progressive hereditary sensorimotor polyneuropathy. CSA and OSAH have been described in subjects with CMT types 1 and 2 having neither sleep nor respiratory complaints. The origin of OSAH in CMT is probably related to pharyngeal or laryngeal neuropathy, because some subjects have dysphagia or stridor secondary to vocal cord abductor paresis. Phrenic neuropathy leading to alveolar hypoventilation is associated with CSA.

♦ Laryngeal Obstructive Sleep Apnea/Hypopnea Syndrome

Primary

Most patients with obstructive sleep apnea/hypopnea syndrome (OSAHS) have increased collapsibility and anatomic abnormalities at the level of the pharynx. However, some subjects with OSAHS with normal pharyngeal function and anatomy exhibit paradoxical idiopathic glottic narrowing during inspiration[24] or inspiratory prolapse of an abnormal flaccid and long epiglottis toward the glottis,[25] both predisposing to obstruction of the larynx. In subjects with paradoxical glottic narrowing, CPAP may prevent apneas distending the upper airway at the level of the larynx. In subjects with epiglottic prolapse, epiglottidectomy may be beneficial, and CPAP is contraindicated because the epiglottis may be displaced downward increasing the upper airway obstruction. Although uncommon, the occurrence of sleep apnea as a result of laryngeal obstruction emphasizes the importance of a complete examination of the upper airway including the larynx in subjects evaluated for OSAHS.

Secondary

Secondary OSAHS is a rare condition that has been described in subjects with (1) iatrogenic bilateral vocal cord abductor paralysis after mediastinal surgery[26]; (2) laryngeal structural lesions reducing the glottic area, such as neoplasms, sarcoidosis, myxomas, granulomas, angiofibromas, lymphatic malformations, cysts, polyps, papillomas, or redundant supraglottic mucosa; (3) congenital abnormalities such as laryngomalacia causing supraglottic prolapse; and (4) after head and neck surgery and radiation. OSAHS due to vocal cord abductor paralysis after mediastinal surgery may be resolved with CPAP, arytenoidectomy, or tracheostomy. Laser partial epiglottidectomy is effective in laryngomalacia, particularly in children.

♦ Sleep-Related Laryngospasm[27]

Sleep-related laryngospasm is a rare condition occurring in middle-aged men with gastroesophageal reflux who awaken suddenly from sleep with severe chocking, tachycardia, and anxiety followed by stridor. Episodes last from a few seconds to a few minutes, resolve spontaneously, and occur one to 12 times per month. These episodes also occur during wakefulness. Laryngoscopy during wakefulness shows normal motility. Nocturnal polysomnography shows no evidence of significant upper airway obstruction. Acute spasms of the vocal cords have been identified in a few cases, and one episode has been documented to occur during stage 3 of NREM sleep. The episodes respond to antireflux treatment. Although the pathogenesis is still unknown, it has been speculated that they may result from laryngeal irritability and reflex central apnea secondary to aspiration of gastric content in the larynx.

References

1. Megirian D, Sherry JH. Respiratory functions of the laryngeal muscles during sleep. Sleep 1980;3:289–298
2. Orem J, Lovering AT, Dunin-Barkowski W, Vidruk EH. Tonic activity in the respiratory system in wakefulness, NREM and REM sleep. Sleep 2002;25:488–496
3. Isozaki E, Naito A, Horiguchi S, Kawamura R, Hayashida T, Tanabe H. Early diagnosis and stage classification of vocal cord abductor paralysis in patients with multiple system atrophy. J Neurol Neurosurg Psychiatry 1996;60:399–402
4. Quinn N. Multiple system atrophy-the nature of the beast. J Neurol Neurosurg Psychiatry 1989;52(Suppl):78–89
5. Silber MH. Sleep dysfunction in Parkinson's plus syndrome. In: Chokroverty S, Hening WA, Walters AS, eds. Sleep and Movement Disorders. Philadelphia: Butterworth Heinemann; 2003:489–494
6. Silber MH, Levine S. Stridor and death in multiple system atrophy. Mov Disord 2000;15:699–704
7. Iranzo A, Santamaría J, Tolosa E, et al. Long-term effect of CPAP in the treatment of nocturnal stridor in multiple system atrophy. Neurology 2004;63:930–932
8. Ikeda K, Iwasaki Y, Kuwajima A, et al. Preservation of branchimotor neurons of the nucleus ambiguus in multiple system atrophy (reply letter). Neurology 2003;61:722–723
9. Isozaki E, Naito R, Kanda T, Mizutani T, Hirai S. Different mechanism of vocal cord paralysis between spinocerebellar ataxia (SCA 1 and 3) and multiple system atrophy. J Neurol Sci 2002;197:37–43
10. Isozaki E, Shimizu T, Takamoto K, et al. Vocal abductor paralysis (VCAP) in Parkinson's disease: difference from VCAP in multiple system atrophy. J Neurol Sci 1995;130:197–202
11. Benarroch EE, Schmeichel AM, Parisi JE. Preservation of branchimotor neurons of the nucleus ambiguus in multiple system atrophy. Neurology 2003;60:115–117
12. Isono S, Shiba K, Yamaguchi M, et al. Pathogenesis of laryngeal narrowing in patients with multiple system atrophy. J Physiol 2001;536:237–249
13. Merlo IM, Occhini A, Pacchetti C, Alfonsini E. Not paralysis, but dystonia causes stridor in multiple system atrophy. Neurology 2002;58:649–652
14. Kenyon GS, Apps MCP, Traub M. Stridor and obstructive sleep apnea in Shy-Drager syndrome treated by laringofissure and cord lateralization. Laryngoscope 1984;94:1106–1108
15. Iranzo A, Santamaría J, Tolosa E. Continuous positive airway pressure eliminates nocturnal stridor in multiple system atrophy. Lancet 2000;356:1329–1330
16. Iranzo A, Muñoz E, Santamaría J, Vilaseca I, Milà M, Tolosa E. REM sleep behavior disorder and vocal cord paralysis in Machado-Joseph disease. Mov Disord 2003;18:1179–1183
17. Isozaki E, Hayashi M, Hayashida T, Osa M, Hirai S. Myopathology of the intrinsic laryngeal muscles, with reference to the mechanism of vocal cord paralysis. Rinsho Shinkeigaku 1998;38:711–718
18. Vincken WG, Gauthier SG, Dollfuss RE, Hanson RE, Darauay CM, Cosio MG. Involvement of upper-airway muscles in extrapyramidal disorders. N Engl J Med 1984;311:438–442
19. Nogués M, Gené R, Benarroch E, et al. Respiratory disturbances during sleep in syringomyelia and syringobulbia. Neurology 1999;52:1777–1783
20. Hillel A, Dray T, Miller R, et al. Presentation of ALS to the otolaryngologist/head and neck surgeon: getting to the neurologist. Neurology 1999;53(8, Suppl 5)S22–S25
21. Lyall RA, Donaldson N, Polkey MI, Moxham J. Respiratory muscle strength and ventilatory failure in amyotrophic lateral sclerosis. Brain 2001;124:2000–2013
22. Dyck PJ, Litchy WJ, Minnerath S, et al. Hereditary motor and sensory neuropathy with diaphragm and vocal cord paresis. Ann Neurol 1994;35:608–615
23. Dematteis M, Pepin JL, Jeanmart M, Deschaux C, Labarre A, Levy P. Charcot-Marie-Tooth disease and sleep apnea syndrome: a family study. Lancet 2001;357:267–272
24. Rubinstein I, Slutsky AS, Zamel N, Hoffstein V. Paradoxical glottic narrowing in patients with severe obstructive sleep apnea. J Clin Invest 1988;81:1051–1055
25. Catalfumo FJ, Golz A, Westerman ST, Gilbert LM, Joachims HZ, Goldenberg D. The epiglottis and obstructive sleep apnoea syndrome. J Laryngol Otol 1998;112:940–943
26. Li HY, Wang PC, Hsu CY, Chen NH, Fang TJ. Changes of sleep disordered breathing after laryngeal surgery in patients with bilateral vocal fold paralysis. Eur Arch Otorhinolaryngol Head 2004 (published on line)
27. Thurnheer R, Henz S, Knoblauch A. Sleep-related laryngospasm. Eur Respir J 1997;10:2084–2086

Chapter 9

Acoustic Assessment of Vocal Function

Eugene H. Buder and Michael P. Cannito

Acoustic voice analysis was first applied to neurologic disease early in the previous century.[1] Over the last few decades into the new millennium, however, the proliferation of microcomputer-based technology has led to widespread applications of acoustical analysis methods to neurologically disordered voices. As represented below, the majority of these studies have employed measures of vocal fundamental frequency (the primary physical basis for perceived pitch), sound pressure (the primary basis for perceived loudness), and measures of cycle-to-cycle perturbations in frequency and amplitude in efforts to diagnose and assess neurologic voice disorders, and to track treatment efficacy. A smaller number of reports have also used similar measures to search for early identification of the disorders and to track disease progression. These types of acoustic research are contributing significantly toward the current development of evidence-based practice. In addition, acoustics methods contribute to intervention in the form of biofeedback signals that are used as integral components of treatment delivery.

It nonetheless seems that vocal acoustic analysis techniques, as nonintrusive yet highly sensitive signs of neurologic status, are on the verge of far greater ranges of utility and acceptance. The tools for such techniques are relatively inexpensive, requiring minimally only a microphone, microcomputer, and software (some of which is even free). Several other factors may still limit the range of applications: (1) Training and expertise in the appropriate and valid processing of acoustic measures remain limited, even among speech-language pathologists, and reasoning from acoustic measure to neurophysiology is indeed fraught with many complicated inferential possibilities. (2) Too often it is assumed that acoustic measures are only confirmatory of the diagnostician's perceptions; hence, they are considered secondary or even redundant, even though acoustic analysis can offer far greater potential for discovering and quantifying phenomena that may be difficult to perceive, that are preclinical, or that are even subliminal. (3) Analysis algorithms have traditionally relied on the automatic detection of fundamental frequency as the "normative" basis from which deviations are assessed, but such detection is highly problematic in abnormal voices. (4) Most current acoustic techniques fail to target vocal phenomena that can be clearly associated with neurophysiologic status. (5) Most such techniques are applicable to samples, such as sustained vowel phonation, that may or may not represent the in situ impairments as they affect spontaneous connected speech. This chapter does not attempt to address all of these limitations, but rather introduces the neurologist, otolaryngologist, or speech-language pathologist to some resources, techniques, and ideas that should lead to improved understanding of laryngeal status via acoustic analysis.

♦ Considerations When Evaluating Acoustic Measures of Voice

Any measurement strategy is only as good as the user's theoretical understanding of the object of measurement. This basic epistemologic problem is compounded manyfold in the use of acoustic measures of voice to infer neurologic status because a long chain of inference is required. For example, in the computerized analysis of the class of cycle-to-cycle period perturbations classified under the rubric of "jitter," before direct contemplation of neurologic status, the analyst should consider (1) the nature of the algorithm used to calculate jitter, (2) any limitations imposed by the digital representation of the signal, (3) the quality of the recording equipment and environment, (4) the task performed and its elicitation, (5) the acoustic effects of vocal tract resonances that will have transformed the original laryngeal output, (6) the aerodynamic principles by which glottal flow yields an acoustic product, (7) the interaction of vocal fold movement with aerodynamic forces, (8) nonmuscular tissue characteristics of the vocal folds, and (9) the variety and complex interactions among muscle activations affecting vocal fold configuration. Each of these considerations is vital to a thorough application of acoustic analysis; although this chapter cannot provide detailed information on each of these aspects, the reader can consult a wealth of resources for expanded information.[2-14] The following section provides some practical advice on acquisition and analysis of acoustic voice signals, with special attention to considerations such as those listed above.

♦ Acquisition Strategies

Figure 9.1 depicts some elements of a desirable recording configuration for acoustic voice evaluation, with an emphasis on requirements for meaningful representation of the sound pressure level (SPL) of vocal output. This acoustic parameter is especially important in neurologic disorders because (1) it can be of central importance in relation to many other performance variables in an assessment protocol,[15,16] and (2) other acoustic parameters may systematically vary in association with SPL.[17–19] As detailed in the following discussion, the figure represents a relatively simple and inexpensive protocol that approximates more elaborate procedures described elsewhere.[20]

For samples to be readily compared, it is important that the microphone be maintained at a consistent distance from the speaker's mouth, but far enough away from oral and nasal airstreams so as not to be perturbed by aerodynamic effects. Head-worn microphones are especially ideal for these reasons, but they should be of high quality with a broad and flat frequency response.[21] The inverse square law, which describes an exponential relation between distance from source and detected SPL, predicts an especially exquisite sensitivity at close distances to variations in microphone-to-mouth distances. Other factors, such as gain levels on recording devices, inevitably vary from session to session and patient to patient, and it is advisable to optimize gain settings during each recording to accommodate louder or softer voices. It is therefore impossible, but also undesirable, to maintain consistent settings for all the factors that affect the actual amplitude of a recorded signal, necessitating the use of a recorded signal of known intensity against which to calibrate the recorded signals.

Figure 9.1 depicts the use of a calibration tone-generator with an output speaker that is ideally positioned in close proximity to the patient's mouth. Just prior to the patient's vocal productions, the elicitor should take a reading of this calibration tone from an SPL meter, again taking care to position this meter at a fixed and consistent distance from the output speaker for all samples to be compared (i.e., across sessions and/or patients). Community standards have come to consider relatively inexpensive SPL meters to be acceptable for clinical purposes. The waveforms and accompanying text labels in **Fig. 9.1** indicate how the three resources produced by this protocol are assembled to allow the actual recorded tasks (which, in their raw computer-stored form, will be on a linear volts scale) to be placed on a standard decibel (dB) SPL metric: (1) the integrated (root-mean-square [RMS]) voltage of the calibration tone is measured from its recording, (2) the RMS quantities of interest are measured from the recorded voice samples and placed on a dB SPL scale relative to the calibration tone ($20 \times \log(\mathrm{RMS}_{voice}/\mathrm{RMS}_{cal})$), and (3) the dB value observed on the SPL meter during the calibration tone presentation is added to the dB value or values produced in step 2.

A completely different source of variation that may interfere with valid comparisons between sessions comes from patients and their varying construals or performances of the desired task. Indeed, general issues of task selection and performance merit far more consideration than can be included in this chapter, affecting not just the value and

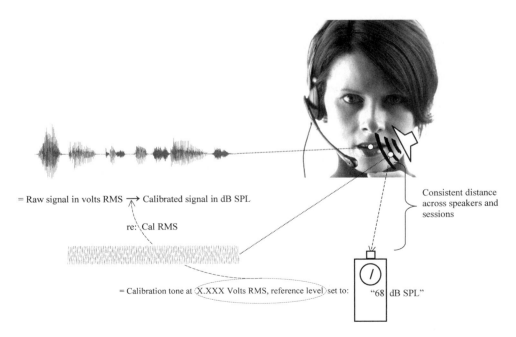

Fig. 9.1 Basic elements required to quantify sound pressure levels (see text for detailed description).

meaning of acoustic parameters but the general interpretive goals of phonatory assessments. These issues are all too often overlooked and should invoke careful consideration by otolaryngologists and speech-language pathologists. The most important consideration in general acoustic terms is the fact that most acoustic measures will co-vary to some degree with the basic parameters of f_0 and SPL. The voice range profile (or "phonetogram"), by which the client's abilities to vary intensity across the entire range of physiologically available fundamental frequencies can be mapped, can be a very useful procedure,[22] but for many purposes it is simply impractical. The procedure is very time-consuming and potentially too fatiguing and laborious for the patients, especially if they suffer from neurologic deficits. The different f_0/SPL combinations produced by a given individual do in fact yield varying and potentially informative acoustic qualities,[18,23] but the amount of measurement and resulting data may also be too laborious for the analyst (not to mention the patient), and overwhelming for the interpreter.

Figure 9.2 outlines a procedure that can be followed as an abbreviated voice range profile to assay basic effects of f_0 and SPL changes on vocal qualities such as jitter, shimmer, and tremors. It is especially simple in conjunction with a real-time pitch and energy program (such as KayPENTAX's [Lincoln, NJ] Real-Time Pitch™ software[24]), as the protocol begins with a quick sampling of the patient's preferred pitch and loudness settings (as obtained from repetitions of a brief sentence, for example). The real-time visual program can then be used to help the patient produce samples that deviate systematically from this central setting. The values depicted in **Fig. 9.2** (one octave up, 10 dB up, three semitones down, and a "soft but high pitch") are reasonable targets for speakers with unimpaired laryngeal control (so failure to achieve them may itself be diagnostic), and the tasks therefore allow a quick assessment of both the control limitations experienced by an impaired individual and the variations in quality that these tasks generally elicit. Although these tasks may also be accompanied by other standard tasks, such as a self-selected maximum sustained vowel production, the protocol should suppress the tendencies for such vowel productions to deviate from habitual spoken levels, to be "sung," or to vary excessively across sessions and patients. The target of high f_0/low SPL is especially valuable as a representation of vocal fold vibratory status at phonation threshold in a loft register. Productions under such "borderline" conditions can reveal laryngeal control difficulties that may not occur at the patient's self-selected levels.

◆ Analysis Strategies

Among the most widely used tools for acoustic voice analysis is the KayPENTAX Multi-Dimensional Voice Program™.[25] Numerous normative and pathologic databases have been collected using this program and collated along with application notes relevant to neurologic disorders of the larynx.[26] Along with the program manual itself and related statements issued by the National Center for Voice and Speech (NCVS),[12] users of this program now have many resources for optimal application of the instrument. Nonetheless, other practical experiences in our laboratories and elsewhere are not consistently reflected in those resources, and so we provide a list of pointers: (1) To implement NCVS standards, one must select the "MDVP Advanced" version of the program that is automatically installed along with the standard version. (2) Clarity in task instructions is critical, especially in neurologic assessments; for example, it seems difficult even for unaffected individuals to produce steady vocal amplitude (to the normative threshold implemented in the program) unless specifically concentrating on this aspect of vocal performance. (3) It should be noted that default normative samples built in to the program database were collected with an (unspecified) target SPL level that is audibly high, often causing an apparently abnormal "soft phonation index" report when patients self-select low-amplitude phonation (and probably also lowering the normative amplitude modulation criterion[13]). (4) Following NCVS standards, the analyst should obtain and average multiple samples (at least five), continuously filling the 3-second waveform panel whenever physiologically possible, and scrutinizing each sample to exclude those with variations

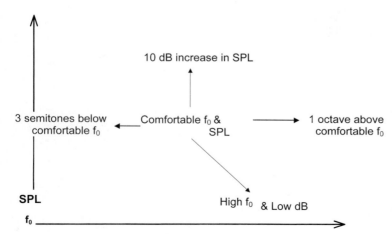

Fig. 9.2 A scheme for sampling the voice range anchored to a given patient's self-selected comfortable f0 and sound pressure level (SPL).

that can be ascribed to anomalous or nonrepresentative productions. (5) The default compact "radial" display, albeit alluring, produces distracting visual elements, obscuring logical groupings of parameters and also the visual salience of values that are significantly lower than, rather than higher than, accepted norms, and also bypassing the explicit step of selecting appropriate gender norms. Analysts are therefore strongly advised to select the "normative bars" graphic display type under the "Options, MDVP" menu. (6) It is critical to inspect the "View B" display of f_0 and peak-to-peak amplitude analysis and verify optimal analysis. Under some circumstances a repeat analysis implementing optional upper and lower pitch analysis range limits is required to avoid erroneous f_0 determinations. (7) Community standards seem unclear regarding whether the cycle-to-cycle pitch and amplitude variations, generally known respectively as jitter and shimmer, should incorporate the deterministic cycle-to-cycle variations caused by subharmonics or focus exclusively on the random variations that are probably more clearly associated with neurologic sources,[27–29] but it is clear that inclusion of subharmonics generally overwhelms typically lower-level random variations in the final jitter and shimmer metrics.[30] Although laborious, it may therefore be advisable to excise visible episodes of subharmonic vibratory patterns from waveforms in order to obtain more focused jitter and shimmer samples. (8) Not all MDVP parameters are uniquely informative. The normative bars display (see point 5, above) are arranged in logical groupings. As supported by factor analyses of MDVP output,[31] analysts should observe these groupings and recognize that many items within the groups vary primarily only in technical aspects of the underlying algorithm and that they may not therefore target distinct aspects of laryngeal function. For example, general standards (as discussed in the program documentation itself) favor relative average perturbation (RAP) among the various jitter metrics and amplitude perturbation quotient (APQ) among the various shimmer metrics provided by the program. (9) Of special interest in many neurologic disorders, the frequencies and modulation depths of both f_0 and SPL tremors may be presented in MDVP output (if they exceed detection thresholds), but analysts may not always avail themselves of the program controls (specifically in "View D" displaying "f_0 and Amplitude Modulation Components") that can be used to override automatic selections in favor of the modulation frequencies of greatest interest. For example, the dominant modulation frequencies seen in untreated essential tremor may not always be the dominant frequencies posttreatment, though it may nonetheless be of greatest clinical value to focus on identical frequencies when sampling across such sessions.[32]

♦ Literature Review

Acoustical studies of neurologically disordered voices may be divided into three major categories: (1) assessment and diagnosis, (2) onset and long-term course, and (3) treatment outcome. Selected studies representing these categories are provided in **Tables 9.1** to **9.3**, in which they are characterized

Table 9.1 Studies of Assessment and Differential Diagnosis of Neurologically Disordered Voices

Reference	Measure	Disorder
Rahn, Chou, Jiang, Zhang (2007)[53]	jitter, shimmer, NLD	PD
Zhang, Jiang, Biazzo, Jorgenson (2005)[54]	jitter, shimmer, NLD	VFP
Feijó, Parente, Behlau, Haussen, De Veccino, Martignago (2004)[55]	spectrography, f_0 var, shimmer, jitter	MS
Lundy, Roy, Xue, Casiano, Jassir (2004)[56]	f_0 mean/var, f_0/SPL modulations	ALS, SD, ET
Dromey (2003)[57]	f_0 mean/var, SPL, jitter, shimmer, HNR, LTAS	Hypokinet. Dys.
Kelchner, Lee, Stemple (2003)[58]	f_0 mean, SPL, NHR	VFP
Heman-Ackah, Michael, Goding (2002)[59]	jitter, shimmer, NHR, CPP	Dysphonia
Hanson, Stevens, Kuo, Chen, Slifka (2001)[7]	harmonic amplitudes	Spasticity, Ataxic, Athet. Dys.
Morsomme, Jamart, Wéry, Giovanni, Remacle (2001)[60]	f_0/SPL mean/var, shimmer, and jitter	VFP
Jiang, Lin, Hanson (2000)[61]	SPL modulations	PD, Cerebell., UMND, ET
Kent, Kent, Duffy, Thomas, Wiesmer, Stuntebeck (2000)[62]	f_0 mean/var, SPL var, jitter, shimmer	Atax. Dys.
Murry, Sapienza, Walton (2000)[63]	dynamics	SD, MTD
Sherrard, Marquardt, Cannito (2000)[64]	jitter, shimmer, HNR, f_0 var, breaks	SD, PBD
Kent, Vorperian, Duffy (1999)[65]	MDVP	CVA, PD, etc.
Sapienza, Walton, Murry (1999)[66]	dynamics	SD
Robert, Pouget, Giovanni, Azulay, Triglia (1999)[67]	f_0 mean/var, SPL, jitter, shimmer	ALS
Eckley, Sataloff, Hawkshaw, Speigel, Mandel (1998)[68]	f_0 var	VFP
Le Dorze, Ryalls, Brassard, Boulanger, Ratte (1998)[69]	f_0 mean/var	PD, Friedreich's
Gamboa, Jiménez-Jiménez, Nieto, et al (1998)[70]	f_0 mean/var, jitter, shimmer, HNR	ET
Gamboa, Jiménez-Jiménez, Nieto, et al (1997)[71]	f_0 mean/var, jitter, shimmer, HNR	PD

(Continued on page 78)

Table 9.1 *(Continued)* Studies of Assessment and Differential Diagnosis of Neurologically Disordered Voices

Reference	Measure	Disorder
Hertrich, Lutzenberger, Spieker, Ackermann (1997)[72]	fractal dimension	PD, cerebell.
Walker (1997)[73]	f_0 var	MG
Doyle, Raade, St. Pierre, Desai (1995)[74]	f_0 mean/var	Hypokinet. Dys.
Hertrich, Ackermann (1995)[75]	f_0 mean, jitter, shimmer, HNR	PD, HD
Murry, Brown, Morris (1995)[76]	f_0 mean/var	VFP
Ackermann, Ziegler (1994)[77]	f_0 mean/var, jitter	Atax. dys., dysphonia
Strand, Buder, Yorkston, Ramig (1994)[78]	f_0 mean/var, jitter, shimmer, SNR	ALS
Hertrich, Ackermann (1994)[79]	f_0/SPL var	Friedreich's
Zwirner, Murry, Woodson (1993)[80]	f_0 mean/var, jitter, shimmer, SNR	SD
Aronson, Ramig, Winholtz, Silber (1992)[81]	f_0/SPL modulations	ALS
Zwirner, Murry, Woodson (1991)[82]	f_0 mean/var, jitter, shimmer, SNR	PD, HD, Cerebell.
Rosenfield, Viswanath, Herbrich, Nudelman (1991)[83]	f_0 var	ALS
Klingholz (1990)[18]	f_0/SPL/SNR covariations	VFP
Klingholz and Martin (1989)[19]	SPL var	VFP
Philippbar, Robin, Luschei (1989)[84]	f_0 modulations	PD
Fukazawa, Blaugrund, El-Assuooty, Gould (1988)[85]	spectral analysis	VFP
Hartman, Abbs, Vishwanat (1988)[86]	shimmer, amplitude modulations	SD
Ramig, Shipp (1987)[87]	f_0/SPL modulations, jitter, shimmer	PD, ALS, SD
Ludlow, Connor (1987)[88]	f_0/SPL mean/var	SD
Hirano, Hibi, Terasawa, and Fujiu (1986)[89]	f_0/SPL mean/var, SNR, harmonic amplitudes	VFP
Kasuya, Ogawa, Mashima, Ebihara (1986)[90]	spectral noise	VFP
Hartmann, von Cramon (1984)[91]	f_0, jitter, shimmer, spectral analysis, dynamics	TBI
Ludlow, Bassich (1983)[92]	f_0/SPL mean/var, jitter	PD, Shy-Drager
Rontal, Rontal, Leuchter, Rolnick (1978)[93]	descriptive spectrography	MG
Iwata (1972)[94]	waveform analysis	VFP
Koike (1968)[95]	waveform perturbations	VFP
Brown, Simonson (1963)[33]	SPL modulations	ET

Key for measure abbreviations appearing in Tables 9.1 to 9.3: breaks, occurrences of voice cessation; covariations, a map of two parameters (e.g., voice range profile); CPP, cepstral peak prominence; dynamics, measures associated with abrupt glottal changes; f_0, fundamental frequency; f_0 breaks, occurrences of sudden unintended changes in f_0; f_0 mean, overall central tendency in fundamental frequency; f_0 var, overall variability in fundamental frequency; HNR, harmonics-to-noise ratio; jitter, cycle-to-cycle variability in glottal wave frequency; LTAS, long-term average spectrum; MDVP, measures from the Multi-Dimensional Voice Program[25]; modulation, longer-term variation, such as a tremor; NHR, noise-to harmonics ratio; NLD, nonlinear dynamic measures; SH, subharmonics; shimmer, cycle-to-cycle variability in glottal wave amplitude; SNR, signal-to-noise ratio; SPL, sound pressure level; SPL mean, overall central tendency in sound pressure level; SPL var, overall variability in sound pressure level.

Key for disorders abbreviations appearing in Tables 9.1 to 9.3: ALS, amyotrophic lateral sclerosis; Atax. Dys., ataxic dysarthria; Athet. Dys., athetoid dysarthria; Cerebell, cerebellar disease; CVA, cerebrovascular accident; ET, essential tremor; Friedreich's, Friedreich's ataxia; HD, Huntington's disease; Hypokinet. Dys., hypokinetic dysarthria; MG, myasthenia gravis; MS multiple sclerosis; MTD, muscle tension dysphonia; PD, Parkinson disease; PBD, pseudobulbar dysarthria; SD, spasmodic dysphonia; Spast. Dys., spastic dysarthria; TBI, traumatic brain injury; UMND, upper motor neuron disease; VFP, vocal fold paralysis.

Note: Entries in these tables are selected to represent measures and disorders broadly, and not as an exclusive survey.

in terms of both acoustic measures employed and the neurodiagnostic samples represented. Studies of assessment and diagnosis **(Table 9.1)** are most numerous. They focus mainly on characterizing the acoustic voice characteristics of specific neurologic disorders such as Parkinson disease or cerebellar ataxia. Some also quantify the severity of phonatory dysfunction within a specific disorder. A few studies have attempted to diagnostically differentiate between neurodiagnostic subgroups or to differentiate neurodiagnostic subgroups from other nonneurologic etiologies, based on acoustic voice parameters, with varying degrees of success.

Studies of onset and course of pathology **(Table 9.2)** are the least numerous and represent an area in need of greater research endeavor. Existing studies focus on early identification of vocal markers of neuropathology, as well as longitudinal studies of vocal deterioration in degenerative disorders. These have thus far included Parkinson disease, Huntington disease, multiple sclerosis (MS), amyotrophic lateral sclerosis (ALS), and laryngeal dystonia (spasmodic dysphonia). Early identification appears to be a highly promising area for future investigation involving acoustic measures.

Studies evaluating the effects of treatment **(Table 9.3)** are the second most common category. These studies have examined a broad spectrum of behavioral and medical interventions in a variety of neurologic disorders including Parkinson disease, cerebellar ataxia, laryngeal dystonia (spasmodic dysphonia), essential tremor, and vocal fold

9 Acoustic Assessment of Vocal Function

Table 9.2 Studies of Onset and Course of Neurologic Voice Disorders

Reference	Measure	Disorder
Early Identification		
Harel, Cannizzaro, Snyder (2004)[96]	f_0 var	PD
Silbergleit, Johnson, Jacobson (1997)[97]	f_0 var, jitter, shimmer, SNR	ALS
Hartelius, Buder, Strand (1997)[36]	f_0/SPL modulations	MS
Ramig, Scherer, Titze, Ringel (1988)[98]	f_0 mean/var jitter, shimmer, HNR, tremor	HD, PD, ALS
Wolfe, Ratusnik, Feldman (1979)[99]	descriptive spectrography	SD
Disease Progression/Deterioration		
Leeper, Millard, Bandur, Hudson (1996)[100]	f_0 mean/var, SPL var, jitter, shimmer, SNR	ALS
Kent, Sufit, Rosenbek, et al (1991)[101]	f_0, jitter, shimmer, SNR	ALS
Ramig, Scherer, Klasner, Titze, Horii (1990)[102]	f_0 mean/SD, shimmer, jitter, HNR	ALS
Ramig (1986)[103]	f_0, SH, breaks dynamics	HD

paralysis, to name a few. Interventions have included voice therapy (e.g., Lee Silverman Voice Treatment [LSVT]), pharmacologic therapy, botulinum toxin injection of the vocal folds, vocal fold medialization surgery, subthalamic nucleus stimulation, and pallidotomy.

Reviewing these tables, one is struck by the wide range of neurologic disorders to which acoustic analysis has been applied; however, it is also clear that measurements based on automated f_0 extraction (e.g., mean f_0, jitter, shimmer, harmonics-to-noise ratio [HNR]) have dominated these assessments. Given the extreme aperiodicity of many neurologically disordered voices, more widespread application of measures that are specifically not derived from automated extraction of the fundamental period should be applied to the broader spectrum of neurologic disorders. Such measures include spectral amplitude measures (e.g., long-term average

Table 9.3 Studies of Treatment Outcome for Neurologically Disordered Voices

Reference	Measure	Disorder
Goberman, Blomgren (2008)[104]	f_0 dynamics	PD
Sewall, Jiang, Ford (2006)[105]	SPL, f_0 range	PD
Cannito, Buder, Chorna (2005)[106]	f_0, SPL, LTAS, harmonic amplitudes	SD
Adler, Bansberg, Hentz, et al (2004)[32]	f_0 mean/var, f_0/SPL modulations	ET
Sapir, Spielman, Ramig, et al (2003)[107]	SPL, f_0 mean/var	Atax. Dys.
Wang, Metman, Bakay, Arzbaecher, Bernard (2003)[108]	SPL, f_0 mean, jitter	PD
Kersing, Dejonckere, van der Aa, Buschman (2002)[109]	MDVP, dynamics	Epilepsy (vagus stimulation)
Sapienza, Cannito, Murry, Branski, Woodson (2002)[110]	dynamic measures	SD
Goberman, Coelho (2002)[111]	f_0 mean/var, SPL range	PD
McHenry, Whatman, Pou (2002)[112]	f_0, jitter, shimmer, NHR	Spast. Dys.
Shin, Nam, Yoo, Kim (2002)[113]	f_0, jitter, shimmer, NHR	VFP
Langeveld, van Rossum, Houtman, Zwinderman, Briaire, Baatenburg de Jong (2001)[114]	f_0/SPL mean/var, aperiodicity, dynamics	SD
Mehta, Goldman, Orloff (2001)[115]	f_0 mean/var, jitter, shimmer, SNR	SD
Sapir, Pawlas, Ramig, Seely, Fox, Corboy (2001)[116]	SPL	MS
Dromey, Kumar, Lang, Lozano (2000)[117]	f_0 mean/var, SPL, tremor	PD
Hartl, Hans, Vaissiere, Riquet, Brasnu (2000)[118]	MDVP, CPP, harmonic amplitudes, LTAS	VFP
Schulz, Greer, Friedman (2000)[119]	SPL	PD
Jiang, Lin, Wang, Hanson (1999)[120]	jitter, shimmer, amplitude tremor	PD
Schulz, Peterson, Sapienza, Greer, Friedman (1999)[121]	f_0, SPL	PD
Lu, Casiano, Lundy, Xue (1996)[122]	f_0, jitter, shimmer, HNR	VFP
Bielamowicz, Berke, Gerratt (1995)[123]	jitter, shimmer, HNR	VFP
Bouglé, Ryalls, Le Dorze (1995)[124]	f_0 var	TBI
Adams, Hunt, Charles, Lang (1993)[125]	f_0, jitter, shimmer, breaks	SD
Truong, Rontal, Rolnick, Aronson, Mistura (1991)[126]	f_0, jitter, shimmer, breaks	SD
Zwirner, Murry, Swenson, Woodson (1991)[127]	f_0 SD, jitter, shimmer, SNR, breaks	SD

80 II Clinical Evaluation

spectrum (LTAS) and harmonic amplitudes) as well as direct waveform inspection for dynamic voice features, nonlinear dynamic methods, and extraction of low-frequency modulations of f_0 and SPL, (e.g., tremor, wow, flutter, as detailed further in the following section). Direct measurement of voice intensity (SPL), especially in response to treatment, has been mainly applied to Parkinson disease, but also promises to be of value in determining treatment outcomes in other populations.

♦ Modulation Analysis

Vocal tremor had been one of the earliest neurologic signs to be manifest through the larynx and quantified acoustically,[33,34] and subtle aspects of the disorder are still being revealed through inspection of f_0 and SPL modulations.[32] Recent developments in the visual display and quantification of these modulations suggest that the traditional concept of tremor should be considered in relation to faster modulations such as flutter and slower modulations termed wow.[35] Increased attention to such phenomena may ameliorate the paucity of studies and diagnostic tools applicable to subclinical signs accompanying the early onset of neurologic impairments of laryngeal function,[36] and aid in differential diagnoses or subclassifications in heterogeneous disorders such as multiple sclerosis, which may or may not affect cerebellar systems of laryngeal control.[37]

Figure 9.3 illustrates the prospects of modulation analysis for the observation of subtle signs accompanying the progressive course of ALS. As part of a longitudinal study,[38] sustained vowel phonations were elicited from a 65-year-old woman with ALS 3 months after onset of bulbar symptoms and then again 4 months later. The displays are called "modulograms,"[35] and there are two modulograms displayed in the figure: the first sample (**Fig. 9.3A**), and the second sample (**Fig. 9.3B**). Each modulogram depicts a set of SPL modulations (based on a dB trace) and a set of f_0 modulations. For each set, the trace is displayed below three panels; each panel is effectively a low-frequency spectrogram that, instead of depicting time-varying intensities of acoustic frequencies,

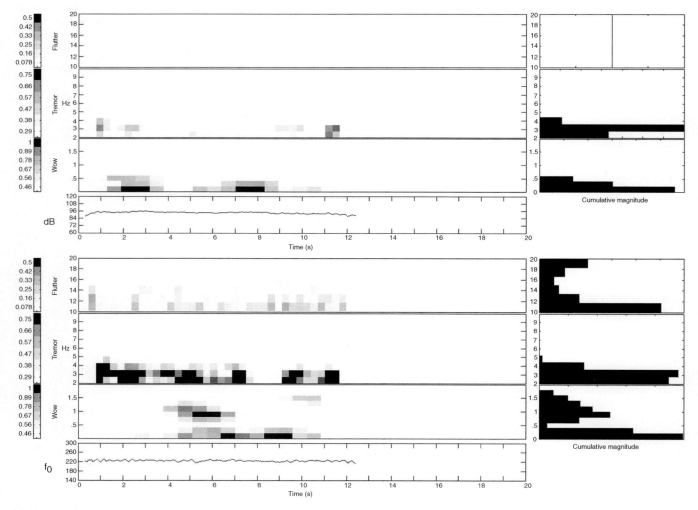

Fig. 9.3 (A, B) Modulograms of two sustained phonations by a woman with amyotrophic lateral sclerosis (ALS), illustrating disease progression (see text for detailed description).

depicts time-varying depths of SPL or f_0 modulations. In each set of three such panels, the lowest panel displays "wow" modulations (from 0.1 to 2.0 Hz), the middle panel displays "tremor" modulations (from 2.0 to 10 Hz), and the uppermost panel displays "flutter" modulations (from 10 to 20 Hz). Histograms along the right panel edges depict time-cumulated observations of modulation; further explanations of the graphic and numerical elements of this display protocol can be found in the source reference. The main observations this figure should support are as follows: the patient clearly has a low-frequency tremor of fundamental frequency in the first sample. Four months later, as seen in the modulogram of **Fig. 9.3B**, this tremor is somewhat exacerbated. Of greatest interest, however, are the degrees of f_0 wow and flutter that have appeared, even while her SPL trace remains relatively stable. This technique therefore illustrates that the course of this woman's phonatory deterioration is more complicated than a simple increase of vocal instability, but rather entails the appearance of new types of instability that are likely to have distinct neurologic sources.

♦ Conclusion

In addition to those measures mentioned here, there are other more basic neuro-diagnostic vocal tasks that can be recorded and assessed most accurately using simple acoustic tools, including maximum phonation time,[39] s/z ratios,[40] and laryngeal diadochokinesis (attempts to rapidly and regularly repeat quick vowel or /ha/ productions, therefore taxing laryngeal adductor and abductor motions).[41] Such measures are facilitated by the use of protocol-driven software tools such as the KayPENTAX Motor Speech Profile™ system.[42] Indeed, diagnostic batteries including sets of laryngeal tasks and measures, along with related assessments such as aerodynamics, are clearly important[43–46] but perhaps underrepresented in the literature as reviewed here, and in need of further testing and standardization. Such efforts would ideally proceed in research programs that incorporate multiple disorders.[47]

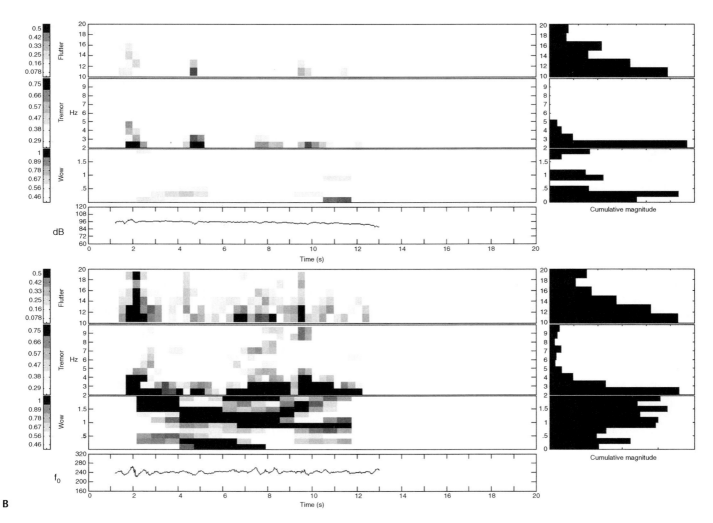

Fig. 9.3 (Continued)

In reviewing the literature tabulated here, it is clear again that the default acoustic assessment of vocal pathology involves the basic set of parameters of f_0, SPL, jitter, and shimmer. The validity of this set is mitigated, however, by problems that are well documented in the literature regarding adequate detection of periodicity-based measures (f_0, jitter, and shimmer),[3,12] some inattention to technical difficulties reviewed here with the use of SPL to compare across patients and sessions, and a growing understanding of the nondeterministic behaviors of vocal fold motion that cause difficulties with inferring neurologic status from vibratory patterns.[13,14] Problems with traditional periodicity-based measures may be alleviated as acoustic analysis tools based on nonlinear dynamic measures continue to be developed and documented in the literature on neurologic dysphonias.[48] Finally, it is clear that methodological difficulties associated with the application of acoustic measures to running conversational speech need to be overcome. Clinical assessments and functional outcomes could then be based on the full dynamics of speech-related vocal behaviors as presented in such materials. Recent studies in this area indicate that a return to basics, such as the essential role of fundamental voice frequency, will be fruitful.[49-52]

References

1. Scripture EW. Records of speech in disseminated sclerosis. Brain 1916;39:455–477
2. Awan SN. The Voice Diagnostic Profile: A Practical Guide to the Diagnosis of Voice Disorders. Gaithersburg, MD: Aspen; 2001
3. Baken RJ, Orlikoff RF. Clinical Measurement of Speech and Voice. San Diego: Singular; 2000
4. Buder EH. Acoustic analysis of voice quality: A tabulation of algorithms 1902–1990. In: Kent RD, Ball MJ, eds. Voice Quality Measurement. San Diego: Singular; 2000:119–244
5. Fant G. Glottal flow: models and interaction. J Phon 1986;14:393–399 (reprinted in Kent RD, Atal BS, Miller JL, eds. Papers in Speech Communication: Speech Production. Woodbury, NY: Acoustical Society of America; 1991:139–146
6. KayPENTAX. Multi-Dimensional Voice Program (MDVP), Model 5105 [computer program]. Lincoln Park, NJ: KayPENTAX; 1993
7. Hanson HM, Stevens KN, Kuo HJ, Chen MY, Slifka J. Towards models of phonation. J Phon 2001;29:451–480
8. Hirano M. Clinical Examination of Voice. Vienna: Springer-Verlag; 1981
9. Kent RD, Ball MJ, eds. Voice Quality Measurement. San Diego, CA: Singular; 2000
10. Ní Chasaide A, Gobl C. Voice source variation. In: Laver J, ed. The Handbook of Phonetic Sciences. Oxford, UK: Blackwell; 1997: 427–461
11. Titze IR. Principles of Voice Production. Englewood Cliffs, NJ: Prentice Hall; 1994
12. Titze IR. Workshop on acoustic voice analysis: summary statement, Iowa City, IA, National Center for Voice and Speech, 1995
13. Buder EH. Voice production and dysfunction in motor speech disorders. In: Weismer G, ed. Motor Speech Disorders: Essays for Ray Kent. San Diego: Plural; 2006:121–150
14. Titze IR. The Myoelastic Aerodynamic Theory of Phonation. Iowa City, IA: National Center for Voice and Speech; 2006
15. Dromey C, Ramig LO. Intentional changes in sound pressure level and rate: Their impact on measures of respiration, phonation, and articulation. J Speech Lang Hear Res 1998;41:1003–1018
16. Dromey C, Ramig LO, Johnson AB. Phonatory and articulatory changes associated with increased vocal intensity in Parkinson disease: a case study. J Speech Hear Res 1995;38:751–764
17. Orlikoff RF, Kahane JC. Influence of mean sound pressure level on jitter and shimmer measures. J Voice 1991;5:113–119
18. Klingholz F. Acoustic representation of speaking-voice quality. J Voice 1990;4:213–219
19. Klingholz F, Martin F. Distribution of the amplitude in the pathologic voice signal. Folia Phoniatr (Basel) 1989;41:23–29
20. Winholtz WS, Titze IR. Conversion of a head-mounted microphone signal into calibrated SPL units. J Voice 1997;11:417–421
21. Winholtz WS, Titze IR. Miniature head-mounted microphone for voice perturbation analysis. J Speech Lang Hear Res 1997;40:894–899
22. Coleman RF. Sources of variation in phonetograms. J Voice 1993; 7:1–14
23. Pabon JPH. Objective acoustic voice-quality parameters in the computer phonetogram. J Voice 1991;5:203–216
24. KayPENTAX. Real Time Pitch (RTP), Model 5121 [computer program]. Lincoln, NJ: KayPENTAX; 2005
25. KayPENTAX. Multi-Dimensional Voice Program (MDVP), Model 5105 [computer program]. Lincoln Park, NJ: KayPENTAX; 2005
26. Kent RD, Vorperian HK, Kent JF, Duffy JR. Voice dysfunction in dysarthria: application of the Multi-Dimensional Voice Program. J Commun Disord 2003;36:281–306
27. Titze IR. A model for neurologic sources of aperiodicity in vocal fold vibration. J Speech Hear Res 1991;34:460–472
28. Larson CR, Kempster G, Kistler M. Changes in voice fundamental frequency following discharge of single motor units in cricothyroid and thyroarytenoid muscles. J Speech Hear Res 1987;30:552–558
29. Baer T. Vocal jitter: a neuromuscular explanation. In: Weinberg B, ed. Transcripts of the Eighth Symposium: Care of the Professional Voice. Part I: Physical Factors in Voice, Vibrato, Registers. New York: The Voice Foundation; 1980:19–24
30. Buder EH. Acoustic assessment of voice. In: Kent RD, ed. MIT Encyclopedia of Communication Disorders. Cambridge, MA: MIT Press; 2003
31. Pützer M. Multiparametrische Stimmqualitätserfassung männlicher und weiblicher Normalstimmen. Folia Phoniatr Logop 2001;53:73–84
32. Adler CH, Bansberg SF, Hentz JG, et al. Botulinum toxin type A for treating voice tremor. Arch Neurol 2004;61:1416–1420
33. Brown JR, Simonson J. Organic voice tremor. Neurology 1963;13: 520–525
34. Critchley M. Observations on essential (heredofamilial) tremor. Brain 1949;72:113–139
35. Buder EH, Strand EA. Quantitative and graphic acoustic analysis of phonatory modulations: The modulogram. J Speech Lang Hear Res 2003;46:475–490
36. Hartelius L, Buder EH, Strand EA. Long-term phonatory instability in individuals with multiple sclerosis. J Speech Lang Hear Res 1997; 40:1056–1072
37. Hartelius L, Buder EH. Phonatory characteristics in individuals with multiple sclerosis with and without cerebellar symptomatology. In: Peters HF, ed. Proceedings of the XXIVth World Congress of the International Association of Logopedics and Phoniatrics, Vol. 2. Nijmegan, Netherlands: Nijmegan University Press; 1999:602–605

38. Britton D, Buder EH, Strand EA. Longitudinal patterns of long-term phonatory instability in amyotrophic lateral sclerosis. Paper presented at American Speech-Language Hearing Association, 1997, San Francisco
39. Kent RD, Kent JF, Rosenbeck JC. Maximum performance tests of speech production. J Speech Hear Disord 1987;52:367–387
40. Eckel FC, Boone DR. The s/z ratio as an indicator of laryngeal pathology. J Speech Hear Disord 1981;46:147–149
41. Ludlow CL, Connor NP, Bassich CJ. Speech timing in Parkinson's and Huntington's disease. Brain Lang 1987;32:195–214
42. KayPENTAX. Motor Speech Profile (MSP) Model 5141 [computer program]. Lincoln, NJ; KayPENTAX; 2005
43. Bielamowicz S, Stager SV. Diagnosis of unilateral recurrent laryngeal nerve paralysis: laryngeal electromyography, subjective rating scales, acoustic and aerodynamic measures. Laryngoscope 2006;116:359–364
44. Verdolini K, Palmer PM. Assessment of a "profiles" approach to voice screening. J Med Speech-Lang Pathol 1997;5:217–232
45. Kent RD, Kent JF. Task-based profiles of the dysarthrias. Folia Phoniatr Logop 2000;52:48–53
46. Kent RD, Kent JF, Duffy J, Weismer G. The dysarthrias: speech-voice profiles, related dysfunctions, and neuropathology. J Med Speech-Lang Pathol 1998;6:165–211
47. Kent RD, Kim H, Weismer G, et al. Laryngeal dysfunction in neurological disease: amyotrophic lateral sclerosis, Parkinson's disease, and stroke. J Med Speech-Lang Pathol 1994;2:157–176
48. Jiang JJ, Zhang Y, McGilligan C. Chaos in voice, from modeling to measurement. J Voice 2006;20:2–17
49. Bunton K. Fundamental frequency as a perceptual cue for vowel identification in speakers with Parkinson's disease. Folia Phoniatr Logop 2006;58:323–339
50. Goberman AM, Elmer LW. Acoustic analysis of clear versus conversational speech in individuals with Parkinson disease. J Commun Disord 2005;38:215–230
51. Rosen KM, Kent RD, Delaney AL. Parametric quantitative acoustic analysis of conversation produced by speakers with dysarthria and healthy speakers. J Speech Lang Hear Res 2006;49:395–411
52. Zhang Y, Jiang JJ. Acoustic analyses of sustained and running voices from patients with laryngeal pathologies. J Voice 2008;22:1–9
53. Rahn DA III, Chou M, Jiang JJ, Zhang Y. Phonatory impairment in Parkinson's disease: evidence from nonlinear dynamic analysis and perturbation analysis. J Voice 2007;21:64–71
54. Zhang Y, Jiang JJ, Biazzo L, Jorgensen M. Perturbation and nonlinear dynamic analysis of voices from patients with unilateral laryngeal paralysis. J Voice 2005;19:519–528
55. Feijó AV, Parente MA, Behlau M, Haussen S, de Veccino MC, Martignago BC. Acoustic analysis of voice in multiple sclerosis patients. J Voice 2004;18:341–347
56. Lundy DS, Roy S, Xue JW, Casiano RR, Jassir D. Spastic/spasmodic vs. tremulous vocal quality: motor speech profile analysis. J Voice 2004;18:146–152
57. Dromey C. Spectral measures and perceptual ratings of hypokinetic dysarthria. J Med Speech-Lang Pathol 2003;11:85–94
58. Kelchner LN, Lee L, Stemple JC. Laryngeal function and vocal fatigue after prolonged reading in individuals with unilateral vocal fold paralysis. J Voice 2003;17:513–528
59. Heman-Ackah YD, Michael DD, Goding GS Jr. The relationship between cepstral and peak prominence and selected parameters of dysphonia. J Voice 2002;16:20–27
60. Morsomme D, Jamart J, Wéry C, Giovanni A, Remacle M. Comparison between the GIRBAS scale and the aerodynamic measures provided by EVA for the assessment of dysphonia following Unilateral Vocal Fold Paralysis. Folia Phoniatr Logop 2001;53:3 17–325
61. Jiang J, Lin E, Hanson DG. Acoustic and airflow spectral analysis of voice tremor. J Speech Lang Hear Res 2000;43:191–204
62. Kent RD, Kent JF, Duffy JR, Thomas JE, Weismer G, Stuntebeck S. Ataxic dysarthria. J Speech Lang Hear Res 2000;43:1275–1289
63. Murry T, Sapienza CM, Walton S. Adductor spasmodic dysphonia and muscular tension dysphonia: Acoustic analysis of sustained phonation and reading. J Voice 2000;14:502–520
64. Sherrard KC, Marquardt TP, Cannito MP. Phonatory and temporal aspects of spasmodic dysphonia and pseudobulbar dysarthria: an acoustic analysis. J Med Speech-Lang Pathol 2000;8:271–277
65. Kent RD, Vorperian HK, Duffy JR. Reliability of the Multi-Dimensional Voice Program. Am J Speech Lang Pathol 1999;8:129–136
66. Sapienza CM, Walton S, Murry T. Acoustic variations in adductor spasmodic dysphonia as a function of speech task. J Speech Lang Hear Res 1999;42:127–140
67. Robert D, Pouget J, Giovanni A, Azulay J-P, Triglia J-M. Quantitative voice analysis in the assessment of bulbar involvement in amyotrophic lateral sclerosis. Acta Otolaryngol 1999;119:724–731
68. Eckley CA, Sataloff RT, Hawkshaw M, Speigel JR, Mandel S. Voice range in superior laryngeal nerve paresis and paralysis. J Voice 1998;12:340–348
69. Le Dorze G, Ryalls J, Brassard C, Boulanger N, Ratte D. A comparison of the prosodic characteristics of the speech of people with Parkinson's disease and Friedreich's ataxia with neurologically normal speakers. Folia Phoniatr Logop 1998;50:1–9
70. Gamboa J, Jiménez-Jiménez FJ, Nieto A, et al. Acoustic voice analysis in patients with essential tremor. J Voice 1998;12:444–452
71. Gamboa J, Jiménez-Jiménez FJ, Nieto A, et al. Acoustic voice analysis in patients with Parkinson's disease treated with dopaminergic drugs. J Voice 1997;11:314–320
72. Hertrich I, Lutzenberger W, Spieker S, Ackermann H. Fractal dimension of sustained vowel productions in neurological dysphonias: an acoustic and electroglottographic analysis. J Acoust Soc Am 1997;102:652–654
73. Walker FO. Voice fatigue in myasthenia gravis: The sinking pitch sign. Neurology 1997;48:1135–1136
74. Doyle PC, Raade AS, St. Pierre A, Desai S. Fundamental frequency and acoustic variability associated with production of sustained vowels by speakers with hypokinetic dysarthria. J Med Speech-Lang Pathol 1995;3:41–50
75. Hertrich I, Ackermann H. Gender-specific vocal dysfunctions in Parkinson's disease: electroglottographic and acoustic analyses. Ann Otol Rhinol Laryngol 1995;104:197–202
76. Murry T, Brown WS Jr, Morris RJ. Patterns of fundamental frequency for three types of voice samples. J Voice 1995;9:282–289
77. Ackermann H, Ziegler W. Acoustic analysis of vocal instability in cerebellar dysfunctions. Ann Otol Rhinol Laryngol 1994;103:98–104
78. Strand EA, Buder EH, Yorkston KM, Ramig LO. Differential phonatory characteristics of four women with amyotrophic lateral sclerosis. J Voice 1994;8:327–339
79. Hertrich I, Ackermann H. Acoustic analysis of speech timing in Huntington's disease. Brain Lang 1994;47:182–196
80. Zwirner P, Murry T, Woodson GE. Perceptual-acoustic relationships in spasmodic dysphonia. J Voice 1993;7:165–171
81. Aronson AE, Ramig LO, Winholtz WS, Silber SR. Rapid voice tremor, or "flutter," in amyotrophic lateral sclerosis. Ann Otol Rhinol Laryngol 1992;101:511–518
82. Zwirner P, Murry T, Woodson GE. Phonatory function of neurologically impaired patients. J Commun Disord 1991;24:287–300
83. Rosenfield DB, Viswanath N, Herbrich KE, Nudelman HB. Evaluation of the speech motor control system in amyotrophic lateral sclerosis. J Voice 1991;5:224–230
84. Philippbar SA, Robin DA, Luschei ES. Limb, jaw, and vocal tremor in Parkinson's individuals. In: Beukelman DR, ed. Recent Advances in Clinical Dysarthria. Boston: College-Hill Press; 1989:165–197
85. Fukazawa T, Blaugrund SM, El-Assuooty A, Gould WJ. Acoustic analysis of hoarse voice: a preliminary report. J Voice 1988;2:127–131

86. Hartman DE, Abbs JH, Vishwanat B. Clinical investigations of adductor spastic dysphonia. Ann Otol Rhinol Laryngol 1988;97:247–252

87. Ramig LO, Shipp T. Comparative measures of vocal tremor and vocal vibrato. J Voice 1987;1:162–167

88. Ludlow CL, Connor NP. Dynamic aspects of phonatory control in spasmodic dysphonia. J Speech Hear Res 1987;30:197–206

89. Hirano M, Hibi S, Terasawa R, Fujiu M. Relationship between aerodynamic, vibratory, acoustic and psychoacoustic correlates in dysphonia. J Phon 1986;14:445–456

90. Kasuya H, Ogawa S, Mashima K, Ebihara S. Normalized noise energy as an acoustic measure to evaluate pathologic voice. J Acoust Soc Am 1986;80:1329–1334

91. Hartmann E, von Cramon D. Acoustic measurement of voice quality in central dysphonia. J Commun Disord 1984;17:425–440

92. Ludlow CL, Bassich CJ. The results of acoustic and perceptual assessment of two types of dysarthria. In: Berry WR, ed. Clinical Dysarthria. San Diego: College Hill Press; 1983:121–153

93. Rontal M, Rontal E, Leuchter W, Rolnick M. Voice spectrography in the evaluation of myasthenia gravis of the larynx. Ann Otol Rhinol Laryngol 1978;87:722–728

94. Iwata S. Periodicities of pitch perturbations in normal and pathologic larynges. Laryngoscope 1972;82:87–96

95. Koike Y. Vowel amplitude modulations in patients with laryngeal diseases. J Acoust Soc Am 1969;45:839–844

96. Harel B, Cannizzaro M, Snyder PJ. Variability in fundamental frequency during speech in prodromal and incipient Parkinson's disease: a longitudinal case study. Brain Cogn 2004;56:24–29

97. Silbergleit AK, Johnson A, Jacobson B. Acoustic analysis of voice in individuals with amyotrophic lateral sclerosis and perceptually normal voice quality. J Voice 1997;11:222–231

98. Ramig LA, Scherer RC, Titze IR, Ringel SP. Acoustic analysis of voices of patients with neurologic disease: rationale and preliminary data. Ann Otol Rhinol Laryngol 1988;97:164–172

99. Wolfe VI, Ratusnik DL, Feldman H. Acoustic and perceptual comparison of chronic and incipient spastic dysphonia. Laryngoscope 1979;89:1478–1486

100. Leeper HA, Millard KM, Bandur DL, Hudson AJ. An investigation of deterioration of vocal function in subgroups of individuals with ALS. J Med Speech-Lang Pathol 1996;4:163–181

101. Kent RD, Sufit RL, Rosenbek JC, et al. Speech deterioration in amyotrophic lateral sclerosis: a case study. J Speech Hear Res 1991;34:1269–1275

102. Ramig LO, Scherer RC, Klasner ER, Titze IR, Horii Y. Acoustic analysis of voice in amyotrophic lateral sclerosis: A longitudinal case study. J Speech Hear Disord 1990;55:2–14

103. Ramig LA. Acoustic analyses of phonation in patients with Huntington's disease: preliminary report. Ann Otol Rhinol Laryngol 1986;95:288–293

104. Goberman AM, Blomgren M. Fundamental frequency change during offset and onset of voicing in individuals with Parkinson disease. J Voice 2008;22:178–191

105. Sewall GK, Jiang J, Ford CN. Clinical evaluation of Parkinson's-related dysphonia. Laryngoscope 2006;116:1740–1744

106. Cannito MP, Buder EH, Chorna LB. Spectral amplitude measures of adductor spasmodic dysphonic speech. J Voice 2005;19:391–410

107. Sapir S, Spielman J, Ramig LO, et al. Effects of intensive voice treatment (the Lee Silverman Voice Treatment [LSVT]) on ataxic dysarthria: a case study. Am J Speech Lang Pathol 2003;12:387–399

108. Wang E, Metman LV, Bakay R, Arzbaecher J, Bernard B. The effect of unilateral electrostimulation of the subthalamic nucleus on respiratory/phonatory subsystems of speech production in Parkinson's disease—a preliminary report. Clin Linguist Phon 2003;17:283–289

109. Kersing W, Dejonckere PH, van der Aa H, Buschman HPJ. Laryngeal and vocal changes during vagus nerve stimulation in epileptic patients. J Voice 2002;16:251–257

110. Sapienza CM, Cannito MP, Murry T, Branski R, Woodson G. Acoustic variations in reading produced by speakers with spasmodic dysphonia pre-botox injection and within early stages of post-botox injection. J Speech Lang Hear Res 2002;45:830–843

111. Goberman AM, Coelho C. Acoustic analysis of parkinsonian speech II: L-Dopa related fluctuations and methodological issues. NeuroRehabilitation 2002;17:247–254

112. McHenry M, Whatman J, Pou A. The effect of botulinum toxin A on the vocal symptoms of spastic dysarthria: a case study. J Voice 2002;16:124–131

113. Shin J-E, Nam SY, Yoo SJ, Kim SY. Analysis of voice and quantitative measurement of glottal gap after thyroplasty type I in the treatment of unilateral voice paralysis. J Voice 2002;16:136–142

114. Langeveld TPM, van Rossum M, Houtman EH, Zwinderman AH, Briaire JJ, Baatenburg de Jong RJ. Evaluation of voice quality in adductor spasmodic dysphonia before and after botulinum toxin treatment. Ann Otol Rhinol Laryngol 2001;110:627–634

115. Mehta RP, Goldman SN, Orloff LA. Long-term therapy of spasmodic dysphonia. Arch Otolaryngol Head Neck Surg 2001;127:393–399

116. Sapir S, Pawlas AA, Ramig LO, Seely E, Fox C, Corboy J. Effects of intensive phonatory-respiratory treatment (LSVT) on voice in two individuals with multiple sclerosis. J Med Speech-Lang Pathol 2001;9:141–151

117. Dromey C, Kumar R, Lang AE, Lozano AM. An investigation of the effects of subthalamic nucleus stimulation on acoustic measures of voice. Mov Disord 2000;15:1132–1138

118. Hartl DM, Hans S, Vaissiere J, Riquet M, Brasnu DF. Objective voice quality analysis before and after onset of unilateral vocal fold paralysis. J Voice 2001;15:351–361

119. Schulz GM, Greer M, Friedman W. Changes in vocal intensity in Parkinson's disease following pallidotomy surgery. J Voice 2000;14:589–606

120. Jiang J, Lin E, Wang J, Hanson DG. Glottographic measures before and after Levodopa treatment in Parkinson's disease. Laryngoscope 1999;109:1287–1294

121. Schulz GM, Peterson T, Sapienza CM, Greer M, Friedman W. Voice and speech characteristics of persons with Parkinson's disease pre- and post-pallidotomy surgery: Preliminary findings. J Speech Lang Hear Res 1999;42:1176–1194

122. Lu F-L, Casiano RR, Lundy DS, Xue JW. Longitudinal evaluation of vocal function after thryroplasty type I in the treatment of unilateral vocal paralysis. Laryngoscope 1996;106:573–577

123. Bielamowicz S, Berke GS, Gerratt BR. A comparison of type I thyroplasty and arytenoid adduction. J Voice 1995;9:466–472

124. Bouglé F, Ryalls J, Le Dorze G. Improving fundamental frequency modulation in head trauma patients: a preliminary comparison of speech-language therapy conducted with and without IBM's SpeechViewer. Folia Phoniatr Logop 1995;47:24–32

125. Adams SG, Hunt EJ, Charles DA, Lang AE. Unilateral versus bilateral botulinum toxin injections in spasmodic dysphonia: acoustic and perceptual results. J Otolaryngol 1993;22:171–175

126. Troung DD, Rontal M, Rolnick M, Aronson AE, Mistura K. Double-blind controlled study of botulinum toxin in adductor spasmodic dysphonia. Laryngoscope 1991;101:630–634

127. Zwirner P, Murry T, Swenson M, Woodson GE. Acoustic changes in spasmodic dysphonia after botulinum toxin injection. J Voice 1991;5:78–84

Chapter 10

Stroboscopic Examination of the Normal Larynx

Minoru Hirano

Stroboscopic examination of the larynx is one of the minimum essential procedures of modern laryngologic practice. The key event in voice production is vibration of the vocal folds. The vibratory behavior of the vocal folds is one of the most important and crucial determinants of the voice character. Abnormal voices are always associated with abnormal vibratory patterns of the vocal fold. Examination of vocal fold vibration, therefore, is necessary and essential to determine the cause and mechanism of abnormal voices. Stroboscopy is the only existing modality to observe vocal fold vibration that is available for clinical purposes.

♦ How Stroboscopic Images of Vocal Fold Vibrations Are Obtained

Stroboscopic light sources produce intermittent flashes of light that are synchronous with the vibratory cycles of the vocal folds. The waveform of the patient's voice picked up with a microphone triggers the light source. When the frequency of the light flashes emitted is the same as that of the vocal fold vibration, a clear still image of the vocal folds at a given phase point is observed (**Fig. 10.1A**). When the frequency of the flashes is slightly less than that of the vocal fold vibration, resulting in a systematic phase delay of the consecutive light flashes, a slow motion effect is obtained (**Fig. 10.1B**). Stroboscopy cannot demonstrate fine details of each individual vibratory cycle, but it depicts a vibratory mode averaged over many successive vibratory cycles. If successive vibrations are completely periodic and the vibratory behavior is perfectly uniform, the stroboscopic images reflect precisely the slow-motion images of each vibratory cycle. In humans, however, successive vibrations are aperiodic to a greater or lesser extent. Nevertheless, it is extremely useful for clinical purposes.

♦ Normal Vibratory Pattern of Vocal Folds

Figure 10.2 schematically depicts normal vibratory pattern of the vocal fold in modal register and **Fig. 10.3** shows vibratory phases in one vibratory cycle. The vibratory cycle consists of three phases: the opening phase, in which the vocal fold edges move laterally; the closing phase, in which the vocal edges move medially; and the closed phase, in which the bilateral vocal folds are in contact with each other.

Typically, two wave peaks are observed on the vocal folds. They are referred to as the upper and lower lips. The upper and lower lips are not structures that are located at consistent places of the vocal fold, but they are the peaks of waves that travel on the vocal fold mucosa.

At the end of the closed phase, the vocal folds are in contact with each other only at the upper lip (**Fig. 10.2A**). During the early stage of the opening phase, the entire vocal fold shifts laterally (**Fig. 10.2B**). At the maximum opening the upper and lower lips are lined up on the same plane (**Fig. 10.2C**). In the early stage of the closing phase, the lower lips move medially whereas the upper lips still move laterally (**Fig. 10.2D**). During the late stage of the closing phase, both upper and lower lips move medially (**Fig. 10.2E,F**). The lower lips usually meet first at the end of the closing phase or at the beginning of the closed phase (**Fig. 10.2G**). In the early stage of the closed phase, the contact area of the two vocal folds increases (**Fig. 10.2H**). After

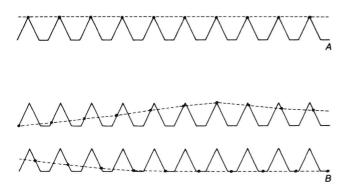

Fig. 10.1 Schematic presentation of the principle of stroboscopy. (From Hirano M. *Clinical Examination of Voice.* Vienna–New York: Springer Verlag; 1981. Reprinted with permission.)

86 II Clinical Evaluation

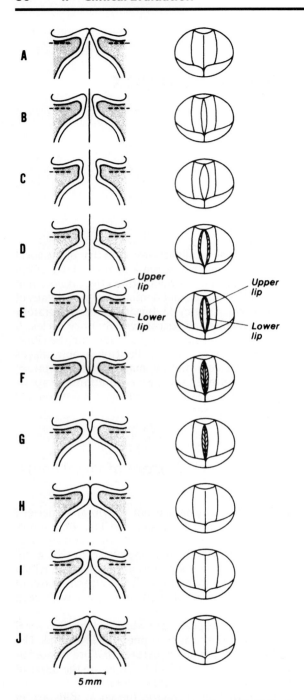

Fig. 10.2 Schematic presentation of normal vocal fold vibration. (From Hirano M. *Clinical Examination of Voice.* Vienna–New York: Springer Verlag; 1981. Reprinted with permission.)

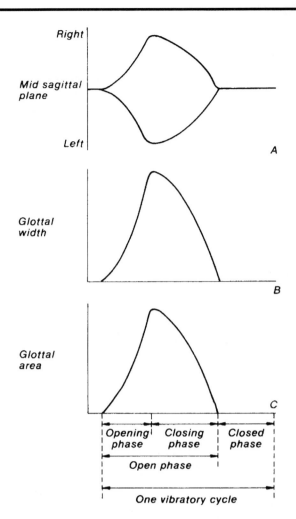

Fig. 10.3 Phases in one vibratory cycle. **(A)** Horizontal excursion. **(B)** Glottal width. **(C)** Glottal area. (From Hirano M. *Clinical Examination of Voice.* Vienna–New York: Springer Verlag; 1981. Reprinted with permission.)

the maximum contact, the vocal folds start separating from each other. The separation usually proceeds from the bottom to the top (**Fig. 10.2I, J**).

The vocal fold edge viewed from above, therefore, is the tip of the upper lip from the late stage of the closed phase through the opening phase, whereas it is the tip of the lower lip during the closing phase and the early stage of the closed phase.

♦ Parameters for Stroboscopic Examination of Vocal Fold Vibrations

The following parameters should be examined during stroboscopy and documented:

Fundamental frequency (F_o): F_o is shown on the F_o indicator embedded in stroboscopes.

Symmetry of movements of the bilateral vocal folds: The symmetry should be checked whether or not the movements of the bilateral vocal folds are symmetrical. Normally they look symmetrical in stroboscopy. Asymmetry, when noted, should be described in terms of amplitude and phase.

Regularity or periodicity of successive vibrations: The regularity implies how uniform the successive vibratory movements are. Normally they look regular or periodic in stroboscopy.

Glottic closure: The clinician should determine if a complete glottic closure takes place during the vibratory cycle. Normally it takes place at the intermembranous portion of the glottis. At the intercartilaginous portion, the glottis closes completely in most normal patients, but in some patients it does not always completely close.

Amplitude: The maximum amplitude of the horizontal excursion of the edges of the vocal folds is evaluated subjectively and qualitatively. It is described as "greater than normal," "normal," "smaller than normal," or "zero." Typically, the amplitude is approximately one third of the width of the vocal fold in normal patients. Differences in the amplitude of the two vocal folds are also examined.

Mucosal wave: The size and extent of the mucosal wave that travels on the vocal fold are evaluated subjectively and qualitatively. It is described as "greater than normal," "normal," "smaller than normal," or "none." Differences in the mucosal wave between the two vocal folds are also examined.

Nonvibrating portion: If there is any portion of the vocal fold that does not vibrate, in other words, that remains still during phonation, this should be specified. The absence of vibratory movement can occur either occasionally or always, and either partially or entirely.

Other findings: If any other findings are noted, they should be described.

Table 10.1 presents an example of a form of stroboscopic record.

♦ Normal Variations in Vocal Fold Vibrations

The vibratory behavior of the vocal folds varies significantly depending on the F_o and sound pressure level (SPL) of phonation, vocal register, and phonatory mode. The following general tendencies occur:

1. As the F_o increases, the amplitude, mucosal wave, and relative length of the closed phase decrease.
2. As the SPL increases, the amplitude, mucosal wave, and relative length of the closed phase increase.
3. In the falsetto register, the amplitude is small, little mucosal wave is noted, and the membranous portion of the glottis does not completely close.

Table 10.1 A Form for the Recording of Stroboscopic Findings

1. Fundamental frequency ____ Hz
2. Symmetry
   a. Symmetrical
   b. Asymmetrical
      (1) In amplitude (+, −)
      (2) In phase (+, −)
3. Regularity (periodicity)
   a. Regular (periodic)
   b. Inconsistent (sometimes regular, sometimes irregular)
   c. Irregular (aperiodic)
4. Glottic closure
   a. Complete
   b. Inconsistent (sometimes complete, sometimes incomplete)
   c. Incomplete
      (1) Along entire length
      (2) Spindle shape
      (3) Sandglass shape
      (4) Irregular shape
      (5) Anterior portion
      (6) Posterior portion of intermembranous glottis
      (7) Intercartilaginous portion
      (8) 6 and 7
      (9) Others; specify
5. Amplitude
   a. Right: (1) great (2) normal (3) small (4) zero
   b. Left: (1) great (2) normal (3) small (4) zero
      (1) Right > Left
      (2) Right = Left
      (3) Right < Left
6. Mucosal wave
   a. Right: (1) great (2) normal (3) small (4) absent
   b. Left: (1) great (2) normal (3) small (4) absent
      (1) Right > Left
      (2) Right = Left
      (3) Right < Left
7. Nonvibrating portion
   a. Right: (1) none (2) occasionally, partially (3) always, partially, (4) occasionally, entirely, (5) always, entirely
   b. Left: (1) none (2) occasionally, partially (3) always, partially, (4) occasionally, entirely, (5) always, entirely
8. Other findings
   a. None
   b. Noted; specify

Note: (1) When the amplitude is zero, the nonvibrating portion should be assigned to be "always, entirely." (2) When the amplitude or the mucosal wave differs at different places of one vocal fold, specify the details. (3) When the amplitude or the mucosal wave changes during phonation, specify the details. (4) When the amplitude or the mucosal wave differs among varying phonatory conditions, specify the details.

4. Hyperfunctional or strained phonation is associated with a long closed phase, whereas hypofunctional or asthenic phonation is accompanied by a short or no closed phase.

♦ Video Recording of Stroboscopic Images

Stroboscopy was originally based on a completely subjective evaluation. Recently, video recordings of stroboscopic images have become feasible and, in fact, are employed in many laryngologic clinics. Stroboscopic images are recorded on videotape usually by means of a fiberscope or a telescope connected to a video camera. A microscope in which a stroboscopic light source is embedded can also be used. Video recordings of stroboscopic images have made stroboscopy a more objective and reliable procedure.

Chapter 11

Flexible Endoscopic Evaluation of Swallowing with Sensory Testing (FEESST)

Jonathan E. Aviv and Thomas Murry

Flexible endoscopic evaluation of swallowing with sensory testing (FEESST) is a technique used to evaluate the patient with dysphagia, or difficulty swallowing. Dysphagia is one of the most common problems affecting the population as it ages and is one of the most likely reasons why patients consult with an otolaryngologist as they get older. Swallowing should be thought of as an interaction between two related physiologic entities: airway protection and bolus transport.[1] Airway protection is determined by assessment of the sensory component of swallowing, and bolus transport is determined by assessment of the motor component of swallowing. This chapter discusses the magnitude of swallowing problems in the population in general, the likely reasons why individuals have swallowing difficulties, and the diagnostic techniques necessary to fully evaluate the patient with dysphagia. Emphasis is placed on the FEESST technique to assess the severity of dysphagia.

♦ Epidemiology of Dysphagia

The ubiquitous nature of swallowing problems is demonstrated by examining the incidence of swallowing problems after stroke. Stroke affects 400,000 people a year and results in an incidence of dysphagia ranging from 35 to 47%.[2,3] Patients succumb after a stroke primarily because of pulmonary complications, specifically aspiration pneumonia. Approximately 50,000 people die each year as a result of aspiration pneumonia after stroke.[4,5] Although the development of aspiration pneumonia is a multifactorial process, several studies have demonstrated a significant association between dysphagia and aspiration pneumonia. Dysphagia often results in difficulty handling food and secretions, a consequence of which is foreign material soiling the lungs.[6-10]

Aspiration pneumonia is also a significant cause of chronic illness in the elderly residing in United States nursing homes and is the most common reason why residents of nursing homes are transferred to a hospital.[11,12] In U.S. nursing homes the prevalence of aspiration pneumonia has been reported to be as high as 8%.[13-16] The cost of treating a single episode of pneumonia in a hospital, including intravenous antibiotics and a stay in an intensive care unit, with or without respiratory support, averaged $30,400 in 2008.[17] This treatment cost has escalated in proportion to other medical costs since that time. Extrapolating to the current population of 2 million people in nursing homes, the annual health care costs related to aspiration pneumonia from the nursing home population is over $3 billion per year. Although the mortality from aspiration pneumonia can approach 40%, it is not the first episode of pneumonia that results in demise; rather, it is recurrent pneumonia over a several-year period that is so deadly and so costly.[4,5]

♦ Etiology of Dysphagia

As one ages, dysphagia and aspiration during swallowing are more likely to occur.[18,19] The primary explanations for these observations have been oral and pharyngeal motor dysfunctions such as abnormal lingual activity, poor lingual–palatal seal, and pharyngeal pooling.[18,20] Although oropharyngeal motor dysfunction contributes to swallowing difficulties, it has also been shown that oral cavity sensory discriminatory ability diminishes with advancing age.[21,22] Over the past decade laryngopharyngeal sensory capacity has been studied in the elderly, and it has been demonstrated that airway protective capacity also diminishes as people age. Specifically, with aging there is a progressive increase in the stimuli required to elicit fundamental airway protective reflexes, with patients 61 years and older requiring a more intense stimuli than those 60 and younger.[23] In a study of fresh human cadavers, changes in sensory nerve composition that take place with increasing age in the human superior laryngeal nerve (SLN) were examined.[24] It was found that there is an extensive and statistically significant decrease in the number of sensory nerve fibers in subjects over 60 years of age.[24] Because it is the SLN that provides afferent fibers to the hypopharynx from the laryngeal surface of the epiglottis to the level of the true vocal folds, this basic science work supports the aforementioned clinical studies.

Although the healthy elderly develop a progressive diminution in both airway protective capacity and motor capabilities as they age, the unhealthy elderly, such as those who suffer from stroke, progressive neuromuscular diseases, diabetes, and a general decline in health status, suffer even more of an assault to their airway protective capacity and muscular coordination.[25-27] Studies evaluating sensory capacity of the laryngopharynx in supratentorial and brainstem stroke patients who presented with dysphagia showed that stroke patients had either unilateral or bilateral laryngopharyngeal sensory deficits.[25] These sensory deficits were significantly greater than in age-matched controls, and thus these studies provide evidence that impairment of airway protective capacity contributes to dysphagia after stroke. The point of these studies is that in patients with swallowing problems, attention must be paid to how patients sense the food in the upper aerodigestive tract and to how food moves from the lips into the esophagus. Without a precise understanding of patients' ability to sense the food bolus, clinicians can only guess, at best, if patients can swallow safely.

♦ Diagnostic Techniques of Dysphagia

Knowing why a patient is having a swallowing problem is essential in formulating an appropriate treatment plan. Therefore, the diagnostic technique that is chosen to help determine what is functionally wrong with the swallow is of paramount importance. There are non–instrument-based and instrument-based methods of determining what is taking place when a patient swallows. The non–instrument-based test of swallowing is an observation of how a patient reacts when swallowing solid or liquid food: does the patient cough, choke, or otherwise react to the presented bolus? Because of the limited nature of reliable information obtainable with such a "hands-off" observational technique, a bedside swallowing evaluation is a gross screening tool for the patient with dysphagia.[28-30]

The instrument-based swallowing tests use either x-rays or a flexible endoscope. The x-ray–based test is known as the modified barium swallow (MBS) or videofluoroscopy.[31,32] The endoscopic tests are known as fiberoptic endoscopic examination of swallowing (FEES)[33-35] and flexible endoscopic evaluation of swallowing with sensory testing (FEESST).[36,37] The MBS, FEES, and FEESST all provide detailed functional and physiologic information regarding the swallow.

Unlike the MBS, the FEES and FEESST do not involve x-ray exposure or barium administration, or require the presence of a radiologist or a radiology technician. FEES and FEESST involve endoscopy, and provide direct evidence regarding the handling of secretions.[38] FEESST specifically provides an objective assessment of hypopharyngeal sensitivity, which, in turn, gives the clinician information regarding patients' ability to protect their airway during the ingestion of food.

In addition, FEESST does not require the patient to sit in a particular position or posture during the exam, which is an important consideration when examining a patient with neurologic disease. The exam can be readily performed with the patient sitting on a bed. All the instrument-based swallowing tests involve the active participation of a speech-language pathologist (SLP) who works with the physician to determine behavioral and dietary modifications that will ensure a safe swallow.

The importance of sensation as it relates to swallowing and airway protection in healthy individuals has been studied extensively.[39,40] The concept that sensation plays a determining role in the outcome of a swallow was first studied by Kidd et al,[41] who demonstrated that impaired pharyngeal sensation is related to the development of pneumonia after stroke. Kidd et al assessed pharyngeal sensation by placing a wooden probe via the mouth and tapping the posterior pharyngeal wall to elicit a gag reflex from the patient. Although this was a rudimentary approach to measuring sensory thresholds, it was a start in the right direction. A more precise method of pharyngeal sensory assessment was subsequently developed that avoided the mouth with the transnasal passage of a flexible endoscope to the laryngopharynx. Through either a port in the endoscope or via an endosheath covering the endoscope, a discrete pulse of air is delivered to the epithelium innervated by the SLN to elicit the laryngeal adductor reflex (LAR). The LAR is a brainstem-mediated, fundamental sensorimotor airway protective reflex.[39,42] Once sensory thresholds are determined, the patient is then given varying consistencies and volumes of food containing green food coloring for contrast with the surrounding pink hypopharyngeal lining. The entire examination is recorded using either digital or analog technology. FEESST combines the elicitation of the LAR with food administration trials so that both the sensory and motor components of the swallow can be analyzed. The radical concept here is to assess airway protective capacity before giving a potential foreign body to the larynx.

The FEESST is a versatile, efficient, and portable method to assess swallowing problems in a variety of patient settings.[43] A prospective, randomized outcome study investigating whether FEESST or MBS was superior as the diagnostic test for evaluating and guiding the behavioral and dietary management of patients with dysphagia has shown that the overall pneumonia incidence and pneumonia-free interval are essentially the same using either technique.[44] The only difference in outcomes was seen in a small cohort of patients with stroke whose pneumonia incidence was less in those whose management was guided by FEESST.

There are two possible reasons why dietary and behavioral management of stroke patients guided by FEESST resulted in better outcomes than those seen in patients whose management was guided by MBS. One reason is related to the greater amount of time that is allowed for a FEESST relative to a MBS, so that patient fatigue and its sequelae are more readily identified and managed. Fatigue as a meal progresses is not unusual in the geriatric patient in general, and can be severely exacerbated after stroke.

Patients with stroke have been shown to experience fatigue of the pharyngeal phase of swallowing as they progress through a meal.[26,27] The other reason for the marked difference in stroke patient outcomes may be related to the fact that information regarding the sensory or afferent component of the swallow is rigorously assayed with FEESST, whereas it is only indirectly addressed with MBS. As a result, the clinician using FEESST has a heightened awareness of potential aspiration and pneumonia risks that might otherwise have been overlooked.

♦ Conclusion

Comprehensive, instrument-based management of the patient with a swallowing disorder provides nutritional, rehabilitative, and social benefits to patients. In all cases of patients with swallowing disorders, the first concern is swallow safety, which begins with the functional assessment of the sensory and motor components of swallowing.

References

1. Zamir Z, Ren J, Hogan W, Shaker R. Coordination of deglutitive vocal cord closure and oral-pharyngeal swallowing events in the elderly. Eur J Gastroenterol Hepatol 1996;8:425–429
2. Veis SL, Logemann J. Swallowing disorders in persons with cerebral vascular accident. Arch Phys Med Rehabil 1985;66:372–375
3. Horner J, Massey EW, Riski JE, Lathrop DL, Chase KN. Aspiration following stroke: clinical correlates and outcome. Neurology 1988;38:1359–1362
4. Brown M, Glassenberg M. Mortality factors in patients with acute stroke. JAMA 1973;224:1493–1495
5. Scmidt EV, Smirnov VE, Ryabova VS. Results of the Seven Year Prospective Study of Stroke Patients. Stroke 1988;19:942–949
6. Schmidt J, Holas M, Halvorson K, Reding M. Video-fluoroscopic evidence of aspiration predicts pneumonia but not dehydration following stroke. Dysphagia 1994;9:7–11
7. Martin BJW, Corlew MM, Wood H, et al. The association of swallowing dysfunction and aspiration pneumonia. Dysphagia 1994;9:1–6
8. Johnson ER, McKenzie SW, Sievers A. Aspiration pneumonia in stroke. Arch Phys Med Rehabil 1993;74:973–976
9. Holas MA, DePippo KL, Reding MJ. Aspiration and relative risk of medical complications following stroke. Arch Neurol 1994;51:1051–1053
10. Smithard DG, O'Neill PA, Park C, et al. Complications and outcome after acute stroke. Does dysphagia matter? Stroke 1996;27:1200–1204
11. Marrie TJ, Durant H, Kwan C. Nursing home-acquired pneumonia. J Am Geriatr Soc 1986;34:697–702
12. Norman DC, Castle SC, Cantrell M. Infections in the nursing home. J Am Geriatr Soc 1987;35:796–805
13. Alvarez S, Shell CG, Woolley TW, Berk SL, Smith JK. Nosocomial infections in long-term facilities. J Gerontol 1988;43:M9–M17
14. Beck-Sague C, Villarino E, Giuliano D, et al. Infectious diseases and death among nursing home residents: results of surveillance in 13 nursing homes. Infect Control Hosp Epidemiol 1994;15:494–496
15. Scheckler WE, Peterson PJ. Infections and infection control among residents of eight rural Wisconsin nursing homes. Arch Intern Med 1986;146:1981–1984
16. Hoffman N, Jenkins R, Putney K. Nosocomial infection rates during a one-year period in a nursing home care unit of a Veterans Administration hospital. Am J Infect Control 1990;18:55–63
17. Boyce JM, Potter-Boyne G, Dziobek L, Solomon SL. Nosocomial pneumonia in Medicare patients: hospital costs and reimbursement under the prospective payment system. Arch Intern Med 1991;151:1109–1114
18. Feinberg MJ, Ekberg O. Videofluoroscopy in elderly patients with aspiration: importance of evaluating both oral and pharyngeal stages of deglutition. AJR Am J Roentgenol 1991;156:293–296
19. Zavala DC. The threat of aspiration pneumonia in the aged. Geriatrics 1977;32:46–51
20. Feinberg MJ, Knebl J, Tully J. Prandial aspiration and pneumonia in an elderly population followed over 3 years. Dysphagia 1996;11:104–109
21. Aviv JE, Hecht C, Weinberg H, Dalton JF, Urken ML. Surface sensibility of the floor of mouth and tongue in healthy controls and radiated patients. Otolaryngol Head Neck Surg 1992;107:418–423
22. Calhoun KH, Gibson B, Hartley L, Minton J, Hokanson JA. Age-related changes in oral sensation. Laryngoscope 1992;102:109–116
23. Aviv JE, Martin JH, Jones ME, et al. Age related changes in pharyngeal and supraglottic sensation. Ann Otol Rhinol Laryngol 1994;103:749–752
24. Mortelliti AJ, Malmgren LT, Gacek RR. Ultrastructural changes with age in the human superior laryngeal nerve. Arch Otolaryngol Head Neck Surg 1990;116:1062–1068
25. Aviv JE, Martin JH, Sacco RL, et al. Supraglottic and pharyngeal sensory abnormalities in stroke patients with dysphagia. Ann Otol Rhinol Laryngol 1996;105:92–97
26. Hamdy S, Aziz Q, Rothwell JC, et al. Explaining oropharyngeal dysphagia after unilateral hemispheric stroke. Lancet 1997;350:686–692
27. Hamdy S, Aziz Q, Rothwell JC, et al. The cortical topography of human swallowing musculature in health and disease. Nat Med 1996;2:1217–1224
28. Leder SB, Espinosa JF. Aspiration risk after acute stroke: comparison of clinical examination and fiberoptic endoscopic evaluation of swallowing. Dysphagia 2002;17:214–218
29. Aviv JE. The bedside swallowing evaluation when endoscopy is an option: what would you choose? Dysphagia 2002;17:219
30. Splaingard ML, Hutchins B, Sulton L, Chaudhuri G. Aspiration in rehabilitation patients: videofluoroscopy vs. bedside clinical assessment. Arch Phys Med Rehabil 1988;69:637–640
31. McConnel FMS, Cerenko D, Hersh T, Weil LJ. Evaluation of pharyngeal dysphagia with manofluorography. Dysphagia 1988;2:187–195
32. Logemann JE. Evaluation and Treatment of Swallowing Disorders. San Diego: College Hill Press; 1983:214–227
33. Langmore SE, Schatz K, Olsen N. Fiberoptic endoscopic examination of swallowing safety: a new procedure. Dysphagia 1988;2:216–219
34. Bastian RW. Videoendoscopic evaluation of patients with dysphagia: an adjunct to modified barium swallow. Otolaryngol Head Neck Surg 1991;104:339–350
35. Hiss SG, Postma GN. Fiberoptic endoscopic evaluation of swallowing. Laryngoscope 2003;113:1386–1393
36. Setzen M, Cohen MA, Mattucci KF, Perlman PW, Ditkoff MK. Laryngopharyngeal sensory deficits as a predictor of aspiration. Otolaryngol Head Neck Surg 2001;124:622–624

37. Aviv JE, Johnson LF. Flexible endoscopic evaluation of swallowing with sensory testing (FEESST) to diagnose and manage patients with pharyngeal dysphagia. Pract Gastroenterol 2000;24:52–59

38. Murray J, Langmore SE, Ginsberg S, Dostie A. The significance of accumulated oropharyngeal secretions and swallowing frequency in predicting aspiration. Dysphagia 1996;11:99–103

39. Jafari S, Prince RA, Kim DK, Paydarfar D. Sensory regulation of swallowing and airway protection: a role for the internal superior laryngeal nerve in humans. J Physiol 2003;550:287–304

40. Sulica L, Hembree A, Blitzer A. Sensation and swallowing: endoscopic evaluation of deglutition in the anesthetized larynx. Ann Otol Rhinol Laryngol 2002;111:291–294

41. Kidd D, Lawson J, Macmahon J. Aspiration in acute stroke: a clinical study with videofluoroscopy. Q J Med 1993;86:825–829

42. Aviv JE, Martin JH, Kim T, et al. Laryngopharyngeal sensory discrimination testing and the laryngeal adductor reflex. Ann Otol Rhinol Laryngol 1999;108:725–730

43. Spiegel JR, Selber JC, Creed J. A functional diagnosis of dysphagia using videoendoscopy. Ear Nose Throat J 1998;77:628–632

44. Aviv JE. Prospective, randomized outcome study of endoscopy versus modified barium swallow in patients with dysphagia. Laryngoscope 2000;110:563–574

Section III

Diseases and Treatment

Chapter 12

Speech Treatment for Neurologic Disorders

Shimon Sapir, Lorraine O. Ramig, and Cynthia M. Fox

Speech treatment is essential for overall management of patients with speech and voice disorders secondary to neurologic conditions. Speech treatment may occur in conjunction with medical (surgical, pharmacologic) intervention or as a separate entity. Whatever the case, speech treatment can facilitate maximum improvement in speech intelligibility, acceptability, functional communication, and overall quality of life. The speech pathologist, neurologist, and otolaryngologist function as a team to provide comprehensive diagnosis and management of patients with neurologic disorders of the larynx.

Historically, speech treatment of individuals with neurologic voice disorders, especially those associated with degenerative diseases, has been challenging.[1] These individuals often have complex disorders that are progressive and involve multiple systems, including cognitive, sensory, and motor problems, as well as attention, vigilance, learning, and memory challenges.[1-4] These limitations can make it difficult to obtain successful treatment outcomes.

Recently, it has been demonstrated in humans and animals, through clinical and experimental studies, that effective exercise-based behavioral treatment of neurologically based motor disorders, including motor speech disorders (dysarthria), is possible.[2,5-9] Among the key elements of such successful treatment are intensive training, increased practice, and active engagement in tasks (salience). These key elements have also been shown to contribute to neural plasticity, brain reorganization, and neural protection, as evident in molecular and cellular studies in animals[10,11] and brain imaging and electrophysiologic studies in humans.[6,12-14] Importantly, the impact of such exercise has maximum effects when delivered early in the disease process. It has also been suggested that exercise could reactivate mechanisms of plasticity and enhance treatment of functional deficits. Given these facts, the impact of exercise, and its potential to promote or sustain brain plasticity, has moved to the forefront in management of symptoms accompanying neurologic disorders.

Our ability to embrace these principles of neural plasticity in the design of our speech treatments for individuals with neurologic voice disorders may allow us to optimize outcomes with these complex and challenging patients. Evidence to support that notion comes from outcome data of Lee Silverman Voice Treatment (LSVT)® LOUD, an intensive, high-effort voice treatment program that embraces many of the plasticity-inducing principles. LSVT LOUD has generated the first level-one evidence for a speech treatment for Parkinson disease through a series of randomized trials (RTCs).[2-4] Case studies also indicate effective treatment of speech disorders in other neurologic conditions such as multiple sclerosis,[15] cerebellar dysfunction,[16] stroke,[17] Down syndrome,[18] and cerebral palsy.[19] If we are to make a significant and lasting impact on speech and voice production in individuals with neurologic voice disorders, we may need to change our conventional treatment paradigms and embrace principles of neural plasticity in the design of our interventions.[20] Furthermore, to deliver treatment consistent with the plasticity-inducing intensity and dosage, we may need to turn to technology (Webcam, software, personal digital assistant [PDA]) to offer our patients feasible and adequate access to support learning and long-term maintenance. Some studies in these directions are already being conducted.[21,22]

♦ Speech Therapy Approaches for Laryngeal Disorders that Are Secondary to Neurologic Disorders

The speech therapy approaches presented in this chapter are mainly organized in relation to laryngeal dysfunction, rather than being associated with a specific neurologic condition, as has been done traditionally.[23,24] We assume that a direct relationship exists between the laryngeal dysfunction and the resulting sound of the voice and therefore the approach to treatment. We believe that this approach establishes the most direct path to improving the sound of the voice. This approach also accommodates the numerous sources of variation in voice characteristics accompanying neurologic disorders, such as compensatory behaviors, multiple neural pathologies, and neuropharmacologic effects. It also facilitates application of principles of normal laryngeal function to treatment. Specific information about the neurologic disorder is included when it is relevant for determining the most efficacious method to address the disorder.

Table 12.1 Summary of Laryngeal Disorders with Examples of Associated Neurologic Disorders, Perceptual Characteristics, and Therapy Goals and Techniques

Laryngeal Disorder	Examples of Associated Neurologic Disorder	Perceptual Characteristics	Therapy Goals and Techniques
Hypoadduction	Laryngeal nerve paralysis; Parkinson disease	Reduced loudness; breathy, hoarse quality	Increase loudness; increase adduction and respiratory support
Hyperadduction	Spasticity; extrapyramidal disorders	Pressed, harsh, strain-strangled quality	Reduce strained quality; relax laryngeal and respiratory musculature
Phonatory instability	Most neurologic disorders of the larynx	Tremorous, rough hoarse quality; pitch breaks; glottal fry	Increase steady, clear phonation; maximize respiratory and laryngeal coordination
Phonatory incoordination and prosody	Parkinson disease; ataxia	Reduced melody of speech; excessive melody of speech	Stimulate improved melody of speech; rate control
Voice-voiceless contrast	Parkinson disease	Continuous voicing	Emphasize other aspects of voicing contrasts, e.g., aspiration

When laryngeal dysfunction is a primary contributor to reduced speech intelligibility, speech therapy is designed to improve or compensate for the underlying disordered laryngeal physiology. Laryngeal dysfunctions in patients with neurologic disorders include problems in adducting the vocal folds (hypoadduction, hyperadduction), producing a stable voice (phonatory instability), and coordinating movements (respiratory-phonatory and phonatory-articulatory incoordination). These dysfunctions may reduce speech intelligibility by affecting the perceptual characteristics of voice pitch, loudness, quality, intonation (prosodic modulation of pitch), and voice-voiceless contrasts **(Table 12.1)**.[25]

When laryngeal function is affected due to a neurologic disorder, other components of the speech production system are frequently affected as well.[23,24] Therefore, it is important to assess laryngeal function and apply treatment strategies within the framework of the entire speech mechanism. One such framework includes the following functional components that are primarily responsible for producing speech: the abdominal muscles, diaphragm, rib cage and associated muscles, larynx, velopharynx, tongue-pharynx, middle portion of the tongue, anterior portion of the tongue, jaw, and lips. **(Fig. 12.1)**.[26] Using a sampling of perceptual, acoustic, aerodynamic, and physiologic measures, the speech pathologist evaluates the individual and the interactive contribution of all components of the speech production system to a reduction in speech intelligibility, and makes hypotheses about the disordered physiology underlying the speech problem **(Fig. 12.2)**.[27] This information, used in combination with otolaryngologic and neurologic findings, is likely to result in a program of speech therapy that maximizes treatment outcomes for each patient.

type and extent of hypoadduction may be associated with the site and extent of the related neurologic damage.[24] Hypoadduction is typically associated with lower motor neuron involvement, which is characterized by flaccid paresis (weakness) or paralysis (immobility), atrophy (in the case of amyotrophic lateral sclerosis), or fatigue (in the case of myasthenia gravis).

Some patients do not adduct the vocal folds and are unable to produce phonation voluntarily. Common etiologies for this form of hypoadduction are closed head injury with brainstem contusion[28,29] and brainstem cerebrovascular accident (CVA). Other patients can only partially

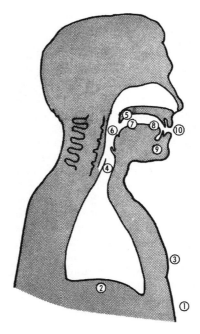

Fig. 12.1 Functional components of the speaking mechanism, showing areas where the airstream may be valved.
(From Netsell R. Lip electromyography in the dysarthrias. Paper presented at the American Speech and Hearing Association, San Francisco, 1972. Adapted with permission.)

◆ Problems with Vocal Fold Adduction

Hypoadduction

Certain neurologic disorders are accompanied by inadequate vocal fold adduction or hypoadduction. The particular

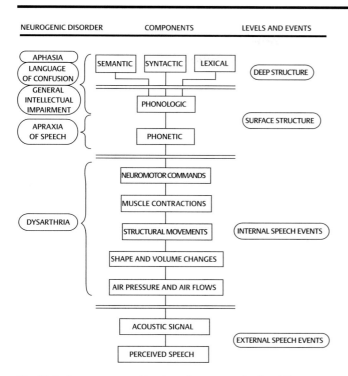

Fig. 12.2 Components and levels and events involved in different neuropathologies of speech and language.
(From Kent R. Study of vocal tract characteristics in the dysarthrias. Paper presented at the Veterans Administration Workshop on Motor Speech Disorders, Madison, WI, 1976. Adapted with permission.)

adduct their vocal folds during speech. This may be unilateral or bilateral and result from damage to (or a disease of) the laryngeal adductor muscles (lateral cricoarytenoid and interarytenoids), to the nerve that innervates them (recurrent laryngeal nerve branch of the vagus),[30] or to a disease of brainstem motor neurons, such as flaccid forms of amyotrophic lateral sclerosis.[24,31] Other patients may adduct their vocal folds posteriorly, but the folds do not close medially and are said to be bowed. This form of hypoadduction has been associated with bilateral superior laryngeal nerve paralysis[24,32] and Parkinson disease (PD).[33] Progressive hypoadduction involving restriction of adductor-abductor movements, associated with fatigue accompanying continuous talking, has been observed in patients with myasthenia gravis.[32]

The major effects of hypoadduction on speech intelligibility are reduced loudness, breathy or hoarse voice quality, and, in some cases, diplophonia (the perception of two pitches). Aerodynamic and acoustic data may show high airflow, short or absent closed phase, low signal-to-noise ratio, reduced intensity range, and short maximum duration.[34,35] In certain cases of hypoadduction, patients may be unable to produce adequate voice–voiceless contrasts. Hypernasality and nasal air escape may accompany laryngeal paralysis or paresis if the pharyngeal branch of the motor vagus is affected. Thus, careful examination of the velopharyngeal system is necessary whenever hypoadduction of the vocal folds is present.[24]

Speech Therapy

Laryngeal The primary focus of voice therapy for patients without voluntary phonation is to obtain regular vocal fold vibration (voicing) through adduction of the vocal folds with sufficient subglottal air pressure.[36] This may be accomplished by attempting to elicit emotive or primitive phonatory behaviors (i.e., laughing, coughing) on a repetitive basis with simultaneous stimulation of subglottal pressure using externally applied abdominal pressure.[37] Sapir and Aronson[38] reported that digital manipulation of the larynx, stimulated coughing, and prodding to phonate successfully elicited phonation in two patients with whispered phonation accompanying closed head injury. The larynx in these individuals was intact and functional for swallowing and other vegetative functions, suggesting that the abnormal voice was related to limbic–prefrontal lobe dysfunction rather than true paralysis or apraxia of the vocal folds. For patients with reduced adduction accompanying muscle or nerve damage, the primary goal is to increase loudness and reduce breathy, hoarse voice quality by increasing vocal fold adduction and reducing undue vocal fold tension. Procedures to accomplish this are probably the best referenced of all techniques in the area of neurologic voice disorders. The techniques include pushing, pulling, and lifting while phonating.[36] When done as a systematic exercise, progressing from vowels to syllables to words to phrases, pushing helps to strengthen the muscles of adduction. In certain cases, these adduction exercises are included as part of LSVT LOUD (described below) to increase loudness in patients with bowed vocal folds accompanying PD.[39,40] Other adduction enhancing techniques include hard glottal attack, turning the head to one side or the other (to increase tension on the paralyzed fold), digital manipulation of the thyroid cartilage (to approximate the vocal folds more closely),[24] and speaking at a higher or lower pitch (to make use of the adductory function of the cricothyroid muscle).[36] Some of these techniques are combined with auditory training and kinesthetic feedback so that the patient can learn how to keep the vocal folds adducted by maintaining audible phonation with good voice quality. Such auditory and kinesthetic monitoring and training[41] are facilitated through various forms of biofeedback, including visual feedback of vocal fold adduction through videoendoscopy,[42,43] or intensity feedback through a voice light or Visi-Pitch.

Support Systems To facilitate the goal of increased loudness and improved quality, the respiratory system is often a focus of treatment. The goal is to achieve a consistent subglottal pressure during speech that is produced with minimal fatigue and appropriate breath group lengths.[44] The first step may be to stabilize body posture.[45] This may involve the use of support devices such as neck braces, girdling, expiratory boards, or paddles that are implemented in collaboration with the physical therapist and physician. For some patients, working on respiratory support from the supine position is most effective.[46]

Once the patients' postural support is maximized, they are instructed, through a hierarchical schedule, to optimally inhale and increase air intake, sustain expiratory airflow for as long as possible, control the rate of expiratory air flow, and produce various levels of subglottal pressure. Various procedures assist patients in increasing systematically the duration and the level of air pressure they can sustain.[47] Other techniques to strengthen respiratory muscles include exercises against a resistive load, tracking of a visible analogue of respiratory behavior, and controlled exhalation.[48] A 4-week, daily intensive respiratory training with a pressure threshold device and with a regimented treatment protocol based on principles of neural plasticity training has been shown to markedly improve expiratory muscle strength in patients with multiple sclerosis and spinal cord injury.[49]

To train improved coordination of respiration and phonation, various techniques such as maximum duration vowel phonation[39,40] and phonation with simultaneous respiratory (e.g., Respitrace) and vocal (e.g., Visi-Pitch) feedback have been suggested.[50] During speech tasks, patients are encouraged to take breaths more often, produce fewer syllables on each exhalation,[41,51] and initiate phonation at the beginning of exhalation.[37] The goal is to assist patients in organizing their linguistic output into units that are manageable by patients' peripheral speech mechanism[41] and that afford them the greatest gains in speech intelligibility. Patients with hypoadduction may also be encouraged to maximize oral resonance to increase loudness and quality. Linguistically appropriate pauses may help breathing, speech perception, and intelligibility. The use of articulatory gestures to increase vocal loudness is also justified by evidence for orofacial biomechanical and sensorimotor (reflexogenic) influences on vocal folds closure and muscle tone.[52]

In the case of velopharyngeal insufficiency associated with vagus motor impairment, surgical or prosthetic intervention may be necessary to provide adequate physiologic support, after which speech therapy is initiated.[41] Management of the velopharyngeal and articulatory mechanisms are summarized elsewhere.[53,54]

Speech Therapy and Medical Management in Combination for Hypoadduction

In certain cases of hypoadduction, a combination of medical management and voice/speech therapy offers maximum results. Voice therapy may precede surgery, or vice versa, for optimal management. After such surgery, speech therapy teaches patients how to achieve maximum vocal efficiency and optimal voice quality and prosody within the new range of function afforded by their modified laryngeal mechanism. In cases where the paralysis is at a paramedian position, with the voice being only moderately affected, it is suggested that the physician and voice clinician should prescribe voice therapy; surgery should be considered only if there is no significant improvement.[55,56] In other cases, such as in myasthenia gravis, the primary improvement in voice production may occur with medical management (thymectomy or anticholinesterase drugs)[57]; intensive exercises to increase vocal fold adduction should not be attempted. To prevent fatigue in these patients, speech therapy may help them learn to economize air intake and use and to minimize vocal effort by using short phrases. Before medical management or speech therapy, or when neither provides the necessary gains in speech intelligibility, augmentative forms of communication (discussed below) may be useful.

Hypophonia and dysphonia in individuals with PD have been shown to improve in small pilot studies with repetitive transcranial magnetic stimulation (rTMS) of the primary motor cortex (M1)–mouth area[58] and transoral vocal fold collagen injection.[59] Hypophonia and dysphonia in other neurologic diseases affecting the laryngeal nerves may also benefit from surgical and prosthetic medialization of the vocal folds.[60]

Case Example Mr. J., a 60-year-old man, was diagnosed with PD 3 years ago. One of his first complaints was the inability to project his voice. Speech assessment revealed that reduced loudness and a breathy, hoarse voice quality were the characteristics that reduced his speech intelligibility most significantly. His intonation was characterized as flat. Acoustic data supported these perceptual observations. Laryngologic examination revealed moderately bowed vocal folds. An intensive (daily) program of speech therapy (LSVT LOUD) was initiated, which focused on increasing vocal loudness and sensory retraining. Techniques included optimizing vocal fold adduction through increasing vocal loudness, maximizing respiratory and phonatory coordination and phonatory stability by practicing maximum duration sustained vowel phonation and generalizing this louder voice into speech tasks. At the end of 1 month of intensive therapy, Mr. J.'s speech intelligibility improved; his voice was louder and steadier, and had greater intonation. Both he and his family noticed that he was much easier to understand. These observations were supported by acoustic measures. Posttreatment laryngeal examination revealed improved vocal fold adduction. It was recommended that Mr. J. continue to engage in daily voice practice at home and remember to "think LOUD."

Hypoadduction may also occur secondary to conversion disorder and other psychological causes. Coexisting neurogenic and psychogenic dysphonia (such as a paralyzed vocal fold in the paramedian position with complete aphonia that is alleviated with one session of voice therapy) may be seen in some patients. Thus, careful differential diagnosis and special therapy methods are needed for treating the dysphonia.[61–63]

Hyperadduction

Certain neurologic disorders result in excess vocal fold adduction, or hyperadduction. In some cases, the ventricular (false) vocal folds may hyperadduct as well.[24,64] The particular type and extent of hyperadduction may be associated with the site and extent of the related neurologic damage. Hyperadduction most frequently occurs in cases of bilateral upper motor neuron system disorders characterized by spasticity or hypertonicity, and extrapyramidal system diseases accompanied by abnormal involuntary movements (e.g., tics, chorea, dystonia) that may be focal or generalized.[24] Hyperadduction may also occur in cases of long-term use of psychotropic and antiparkinson drugs and is then considered a symptom of tardive dyskinesia.[65] In some patients, hyperadduction is so extreme that phonation cannot be initiated or sustained, or can be sustained only with abrupt voice breaks or long duration of aphonia (no voicing). A severe case of adductory laryngospasm associated with adductor spastic dysphonia is an example. Other patients may have moderate hyperadduction, which results in a strained-strangled, harsh voice quality with excessively low pitch and reduced loudness,[24] such as in cases of bilateral stroke (pseudobulbar palsy) and spastic cerebral palsy. Still other patients have a mild, continuous hyperadduction, resulting in pitch breaks and a pressed, strained, harsh quality, such as in cases of spastic amyotrophic lateral sclerosis.[24] When random periods or "bursts" of hyperadduction or hypoadduction occur, they are frequently associated with dyskinesias such as those associated with Huntington disease, dystonia, and myoclonus. The resulting periods of adductory or abductory laryngeal spasm may generate random, intermittent periods of spastic or breathy voice arrest, respectively.[24,66,67] In the case of myoclonus or severe tremor, vocal arrests may be rhythmical.[24]

It should be pointed out that hyperadduction may be compensatory. For example, a patient may have weak respiratory support or velopharyngeal closure and hyperadduct to manage the airstream for adequate loudness.[48] The harsh, high-pitched voice with reduced loudness and pitch variations observed in patients with spinal forms of multiple sclerosis has been associated with the extreme neck and laryngeal tension and upper thoracic and clavicular breathing adopted by these patients in an attempt to produce phrases of normal length.[25]

The major effect of hyperadduction on speech intelligibility is a quality disorder ranging from a pressed, strained, harsh voice to inaudible speech. Smitheran and Hixon[68] reported extremely high measures of laryngeal resistance for a speaker who had a strained-strangled voice quality after multiple, bilateral cerebrovascular accidents. Aerodynamic and acoustic data reveal decreased mean airflow rate[69] and reduced fundamental frequency and fundamental frequency range associated with such hyperadduction.

Speech Therapy

Laryngeal The primary focus of voice therapy for patients with hyperadduction is to decrease the pressed, strained voice by reducing vocal fold hyperadduction. Behavioral procedures to accomplish this include those designed to relax laryngeal musculature and facilitate easy voice onset. These techniques frequently begin with progressive whole-body relaxation[70] and then focus on relaxing laryngeal musculature. Humming, confidential speech, chanting, and other types of vocalizations mentioned below may help reduce hyperadduction. Techniques of biofeedback-enhanced relaxation have been applied to laryngeal musculature.[71,72] The specific form of feedback may be electromyographic or visual (videoendoscopy). Another approach for relaxing laryngeal muscle tension and thereby hyperadduction includes manual massage of extrinsic laryngeal muscles.[24,25]

Some approaches such as "chewing," "yawn-sigh," chanting, and delayed auditory feedback have been used to teach more relaxed and less hyperadducted phonation.[36] This relaxed voice production is then shaped into more natural sounding conversational speech. The breathy sigh can be shaped into a relaxed vowel, then to single-syllable words beginning with "H," followed by open mouth vowels and a nasal consonant or continuant, followed by short duration nasal humming.[73]

Improved voice quality has been reported in a strained-strangled voice when a speaker raises his pitch, rotates his head backward, and initiates utterances from a high lung volume; these behaviors are associated with decreased airway resistance.[68] It was suggested that improved voice quality was the result of passive abduction or relaxation of the vocal folds brought about by the tracheal tug associated with a lower diaphragm position at a higher lung volume level.[68]

Support Systems To facilitate improved voice quality, the respiratory system is often a focus of treatment in patients with hyperadduction. The goal of respiratory treatment is to achieve consistent, steady airflow with relaxed respiratory musculature.[73] The first step may be stabilization of posture. Supporting the abdominal musculature with an elastic band or selective positioning in a reclining wheelchair has helped some patients with spastic dysarthria produce better air flow with less effort and reduced strained-strangled phonation.[73] Once the patients' postural support is maximized, they may then be instructed in procedures of relaxed abdominal breathing[73] to provide the greatest respiratory support with the minimum muscle tension throughout the speech mechanism. These activities may be combined with the progressive relaxation procedures referenced earlier. To remove the laryngeal focus and encourage reduced hyperadduction, some clinicians[74] encourage "placement" of the vocal resonance in the frontal nasal area (also called "tone focus" or "mask area"). A modest improvement in articulatory precision without overflow of tension into the oral or laryngeal/respiratory musculature also has been suggested to improve overall speech intelligibility.[73]

Speech Therapy and Medical Management in Combination

In some patients with hyperadduction, a combination of voice/speech therapy and medical management affords the greatest vocal outcome. For example, adductor spastic dysphonia is a disorder of hyperadduction that has a reputation of being especially resistant to speech therapy.[24] In most patients with adductor spastic dysphonia, the dysphonia is symptomatic of neurologic disorders such as laryngeal dystonia or tremor.[24] However, the dysphonia may be simulated by nonorganic mechanisms such as conversion disorder and musculoskeletal tension disorder. Thus, careful differential diagnosis is important.[24,37,61] Also, these etiologies have different prognoses, with psychogenic spasmodic dysphonia responding favorably, and neurologically based spasmodic dysphonia responding less favorably or not at all to behavioral voice therapy. The following approaches have been suggested[24]: (1) symptomatic voice therapy including musculoskeletal tension reduction, establishing natural pitch, "tone focus in the mask area," and abdominal breathing[74] when the spastic dysphonia is due to excess muscular tension; (2) symptomatic voice therapy followed by psychotherapy when the spastic dysphonia is due to a conversion disorder or other psychogenic causes[37,61]; and (3) medical management such as recurrent laryngeal nerve section or avulsion[75] and botulinum toxin injection[76] when the disorder is associated with a neurologic disorder.

When medical intervention for hyperadduction is performed,[75,76] voice/speech therapy procedures designed to maximize vocal efficiency are recommended. For example, if the postsurgical voice is breathy, techniques to elevate the pitch and increase glottal adduction have been suggested.[36]

Certain forms of hyperadduction accompanying extrapyramidal disorders (e.g., Huntington disease) appear resistant to voice/speech therapy. The primary treatment approaches for individuals with such hyperkinesias involve medical (pharmacologic and surgical intervention) rather than behavioral management.[77] Because the speech symptoms are so closely related to the underlying movement disorder, any improvement in speech symptoms depends on modification of the severity of the movement disorder.[77] The primary voice/speech therapy for these patients may involve instructions about managing verbal interactions, such as (1) maintaining eye contact, (2) asking listeners to inform the patient when he has not been understood, (3) repeating a word when an abnormal movement has interfered, and (4) introducing the topic of conversation. For certain of these patients, it may be appropriate to consider augmentative forms of communication (see below).

♦ Problems with Phonatory Stability

Phonatory Stability and Voice Production

The ability to produce a tonal, pleasant voice, with smooth changes in pitch and loudness depends on the symmetry of the vocal folds, vocal fold tissue mass and stiffness distribution, vocal fold closure, and the three-dimensional configuration of the vocal folds. Biomechanical asymmetries (such as unilateral tissue changes) may give rise to significant vocal fold motion asymmetries.[78] Neuromuscular innervation abnormalities may give rise to laryngeal muscle perturbations,[79] abnormal glottal adduction behavior, airflow disturbances from abnormal respiratory muscle function, and vocal tract tissue oscillations. Mucus accumulation on the vocal folds can give rise to transients that sound like sharp "bubbling." Turbulent airflow through the glottis is an aperiodic noise source that causes the perception of breathiness.

The regularity of phonation can be measured or inferred from visual recordings (e.g., from high-speed photography),[69] or from signals related to vocal fold movement such as the electroglottograph signal[80] and the photoglottograph signal.[81] Typically, however, perturbation measures have been from an accelerometer or a microphone (airborne acoustic) signal.[82]

Increased Phonatory Instability

Certain neurologic disorders are accompanied by increased phonatory instability. The particular type, extent, and regularity of instability may be associated with the site and extent of the related neurologic damage.[83] Long-term fluctuations (generally 5- to 12-Hz fluctuations in pitch or loudness) and short-term changes (cycle-to-cycle fluctuations) can occur as well as random or continuous use of alternative modes of voicing such as ventricular phonation, glottal fry, or diplophonia.[24] These forms of instability may occur singly or in combination and may be related to the problems of adduction discussed previously.

One type of long-term phonatory instability is vocal tremor. Vocal tremor has been associated with oscillations in the adductory-abductory system, in cricothyroid muscle activity, in the activity of extrinsic laryngeal muscles (indirectly), and in ventricular fold activity.[84,85] Frequently, tremor may occur simultaneously in respiratory, laryngeal, and orofacial musculature.[23] The neurologic origin of tremor is thought to be a central tremor generator located in the cerebellum, basal ganglia, subthalamic nucleus, or thalamus, or a peripheral stretch reflex.[86] Vocal tremor has been observed in many neurologic diseases such as PD,[24,83] postencephalitic parkinsonism,[87] essential tremor,[24,88] ataxia,[89] and spinal muscular atrophy.[88] The major effect of long-term instabilities on speech intelligibility is perceived tremor, shakiness, or quivering in the voice. Acoustic data reveal frequency and amplitude oscillations ranging from 5 to 12 Hz.[24,88]

Short-term phonatory instabilities have been related to cycle-to-cycle irregularities in the adductor-abductor system or to irregularities in vocal fold elasticity.[90] Although the neural bases of short-term instabilities are not well understood, they have been associated with variations in single motor unit activity.[91] The major effect of short-term instabilities on speech intelligibility is a perceived hoarse or rough voice quality.[92] Acoustic data show abnormally high measures of cycle-to-cycle differences in amplitude (shimmer) and time (jitter) in neurologic diseases such as myotonic muscular dystrophy,[83] PD,[83] and amyotrophic lateral sclerosis.[31]

Ventricular (false) fold phonation, glottal fry phonation, and diplophonia are forms of phonatory instability accompanying several neurologic disorders of the larynx such as Huntington disease,[66] adductor spastic dysphonia,[24] and unilateral nerve paralysis.[24] Ventricular phonation, which may develop as a result of excess muscular tension or as a compensatory form of phonation,[24] is hoarse and low-pitched, with restricted pitch and loudness ranges. Glottal fry, which may be produced by the true or ventricular folds or both in combination, may be produced under conditions of extreme glottal resistance (tension)[93] or with flaccid (relaxed) vocal folds approximated tightly with very little airflow and very little subglottal pressure.[94] Diplophonia, which is the simultaneous production of two pitches, may occur in cases of unilateral vocal fold paralysis when each vocal fold apparently vibrates at a different frequency or in cases where both the ventricular folds and the true folds vibrate.[24,95] All of these instabilities adversely affect the quality of voice and reduce speech intelligibility.

Speech Therapy

The major focus of voice/speech therapy for patients with phonatory instability is to reduce the unsteady, hoarse, rough voice quality by targeting steady, clear phonation. Patients are encouraged to maximize respiratory and laryngeal coordination, as discussed previously, to sustain steady voicing with consistently good quality. Treatments discussed earlier to promote more efficient vocal fold adduction have been reported to have positive effects on phonatory stability as well. For example, improved voice quality and reduced acoustic measures of phonatory instability (jitter and shimmer) have been measured in patients with PD after therapy designed to increase vocal loudness and increased adduction.[39-41,96] Speaking on inhalation has been suggested as a technique to temporarily facilitate true vocal fold vibration in patients using ventricular phonation.[97] In some patients, excess saliva may interfere with stability of voice production, and reminders to swallow or drink water before speaking may be helpful.

Vocal instability (especially short-term) is likely to occur when the vocal folds are not optimally adducted, when there is asymmetry in tension in the vocal folds, when the vocal folds are highly stiff, when airflow between the vocal fold is rapid, or a combination of these.[98] Such conditions often occur with vocal fold paralysis and when the patient attempts to force the voice out. One way to reduce this effect is to teach the patient to produce a more relaxed phonation, through humming, chanting, confidential speech, or yawn-sigh techniques. As the patient learns to improve voice quality, treatment is geared toward gradually increasing voice intensity toward normalcy, but without deterioration in voice quality.

Auditory training (e.g., differentiating between tonal and hoarse, breathy harsh voice), and enhanced auditory and visual feedback (e.g., language master, tape recorder, Kay Elemetrics Inc. [Lincoln Park, NJ] Visi-Pitch) might help the patient in monitoring his voice quality. Visual feedback (videoendoscopy) has been useful in elimination of ventricular fold phonation.[43,99]

Speech Therapy and Medical Intervention in Combination

In certain cases of phonatory instability, optimum voice is obtained through a combination of voice/speech therapy and medical management. For example, pharmacologic treatment may provide the necessary changes in underlying laryngeal physiology to generate a more stable voice with the assistance of voice/speech therapy. In some patients with PD, changes in phonatory stability appear to be related to neuropharmacologic treatment.[100,101]

Although enhanced respiratory and phonatory interaction may positively affect secondary (compensatory) behaviors accompanying vocal tremor, voice/speech therapy techniques have not been effective in reducing the primary symptom of vocal tremor.[24] Medical intervention (surgical or pharmacologic) may offer some relief.[100,101]

♦ Problems with Prosody

Many neurologic disorders are accompanied by disordered prosody,[23,37] which includes problems with stress patterning, intonation, and rate-rhythm.[102] The vocal control prerequisites for prosody include loudness variation, adequate duration of phonation, appropriate pitch level, pitch variation, and acceptable voice quality.[102] The particular type and extent of the disordered prosody may be associated with the site and extent of the related neurologic disorder.[103] For example, reduced prosody, or "aprosody," has been reported in patients with PD or right hemisphere damage,[103] and has been characterized by reduced loudness, monopitch, diminished stress contrasts, and rate abnormalities.[23] In contrast, disordered prosody, has been observed in patients with ataxic dysarthria, hyperkinetic dysarthria, and apraxia of speech, and has been characterized by excessive sweeps of fundamental frequency, scanning, staccato, dissociated, and segregated patterns.[23,103] Because disordered prosody interferes with speech intelligibility and acceptability in many patients,[37,104] speech therapy procedures have been designed to improve prosodic disorders.

Speech Therapy

For patients with reduced prosody or aprosody, the goal is to heighten the relationship between the meaning and production of an utterance.[37] If a patient understands the meaning of the utterance yet cannot signal linguistic stress, treatment should involve identifying the components of stress that the speaker can control.[37] In one study, increased F_o variation in reading was measured in a group of individuals with PD after 1 month of therapy directed toward stimulating the vocal production prerequisites underlying prosody.[39,40] The results of therapy were increases in maximum duration of phonation, maximum fundamental frequency range, phonatory stability, and intelligibility.[39,40,66] For individuals with PD with excessive speaking rates, rate control also may be an effective way to improve prosody.[105] Gesturing, such as touching a place on a pacing board with the production of each syllable, has been suggested for modifying rate and stress.[106] This gestural accompaniment may allow a speaker to slow the rate and use appropriate stress to improve intelligibility.[106]

For patients with disordered or excessive prosody, which is frequently seen in ataxic patients, it has been suggested that treatment should generally involve reducing excessive fundamental frequency and intensity variations and increased use of duration adjustments such as vowel prolongations and pausing.[41,107] Use of breath grouping,[37] contrastive stress drills,[41,66] contrastive intonation contour drills,[108] loudness manipulation,[41] and various forms of visual feedback (e.g., with the use of the Visi-Pitch) have been suggested as useful therapy approaches.

The LSVT LOUD (Lee Silverman Voice Treatment) Within the past 20 years, a voice treatment method known as the LSVT LOUD and developed by Ramig and colleagues[40] has generated much interest among clinicians and researchers because of its powerful effects on various aspects of voice and speech in individuals with neurologic disorders, and because of the extensive research studies that have documented its therapeutic effects, by comparing it to an alternative speech therapy, or to no therapy.[2,3,8,109,110] The LSVT LOUD was developed as a PD-specific approach that trains amplitude (increased vocal loudness) as a single motor control parameter, thereby targeting the proposed pathophysiologic mechanisms underlying bradykinesia/hypokinesia—mainly inadequate scaling of agonist muscle activation.[111] LSVT LOUD also trains individuals with PD to recalibrate their motor and perceptual systems so that they are less inclined to downscale (reduce amplitude) speech movement parameters. As well, it is geared toward overcoming or compensating for deficits in internal cuing and self-regulation of vocal effort during speech production. The LSVT LOUD is delivered in a manner consistent with theories of motor learning[45] and skill acquisition, as well as principles of neural plasticity (e.g., intensity, complexity, saliency).[2,20]

In brief, the LSVT LOUD uses high-effort healthy loud phonation to encourage maximum phonatory efficiency and coactivation and coordination of speech subsystems.[3,52] Patients are taken through exercises on a daily basis, repeatedly practicing and emphasizing maximum-duration loud phonations, maximum high- and low-pitch phonations, and speech exercises with improved loudness. This improved phonation is then carried over into speech and conversation following a standardized hierarchy, with focus on monitoring the amount of effort required to sustain sufficient vocal loudness (calibration). No direct attention is given to speech rate, prosodic pitch inflection, or articulation. Therapy is administered four times per week over four successive weeks, each session lasting 50 to 60 minutes. In addition, there are daily homework exercises (on treatment and nontreatment days) and daily assignments to use the louder voice with other speakers in daily living.

To date, physiologic, acoustic, perceptual, and clinical trial studies involving over 200 individuals with PD (included are those treated by LSVT LOUD, those treated by an alternative speech therapy, and those awaiting therapy) and 40 healthy controls (receiving no treatment) have documented widespread, long-term, therapeutic effects of LSVT LOUD on respiratory- laryngeal[112,113] and orofacial functions,[52,114-117] with evidence of improved vocal loudness,[110,118] voice quality,[96] prosodic pitch inflection,[118] speech articulation,[52] and overall speech quality[110] and intelligibility.[25] Improvements in tongue motility and strength,[117] swallowing,[115] and facial expression[116] with LSVT LOUD have also been reported, even though these functions were not directly targeted for therapy. Brain imaging studies using ^{15}O positron emission tomography have also documented marked changes in brain function consistent with speech improvement following LSVT LOUD.[12,14] Specifically, although stimulated loud phonation prior to the administration of LSVT LOUD activated cortical premotor areas, particularly the supplementary motor area (SMA), after the completion of the LSVT LOUD program, SMA activity was normalized, and increased activity in the basal ganglia (right putamen) suggested a shift from abnormal cortical motor activation to normal subcortical organization of speech-motor output. The LSVT LOUD-induced changes also indicated an increase in activity in right anterior insula and right dorsolateral prefrontal cortex, suggesting that LSVT LOUD recruits a phylogenetically old, preverbal communication system involved in vocalization and emotional communication (consistent with multisystem effects of LSVT LOUD). Another interpretation is that the LSVT LOUD improves vocal vigilance and attention to action, which are necessary to overcome the hypophonia and to maintain long-term treatment gains. Excessive activity in the auditory cortex prior to LSVT LOUD and its marked reduction to normal levels after LSVT LOUD also suggests improvement in brain function. In a recent review of treatment of dysarthria, the members of the U.S. Academy of Neurologic Communications Disorders and Sciences (ANCDS) considered the LSVT LOUD to be the most efficacious behavioral method to improve voice and speech and related orofacial functions such as swallowing and facial expression in individuals with PD, and to have marked therapeutic effects on voice and speech in individuals with other neurologic diseases, such as multiple sclerosis, cerebellar dysfunction, cerebral palsy, and stroke.[119]

The treatment is specifically aimed at the most likely etiologic factors in speech deficits in PD patients, namely, deficits in sensorimotor gating and internal cuing, scaling of agonist muscle activation and movement amplitude, and auditory perception and self-regulation of vocal effort. Follow-up studies indicate that the therapeutic effects of the LSVT LOUD are maintained even 1[110] and 2 years posttreatment.[120] These findings, along with the intensive, repetitive, and cognitively nondemanding features of the LSVT LOUD, strongly suggest that this behavioral treatment can potentially play an important role in neural plasticity and possibly in neural protection.[2,20]

We discussed the LSVT LOUD separately from the other therapeutic methods because of its spreads of effects, unlike the other methods, which have more localized therapeutic effects. The LSVT LOUD is powerful not only because of its global effects, but also because of its maintenance of therapeutic effects over a long time period and in the context of a degenerative disease. Much more has to be learned about the neuropsychological mechanisms underlying the effects of LSVT LOUD. There are ongoing studies aimed at elucidating these mechanisms. Computer technology—such as the PDA, virtual reality, and telehealth systems—is being developed and tested to make treatments with intensive dosage, such as LSVT LOUD, accessible to patients with PD, and to optimize home practice.[21,22,121] The results from these pilot studies support the use of such technology, in terms of its therapeutic effects, cost-effectiveness, and potential availability to a large number of individuals. For PD patients who cannot adhere to the tight schedule of the LSVT LOUD, an alternative program, an extended version of the LSVT, or LSVT-X, spreads the treatment over 8 weeks (2 days of treatment with the clinician and 2 days of extensive home practice per week), instead of the classical 4 weeks program (4 days of treatment with the clinician per week). The results from the LSVT-X are similar to the classical program in terms of increased voice sound pressure level, decreased perceived voice handicap, and improved functional speech.[122] However, more research is needed to assess the LSVT-X benefits compared with those of the LSVT.

The effectiveness of the LSVT LOUD program may be compromised by several factors, including severe depression, dementia, atypical parkinsonism, or side effects of medication and neurosurgery.

♦ Augmentative Communication

When voice/speech therapy and medical management are unable to offer patients a level of communication intelligibility adequate for their needs, an augmentative communication system should be considered.[123] If the patient has only laryngeal pathology primarily affecting loudness, then an amplification system[124] or artificial larynx[125] may be useful. When other components of the speech mechanism are affected so that intelligible articulation is impossible, more sophisticated forms of augmentative communication systems may be appropriate.[126] These systems range from alphabet and word boards to computer-based systems.[37] Selection of the appropriate system for each patient is based on his or her cognitive, language, and motor skill abilities,[37] which actually may improve with the use of an augmentative system.[123] Issues related to augmentative systems are summarized elsewhere.[126]

♦ Other Considerations in Speech Therapy

Because the underlying physiologic breakdowns in patients with neurologic disorders are often severe and sometimes degenerative, the most realistic therapy goal may be compensated communication intelligibility,[25,41] rather than returning the speaker to normal communication.[24] In the case of degenerative diseases, the therapy goals may change as the disease progresses; thus, short-term and long-term goals and objectives should be consistent with the prognosis for the disorder, with the intent of maximizing communication effectiveness. Age, educational and vocational status, home environment, and communicative needs should be considered in the establishment of therapy goals.

Speech therapy for patients with some neurologic diseases, but not all (e.g., myasthenia gravis, amyotrophic lateral sclerosis), should be intensive, vigilant, and coordinated with other forms of treatment. Intensive therapy, with a direct focus on underlying laryngeal pathophysiology, offered maximum gains in speech intelligibility to a group of patients with PD[39,40,66] and other neurologic disorders, such as multiple sclerosis,[15] cerebellar dysfunction,[16] cerebral palsy,[19] and stroke.[17]

Today our approaches to voice/speech therapy for neurologic disorders of the larynx are based on systematic application of principles of normal laryngeal function[127,128] and generalization of techniques used in the treatment of patients with functional voice disorders[24,36] and dysarthrias.[25,37] Research that advances our knowledge of the relationship between voice characteristics and underlying laryngeal pathophysiologies will contribute to our future treatment success.

♦ Conclusion

The ability to generate maximally intelligible speech affords great psychological and communicative benefits to the patient with a neurologic disorder of the larynx. The combined services of the speech pathologist, neurologist, and otolaryngologist can provide the patient with optimal speech intelligibility. Because speech pathologists understand the production and rehabilitation of communication skills, they make an effective and necessary contribution to diagnosis and treatment of patients with neurologic disorders of the larynx.

It has been pointed out that most treatment methods for neurologically based voice and speech disorders have not been investigated scientifically and vigorously to assess their efficacy. The LSVT LOUD might be an exception to this observation, inasmuch as it has been extensively studied in a series of randomized control trials (RCTs) principles. The insights gained from these studies are significant, yet further research studies of the LSVT LOUD and other therapy methods should be performed to enhance our understanding of the mechanisms underlying the therapeutic effects, and to improve communication and quality of life in patients, their families, and society at large.

In the study, diagnosis, and treatment of dysphonia, we must not lose sight of the patient, for whom the impact of the dysphonia on communication, work, socialization, psychological well-being, and quality of life may be devastating.

Acknowledgment We gratefully acknowledge support from the National Institutes of Health, National Institute of Deafness and Other Communication Disorders (NIH NIDCD; grant RO1 DCO-1150).

Disclosure Lorraine O. Ramig and Cynthia M. Fox receive a lecturer honorarium and have ownership interest in LSVT Global (for-profit organization that runs training courses and sells products related to LSVT).

References

1. Trail M, Fox C, Ramig LO, Sapir S, Howard J, Lai EC. Speech treatment for Parkinson's disease. NeuroRehabilitation 2005;20:205–221

2. Fox CM, Ramig LO, Ciucci MR, Sapir S, McFarland DH, Farley BG. The science and practice of LSVT/LOUD: neural plasticity-principled approach to treating individuals with Parkinson disease and other neurological disorders. Semin Speech Lang 2006;27:283–299

3. Ramig LO, Fox C, Sapir S. Speech treatment for Parkinson's disease. Expert Rev Neurother 2008;8:297–309

4. Sapir S, Ramig L, Fox C. The Lee Silverman Voice Treatment [LSVT®] for voice, speech, and other orofacial disorders in people with Parkinson's disease. Future Neurol 2006;1:563–570

5. Kleim JA, Jones TA, Schallert T. Motor enrichment and the induction of plasticity before or after brain injury. Neurochem Res 2003;28:1757–1769

6. Liepert J, Miltner WH, Bauder H, et al. Motor cortex plasticity during constraint-induced movement therapy in stroke patients. Neurosci Lett 1998;250:5–8

7. Ramig LO, Countryman S, Thompson L, Horii Y. A comparison of two forms of intensive speech treatment for Parkinson disease. J Speech Hear Res 1995;38:1232–1251

8. Sapir S, Ramig L, Countryman S, Fox C. Voice, speech, and swallowing disorders. In: Factor S, Weiner F, eds. Parkinson Disease: Diagnosis and Clinical Management. 2nd ed. New York: Demos; 2008:77–97

9. Taub E. Harnessing brain plasticity through behavioral techniques to produce new treatments in neurorehabilitation. Am Psychol 2004;59:692–704

10. Tillerson JL, Cohen AD, Philhower J, Miller GW, Zigmond MJ, Schallert T. Forced limb-use effects on the behavioral and neurochemical effects of 6-hydroxydopamine. J Neurosci 2001;21:4427–4435

11. Tillerson JL, Caudle WM, Reveron ME, Miller GW. Exercise induces behavioral recovery and attenuates neurochemical deficits in rodent models of Parkinson's disease. Neuroscience 2003;119:899–911

12. Narayana S, Vogel D, Brown S, et al. Mechanism of action of voice therapy in Parkinson's hypophonia—a PET study. A poster presented at the 11th Annual Meeting of the Organization for Human Brain Mapping, Toronto, Ontario, Canada, 2005

13. Liotti M, Vogel D, Sapir S, Ramig L, New P, Fox P. Abnormal auditory gating in Parkinson's disease before and after LSVT. Paper presented at the Annual Meeting of the American Speech, Language and Hearing Association, Washington, DC, November 2000

14. Liotti M, Ramig LO, Vogel D, et al. Hypophonia in Parkinson's disease: neural correlates of voice treatment revealed by PET. Neurology 2003;60:432–440

15. Sapir S, Pawlas A, Ramig L, Seeley E, Fox C, Corboy J. Effects of intensive phonatory-respiratory treatment (LSVT®) on voice in two individuals with multiple sclerosis. J Med Speech-Lang Pathol 2001;9:141–151

16. Sapir S, Spielman J, Ramig LO, et al. Effects of intensive voice treatment (the Lee Silverman Voice Treatment [LSVT]) on ataxic dysarthria: a case study. Am J Speech Lang Pathol 2003;12:387–399

17. Mahler L, Ramig LO, Fox C. Intensive voice treatment (LSVT® LOUD) for dysarthria secondary to stroke. J Med Speech-Language Pathol in submission

18. Boliek CA, Wilson L, Smith J, et al. LSVT®: applications to the Down syndrome population. Am J Speech Lang Pathol, in preparation

19. Fox C, Boliek C. Intensive voice treatment for children with spastic cerebral palsy. J Speech Lang Hear Res, in revision

20. Ludlow CL, Hoit J, Kent R, et al. Translating principles of neural plasticity into research on speech motor control recovery and rehabilitation. J Speech Lang Hear Res 2008;51:S240–S258

21. Halpern AE, Matos C, Ramig LO, Petska J, Spielman J. LSVTC—a PDA supported speech treatment for Parkinson's disease. Paper presented at the Annual American Speech-Language-Hearing Association Meeting, Philadelphia, 2004

22. Halpern A, Matos C, Ramig L, Petska J, Spielman J, Bennett J. LSVTC—a PDA supported speech treatment for Parkinson's disease. Paper presented at the 9th International Congress of Parkinson's Disease and Movement Disorders, New Orleans, 2005

23. Duffy J. Motor Speech Disorders: Substrates, Differential Diagnosis, and Management. 2nd revised ed. New York: Elsevier Health Sciences; 2005

24. Aronson A. Clinical Voice Disorders: An Interdisciplinary Approach. New York: Thieme-Stratton; 1980

25. Ramig LO. The role of phonation in speech intelligibility: a review and preliminary data from patients with Parkinson's disease. In: Kent R, ed. Intelligibility in Speech Disorders: Theory, Measurement and Management. Amsterdam: John Benjamin, 1992

26. Netsell R. Speech physiology. In: Minifie FD, Hixon TJ, Williams F, eds. Normal Aspects of Speech, Hearing, and Language. Englewood Cliffs, NJ: Prentice-Hall; 1973

27. Kent RD. Study of vocal tract characteristics in the dysarthrias. Paper presented at the Veterans Administration Workshop on Motor Speech Disorders, Madison, WI, 1976

28. Von Cramon D. Traumatic mutism and the subsequent reorganization of speech functions. Neuropsychologia 1981;19:801–805

29. Vogel M, Von Cramon D. Dysphonia after traumatic midbrain damage: a follow-up study. Folia Phoniatr (Basel) 1982;34:150–159

30. Tucker HM. Vocal cord paralysis—1979: etiology and management. Laryngoscope 1980;90:585–590

31. Ramig LO, Scherer RC, Burton E, Titze IR, Horii Y. Acoustic analysis of voice in amyotrophic lateral sclerosis: a longitudinal case study. J Speech Hear Disord 1990;55:2–14

32. Neiman RF, Mountjoy JR, Alien EL. Myasthenia gravis focal to the larynx. Arch Otolaryngol 1975;101:569–570

33. Blumin JH, Pcolinsky DE, Atkins JP. Laryngeal findings in advanced Parkinson's disease. Ann Otol Rhinol Laryngol 2004;113:253–258

34. Bless DM. Voice disorders in the adult: treatment. In: Yoder DE, Kent RD, eds. Decision Making in Speech-Language Pathology. Philadelphia: BC Decker; 1988:140–143

35. Hirano M, Koike Y, von Leden H. Maximum phonation time and air usage during phonation. Clinical study. Folia Phoniatr (Basel) 1968;20:185–201

36. Boone DR, McFarlane SC. The Voice and Voice Therapy. 4th ed. Englewood Cliffs, NJ: Prentice-Hall; 1988

37. Yorkston KM, Beukelman DR, Bell KR. Clinical Management of Dysarthric Speakers. Boston: College-Hill Press; 1988

38. Sapir S, Aronson AE. Aphonia after closed head injury: aetiologic considerations. Br J Disord Commun 1985;20:289–296

39. Ramig LA, Mead CL, Scherer RC, Horii Y, Larson K, Kohler D. Voice therapy and Parkinson's disease: a longitudinal study of efficacy. Paper presented at the Clinical Dysarthria Conference, San Diego, 1988

40. Ramig LA, Mead CL, Winholtz W. Speech therapy: Parkinson's disease. A videotape of speech treatment for patients with Parkinson's disease. Produced by the Recording and Research Center of the Denver Center for the Performing Arts and the Lee Silverman Center for Parkinson's, 1988

41. Linebaugh CW. Treatment of flaccid dysarthria. In: Perkins WH, ed. Current Therapy of Communication Disorders: Dysarthria and Apraxia. New York: Thieme; 1983:59–67

42. McFarlane SC, Lavorato AS. The use of video endoscopy in the evaluation and treatment of dysphonia. Commun Disord 1984;9:117–126

43. Bastian R. Laryngeal image feedback for voice disorder patients. J Voice 1987;1/3:279–282

44. Netsell R, Daniel B. Dysarthria in adults: physiologic approach to rehabilitation. Arch Phys Med Rehabil 1979;60:502–508

45. Porter PB, Wurth B, Stowers S. Seating and positioning for communication. In: Yoder DE, Kent RD, eds. Decision Making in Speech-Language Pathology. Philadelphia: BC Decker; 1988:186–187

46. Hardy J. Cerebral Palsy. Englewood Cliffs, NJ: Prentice-Hall; 1983

47. Hixon TJ, Hawley JL, Wilson JL. An around-the-house device for the clinical determination of respiratory driving pressure: a note on making simple even simpler. J Speech Hear Disord 1982;47:413–415

48. Putnam AHB. Respiratory dysfunction: management. In: Yoder DE, Kent RD, eds. Decision Making in Speech-Language Pathology. Philadelphia: BC Decker; 1988:128–131

49. Sapienza CM, Wheeler K. Respiratory muscle strength training: functional outcomes versus plasticity. Semin Speech Lang 2006;27:236–244

50. Kent RD, Kent JF, Rosenbek JC. Maximum performance tests of speech production. J Speech Hear Disord 1987;52:367–387

51. Rubow R, Swift E. Microcomputer-based wearable biofeedback device to improve treatment carry-over in parkinsonian dysarthria. J Speech Hear Disord 1985;50:178–185

52. Sapir S, Spielman JL, Ramig LO, Story BH, Fox C. Effects of intensive voice treatment (the Lee Silverman Voice Treatment [LSVT]) on vowel articulation in dysarthric individuals with idiopathic Parkinson disease: acoustic and perceptual findings. J Speech Lang Hear Res 2007;50:899–912

53. Netsell R. Velopharyngeal dysfunction. In: Yoder DE, Kent RD, eds. Decision Making in Speech-Language Pathology. Philadelphia: BC Decker; 1988:150–151

54. Johns DF. Surgical and prosthetic management of neurogenic velopharyngeal incompetency in dysarthria. In: Johns DF, ed. Clinical Management of Neurogenic Communicative Disorders. Boston: Little, Brown; 1985

55. D'Alatri L, Galla S, Rigante M, Antonelli O, Buldrini S, Marchese MR. Role of early voice therapy in patients affected by unilateral vocal fold paralysis. J Laryngol Otol 2008;122:936–941

56. Miller S. Voice therapy for vocal fold paralysis. Otolaryngol Clin North Am 2004;37:105–119

57. Rontal M, Rontal E, Leuchter W, Rolnick M. Voice spectrography in the evaluation of myasthenia gravis of the larynx. Ann Otol Rhinol Laryngol 1978;87:722–728

58. Dias AE, Barbosa ER, Coracini K, Maia F, Marcolin MA, Fregni F. Effects of repetitive transcranial magnetic stimulation on voice and speech in Parkinson's disease. Acta Neurol Scand 2006;113:92–99

59. Sewall GK, Jiang J, Ford CN. Clinical evaluation of Parkinson's-related dysphonia. Laryngoscope 2006;116:1740–1744

60. Sapir S. Medical, surgical, and behavioral approaches to vocal therapeutics. Curr Opin Otolaryngol Head Neck Surg 1994;2:247–251

61. Sapir S. Psychogenic spasmodic dysphonia: a case study with expert opinions. J Voice 1995;9:270–281

62. Sapir S, Aronson AE. Coexisting psychogenic and neurogenic dysphonia: a source of diagnostic confusion. Br J Disord Commun 1987; 22:73–80

63. Sapir S, Aronson A. The relationship between psychopathology and speech and language disorders in neurologic patients. J Speech Hear Disord 1990;55:503–509

64. Davis P, Boone D, Carroll RL, Darvenzia P, Harrison G. Adductor spastic dysphonia: heterogeneity of physiological and phonatory characteristics. Ann Otol Rhinol Laryngol 1987;97:179–185

65. Portnoy RA. Hyperkinetic dysarthria as an early indicator of impending tardive dyskinesia. J Speech Hear Disord 1979;44:214–219

66. Ramig LA. Acoustic analysis of phonation in patients with Huntington's disease: preliminary report. Ann Otol Rhinol Laryngol 1986;95: 288–293

67. Shipp T, Mueller P, Zwitman D. Intermittent abductory dysphonia. J Speech Hear Disord 1980;45:281

68. Smitheran J, Hixon T. A clinical method for estimating laryngeal airway resistance during vowel production. J Speech Hear Disord 1981; 46:138–146

69. von Leden H. Objective measures of laryngeal function and phonation. Ann N Y Acad Sci 1968;155:56–67

70. McClosky DG. General techniques and specific procedures for certain voice problems. In: Cooper M, Cooper MH, eds. Approaches to Vocal Rehabilitation. Springfield, IL: Charles C Thomas; 1977: 138–152

71. Prosek RA, Montogomery AA, Walden BE, Schwartz DM. EMG biofeedback in the treatment of hyperfunctional voice disorders. J Speech Hear Disord 1978;43:282–294

72. Stemple JC, Weiler E, Whitehead W, Komray R. Electromyographic biofeedback training with patients exhibiting a hyperfunctional voice disorder. Laryngoscope 1980;90:471–475

73. Aten JL. Treatment of spastic dysarthria. In: Perkins WH, ed. Current Therapy of Communication Disorders: Dysarthria and Apraxia. New York: Thieme; 1983:69–78

74. Cooper M, Cooper MH. Approaches to Vocal Rehabilitation. Springfield, IL: Charles C Thomas; 1977

75. Netterville JL, Stone RE, Rainey C, Zealer D, Ossoff RH. Recurrent laryngeal nerve avulsion for the treatment of spastic dysphonia. Ann Otol Rhinol Laryngol 1991;100:10–14

76. Blitzer A, Brin M, Fahn S, Lovelace R. Localized injections of botulinum toxin for the treatment of focal laryngeal dystonia (spastic dysphonia). Laryngoscope 1988;98:193–197

77. Beukelman D. Treatment of hyperkinetic dysarthria. In: Perkins WH, ed. Current Therapy of Communication Disorders: Dysarthria and Apraxia. New York: Thieme; 1983:101–104

78. Isshiki N, Tanabe M, Ishizaka K, Broad D. Clinical significance of asymmetrical vocal cord tension. Ann Otol Rhinol Laryngol 1977; 86:58–66

79. Titze IR. A model for neurologic sources of aperiodicity in vocal fold vibration. J Speech Hear Res 1991;34:460–472

80. Horiguchi S, Haji T, Baer T, Gould WJ. Comparison of electroglottographic and acoustic waveform perturbation measures. In: Baer T, Sasaki C, Harris K, eds. Laryngeal Function in Phonation and Respiration. Boston: College-Hill Press; Little, Brown; 1987:509–518

81. Garrett BR, Hanson DG, Berke GS. Glottographic measures of laryngeal function in individuals with abnormal motor control. In: Baer T, Sasaki C, Harris K, eds. Laryngeal Function in Phonation and Respiration. Boston: College-Hill Press; Little, Brown; 1987:521–532

82. Horii Y, Fuller BF. Selected acoustic characteristics of voices before intubation and after extubation. J Speech Hear Res 1990;33:505–510

83. Ramig LA, Scherer RC, Titze IR, Ringel SP. Acoustic characteristics of voice of patients with neurological disease: a preliminary report. Ann Otol Rhinol Laryngol 1988;97:164–172

84. Ward PH, Hansen DG, Berci G. Observations on central neurologic etiology for laryngeal dysfunction. Ann Otol Rhinol Laryngol 1981; 90:430–441

85. Perez KS, Ramig LO, Smith ME, Dromey C. The Parkinson larynx: tremor and videostroboscopic findings. J Voice 1996;10:354–361

86. Desmedt J. Physiological tremor, pathological tremor and gradation of muscle force. Prog Clin Neurophysiol Basel: S. Karger. 1979

87. Ward PH, Hanson DG, Berci G. Photographic studies of the larynx in central laryngeal paresis and paralysis. Acta Otolaryngol 1981;91: 353–367

88. Ramig L, Shipp T. Comparative measures of vocal tremor and vocal vibrato. J Voice 1987;1/2:162–167

89. Yorkston KM, Beukelman DR. Ataxic dysarthria: treatment sequences based on intelligibility and prosodic considerations. J Speech Hear Disord 1981;46:398–404

90. Titze IR. Parameterization of the glottal area, glottal flow, and vocal fold contact area. J Acoust Soc Am 1984;75:570–580

91. Titze IR. A model for neurologic sources of aperiodicity in vocal fold vibration. J Speech Hear Res 1991;34:460–472

92. Yumoto E, Gould WJ, Baer T. Harmonics-to-noise ratio as an index of the degree of hoarseness. J Acoust Soc Am 1982;71:1544–1550

93. Case J. Neurogenic voice disorders. In: Case J, ed. Voice Disorders. Rockville, MD: Aspen; 1984
94. Zemlin WR. Speech and Hearing Science: Anatomy and Physiology. 2nd ed. Englewood Cliffs, NJ: Prentice-Hall; 1981
95. Garrett BR, Precoda K, Hansen DG. Diplophonia: features in the time domain. J Am Speech Lang Hear Assoc. 1987;29:91A
96. Baumgartner CA, Sapir S, Ramig LO. Voice quality changes following phonatory-respiratory effort treatment (LSVT) versus respiratory effort treatment for individuals with Parkinson disease. J Voice 2001; 15:105–114
97. Greene MCL. The Voice and Its Disorders. 4th ed. Philadelphia: JB Lippincott; 1980
98. Isshiki N. Progress in laryngeal framework surgery. Acta Otolaryngol 2000;120:120–127
99. D'Antonio L, Lotz W, Chait D, Netsell R. Perceptual-physiologic approach to evaluation and treatment of dysphonia. Ann Otol Rhinol Laryngol 1987;96:187–190
100. Sanabria J, Ruiz PG, Gutierrez R, et al. The effect of levodopa on vocal function in Parkinson's disease. Clin Neuropharmacol 2001;24:99–102
101. Jiang J, Lin E, Wang J, Hanson DG. Glottographic measures before and after levodopa treatment in Parkinson's disease. Laryngoscope 1999;109:1287–1294
102. Kent RD. The dysarthric or apraxic client. In: Yoder DE, Kent RD, eds. Decision Making in Speech-Language Pathology. Philadelphia: BC Decker; 1988:156–157
103. Kent RD, Rosenbek J. Prosodic disturbance and neurogenic lesions. Brain Lang 1982;15:259–291
104. De Bodt MS, Hernández-Díaz HM, Van De Heyning PH. Intelligibility as a linear combination of dimensions in dysarthric speech. J Commun Disord 2002;35:283–292
105. Yorkston KM. Prosody in the adult. In: Yoder DE, Kent RD, eds. Decision Making in Speech-Language Pathology. Philadelphia: BC Decker; 1988:146–147
106. Helm NA. Management of palilalia with a pacing board. J Speech Hear Disord 1979;44:350–353
107. Yorkston KM, Beukelman DR, Minifie FD, Sapir S. Assessment of stress patterning. In: McNeil MR, Rosenbek JC, Aronson AE, eds. The Dysarthrias: Physiology, Acoustics, Perception and Management. San Diego: College-Hill Press; 1984:131–162
108. Murry T. Treatment of ataxia dysarthria. In: Perkins WH, ed. Current Therapy of Communication Disorders: Dysarthria and Apraxia. New York: Thieme; 1983:79–90
109. Ramig LO, Sapir S, Fox C, Countryman S. Changes in vocal loudness following intensive voice treatment (LSVT) in individuals with Parkinson's disease: a comparison with untreated patients and normal age-matched controls. Mov Disord 2001;16:79–83
110. Sapir S, Ramig LO, Hoyt P, Countryman S, O'Brien C, Hoehn M. Speech loudness and quality 12 months after intensive voice treatment (LSVT) for Parkinson's disease: a comparison with an alternative speech treatment. Folia Phoniatr Logop 2002;54:296–303
111. Desmurget M, Grafton ST, Vindras P, Gréa H, Turner RS. The basal ganglia network mediates the planning of movement amplitude. Eur J Neurosci 2004;19:2871–2880
112. Huber J, Stathopoulos E, Ramig L, Lancaster S. Respiratory function and variability in individuals with Parkinson disease: pre and post Lee Silverman Voice Treatment (LSVT®). J Med Speech-Lang Pathol 2003;11:185–201
113. Smith ME, Ramig LO, Dromey C, Perez K, Samandari R. Intensive voice treatment in Parkinson's disease: laryngostroboscopic findings. J Voice 1995;9:453–459
114. de Angelis EC, Mourao LF, Ferraz HB, Behlau MS, Pontes PA, Andrade LA. Effect of voice rehabilitation on oral communication of Parkinson's disease patients. Acta Neurol Scand 1997;96:199–205
115. El Sharkawi A, Ramig L, Logemann JA, et al. Swallowing and voice effects of Lee Silverman Voice Treatment (LSVT): a pilot study. J Neurol Neurosurg Psychiatry 2002;72:31–36
116. Spielman JL, Borod JC, Ramig LO. The effects of intensive voice treatment on facial expressiveness in Parkinson disease: preliminary data. Cogn Behav Neurol 2003;16:177–188
117. Ward E, Theodoros D, Murdoch B, Silburn P. Changes in maximum capacity tongue function following the Lee Silverman Voice Treatment program. J Med Speech-Lang Pathol 2000;8:331–335
118. Ramig LO, Sapir S, Fox C, Countryman S. Changes in vocal intensity following intensive voice treatment (LSVT®) in individuals with Parkinson disease: a comparison with untreated patients and normal age-matched controls. Mov Disord 2001;16:79–83
119. Yorkston KM. The degenerative dysarthrias: a window into critical clinical and research issues. Folia Phoniatr Logop 2007;59:107–117
120. Ramig LO, Sapir S, Countryman S, et al. Intensive voice treatment (LSVT) for patients with Parkinson's disease: a 2 year follow up. J Neurol Neurosurg Psychiatry 2001;71:493–498
121. Theodoros DG, Constantinescu G, Russel T, Ward E, Wilson S, Wootton R. Treating the speech disorder in Parkinson's disease online. J Telemed Telecare 2006;12(suppl 3):88–91
122. Spielman J, Ramig LO, Mahler L, Halpern A, Gavin WJ. Effects of an extended version of the Lee Silverman voice treatment on voice and speech in Parkinson's disease. Am J Speech Lang Pathol 2007; 16:95–107
123. Silverman F. Communication Aids for the Speechless. Englewood Cliffs, NJ: Prentice-Hall; 1980
124. Greene MC, Watson BW. The value of speech amplification in Parkinson's disease patients. Folia Phoniatr (Basel) 1968;20:250–257
125. Blom E. Artificial larynx: past and present. In: Salmon S, Goldstein L, eds. Artificial Larynx Handbook. New York: Grune & Stratton; 1978
126. Beukelman DR, Garrett K. Augmentative communication for adults with acquired severe communication disorders. Augment Altern Commun 1988;4:104–121
127. Titze IR. Biomechanics and distributed mass models of vocal fold vibrations. In: Stevens KN, Hirano M, eds. Vocal Fold Physiology. Tokyo: University of Tokyo Press; 1981:245–264
128. Scherer RC, Gould WJ, Titze IR, Meyers AD, Sataloff RT. Preliminary evaluation of selected acoustic and glottographic measures for clinical phonatory function analysis. J Voice 1988;2/3:230–244

ID # Chapter 13

Diagnosis and Evaluation of Laryngeal Paralysis and Paresis

Alexander T. Hillel, Robin A. Samlan, and Paul W. Flint

In the 4th century B.C. Hippocrates recognized laryngeal paralysis as a cause of aspiration. In the 1860s, Gerhardt, with the help of indirect mirror laryngoscopy, first diagnosed the clinical condition of laryngeal paralysis.[1] Twenty years later, Felix Semon[2] observed a pattern of paramedian fold position in vocal paralysis and hypothesized that abductor nerve fibers were more susceptible to disease than adductor fibers. In the ensuing century otolaryngologists have observed multiple fold positions in laryngeal paralysis and gained a greater understanding of the complexities of the neuromuscular pathophysiology of this condition.

The larynx provides the major functions of airway protection, airway support, and phonation. The nerve supply to the larynx is long and circuitous, highlighted by the left recurrent laryngeal nerve (RLN) coursing around the aortic arch. Complete interruption of laryngeal nerve pathway results in laryngeal paralysis. In the medical lexicon, laryngeal paralysis has evolved to erroneously represent the spectrum of partial to complete nerve deficit. It should be stressed that a true paralysis is a rare condition, and that most patients have a partial nerve deficit, or paresis.

Complete paralysis of the larynx is usually seen with complete transection of the RLN and superior laryngeal nerve (SLN). More often an injury results in neuropraxic damage to a portion of the motor nerve. Other causes of partial deficits include an interrupted vascular supply and nerve regeneration resulting in laryngeal function months after the initial nerve injury. Therefore, most patients present with a paresis. The differential diagnosis and evaluation of vocal fold paralysis and paresis differ based on known or unknown etiology, bilateral versus unilateral disease, and whether the patient is a child or an adult.

◆ Etiology

The etiologies of laryngeal paralysis and paresis are numerous (**Table 13.1**). Trauma (both surgical and nonsurgical), neoplasm, and central nervous system disease are the leading causes in both children and adults (**Table 13.2** and **Table 13.3**). Often after an extensive evaluation a large number of cases remain idiopathic. Comparing unilateral and bilateral vocal fold paresis across age classification demonstrates that adults suffer unilateral paresis more often than bilateral disease.[3-7] In contrast, unilateral and bilateral disease present with a similar prevalence in children.[8-10] In both age groups, left-sided lesions account for around two thirds of unilateral cases, as the long anatomic course of the left RLN is more frequently interrupted during surgery and by pulmonary neoplasm.[3,6-8,10-13]

Across the past three decades the etiology of adult unilateral vocal fold immobility has remained stable. The primary causes are surgical trauma and extralaryngeal malignancy, with pulmonary and mediastinal tumor representing the most common locations. A review of the literature demonstrates that primary lung cancer is not distinguished from metastatic lung cancer.[3,5-7,12-14] The next largest category is idiopathic, ranging from 11 to 42%.[3,5-7,12,13] Central nervous system disorders, nonsurgical trauma, and intubation are common but less frequent causes of unilateral laryngeal nerve deficit.

Iatrogenic injury is the leading cause of adult bilateral vocal fold paralysis. The singular operation responsible for the surgical trauma to both vocal folds is the total thyroidectomy. Fortunately, recent studies demonstrate a decreasing proportion of bilateral vocal fold paralysis due to thyroidectomy, decreasing from 58% to 30%.[3] This decrease may be a function of subspecialization, as endocrine specialists are now primarily responsible for surgical management of thyroid disease. Intubation injuries commonly cause bilateral disease; however, it is rare for a malignancy to affect both RLNs. When malignancies result in bilateral disease, immobility occurs precipitously and is the result of a very aggressive neoplasm, such as an anaplastic thyroid tumor or submucosal tumor extension.

In children and neonates, congenital central nervous system disorders are the leading cause of bilateral paralysis. Arnold-Chiari malformation type II is the most common central nervous system disease. Iatrogenic injury is a leading cause of unilateral vocal fold paralysis in children, with reports as high as 73%.[8] Other causes such as cardiovascular anomalies and surgery are responsible for left vocal fold deficits. In neonates, birth trauma is a common cause of

Table 13.1 Etiology of Vocal Fold Paralysis and Paresis

Central nervous system disorders	Skull base surgery
Cerebrovascular accident	Anterior cervical spine fusion
Arnold-Chiari malformation	Other head and neck surgery
Meningomyelocele	Nonsurgical trauma
Hydrocephalus	Birth trauma
Syringomyelia	Intubation
Concussion	Blunt or sharp trauma
Neurofibromatosis	Idiopathic
Brainstem dysgenesis	Infectious
Kernicterus	Viral
Leukodystrophy	Herpes simplex virus
Encephalocele	Epstein-Barr virus
Neuromuscular disease	Cytomegalovirus
Myasthenia gravis	Postpolio syndrome
Multiple sclerosis	Encephalitis
Amyotrophic lateral sclerosis	Bacterial
Guillain-Barré syndrome	Botulism
Charcot-Marie-Tooth disease	Tetanus
Myopathy	Syphilis
Neoplasm	Rabies
Brain	Lyme disease
Skull base	Mycobacterial
Neck	Other
Lung	Familial
Trauma	Vincristine chemotherapy
Surgical trauma	Aortic aneurysm
Thyroid surgery	Enlargement of the heart
Thoracic surgery	Diabetes mellitus

Source: Data from Hillel AD, Benninger M, Blitzer A, Crumley R, et al. Evaluation and management of bilateral vocal cord immobility. Otolaryngol Head Neck Surg 1999;121:760–765, and Parikh SR. Pediatric unilateral vocal fold immobility. Otolaryngol Clin N Am 2004;37:203–215.

Table 13.2 Etiologies of Laryngeal Paralysis in Adults

Unilateral	Maisel, 1974		Yamada, 1983		Terris, 1992		Rosenthal, 2007		Havas, 1999	
Etiology	No.	%	No.	%	No.	%	No.	%	No.	%
Right Side	54	43	148	29	27	32	247	38	38	35
Left Side	73	57	371	71	57	68	396	62	70	65
Neoplastic	31	25	92	18	34	41	118	18	12	11
(Thoracic[a])	(11)	(9)	(44)	(8)	(14)	(17)	(79)	(12)	(4)	(4)
Surgical Trauma	20	16	116	22	29	35	235	37	43	40
(Thyroid)	(10)	(8)	(62)	(12)	(7)	(8)	(80)	(12)	(29)	(27)
(Nonthyroid)	(10)	(8)	(54)	(10)	(22)	(27)	(155)	(24)	(14)	(13)
Non-Surgical Trauma	13	10	12	2	1	1	39	6	4	4
Intubation	4	3	54	11	6	7	37	6	2	2
CNS	10	8	6	1	2	2	33	5	6	5
Idiopathic	27	21	217	42	9	11	119	19	36	33
Other	22	17	22	4	3	3	62	10	5	5
Total	127	100	519	100	84	100	280	100	108	100

(Continued on page 109)

Table 13.2 *(Continued)* Etiologies of Laryngeal Paralysis in Adults

Bilateral	Maisel, 1974		Holinger, 1976		Rosenthal, 2007	
Etiology	No.	%	No.	%	No.	%
Neoplastic	4	7	16	6	27	14
(Thoracic[a])	(0)	(0)	(0)	(0)	(9)	(5)
Surgical Trauma	23	43	140	59	70	37
(Thyroid)	(22)	(41)	(138)	(58)	(56)	(30)
(Nonthyroid)	(1)	(2)	(2)	(1)	(14)	(7)
Non-Surgical Trauma	15	28	2	1	14	7
Intubation	1	2	0	0	25	13
CNS	4	7	16	7	20	11
Idiopathic	2	4	8	3	21	11
Other	5	9	58	24	12	6
Total	240	100	240	100	189	100

Source: Data from Rosenthal LH, Benninger MS, Deeb RH. Vocal fold immobility: A longitudinal analysis of etiology over 20 years. Laryngoscope 2007;117:1864–1870; Maisel RH, Ogura JH. Evaluation and treatment of vocal cord paralysis. Laryngoscope 1974;84:302–316; Yamada M, Hirano M, Ohkubo H. Recurrent laryngeal nerve paralysis. A 10-year review of 564 patients. Auris Nasus Larynx 1983;10:S1–S15; Havas T, Lowinger D, Priestley J. Unilateral vocal fold paralysis: causes, options and outcomes. Aust N Z J Surg 1999;69:509–513; Terris DJ, Arnstein DP, Nguyen HH. Contemporary evaluation of unilateral vocal cord paralysis. Otolaryngol Head Neck Surg 1992;107:84–90; and Holinger LD, Holinger PC, Holinger PH. Etiology of bilateral abductor vocal cord paralysis. Ann Otol Rhinol Laryngol 1976;85:428–436.

[a]Thoracic neoplasms include pulmonary and mediastinal neoplasms.

Abbreviation: CNS, central nervous system.

Table 13.3 Etiology of Laryngeal Paralysis in Neonates and Children

Unilateral	Cohen et al, 1982		Narcy et al, 1990		Daya et al, 2000	
Etiology	No.	%	No.	%	No.	%
Right side	7	19	36	28	12	23
Left side	26	68	91	72	41	77
Birth trauma	7	19	30	24	0	0
Surgical trauma	5	13	31	24	39	73
Neurologic	5	13	18	14	3	6
Idiopathic	17	45	44	35	10	19
Other	2	3	4	3	1	2
Total	33	100	127	100	53	100

Bilateral	Cohen, 1982		Narcy, 1990[a]		Daya, 2000	
Etiology	No.	%	No.	%	No.	%
Birth trauma	12	18	7	8	5	10
Surgical trauma	4	6	4	4	5	10
Neurologic	27	42	26	28	13	27
Idiopathic	19	29	53	58	26	53
Other	3	5	0	0	0	0
Total	65	100	92	98	49	100

Source: Data from Daya H, Hosni A, Bejar-Solar I, Evans JNG, Bailey CM. Pediatric vocal fold paralysis: a long term retrospective study. Arch Otolaryngol Head Neck Surg 2000;126:21–25; Cohen SR, Birns JW, Geller KA, Thompson JW. Laryngeal paralysis in children: a long-term retrospective study. Ann Otol Rhinol Laryngol 1982;91:417–424; and Narcy P, Contencin P, Viala P. Surgical treatment for laryngeal paralysis in infants and children. Ann Otol Rhinol Laryngol 1990;99:124–8.

[a]Series included two cases with insufficient documentation in chart to assign an etiology.

both bilateral and unilateral paralysis. As in adults, there is a high percentage of unilateral idiopathic laryngeal paresis. On the other hand, bilateral idiopathic paresis, which is rare in adults, is quite common in children.

Viral illness is speculated to cause a large percentage of idiopathic vocal fold paresis. There are many case reports of laryngeal paresis associated with reactivated herpes simplex virus (HSV) and more rarely cytomegalovirus, Epstein-Barr virus, and postpolio patients.[15-19] In a 2001 series Koufman et al[20] presented separate idiopathic and viral etiologies, with the viral cause defined by the patient's report of recent viral upper respiratory infection. This study demonstrated around 40% of previously defined idiopathic cases to be of viral etiology. A series of SLN paresis reported by Dursun et al[21] found a viral etiology in 94% of patients.[21] Although case reports have demonstrated HSV-positive serology, a large-scale study has not been performed.[18-21] If a large series correlates HSV-positive herpes serology in patients with idiopathic vocal fold paresis, antiviral therapy could be implemented as treatment, as is the current practice in subclinical viral labyrinthitis.

Two rare causes of laryngeal paralysis are familial disease and vincristine chemotherapy. The hereditary forms cause bilateral paralysis and include patterns suggesting both an X-linked and autosomal dominant inheritance.[22-24] No gene has been identified at this time. Vincristine's peripheral neurotoxicity has been reported to cause both bilateral and unilateral laryngeal paralysis in children and adults.[25,26] The paralysis usually resolves with discontinuation of chemotherapy.[25,26]

♦ Signs and Symptoms

Neural dysfunction of the larynx can adversely affect voice, ventilation, and airway protection. The resulting clinical manifestations are variable and dependent on the degree of paresis. With regard to voice, dysphonia and vocal fatigue are common. Vocal fatigue is a result of exhausted compensating musculature. A neonate may be unable to cry due to the large glottic gap. Adult patients with unilateral vocal fold immobility frequently present with a weak and breathy voice. In SLN deficit the voice often displays a loss of projection and power, especially noticeable at a high pitch—a result of decreased tension on the affected fold. Koufman et al[4] demonstrated that voice change is present in 100% and vocal fatigue in 76% in a review of 50 patients presenting with paresis. Diplophonia (40%), or two tones produced by different tension of the vocal folds, and pain with phonation (10%) were found to be less frequent.

Exertional phonation in combination with dysphonia, vocal fatigue, and odynophonia is a sign of excessive supraglottic activity.[4,27] This condition is frequently due to abnormal muscle tension in the larynx. Its presence should alert the physician to focus the examination on the glottis, which often reveals incomplete closure. Muscle tension dysphonia usually represents a compensatory behavior for a laryngeal deficit. Although it is important to exclude a nerve injury, the vocal fold weakness may be due to a movement disorder, such as Parkinson disease, a soft tissue deficit or mass, or trauma, as in the case of arytenoid dislocation.

Stridor is often seen in bilateral vocal fold paralysis and causes dyspnea and respiratory distress in a small percentage of adult patients. This is a result of a fixed midline fold position, which preserves voice function and usually prevents aspiration. In children, stridor is the leading symptom and is frequently seen in unilateral disease as well as in bilateral paralysis. Cohen et al[10] reported stridor in 71% and obstruction in 44% of children with laryngeal paralysis. Dysphonia (35%), dysphagia (38%), and aspiration (14%) were encountered less often. Airway distress, cyanosis, and apnea are common in bilateral immobility, though some infants may remain asymptomatic for up to 6 months; however, when their oxygen needs increase, they become symptomatic.

Aspiration may be seen in unilateral vagal or RLN paralysis because the affected fold is often in the paramedian position and cannot fully close. These patients have difficulty protecting the airway and lack a sufficient cough that results in aspiration. Dysphagia is less severe with an RLN injury alone than is a high vagal injury that includes sensory denervation. In newborns, aspiration may manifest as recurrent pneumonia. SLN deficit rarely causes choking and aspiration; when present, these symptoms are a function of sensory deficit from the external nerve branch. Aspiration almost always indicates bilateral SLN denervation, as unilateral sensory deficit is usually compensated by the contralateral sensation.[21,28]

♦ Neuropathology

The four nerve deficits that can cause vocal fold paralysis are central nervous system disorder, high vagal lesion, RLN injury, and SLN injury. Each lesion has a classic pattern of muscle weakness and vocal fold position. Clinically, patients present with variable vocal fold position that is a function of the degree of paresis, the presence of synkinesis, mechanical trauma, and the patient's laryngeal anatomy, which substantially differs between men and women. Although every patient with a specific nerve deficit does not present with the same fold position, these common patterns, if observed, may assist in the diagnosis and evaluation.

Central nervous system injury causing laryngeal paresis usually indicates brainstem dysfunction. Brainstem lesions frequently occur as a result of a stroke or tumor and are associated with involvement of other cranial nerves. The lesion may only affect motor innervation due to injury to the dorsal and ventral nucleus ambiguus. Therefore, the presentation includes motor loss of the pharynx in addition to laryngeal deficit.[29] A distinguishing feature of central nervous system deficit is the lack of a sensory or secretory deficit.[30] As is commonly observed with upper motor neuron deficit, the initial flaccid paresis segues into a spastic paresis with slow laryngeal movement and a decreased range of abductor and adductor function.[31] A shift in the posterior glottis to the normal side with the onset of speech may also be seen.[32] Cortical lesions tend to spare the vocal folds due to diffuse interhemispheric connections that provide bilateral input to laryngeal nerve pathways.

The unique combination of motor, sensory, and secretory deficit usually indicates extracranial vagal injury.[30] This is a result of the combined injury to the recurrent and superior laryngeal nerves pathways within the vagus. In high vagal paralysis, the fold is frequently paramedian, with bowing and atrophic changes resulting in a glottic gap. The two folds are at different levels and in an asymmetric position.[32] In unilateral disease, the healthy fold might cross midline; however, most patients suffer mild to moderate hoarseness due to incomplete glottic closure and vibratory asymmetry. Nerve injury affects the muscles unequally, and the loss of opposing forces results in the vocal process falling anteromedially. More frequently, nerve injury affects the muscles unequally. The loss of opposing forces results in the vocal process falling anteromedially.

An isolated RLN injury is similar to a high vagal lesion with the affected fold(s) in a paramedian position. On the other hand, there is no sensory or secretory deficit and the cricothyroid muscle remains fully innervated. Denervation of the posterior cricoarytenoid alone results in abduction deficit, whereas isolated thyroarytenoid deficit causes atrophy of the affected fold. This paretic condition leads to premature and greater lateralization with an abnormal mucosal wave.[32] As with vagal injury, bilateral deficit does not usually provide enough airway support and necessitates urgent tracheostomy.

An SLN deficit results in ipsilateral cricothyroid muscle weakness. Diplophonia is commonly encountered due to the different vibratory frequency of the affected nerve from the healthy side. The most consistent signs are a shortened bowed vocal fold and sluggish motion.[21] Debate remains on whether a cricothyroid deficit alone can cause a deviation of the larynx toward the affected nerve.[33]

♦ Evaluation

An algorithm can be used for the evaluation of laryngeal paralysis (**Fig. 13.1**). Its purpose is to provide a comprehensive and financially efficient decision tree of diagnostic studies. An extensive evaluation searching for the cause of idiopathic immobility can be expensive, yet often it is clinical suspicion combined with a directed workup that reveals a diagnosis. In a study on the evaluation of unilateral vocal fold paralysis, Terris et al[13] reported that otolaryngologists with greater experience pursue a briefer and less expensive evaluation for unilateral vocal fold paralysis.

The first issue the clinician must address is airway stability. After determining or obtaining airway stability, a useful question to ask the patient is, "Did something happen that caused the problem with your larynx?" A majority of patients present with a known cause of paralysis; studies of unilateral paralysis show that number to be between 57 and 63%.[5,13] Known etiologies frequently include surgical trauma, intubation trauma, blunt trauma, malignancy, and central nervous system disorders. Knowledge or suspicion of an

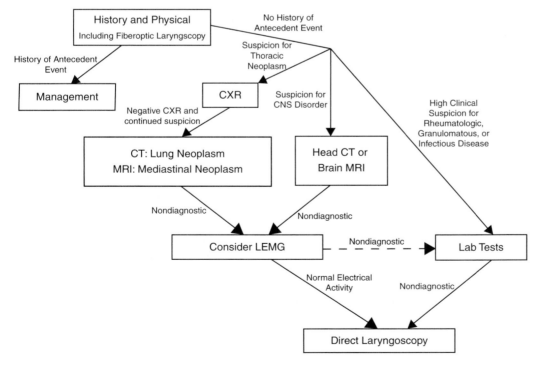

Fig. 13.1 Algorithm for evaluation of laryngeal paralysis and paresis. CT, computed tomography; CXR, chest x-ray; LEMG, laryngeal electromyography; MRI, magnetic resonance imaging.

etiology avoids a potentially lengthy and costly evaluation and allows the physician to proceed to management. If the etiology remains elusive, the clinical assessment should begin with a focused history and physical exam and may ultimately extend to a scheduled operative exam under anesthesia.

History and Physical Examination

Obtaining the history allows the physician to listen to the patient's report of the problem and provides an unobtrusive examination of the sound of their voice, which may reveal tremor or pitch breaks. Though the neonate does not have speech, the cry may disclose vocal fold position before examination. Important questions to address include onset, the frequency of vocal fatigue, relief with rest, associated pain with speaking, exertional intolerance, and effort needed for speech. Associated symptoms such as difficulty swallowing and loss of sensation of food in the mouth and throat may raise suspicion of an SLN component and allow for a more focused examination. The clinician should also obtain a past medical and surgical history. In addition, a thorough family history may reveal a rare hereditary cause of vocal paralysis. A history of smoking combined with weight loss should arouse suspicion for a neoplasm. In children and neonates it is important to obtain from the mother or her physician a history of difficult delivery or birth trauma. The lack of ability to feed and an inappropriate weight and height for age may reveal a failure to thrive. Furthermore, vaccination status helps in the evaluation of possible infectious etiologies.

Thorough cranial nerve, head and neck, and lung exams are vital. The cranial nerve exam may reveal abnormal spontaneous movement or weakness of the tongue, lips, and palate. Neurologic involvement of cranial nerves suggests a brainstem lesion, whereas palpation of solid nodes or masses in the neck suggests tumor impinging the larynges. An important sign in neonates is bulging or full fontanelles that would indicate hydrocephalus. A complete lung examination is recommended, with observation for retractions and use of accessory respiratory muscles, and auscultation of the lungs for respiratory pattern and stridor.

Indirect Laryngoscopy

The next step after a history and physical is to proceed to indirect laryngoscopy. The indirect mirror exam has been superseded by fiberoptic laryngeal examination, which represents today's standard for visualizing the larynx. Every patient with suspected vocal fold immobility should be examined with either flexible or rigid laryngoscopy. Flexible laryngoscopy provides an excellent view of the palatal structures, pharynx, hypopharynx, and, if desired, the subglottic space and the larynx. If pharyngeal constrictor dysfunction is demonstrated, a brainstem deficit should be suspected. In small children flexible fiberoptic laryngoscopy is better tolerated than rigid endoscopy.

During indirect laryngeal exam, abduction and adduction should be observed (**Figs. 13.2** and **13.3**). RLN paralysis may be diagnosed by a lack of motion of the affected vocal fold(s) with phonation or ventilation. However, this may require repetitive vocal fold motion to reveal a partial deficit. In SLN disease, the patient may be unable to increase pitch due to difficulty in lengthening and thinning the affected fold. Two other tests of laryngeal function are recommended during laryngoscopy. First, the patient should be asked to cough, to differentiate functional stridor from vocal fold paralysis.[34] Second, during a sniff or whistle, normal abduction may differentiate a dystonic, malingering, or laryngospastic patient from neurologic paralysis.[35] While visualizing the larynx, the physician should rule out other causes of immobility such as glottic webbing or interarytenoid scars. In addition, subtle arytenoid movement may be detected that rules out cricoarytenoid fixation. This often occurs when an arytenoid in the lateral position is bumped by the contralateral arytenoid.

Videostroboscopy

If the lesion remains undiagnosed by laryngoscopy, videostroboscopy may yield additional information. Videostroboscopy slows the dynamic image of the vocal fold to allow for examination of vibratory patterns of the folds. This is especially useful in recording and diagnosing SLN dysfunction, as a paretic or paralyzed cricothyroid muscle will slow

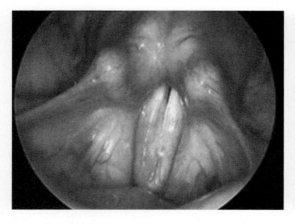
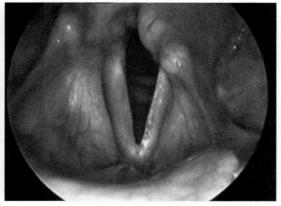

Fig. 13.2 Left unilateral vocal fold paralysis in an abducted **(A)** and adducted **(B)** position. The vocal fold is in a paramedian position with a straight fold edge and upright arytenoid position.

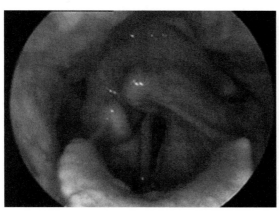 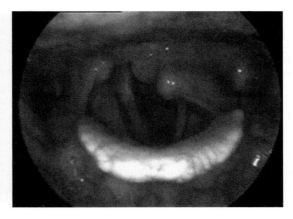

Fig. 13.3 Left paralyzed vocal fold in an abducted **(A)** and adducted **(B)** position. The vocal fold is in a lateral position with a bowed appearance. The left arytenoid is rotated anteromedially, resulting in an asymmetric glottal configuration.

the movement of the ipsilateral vocal fold. Videostroboscopy also evaluates glottic closure and the mucosal wave, which when absent may be associated with denervation. In addition, videostroboscopy has the potential to differentiate high vagal and RLN paralysis.[30] Localizing the anatomic course of nerve paralysis allows the physician to narrow the scope of investigation toward the skull base (high vagal lesion) or neck, lungs, and mediastinum (RLN lesion).[13]

Radiographic Studies

Appropriate radiographic studies are integral in the diagnosis of laryngeal paralysis. In immobility of unknown etiology, most otolaryngologists include a chest x-ray (CXR) in the routine evaluation.[35–37] It is an inexpensive, low-radiation exposure imaging study that may reveal a tumor and clearly demonstrates the course of the trachea. Terris et al[13] found that a CXR is the most useful diagnostic tool in their series **(Table 13.4)**, as it identified a diagnosis in greater than one third of patients with previously undiagnosed unilateral vocal fold immobility.

In patients with vocal fold immobility and a suspected lung malignancy there is debate about whether CXR or computed tomography (CT) is the appropriate study. The thoracic literature reports CT to be better than CXR at detection of small (≤2 cm) lung masses.[38] However, such sensitivity is usually not required in patients with vocal fold immobility due to suspected lung cancer, which is usually at an advanced stage if symptomatic. The high false-positive rate of CT, the low-radiation exposure and low cost of CXR, and the presumably large lung lesion causing vocal fold immobility make CXR a better initial study to rule out lung malignancy.[13,36] Terris et al[13] demonstrated a 48% yield (diagnosis rate per number of tests ordered) when ordering a CXR to evaluate a lung mass in patients with unilateral paralysis **(Table 13.5)**. In children, the CXR has less utility due to the low incidence of pulmonary neoplasm.

Should suspicion of a thoracic malignancy persist after CXR, CT scan or magnetic resonance imaging (MRI) for

Table 13.4 Number and Percentage of Diagnoses Achieved by Study Type in a Series of 84 Patients with Unilateral Vocal Fold Immobility

Diagnostic Test	Number (n = 84)	Percentage	Cumulative Diagnosis (%)
Diagnosis known	48	57	57
CXR	13	15	72
CT	7	8	80
MRI	3	4	84
Other	4	5	89
Unknown diagnosis	9	11	100

Source: Adapted from Terris DJ, Arnstein DP, Nguyen HH. Contemporary evaluation of unilateral vocal cord paralysis. Otolaryngol Head Neck Surg 1992;107:84–90. Adapted with permission.

Abbreviations: CT, computed tomography; CXR, chest x-ray; MRI, magnetic resonance imaging.

Table 13.5 Yield (Percentage of Tests Ordered that Achieved a Diagnosis) of Various Tests from the Group of Patients in which a Workup Was Required (n = 36)

Diagnostic Test	No. of Tests Ordered	No. of Diagnoses Achieved	Yield (%)
MRI scan	5	3	60
CXR	24	13	54
CT scan	20	7	35
Endoscopy	5	1	20
Barium swallow	10	0	0
Thyroid function tests	2	0	0
Skull series	2	0	0
Thyroid scan	1	0	0

Source: Adapted from Terris DJ, Arnstein DP, Nguyen HH. Contemporary evaluation of unilateral vocal cord paralysis. Otolaryngol Head Neck Surg 1992;107:84–90. Adapted with permission.

mediastinal lesions is an appropriate second-line study. The entire course of the vagal and RLN should be imaged to rule out neoplasm. CT represents the best modality and should extend to the aortic arch for left-sided immobility and to the thoracic inlet for right-sided immobility.[39] In bilateral immobility with suspicion of a central nervous system etiology, a CT or MRI of the brain is appropriate. If these studies are unrevealing, Dray et al[39] further recommend a neurologic consultation to formally evaluate potential neurologic causes.

Two other radiographic studies are reported in the literature to assist in the diagnosis of laryngeal paralysis. A simple contrast swallow study can demonstrate subtle swallowing difficulties, which may indicate neurologic etiology.[37] A barium swallow study is useful to demonstrate aspiration, which may be due to afferent laryngeal dysfunction. The efficacy of these two studies is questioned. Terris et al[13] reported a yield of 0% for barium swallow in the diagnosis of unilateral laryngeal immobility.

Laryngeal ultrasound is a modality routinely used to evaluate pediatric vocal fold immobility.[8,40,41] Ultrasound is able to noninvasively image the anatomic structure of the larynx as well as demonstrate vibration echo of the fold.[42] In a prospective trial, Friedman[40] demonstrated laryngeal ultrasound to be a simple, safe, rapid, and reliable method to diagnose vocal fold immobility. Although not a replacement for flexible laryngoscopy, this noninvasive study is a useful adjunct and may be a viable alternative in children who do not tolerate indirect laryngoscopy.[41] Laryngeal ultrasound has little role in the adult evaluation, as other diagnostic tests are well tolerated.

Laryngeal Electromyography

Following unrevealing radiologic tests, laryngeal electromyography (LEMG) is indicated. Electromyography represents the diagnostic gold standard for vocal fold paralysis and paresis.[4] Due to the complex technique, its invasiveness, and its higher cost, LEMG should be performed later in the evaluation if the aforementioned studies are nondiagnostic. LEMG can objectively differentiate between neuromuscular deficit and mechanical fixation of the folds. For this reason LEMG plays a unique role in the evaluation of both unilateral and bilateral vocal fold immobility. Furthermore, LEMG can predict the likelihood of recovery, which assists in developing a treatment plan. In the pediatric evaluation LEMG can be a difficult procedure to perform and is limited to many tertiary care hospitals, though it may be of limited utility due to a high number of false-negative exams.[43] (LEMG is also discussed in Chapter 6.)

Laboratory Studies

A review of the literature shows that blood screening tests should not be ordered routinely without clinical suspicion for infectious, neurologic, rheumatologic, or granulomatous disease.[13,35,39] If a very high suspicion for a disease exists, or following an extensive evaluation with no diagnosis, the physician may consider blood tests for rare causes of laryngeal paralysis, which may help to obviate surgical intervention. For example, fasting blood sugar and Lyme titer will rule out diabetes and Lyme disease, respectively, as causes of peripheral neuropathy. Additionally, an acetylcholine receptor antibody test can help to rule out myasthenia gravis. Sarcoidosis is a rare cause of laryngeal impairment. When it occurs, granulomatous nodules tend to affect the left RLN pathway; however, bilateral disease due to cranial polyneuritis has been reported.[44] If sarcoidosis is suspected, an angiotensin-converting enzyme level should be measured.

Certain rheumatologic diseases are known to cause vocal fold immobility. The current rheumatologic literature describes rare case reports of cricoarytenoid arthritis in systemic lupus erythematosus (SLE), rheumatoid arthritis (RA), and Wegener's granulomatosis.[45] Antinuclear antibodies (ANAs) and anti–double-stranded DNA (dsDNA) antibodies may be tested for SLE, rheumatoid factor should be tested if RA is suspected, and cytoplasmic-staining antineutrophil cytoplasmic antibody (C-ANCA) helps test for Wegener's granulomatosis. Laryngeal involvement is rarely observed in ankylosing spondylitis, gout, Reiter's arthritis, and juvenile rheumatoid arthritis.[45–47] Those diseases with a beneficial laboratory test include ankylosing spondylitis for which human leukocyte antigen (HLA) B27 is recommended, and for pauciarticular juvenile rheumatoid arthritis an ANA panel should be ordered. A focused blood panel is advisable for cost considerations, and if rheumatologic disease is suspected a consultation is recommended for a formal evaluation. Blood tests with little yield include Venereal Disease Research Laboratory (VDRL) testing or fluorescent treponemal antibody absorption (FTA-ABS) testing for syphilis and thyroid function tests.[13]

Direct Laryngoscopy

Direct laryngoscopy under anesthesia is the ultimate step in the evaluation. It is indicated in a patient with an undiagnosed cause of immobility. Palpation of the vocal process under anesthesia is the definitive method to distinguish complicating etiologies such as laryngeal synkinesis, cricoarytenoid joint fixation, and glottic webbing. In cases with a continued suspicion for neoplasia or for a required tissue sample, pan (laryngeal, bronchial, esophageal) endoscopy allows for excellent visualization and the opportunity to biopsy. In patients with unilateral impairment, infiltrating mucosal changes of the larynx should arouse a high suspicion for a subglottic lesion. Therefore, the subglottis in addition to the trachea should be examined for potential abnormalities. Even after this exam the etiology frequently remains idiopathic. In young children and neonates who do not tolerate flexible fiberoptic laryngoscopy, an exam under anesthesia may be necessary to fully evaluate the larynx.

Aerodynamics and Acoustic Analysis

Aerodynamic and acoustic analyses are two ancillary methods that may be used to objectively measure the effects of paresis on vocal function. Subglottal pressure is inferred from intraoral pressure during interruption of phonation and then analyzed together with the airflow rate. Incomplete glottic closure often results in elevated airflow compared to normal subjects. Isolated SLN paresis is associated with high subglottic pressures.[32] Acoustic analysis is used to quantify aspects of voice such as fundamental frequency, perturbation of frequency and amplitude, shimmer and jitter, and spectral analysis.[48] Although these measurements often correspond to the degree of paresis, unfortunately they tend not to correlate to specific nerve abnormalities.[32]

◆ Staging

At this time no uniform staging system exists to evaluate vocal fold paralysis. In 1991 Woo et al[49] suggested a staging system based on objective measurements of phonatory function that correlated to aspiration and dysphonia. This classification encompassed all etiologies and included both unilateral and bilateral vocal fold paralysis. Although Woo et al's system is not commonly implemented, partly because stage category did not correlate to outcomes, it demonstrates an area of future study in laryngology. An accepted uniform staging system would (1) accurately define relative deficits and potential outcomes, (2) provide for clear communication between physicians, and (3) establish a common classification for more accurate study.

◆ Management and Prognosis

Developing a treatment strategy is a critical component of the diagnosis and evaluation of laryngeal paralysis. The management of vocal fold paralysis is described in detail in subsequent chapters. In brief, management should address quality of voice, risk of aspiration, and airway obstruction. The definitive treatment for vocal fold paralysis resulting in airway compromise is immediate tracheotomy. Severe aspiration also demands immediate intervention in the form of intubation. For less critical conditions, factors such as prognosis for recovery, degree of impairment, the overall health of the patient, and the patient's desire and requirement for voice quality influence the timing and type of intervention.[32,35] A patient with uncertain prognosis and mild symptoms of dysphonia may benefit from a period of watchful waiting to allow for spontaneous recovery. On the other hand, an opera singer who fails voice therapy may prefer an earlier intervention.

In general, adults with vocal fold paresis are advised to wait one year before surgical intervention to allow for nerve regrowth and improvement of function. Both the physician and the patient should have patience with voice therapy and medical treatment.[32] If early intervention is chosen, a short-term and potentially reversible treatment is recommended.[50] After one year of nonsurgical treatment or an electromyograph (EMG) predictive of irreversible nerve damage, surgical treatment should be considered.[35] The ultimate step of surgically disrupting the laryngeal tissues should be reserved for patients who have no alternative means of recovery.[35]

Prognosis may be predicted by the etiology and neuropathology of nerve injury. Etiologies with a favorable prognosis for spontaneous recovery include blunt trauma, intubation injury, idiopathic paralysis, and paralysis associated with a viral illness. In a subset of Yamada et al's[7] 1983 study of 563 patients with vocal fold paralysis, 72% (23 of 32) of patients with intubation injury and 49% (54 of 110) of patients with an idiopathic cause of unilateral laryngeal paralysis spontaneously recovered a normal voice. Similarly, in a retrospective series of 102 children with vocal fold paralysis, Daya et al[8] showed a recovery rate of 71% (5 of 7) in children with a neurologic etiology and 64% (18 of 28) with idiopathic paralysis.[8] In contrast, laryngeal paralysis caused by iatrogenic transection of the nerve, tumor invasion of the nerve, thoracic aortic aneurysm, or progressive neurologic disorders have a poor prognosis. Yamada et al reported that 26% (15 of 58) of adults with an iatrogenic etiology regained a normal voice, whereas Daya et al found that 46% (12 of 26) of children with an iatrogenic etiology recovered. With regard to a specific type of nerve injury, SLN deficits have a high rate of recovery, though this may be due to the large percentage of viral disease.[21] High vagal nerve injuries frequently do poorly, likely a function of their comprehensive effect on all the muscles of the larynx.

Management of laryngeal paralysis in children differs from that in adults. In addition to ventilation and airway protection, preserving intelligible speech and feeding and growth are paramount.[51] Children have a higher overall rate of spontaneous recovery than do adults, with rates as high as 55%.[8,10] Spontaneous resolution has been reported to occur as late as 11 years after onset; therefore, it may be advisable to extend the observational period.[8] Furthermore, children adapt well to unilateral vocal fold immobility, compensating with the contralateral fold. These children rarely have permanent dysphonia and exhibit little or no airway deficit. With the exception of severe airway compromise, surgical intervention is not indicated for neonates and young children with unilateral paralysis.[51] Although children with bilateral laryngeal paralysis often require tracheotomy, current recommendations recommend waiting one year before surgical intervention to treat the vocal fold deficit as spontaneous recovery can occur after several years.

References

1. Willat DJ, Stell PM. Vocal cord paralysis. In: Paparella MM, Shumrick DA, Bluckman JL, et al, eds. Otolaryngology. Philadelphia: WB Saunders; 1991:2289–2306
2. Semon F. Clinical remarks. Arch Laryngol 1881;2:197–222
3. Benninger MS, Gillen JB, Altman JS. Changing etiology of vocal fold immobility. Laryngoscope 1998;108:1346–1350
4. Koufman JA, Postma GN, Cummins MM, Blalock DP. Vocal fold paresis. Otolaryngol Head Neck Surg 2000;122:537–541
5. Ramadan HH, Wax MK, Avery S. Outcome and changing cause of unilateral vocal cord paralysis. Otolaryngol Head Neck Surg 1998;118:199–202
6. Maisel RH, Ogura JH. Evaluation and treatment of vocal cord paralysis. Laryngoscope 1974;84:302–316
7. Yamada M, Hirano M, Ohkubo H. Recurrent laryngeal nerve paralysis. A 10-year review of 564 patients. Auris Nasus Larynx 1983;10:S1–S15
8. Daya H, Hosni A, Bejar-Solar I, Evans JNG, Bailey CM. Pediatric vocal fold paralysis: a long term retrospective study. Arch Otolaryngol Head Neck Surg 2000;126:21–25
9. Zbar RI, Smith R. Vocal fold paralysis in infants twelve months of age and younger. Otolaryngol Head Neck Surg 1996;114:18–21
10. Cohen SR, Birns JW, Geller KA, Thompson JW. Laryngeal paralysis in children: a long-term retrospective study. Ann Otol Rhinol Laryngol 1982;91:417–424
11. Narcy P, Contencin P, Viala P. Surgical treatment for laryngeal paralysis in infants and children. Ann Otol Rhinol Laryngol 1990;99:124–128
12. Havas T, Lowinger D, Priestley J. Unilateral vocal fold paralysis: causes, options and outcomes. Aust N Z J Surg 1999;69:509–513
13. Terris DJ, Arnstein DP, Nguyen HH. Contemporary evaluation of unilateral vocal cord paralysis. Otolaryngol Head Neck Surg 1992;107:84–90
14. Holinger LD, Holinger PC, Holinger PH. Etiology of bilateral abductor vocal cord paralysis. Ann Otol Rhinol Laryngol 1976;85:428–436
15. Driscoll BP, Gracco C, Coelho C, et al. Laryngeal function in postpolio patients. Laryngoscope 1995;105:35–41
16. Johns MM, Hogikyan ND. Simultaneous vocal fold and tongue paresis secondary to Epstein-Barr virus infection. Arch Otolaryngol Head Neck Surg 2000;126:1491–1494
17. Small PM, McPhaul LW, Sooy CD, et al. Cytomegalovirus infection of the laryngeal nerve presenting as hoarseness in patients with acquired immunodeficiency syndrome. Am J Med 1989;86:108–110
18. Magnussen CR, Patanella HP. Herpes simplex virus and recurrent laryngeal paralysis. Report of a case and review of the literature. Arch Intern Med 1979;139:1423–1424
19. Bachor E, Bonkowsky V, Hacki T. Herpes simplex virus type 1 reactivation as a cause of a unilateral temporary paralysis of the vagus nerve. Eur Arch Otorhinolaryngol 1996;253:297–300
20. Koufman JA, Postma GN, Whang CS, et al. Diagnostic laryngeal electromyography: the Wake Forest experience 1995–1999. Otolaryngol Head Neck Surg 2001;124:603–606
21. Dursun G, Sataloff RT, Spiegel JR, et al. Superior laryngeal nerve paresis and paralysis. J Voice 1996;10:206–211
22. Grundfast KM, Milmoe G. Congenital hereditary bilateral abductor vocal cord paralysis. Ann Otol Rhinol Laryngol 1982;91:564–566
23. Plott D. Congenital laryngeal-abductor paralysis due to nucleus ambiguous dysgenesis in three brothers. N Engl J Med 1964;271:593–597
24. Gacek RR. Hereditary abductor vocal cord paralysis. Ann Otol Rhinol Laryngol 1976;85:90–93
25. Tobias JD, Bozeman PM. Vincristine-induced recurrent laryngeal nerve paralysis in children. Intensive Care Med 1991;17:304–305
26. Whittaker JA, Griffith IP. Recurrent laryngeal nerve paralysis in patients receiving vincristine and vinblastine. BMJ 1977;1:1251–1252
27. Morrison MD, Nichol H, Rammage LA. Diagnostic criteria in functional dysphonia. Laryngoscope 1986;96:1–8
28. Tucker HM, Lavertu P. Paralysis and paresis of the vocal folds. In: Blitzer A, et al, eds. Neurologic Disorders of the Larynx. New York: Thieme; 1992:182–200
29. Kokesh J, Flint PW, Robinson LR, Cummings CW. Correlation between stroboscopy and electromyography in laryngeal paralysis. Ann Otol Rhinol Laryngol 1993;102:852–857
30. Ward PH, Berci GB. Observations on so-called idiopathic vocal cord paralysis. Ann Otol Rhinol Laryngol 1982;91:558–563
31. Ward PH, Hanson DG, Berci G. Observations on central neurologic etiology for laryngeal dysfunction. Ann Otol Rhinol Laryngol 1981;90:430–441
32. Benninger MS, Crumley RL, Ford CN, et al. Evaluation and treatment of the unilateral paralyzed vocal fold. Otolaryngol Head Neck Surg 1994;111:497–508
33. Woodson GE, Blitzer A. Neurologic evaluation of the larynx and pharynx. In: Cummings C, Haughey BH, Thomas JR, et al, eds. Otolaryngology: Head and Neck Surgery. 4th ed. Philadelphia: Mosby; 2005: 2054–2064
34. Woodson GE, Zwirner P, Murry R, Swenson M. Use of flexible laryngoscopy to assess patients with spasmodic dysphonia. J Voice 1991;5: 85–91
35. Hillel AD, Benninger M, Blitzer A, et al. Evaluation and management of bilateral vocal cord immobility. Otolaryngol Head Neck Surg 1999;121: 760–765
36. Altman JS, Benninger MS. The evaluation of unilateral vocal fold immobility: is chest X-ray enough? J Voice 1997;11:364–367
37. Grundfast KM, Harley E. Vocal cord paralysis. Otolaryngol Clin North Am 1989;22:569–597
38. Jett JR, Midthun DE. Screening for lung cancer: current status and future directions: Thomas A. Neff Lecture. Chest 2004;125:158S–162S
39. Dray TG, Robinson LR, Hillel AD. Idiopathic bilateral vocal fold weakness. Laryngoscope 1999;109:995–1002
40. Friedman EM. Role of ultrasound in the assessment of vocal cord function in infants and children. Ann Otol Rhinol Laryngol 1997;106:199–209
41. Vats A, Worley GA, de Bruyn R, et al. Laryngeal ultrasound to assess vocal fold paralysis in children. J Laryngol Otol 2004;118:429–431
42. Kitamura T, Kaneko T, Asano H, Miura T. Ultrasonoglottography: a preliminary report. Rev Laryngol Otol Rhinol (Bord) 1969;90:190–195
43. Jacobs IN, Finkej RS. Laryngeal electromyography in the management of vocal cord mobility problems in children. Laryngoscope 2002;112: 1243–1248
44. Witt RL. Sarcoidosis presenting as bilateral vocal fold paralysis. J Voice 2003;17:265–268
45. Bandi V, Munnu U, Braman SS. Airway problems in patients with rheumatologic disorders. Crit Care Clin 2002;18:749–765
46. Guttenplan MD, Hendrix RA, Townsend MJ, Balsara G. Laryngeal manifestations of gout. Ann Otol Rhinol Laryngol 1991;100:899–902
47. Teitel AD, MacKenzie CR, Stern R, Paget SA. Laryngeal involvement in systemic lupus erythematosus. Semin Arthritis Rheum 1992;22: 203–214
48. Baken RJ. Clinical Measurements of Speech and Voice. Boston: College-Hill Press; 1987
49. Woo P, Colton R, Brewer D, Casper J. Functional staging for vocal cord paralysis. Otolaryngol Head Neck Surg 1991;105:440–448
50. Benninger MS, Gillen JB, Altman JS. Changing etiology of vocal fold mobility. Laryngoscope 1998;108:1346–1350
51. de Jong AL, Kuppersmith RB, Sulek M, Friedman EM. Vocal cord paralysis in infants and children. Otolaryngol Clin North Am 2000;33: 131–149

Chapter 14

Management of Vocal Fold Incompetence with Vocal Fold Injectable Fillers

Charles N. Ford and Karen A. Cooper

♦ Vocal Fold Incompetence

Etiology

Vocal fold incompetence is a pathologic state characterized by the reduction of efficient vocal fold vibration in the setting of normal aerodynamic support. It can arise from reduced vocal fold adduction, loss of vocal fold volume, alteration of vocal fold viscoelasticity, or from a combination of the three. In all cases the entrained oscillation of the vocal folds is hindered, and increased subglottal pressures and airflow are required to power glottic sound production. Patients complain of vocal fatigue, reduced vocal projection, and a breathy voice quality.[1]

Reduction of glottic closure is commonly seen in unilateral vocal fold paralysis.[2,3] Common causes of this paralysis include iatrogenic injury to the recurrent laryngeal nerve (RLN), viral palsy, and neural compression from intrathoracic processes.[4] The denervation of the intrinsic laryngeal musculature prevents full closure of the glottis during phonation and also introduces viscoelastic asymmetry from the flaccidity of the affected vocal fold.[5] In these cases, injection of filler into the vocal fold can address glottal competence by moving the affected vocal fold medially.[2,3,6-8] However the position of the arytenoid and the issue of viscoelastic asymmetry are difficult to address precisely. Partial immobility of the vocal folds may also result from synkinetic reinnervation of the denervated cricoarytenoid unit, paresis from a partial RLN injury, or paresis from a superior laryngeal nerve (SLN) palsy.[9-11] These conditions produce glottal incompetence with lesser degrees of severity. Given the smaller contribution of arytenoid misplacement, injection techniques may have a more beneficial effect.

Vocal fold immobility may also result from fixation of the cricoarytenoid (CA) joint. Most commonly seen after prolonged intubation and described well by Bastian and Richardson,[12] periarticular fibrosis of the CA joint reduces the abduction and adduction of both CA units, leaving a large gap between both the arytenoid and the musculomembranous segments. Fixed arytenoids can also result from end-stage rheumatoid arthritis, osteoarthritis, or gout within the CA joint, creating an identical dilemma.[13-18] Injection techniques may be of benefit in medializing the anterior (musculomembranous) segment, but they neither restore mobility to the CA joints nor provide closure to the posterior (cartilaginous) segment. Viscoelastic alteration of the vocal folds is generally not an important contributor to glottal incompetence because innervation is intact and tension is maintained.

Neuromuscular discoordination as seen in spasmodic dysphonia and Parkinson disease can also produce glottal incompetence, not from an inability to achieve glottic closure or a change in viscoelasticity but rather from involuntary motion of the CA units. Glottic closure is not well synchronized with respiration, producing untimely exit of air through the glottis and a loss of entrained oscillation. Although neuromuscular discoordination has historically been managed at least in part by open laryngoplastic techniques, injection techniques may be aimed at augmenting the musculomembranous segments to reduce the size of the glottic gap at times of involuntary vocal fold separation, thereby reducing the degree of air loss.[19-21]

Other causes of glottic incompetence are related to actual loss of vocal fold tissue. Often referred to as presbylaryngis, aging changes to the vocal folds produce a loss of volume in the vocal fold cover (lamina propria [LP]).[22,23] The glottic appearance on office endoscopy is that of "bowing," in which a spindle-shaped aperture is described. Despite the adequate adduction of the arytenoids, air loss through this incompetent anterior valve is inevitable. Injection of the musculomembranous segment can produce improved closure by approximation of the oscillating surface and has been used also to replace some of the lamina propria lost in the aging process.[24] Increasing efforts are being made to reconstitute the lamina propria using fillers of appropriate viscoelasticity, either directly introduced or through means of stimulation, such as growth factors and tissue engineering.[25-27] These techniques likely represent the future of vocal fold restitution and are discussed later in the chapter.

Vocal fold tissue can also be lost in extirpative procedures related to cancer or infiltrative processes such as amyloidosis or sarcoidosis.[28-30] These resections, performed either with cold instruments or with CO_2 laser leave fixed focal gaps in the anterior segment of the glottis, creating a constantly inefficient phonatory mechanism. Attempts at closure of these gaps have targeted the medialization of the concave area with injection techniques and open laryngoplasty.[31-33] Restitution of the layered microstructure of the hemilarynx has been performed in animal models using scaffolds of sheeting that allow for influx of regionally appropriate tissue.[34] Repair of macro- and microdefects will certainly be enhanced by using tissue engineering as techniques advance to human trials. Of note, tissue defects from extirpative procedures fill in partially during the healing phase, thereby closing some of the initial defect. However, the native pliable tissue is replaced by scar that has reduced pliability relative to the original tissue. Therefore, even in cases of complete "fill-in" the patient is doomed to have some degree of glottal incompetence due to the side-to-side viscoelastic difference.

The last major contributor to vocal fold incompetence is pure loss of pliability within the lamina propria. This change can result from iatrogenesis, developmental anomalies, and chronic basement membrane zone injury from phonotrauma.[35] Iatrogenic reduction of vocal fold pliability is likely seen most often after repeated treatment of recurrent respiratory papillomatosis.[36] Application of the CO_2 laser has beneficial effects with respect to hemostatic reduction of massive papillomata.[37] However, the surrounding injury zone induces repair with scar, which has reduced viscoelastic qualities relative to native LP. Tissue biopsies that create a defect also induce tissue fill-in with scar, reducing the local pliability. Developmental anomalies such as sulcus vocalis types 2 and 3 produce local loss of pliability by replacing normal tissue with epithelium and scar and by interrupting the mucosal wave as it propagates from the inferior to superior lips of the vocal fold.[38] Treatment strategies have been directed at restoration of a normal vocal fold microstructure and replacement of the dead space with a pliable implant such as alloderm.[39] Injection techniques can introduce fillers but cannot separate the invagination of the vocal fold from the deep ligament. Phonotraumatic lesions of the vocal folds are very common and represent a spectrum of severity that is guided by how much scar has been deposited at the basement membrane zone. Nodules, for example, have been shown histopathologically to represent alteration of the normal microarchitecture with deposition of fibronectin and disruption of the smooth basement membrane.[35]

Patient Findings

Patients with vocal fold incompetence have similar clinical presentations and endoscopic findings. Glottal inefficiency requires increased effort and airflow for voicing. As patients fatigue from speaking, their ability to project is also diminished. Particularly in cases of reduced pliability, the upper singing range may be eliminated.[32] Additional comorbidities (advanced age, malignancy, neurologic weakness) may also contribute to a lack of energy sufficient for respiratory support.

On physical examination, patients with vocal fold incompetence have a reduced maximum phonation time, a breathy voice quality, and possibly compensatory pitch elevation or supraglottic compression. A basic mirror examination proves useful in determining the pathology of gross vocal fold motion and visible mass lesions, but does not sufficiently evaluate pliability changes. Rigid telescopic strobovideolaryngoscopic exam is still the gold standard for evaluation of viscoelastic qualities of the vocal folds and for minor anatomic detail of the epithelium and LP.[40] Digital archiving of the examination allows slow-motion review of gross adduction and abduction and helps reveal the glottal gap uniformly evident in this disorder. For example, in cases of vocal fold atrophy with aging, a spindle-shaped aperture is obvious (**Fig. 14.1**), particularly when compared with a normal subject. It is important to note if there is glottal inefficiency even in the modal range because the vocal folds are less taut and the LP has a greater ability to close. Unilateral defects are also visible in cases of prior biopsy and scarring montage. Here the normal vocal fold propagates to midline but the abnormal stiffness of the affected side reduces adequate entrainment. It is not unusual to have full visualization of the glottis reduced because of compensatory supraglottic compression.

♦ Injection Laryngoplasty for Treatment of Vocal Fold Incompetence

Functional and Anatomic Goals

Perhaps the major appeal of vocal fold injection augmentation is the relative ease of the procedure and the likelihood of immediate symptom relief. Essentially, the procedure involves injection of a substance into the vocal fold to passively displace the leading edge of the affected vocal fold toward the midline. The major goal of injecting filler substances in the vocal fold is achievement of glottic competence with improvement of voice and improved airway protection during swallowing. It is unrealistic to expect most patients to achieve a completely normal voice. Usually the immediate response to restoration of glottic competence is that the patient describes less effortful phonation and production of a louder voice. Perceptually, an improved frequency and intensity range can be appreciated. Injecting a filler substance into the vocal fold is just one of several useful approaches to correcting glottal incompetence. It does not necessarily resolve intrinsic pathologic tissue characteristics, such as scarring or muscle atrophy, nor does it correct neuromuscular alterations like Parkinson disease that might cause glottic insufficiency. In unilateral paralysis, successful injection results in glottic closure occurring during active adduction of the contralateral vocal fold. Using only topical anesthesia, injection augmentation can be easily and quickly performed in an office setting, and it is usually well tolerated by patients.

In cases of routine unilateral vocal fold paralysis, augmentation injection is best accomplished by sculpting the affected side to resemble the contour of the contralateral fold. There are several key points essential for achieving optimal results:

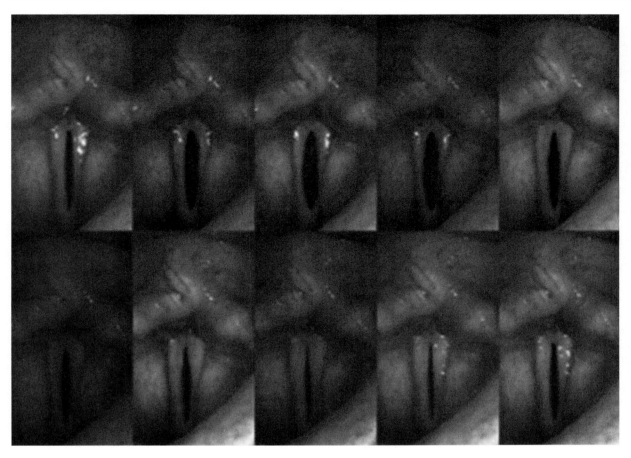

Fig. 14.1 Montage of telescopic rigid strobovideolaryngoscopic images from a patient with bilateral vocal fold atrophy. Note that the vocal folds never achieve complete closure. Also note the longitudinal spindle-shaped glottic aperture characteristic of vocal fold atrophy seen during sustained phonatory tasks.

- Augmentation should be in the same vertical plane as the contralateral fold.
- The leading inferior lip of the vocal fold must be sufficiently displaced because of the important role it plays in initiation of mucosal wave and functional vocal fold entrainment.
- Overfilling the subglottic region does not relieve glottic insufficiency and should be carefully avoided.
- Filling of the anterior vocal fold is usually not helpful and might be counterproductive, as it impacts and impedes oscillation of the opposite fold while failing to correct glottic incompetence in the mid- and post-larynx.

Injection Materials

Although there are many substances to choose from today, such was not always the case. The evolution of injection laryngoplasty began with a simple goal of filling space with an inert substance that could be easily injected to achieve glottic competence. Next we tried bioimplants because they more closely resembled tissues in the vocal fold lamina propria. Rather than posing a risk of granuloma or migration, the bioimplants (collagen, fat, and fascia) tended to be assimilated and replaced with host tissue. Bovine and human-derived materials were introduced including xenographs, homographs, and autogenous material. Historically, in 1911 Brunings injected paraffin via indirect laryngoscopy to medialize an immobile vocal fold. Paraffin allowed for adequate medialization with improved voice but often led to troublesome paraffinomas. Eventually, it was replaced by other inorganic alloplastic materials including silicone, Teflon,[41,42] Bioplastique (a less viscous form), and, more recently, suspended hydroxylapatite Radiesse (Bioform Medical, San Mateo, CA).[43,44] Due to foreign-body reaction granulomas and fibrosis caused by the original alloplasts,[45–49] alternatives were sought. Bioimplants are histologically better tolerated, and typically they in large part become incorporated in the host tissues. The goal in injecting vocal folds with bioimplants is to place a substance that has potential to replace normal lamina propria cells and extracellular matrix. Bioimplants also induce host tissue in growth, avoiding foreign-body granulomatous reactions and favoring restoration of favorable viscoelastic properties. Biologic implants induce this tissue in growth by providing a matrix that facilitates revascularization and in growth of active fibrocytes.[50] In assessing the effect of bioimplants, persistence

Table 14.1 Overview of Injectable Substances

Material	Indication	Characteristics of Implant	Anticipated Problems	Technical Aspects
Teflon/Bioplastique	Large gap, VF paralysis, grave prognosis	Persists, long track record	Granuloma, migration, poor results persist	Deep plane, 19-gauge (g) needle
Calcium Hydroxyapatite, Radiesse (Bioform)	Large gap, VF paralysis	Appears to persist	Uncertain long-term	Deep plane, 19- to 25-g needle
Autologous fat	VF paralysis, paresis, bowing	Low reactivity, inexpensive material, not technically demanding	Unpredictable duration, poor precision, procurement effort, anesthesia, backflow	Must overfill to distortion, 18-g needle
Bovine collagen: Zyderm/Zyplast	Superficial, focal defect, bowing, Parkinson	Temporary filler, softens scar	Unpredictable duration, possible allergic reaction	Superficial and deep plane, 27-g needle
Human collagen: micronized dermis (Cymetra)	Atrophy, bowing, VF paralysis, focal defects	Safe, forgiving, effective in lamina propria or muscle	Unpredictable duration	Superficial and deep plane, 26- to 27-g needle
Gelfoam Radiesse Light*	Temporary filler, test, uncertain diagnosis	Lasts only weeks	Lasts only weeks, availability, preparation time	Inject anywhere, 18-g needle

*Soon-to-be-released product by Bioform Medical, San Mateo, CA.
Abbreviation: VF, vocal fold.

of the correction of vocal fold medialization and function is more relevant than actual persistence of the graft material.

Bovine collagen (Zyderm, Collagen Corp., Palo Alto, CA) was the first bioimplant tried[51]; the cross-linked form (Zyplast, Collagen Corp.) offered decreased risk of allergic reaction but proved less suitable for very superficial use. Both materials appeared to soften scar tissue and were shown to be suitable for small glottic gaps, focal scars, and tissue defects.[24] Autologous collagen (Vocalogen) proved effective and safe,[52] but it required a separate procedure to procure the tissues and long waits for processing the material, and it was costly. It is no longer available. Subsequent bioimplants employed included autogenous fat[7,25,53] and fascia,[54] freeze-dried irradiated human fascia (Fascian, Fascia Biosystems, Beverly Hills, CA), and micronized homologous dermis (Cymetra, Life-Cell Corp., The Woodlands, TX).[8] Concerns of allergic reaction initially limited the use of bovine collagen, but some practitioners still find it useful as a temporary filler and for very superficial applications. Injected fat is difficult to contour in the vocal fold, tends to backflow at the injection site, and requires gross overinjection of material to ensure sufficient correction. It is typically placed throughout the vocal fold tissues, making precise correction of defects difficult. The major problem with currently available bioimplants is their unpredictable persistence. Injection of important extracellular matrix components such as hyaluronic acid (HA) is an attractive option because it is found in normal vocal fold lamina propria.[55] Although HA is also prone to rapid resorption, it can be prepared with varying degrees of cross-linkage to facilitate persistence in the vocal fold; an example is the double cross-linked hyaluronan preparation Hylan B. There is unfortunately an inverse relationship between persistence and the amount of active HA available based on the extent of cross-linkage. Ongoing research is addressing the possible role of active substances that might attract favorable extracellular matrix in growth, and growth factors that induce production of favorable substances in the lamina propria.

At this time there is a spectrum of effective injectable substances that have proven effective and safe. Each substance has a range of indications, unique physical characteristics, and optimal techniques to maximize results. There are also problems encountered with each. **Table 14.1** gives a cursory outline of these features.

Selection of Injection Materials

In choosing a filler substance it is desirable to use one that not only augments but also simulates the physical characteristics of normal vocal fold tissues. Substances that induce fibroplasia or result in fibrous encapsulation must be injected in a deeper plane to preserve the delicate focal fold lamina propria essential to generation of a mucosal wave during phonation. Although several substances thought to be inert have been tried, a major challenge is to provide a substance that matches the viscoelastic properties of lamina propria, or one that promotes generation of substances favorable for normal vocal fold oscillation.

The timing of the intervention is an important factor in selecting the proper material. Factors involved in timing include the etiology of the paralysis, the prognosis for return of function, and the degree of functional impairment. When the prognosis for recovery is poor or functional impairment is severe, such as when patients suffer from aspiration and severe dysphonia, injection may be performed immediately. Teflon (polytef paste) and more recently suspensions of hydroxylapatite microspheres (Radiesse) have proven useful. In situations where recovery is likely, there is usually little harm in immediately using a bioimplant material for injection; it tends to undergo resorption, and even if it does not do so, it does not pose a substantial functional problem if the patient completely recovers from paralysis. When prognosis is uncertain, alloplasts should not be used immediately, as they can lead to irreversible tissue changes and generate symptomatic granulomas. Certainly, in patients with grave prognoses it is often best to proceed with immediate medialization using an alloplastic material. Injection should generally be delayed for patients with a minimal functional impairment and in those with a good prognosis for recovery. Selecting the proper material depends not just on timing. Other important considerations include the actual pathology or injury and the individual patient's needs.

Injection Techniques

Injection can be performed in the operating room under general anesthesia or in the clinic setting with a variety of approaches. Although direct microlaryngoscopy (DML) can provide optimal exposure without requiring patient cooperation, laryngeal anatomy is distorted both by suspension laryngoscopy and the possible presence of an endotracheal tube. In addition, the procedure requires general anesthesia with its associated risks. A major limitation is that the immediate functional outcome (including voice characteristics and impact on vocal fold oscillation or stroboscopically assessed mucosal wave) cannot be determined. In patients who fail to tolerate manipulation, in those with anatomic limitations, and certainly in situations where procurement of bioimplantable tissue is planned, DML under general anesthesia is preferable. Indirect laryngoscopy avoids the risks of general anesthesia and can be done in the office, although visualization is limited to a small nonmagnified mirror image. Telescopic laryngoscopy using only topical anesthesia performed on the awake patient is preferable, especially in a teaching setting; visualization and precision are facilitated by this approach. With the patient awake, incremental placement of the injectate is guided by immediate functional voice assessment possibly aided by videostroboscopy. Transcutaneous injection combined with flexible fiberoptic laryngoscopy can be useful in patients with difficult laryngeal exposure due to such factors as impaired neck extension, uncontrollable gag reflex, omega-shaped epiglottis, or central nervous system movement disorder.[6,56,57] In such cases, a needle is passed through the cricothyroid membrane, or bored through the thyroid cartilage, and directed into the affected vocal fold, with care taken to avoid entering the laryngeal lumen. Although topical laryngeal anesthesia is not necessary, occasionally local anesthesia in the skin at the site of needle insertion might aid in patient tolerance.

When possible, the procedure is best performed in an office or clinic setting, and the exact choice of approach depends largely on patient factors. Exposure and appropriate patient selection are critical to the success of injection augmentation. Generally, the patient should be seated upright and leaning forward with the neck extended **(Fig. 14.2, insert)**. It is helpful to have a telescope equipped for videostroboscopy to evaluate vocal fold function before, possibly during, and immediately after the procedure. A small amount of topical benzocaine is initially sprayed onto the soft palate and tongue base. The patient then protrudes and holds his or her tongue with a 4 × 4 gauze sponge. Topical 4% lidocaine is incrementally dripped onto the tongue base, the laryngeal surface of the epiglottis, supraglottis, and finally on the true vocal folds as the patient phonates **(Fig. 14.2)**. Approximately 0.3 mL is used with each step, and satisfactory anesthesia can be attained with as little as a total of 1.2 mL. Either a laryngeal mirror or the rigid telescope may be used to provide visualization for this step.

During the injection one must be mindful that restoration of proper glottic contour and matching the contralateral vocal fold are the grossly observable goals. The injectate

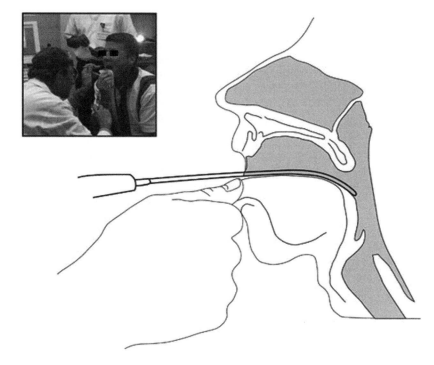

Fig. 14.2 Schematic of a midsagittal cut through the patient's head during an office-based vocal cord injection. The patient's own hand holds out his or her protruded tongue. The surgeon advances a curved metal cannula through which 4% topical lidocaine is dripped onto the tongue base, laryngeal surface of the epiglottis, supraglottis, and true vocal folds as the patient phonates. **Insert:** Optimal patient positioning is produced by seating the patient opposite the physician, upright and leaning forward in sniffing position.

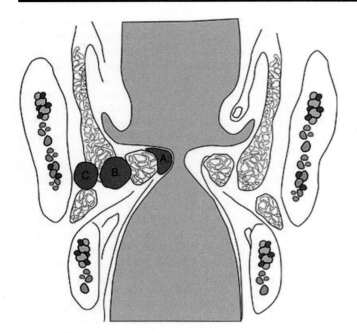

Fig. 14.3 Schematic of a midcoronal section through the larynx. Site A, superficial lamina propria; site B, deep thyroarytenoid muscle; site C, deep paraglottic space.

should provide a smooth medial edge, as the displacement of the affected membranous vocal fold progresses. Essentially it should displace the injected vocal fold to reflect the appearance of the contralateral vocal fold (**Fig. 14.3**). Displacement should be accurately placed in the vertical plane to match the level of the contralateral vocal fold. If only the superior surface of the membranous vocal fold is displaced, the vocal fold can appear adequately medialized when viewed from above, but dynamic assessment reveals adduction off-plane and breathy dysphonia remains. This is in part due to the importance of contact in the infraglottic region for achievement of effective entrainment for oscillation. Efficacy of injection should be judged both on the distance the vocal fold moves to the midline as well as the location along the membranous vocal fold where the movement occurs. Displacement in the anterior one third of the vocal fold can actually impede oscillation of the contralateral fold by premature contact and compression during phonation; this aggravates the dysphonia while failing to correct the glottic insufficiency in the posterior glottis that is important for airway protection. One may attempt to displace the cartilaginous component of the vocal fold (and thus correct posterior glottic insufficiency) by placing relatively dense injectates (e.g., polytef paste or hydroxylapatite suspension) immediately lateral to the vocal process of the arytenoids to achieve medial rotation of the vocal process. Although injection augmentation alters vocal fold viscoelasticity, this can be minimized by limiting dispersion in the superficial lamina propria.

As a rule, alloplastic substances should be placed deep within the thyroarytenoid muscle and paraglottic space to completely avoid the lamina propria (**Fig. 14.3 site C**).

Bioimplants are more forgiving, and although a variety of preferred placements have been described, most can be effective at levels varying from the superficial lamina (**Fig. 14.3 site A**) propria to the deep thyroarytenoid muscle (**Fig. 14.3 site B**). Superficial placement does result in increased stiffness, and for focal surface defects injectate should be placed with accuracy, and care should be taken not to overinject. Deeper injection requires larger amounts and can be effective with less precision, and overcorrection is necessary with bioimplants because of the more rapid resorption from deeper tissues that are more vascular. A Brunings syringe (Storz, St. Louis, MO) with an 18-gauge needle can be used to inject most alloplastics and viscous substances. Teflon is best injected lateral to the vocal ligament, into the thyroarytenoid muscle and paraglottic space. This prevents extrusion of the material, limits distortion of the vocal fold, and minimizes stiffness. Teflon provides excellent medialization, and it is effective in patients with large glottic gaps. Initial underinjection is preferred, with incremental amounts added if necessary based on careful observation, voice assessment, and ideally videostroboscopy. It is effective to begin the injection just anterior and lateral to the tip of the vocal process of the arytenoid. This is often sufficient. If the glottic gap is not adequately corrected, more material may be injected into the mid-membranous vocal fold. Injection into the anterior one third of the vocal fold as well as the subglottis should generally be avoided. In a patient at high risk for aspiration, an effort should be made to correct a posterior glottic gap by placing some material lateral to vocal process. Alloplastics such as Teflon remain an excellent choice for frail elderly patients with a large glottic gap, significant sensory impairment, or a poor prognosis for recovery. Its use is best limited to older or infirm patients in whom optimal voice outcome is not the primary concern. In these cases, the possibility of symptomatic granuloma formation, troublesome foreign-body reaction, and implant migration years later are not likely.

For less viscous injectates (e.g., collagen, Cymetra), superficial injection is often effective and the rate of resorption is reduced. A curved laryngeal injector (Medtronics Xomed, Jacksonville, FL) with a disposable 27-gauge needle is ideal. Keeping in mind the anatomic goals outlined above, one should aim to inject the material at the level of the deep lamina propria, although diffusion throughout the lamina propria is likely. Additional material can be safely injected in the deeper thyroarytenoid muscle tissue, but care must be taken superficially to avoid creation of surface blebs that can cause diplophonia and ruin the voice result. It is useful to begin at the posterior third of the membranous vocal fold.

Approximately 0.3 to 0.8 cm^3 often adequately medializes the membranous vocal fold, but considerably more can be used when placed in deeper planes. The side of the needle may be used to rub and smooth the injected material and to facilitate diffusion into surrounding tissues. If there are persistent focal gaps, further material may be placed into these areas, again with care being taken not to place much material directly into the anterior one third of the vocal fold. The vocal fold should be slightly overmedialized, given the resorption expected with bioimplants. There is more resorption of the portion of material placed deeper in the thyroarytenoid muscle and paraglottic space than with that in the more superficial plane. It appears that most bioimplants are forgiving over time, as success has been reported with a great variety of techniques. In general, bioimplants are best for treating smaller gaps and focal defects, and they are often useful as a temporizing measure while awaiting spontaneous recovery from paralysis.

Outcomes

Improved glottic closure is the expected outcome following augmentation injections. The most common immediate voice result is that patients report being able to produce a louder voice with less effort. More objective assessment of efficacy is facilitated by the use of videostroboscopy to assess vocal fold vibration, mucosal wave pattern, degree of glottic closure, vocal fold symmetry, and supraventricular hyperfunction. Acoustic measures typically reveal improvement in vocal intensity, increased signal-to-noise ratio and frequency range, and decreased perturbation measures such as jitter and shimmer. Aerodynamic changes include increased phonation time and decreased transglottic airflow during phonation. One of the most sensitive indicators of improved aerodynamic efficiency is the phonatory threshold pressure that reflects the minimal pressures necessary to produce phonation. Maximum phonation time is one simple test that the clinician can use to assess the immediate effect of augmentation, but the results are subject to great variability due to patient factors such as pulmonary reserve, practice, and individual effort. Vocal fold scarring and atrophy as well as the patient's neurologic and pulmonary status are important factors that influence voice outcomes.

Unfavorable outcomes and complications do occur. One factor might be failure to displace the affected true vocal fold in the vertical plane of the contralateral vocal fold. In this instance examination may demonstrate apparent medialization on indirect laryngoscopy, but the patient exhibits persistent breathy dysphonia.

Careful examination with videostroboscopy might then reveal that closure is incomplete and off-plane. As mentioned, injection in the anterior one third of the vocal fold can lead to stiffening of the injected side and also decrease the mucosal wave of the opposite vocal fold while possibly worsening the posterior glottic gap, leading to worsening dysphonia. Use of alloplasts such as Teflon is associated with foreign-body reaction, scarring, and granuloma formation as well as migration to distant sites. Virtually all injected Teflon results in a granuloma, but the granuloma is asymptomatic when circumscribed in the paraglottic space. Granulomas impede vocal fold function when involving the superficial layers of the vocal fold and can result in dysphonia and airway compromise. Correcting the problem requires removal of the granuloma. Partial removal can be achieved by transoral direct laryngoscopy, but in our experience the best results are obtained by total removal using an external approach as described by Netterville[58]. Essentially, the technique consists of removal of Teflon granulomas via a lateral laryngotomy and reconstruction of the vocal soft tissues by placement of an inferiorly based sternohyoid muscle flap.

Poor outcomes and complications can be minimized by good visualization and appreciation of the anatomy and the properties of the injection material. Selection of material to inject should be tailored to the individual patient's needs, the nature of the pathology, and the anticipated natural history of the problem. Injectates should not be placed in the false vocal folds, ventricles, subglottis, or the anterior one third of the membranous vocal folds. Precise visualization and placement of the injected material with good visualization is critical. Incremental assessment with videostroboscopy and voice monitoring can be very helpful in ensuring good outcomes.

♦ Frontiers and Research in Repair of Vocal Fold Incompetence

When considering the repair of vocal fold incompetence, it may be useful to consider the history of another laryngeal disorder, specifically glottic stenosis from orotracheal intubation. Scarring freezes the CA joints and we are left to choose between a sufficient airway in the case of abducted vocal folds and sufficient airway protection and voicing in the case of adducted vocal folds, but not both. Only restoration of the mobility of one or both CA joints would restore native function. Moreover, to date repairs of this disorder have involved static manipulation of the tissue in either a destructive or nondestructive pattern. The surgical goal has been guided by tipping the equilibrium either toward the airway or toward deglutition and voicing. Within the heart of every patient and surgeon, however, lies the desire to directly restore function rather than doing so indirectly, in which compromises are made. In the case of vocal fold incompetence the dilemma is not dissimilar. We have moved abnormal vocal folds closer together and injected substances intended to replicate the native tissue, but with sometimes disappointing results. Discovery of materials that are effective, long-lasting, safe, immunologically compatible, easily available, and cost-effective has been a difficult road. Tissue engineering and manipulation at the cellular level, however, offer the body the opportunity to produce what it needs locally through its own means. Recent reports help us see that restoration of the vocal folds may be within reach in this decade.

Although new technologies are promising, a notable challenge of repairing vocal fold incompetence lies partly in the multiplicity of pathophysiologies that create it. Vocal fold immobility, tissue volume loss, and pliability loss are the three main causes. Restoration of vocal fold immobility from neuromuscular causes has begun to be addressed with reconstitution of the recurrent laryngeal nerve.[59,60] Although neural integrity is promising, synkinetic reinnervation where individual laryngeal muscles are appropriately stimulated will remain a challenge. In the case of immobility from fixation, no direct repair of the scarred periarticular region of the CA joint is yet in reach.[12]

Two promising areas of research in tissue engineering relate to simple tissue loss and to tissue pliability. Tissue engineering relies on the effective interaction of a tissue scaffold, cells, and growth factors. Huber et al[34] have examined the dilemma of tissue loss from hemilaryngectomy for cancer. Their solution relies on the introduction of an exogenous tissue scaffold, where local cells and growth factors repair the defect by multilayered "fill-in." In the case of hemilaryngectomy there is a loss not only of epithelium and LP, but also of muscle and surrounding thyroid cartilage. Based on prior studies demonstrating the influx of locally organized and appropriate tissue, Badylak et al[61,62] have demonstrated in a canine model that a scaffold of porcine-derived xenogeneic extracellular matrix can be implanted and shaped to mimic the hemilarynx defect. Furthermore, after 2 months there is histologic evidence that the scaffold sheeting has completely disappeared and has been replaced with a close facsimile of the layered microstructure of the vocal fold, including the thyroid ala cartilage. This approach takes advantage of the phenomenon of organized tissue replacement, directed by the native tissues.

The use of mesenchymal stem cells uses a variant of this approach. Although once thought to be fully differentiated after birth, stem cells present in bone marrow are pleuripotent and can become bone, cartilage, muscle, tendon, adipose, and connective tissue.[63–66] Using a canine model, Kanemaru et al[67] injected surgically injured canine vocal folds with autogenous stem cells and an atelocollagen scaffold carrier. At 2 months, they noted that the vocal folds injected with stem cells and carrier successfully filled in the tissue defect, whereas the vocal folds with carrier only did not. The injected stem cells were noted to be viable. The tissue was not reported to fill in with a layered microstructure. Ongoing work will elucidate the controlling factors in this reparative process.

Restoration of the LP is an area of active research where the application of growth factors offers promise. Wound healing in canine and rabbit vocal folds has been elucidated using histologic, rheometric, and enzyme-linked immunosorbent (ELISA) assays for levels of certain extracellular matrix components. Using a rabbit model for vocal fold scarring after forceps injury, Thibeault et al[68] found an increased level of deposition of collagen, decreased procollagen, and decreased elastin when compared with the uninjured side. Furthermore, rheometric analysis revealed an increased elastic shear modulus and dynamic viscosity on the scarred side. Rousseau et al[69] later corroborated the findings of increased collagen deposition and reduced pliability in the rabbit model. Using a canine model, Hirano et al[70] found that collagen was increased in scarred vocal folds after 2 months and again after 6 months when compared with normals.

In an effort to reduce collagen production during the healing process and thereby enhance pliability, hepatocyte growth factor (HGF) was applied to healing rabbit vocal folds. The vocal folds were then subjected to histologic, rheologic, stroboscopic, and aerodynamic analyses. Treated vocal folds were found to have reduced collagen production, less scar contracture, increased pliability, and improved phonation threshold pressures, glottal closure, and vocal efficiency, when compared with the untreated side.[27] In a similar canine study, Hirano et al[27] examined the effects of HGF with and without the addition of cultured dog fibroblasts (Fb) on wounded vocal folds. After 6 months, similar analyses were conducted revealing that the HGF-treated group had the most dramatic improvement in vibratory and histologic metrics when compared with the sham and HGF/Fb groups. Specifically, there was improved, but not normal, deposition of collagen with reduced scar contracture, improved phonation threshold pressure, and glottal efficiency.[27] Given that HGF was injected at the time of injury in the rabbit model and 1 month postinjury in the canine model, there is evidence that HGF shows promise in the prevention and treatment of vocal fold scarring. Other extracellular components are also targets for reconstitution.

Hyaluronic acid (HA) has been noted to be a major contributor in fetal scarless wound healing. Also, given its presence in human vocal fold LP as an important contributor to normal pliability, its restoration after vocal fold injury has been investigated. Using cultured canine fibroblasts, HGF, epidermal growth factor, basic fibroblast growth factor, and transforming growth factor-β1 all stimulated HA synthesis.[71] Furthermore, HGF stimulated the production of [44]HA and decreased the production of collagen type I from the fibroblasts in Reinke's space in cultured human fibroblasts.[72] Most recently, Hirano et al[73] conducted a study on fibroblasts harvested from young and aged rat vocal folds. They were cultured with or without HGF or basic fibroblast growth factor at different concentrations and subjected to ELISA for production of HA and collagen type I. Basic growth factor was found to have a dramatic result on aged fibroblasts, with a notable decrease in collagen production and increase in HA. Furthermore, the aged fibroblasts themselves grew in size.[73]

Other potential pathways for intervention include gene therapy. These techniques may be used on LP fibroblasts to enhance the profile of collagen, HA, and other extracellular proteins such as elastin and fibronectin. Certainly there is a wealth of possibilities related to possible interventions. During trials of these modalities, there is sure to be an improved understanding of the healing process itself and the relationship of the native cells, extracellular proteins, and growth factors. This clarity will allow more precise and elegant solutions to the multifaceted challenge of vocal fold incompetence.

References

1. Hirano M, Yoshida T, Tanaka S, Hibi S. Sulcus vocalis: functional aspects. Ann Otol Rhinol Laryngol 1990;99(9 Pt 1):679–683
2. Hammarberg B, Fritzell B, Schiratzki H. Teflon injection in 16 patients with paralytic dysphonia: perceptual and acoustic evaluations. J Speech Hear Disord 1984;49:72–82
3. Hartl DM, Hans S, Vaissiere J, Riquet M, Laccourreye O, Brasnu DF. Objective voice analysis after autologous fat injection for unilateral vocal fold paralysis. Ann Otol Rhinol Laryngol 2001;110:229–235
4. Myssiorek D. Recurrent laryngeal nerve paralysis: anatomy and etiology. [Review] [127 refs] Otolaryngol Clin North Am 2004;37:25–44

5. Zeitels SM, Hochman I, Hillman RE. Adduction arytenopexy: a new procedure for paralytic dysphonia with implications for implant medialization. [Review] [110 refs] Ann Otol Rhinol Laryngol Suppl 1998;173:2–24

6. Hirano M, Tanaka S, Tanaka Y, Hibi S. Transcutaneous intrafold injection for unilateral vocal fold paralysis: functional results. Ann Otol Rhinol Laryngol 1990;99:598–604

7. McCulloch TM, Andrews BT, Hoffman HT, Graham SM, Karnell MP, Minnick C. Long-term follow-up of fat injection laryngoplasty for unilateral vocal cord paralysis. Laryngoscope 2002;112(7 Pt 1):1235–1238

8. Lundy DS, Casiano RR, McClinton ME, Xue JW. Early results of transcutaneous injection laryngoplasty with micronized acellular dermis versus type-I thyroplasty for glottic incompetence dysphonia due to unilateral vocal fold paralysis. J Voice 2003;17:589–595

9. Woodson GE. Configuration of the glottis in laryngeal paralysis. I: Clinical study. Laryngoscope 1993;103(11 Pt 1):1227–1234

10. Dursun G, Sataloff RT, Spiegel JR, Mandel S, Heuer RJ, Rosen DC. Superior laryngeal nerve paresis and paralysis. J Voice 1996;10:206–211

11. Eckley CA, Sataloff RT, Hawkshaw M, Spiegel JR, Mandel S. Voice range in superior laryngeal nerve paresis and paralysis. J Voice 1998;12:340–348

12. Bastian RW, Richardson BE. Postintubation phonatory insufficiency: an elusive diagnosis. Otolaryngol Head Neck Surg 2001;124:625–633

13. Montgomery WW. Cricoarytenoid arthritis. Laryngoscope 1963;73:801–836

14. Goodman M, Montgomery W, Minette L. Pathologic findings in gouty cricoarytenoid arthritis. Arch Otolaryngol 1976;102:27–29

15. Montgomery WW, Goodman ML. Rheumatoid cricoarytenoid arthritis complicated by upper esophageal ulcerations. Ann Otol Rhinol Laryngol 1980;89(1 Pt 1):6–8 -Feb.

16. Guttenplan MD, Hendrix RA, Townsend MJ, Balsara G. Laryngeal manifestations of gout. [Review] [17 refs] Ann Otol Rhinol Laryngol 1991;100:899–902

17. Paulsen FP, Tillmann BN. Osteoarthritis in cricoarytenoid joint. Osteoarthritis Cartilage 1999;7:505–514

18. Muller A, Paulsen FP. Impact of vocal cord paralysis on cricoarytenoid joint. Ann Otol Rhinol Laryngol 2002;111:896–901

19. Isshiki N, Tsuji DH, Yamamoto Y, Iizuka Y. Midline lateralization thyroplasty for adductor spasmodic dysphonia. Ann Otol Rhinol Laryngol 2000;109:187–193

20. Isshiki N, Haji T, Yamamoto Y, Mahieu HF. Thyroplasty for adductor spasmodic dysphonia: further experiences. Laryngoscope 2001;111(4 Pt 1):615–621

21. Zeitels SM, Mauri M, Dailey SH. Medialization laryngoplasty with Gore-Tex for voice restoration secondary to glottal incompetence: indications and observations. Ann Otol Rhinol Laryngol 2003;112:180–184

22. Sato K, Hirano M. Age-related changes of the macula flava of the human vocal fold. Ann Otol Rhinol Laryngol 1995;104:839–844

23. Sato K, Hirano M, Nakashima T. Age-related changes of collagenous fibers in the human vocal fold mucosa. Ann Otol Rhinol Laryngol 2002;111:15–20

24. Ford CN, Bless DM, Loftus JM. Role of injectable collagen in the treatment of glottic insufficiency: a study of 119 patients. Ann Otol Rhinol Laryngol 1992;101:237–247

25. Hsiung MW, Woo P, Minasian A, Schaefer MJ. Fat augmentation for glottic insufficiency. Laryngoscope 2000;110:1026–1033

26. Hsiung MW, Lin YS, Su WF, Wang HW. Autogenous fat injection for vocal fold atrophy. Eur Arch Otorhinolaryngol 2003;260:469–474

27. Hirano S, Bless DM, Nagai H, et al. Growth factor therapy for vocal fold scarring in a canine model. Ann Otol Rhinol Laryngol 2004;113:777–785

28. Krespi YP, Mitrani M, Husain S, Meltzer CJ. Treatment of laryngeal sarcoidosis with intralesional steroid injection. Ann Otol Rhinol Laryngol 1987;96:713–715 -Dec.

29. Akst LM, Thompson LD. Larynx amyloidosis. Ear Nose Throat J 2003;82:844–845

30. Zeitels SM, Dailey SH, Burns JA. Technique of en block laser endoscopic frontolateral laryngectomy for glottic cancer. Laryngoscope 2004;114:175–180

31. Zeitels SM, Jarboe J, Franco RA. Phonosurgical reconstruction of early glottic cancer. Laryngoscope 2001;111:1862–1865

32. Zeitels SM, Hillman RE, Franco RA, Bunting GW. Voice and treatment outcome from phonosurgical management of early glottic cancer. Ann Otol Rhinol Laryngol Suppl 2002;190:3–20

33. Zeitels SM. Optimizing voice after endoscopic partial laryngectomy. [Review] [33 refs] Otolaryngol Clin North Am 2004;37:627–636

34. Huber JE, Spievack A, Simmons-Byrd A, Ringel RL, Badylak S. Extracellular matrix as a scaffold for laryngeal reconstruction. Ann Otol Rhinol Laryngol 2003;112:428–433

35. Gray SD, Hammond E, Hanson DF. Benign pathologic responses of the larynx. Ann Otol Rhinol Laryngol 1995;104:13–18

36. Zeitels SM, Franco RA Jr, Dailey SH, Burns JA, Hillman RE, Anderson RR. Office-based treatment of glottal dysplasia and papillomatosis with the 585-nm pulsed dye laser and local anesthesia. Ann Otol Rhinol Laryngol 2004;113:265–276

37. Pasquale K, Wiatrak B, Woolley A, Lewis L. Microdebrider versus CO2 laser removal of recurrent respiratory papillomas: a prospective analysis. Laryngoscope 2003;113:139–143

38. Ford CN, Inagi K, Khidr A, Bless DM, Gilchrist KW. Sulcus vocalis: a rational analytical approach to diagnosis and management. Ann Otol Rhinol Laryngol 1996;105:189–200

39. Welham NV, Rousseau B, Ford CN, Bless DM. Tracking outcomes after phonosurgery for sulcus vocalis: a case report. J Voice 2003;17:571–578

40. Sataloff RT, Spiegel JR, Hawkshaw MJ. Strobovideolaryngoscopy: results and clinical value. Ann Otol Rhinol Laryngol 1991;100(9 Pt 1):725–727

41. Dedo HH, Urrea RD, Lawson L. Intracordal injection of Teflon in the treatment of 135 patients with dysphonia. Ann Otol Rhinol Laryngol 1973;82:661–667

42. Montgomery WW. Laryngeal paralysis–teflon injection. Ann Otol Rhinol Laryngol 1979;88(5 Pt 1):647–657

43. Belafsky PC, Postma GN. Vocal fold augmentation with calcium hydroxylapatite. Otolaryngol Head Neck Surg 2004;131:351–354

44. Rosen CA, Thekdi AA. Vocal fold augmentation with injectable calcium hydroxylapatite: short-term results. J Voice 2004;18:387–391

45. Varvares MA, Montgomery WW, Hillman RE. Teflon granuloma of the larynx: etiology, pathophysiology, and management. Ann Otol Rhinol Laryngol 1995;104:511–515

46. Toomey JM, Brown BS. The histological response to intracordal injection of teflon paste. Laryngoscope 1967;77:110–120

47. Dedo HH, Carlsoo B. Histologic evaluation of Teflon granulomas of human vocal cords. A light and electron microscopic study. Acta Otolaryngol 1982;93:475–484

48. Kasperbauer JL, Slavit DH, Maragos NE. Teflon granulomas and overinjection of Teflon: a therapeutic challenge for the otorhinolaryngologist. Ann Otol Rhinol Laryngol 1993;102:748–751

49. Malizia AA Jr, Reiman HM, Myers RP, et al. Migration and granulomatous reaction after periurethral injection of polytef (Teflon). JAMA 1984;251:3277–3281

50. Ford CN. Histologic studies on the fate of soluble collagen injected into canine vocal folds. Laryngoscope 1986;96:1248–1257

51. Ford CN, Bless DM. Clinical experience with injectable collagen for vocal fold augmentation. Laryngoscope 1986;96:863–869

52. Ford CN, Staskowski PA, Bless DM. Autologous collagen vocal fold injection: a preliminary clinical study. Laryngoscope 1995;105(9 Pt 1):944–948

53. Bauer CA, Valentino J, Hoffman HT. Long-term result of vocal cord augmentation with autogenous fat. Ann Otol Rhinol Laryngol 1995;104:871–874

54. Rihkanen H, Lehikoinen-Soderlund S, Reijonen P. Voice acoustics after autologous fascia injection for vocal fold paralysis. Laryngoscope 1999;109:1854–1858

55. Hertegard S, Dahlqvist A, Laurent C, Borzacchiello A, Ambrosio L. Viscoelastic properties of rabbit vocal folds after augmentation. Otolaryngol Head Neck Surg 2003;128:401–406
56. McCaffrey TV. Transcutaneous Teflon injection for vocal cord paralysis. Otolaryngol Head Neck Surg 1993;109:54–59
57. Ward PH, Hanson DG, Abemayor E. Transcutaneous Teflon injection of the paralyzed vocal cord: a new technique. Laryngoscope 1985;95:644–649
58. Netterville JL, Colemon JR Jr, Chang S, Rainey CL, Reinisch L, Ossoff RH. Lateral laryngotomy for the removal of Teflon granuloma. Ann Otol Rhinol Laryngol 1998;107:735–744
59. Kanemaru S, Nakamura T, Omori K, et al. Recurrent laryngeal nerve regeneration by tissue engineering. Ann Otol Rhinol Laryngol 2003;112:492–498
60. Rubin A, Mobley B, Hogikyan N, et al. Delivery of an adenoviral vector to the crushed recurrent laryngeal nerve. Laryngoscope 2003;113:985–989
61. Badylak SF, Tullius R, Kokini K, et al. The use of xenogeneic small intestinal submucosa as a biomaterial for Achilles tendon repair in a dog model. J Biomed Mater Res 1995;29:977–985
62. Badylak SF, Record R, Lindberg K, Hodde J, Park K. Small intestinal submucosa: a substrate for in vitro cell growth. J Biomater Sci Polym Ed 1998;9:863–878
63. Horwitz EM, Prockop DJ, Fitzpatrick LA, et al. Transplantability and therapeutic effects of bone marrow-derived mesenchymal cells in children with osteogenesis imperfecta. [see comment] Nat Med 1999;5:309–313
64. Pittenger MF, Mackay AM, Beck SC, et al. Multilineage potential of adult human mesenchymal stem cells. Science 1999;284:143–147
65. Deans RJ, Moseley AB. Mesenchymal stem cells: biology and potential clinical uses. [Review] [92 refs] Exp Hematol 2000;28:875–884
66. Woodbury D, Schwarz EJ, Prockop DJ, Black IB. Adult rat and human bone marrow stromal cells differentiate into neurons. J Neurosci Res 2000;61:364–370
67. Kanemaru S, Nakamura T, Omori K, et al. Regeneration of the vocal fold using autologous mesenchymal stem cells. Ann Otol Rhinol Laryngol 2003;112:915–920
68. Thibeault SL, Gray SD, Bless DM, Chan RW, Ford CN. Histologic and rheologic characterization of vocal fold scarring. J Voice 2002;16:96–104
69. Rousseau B, Hirano S, Chan RW, et al. Characterization of chronic vocal fold scarring in a rabbit model. J Voice 2004;18:116–124
70. Hirano S, Bless DM, Rousseau B, Welham N, Scheidt T, Ford CN. Fibronectin and adhesion molecules on canine scarred vocal folds. Laryngoscope 2003;113:966–972
71. Hirano S, Bless DM, Heisey D, Ford CN. Effect of growth factors on hyaluronan production by canine vocal fold fibroblasts. Ann Otol Rhinol Laryngol 2003;112:617–624
72. Hirano S, Bless DM, Massey RJ, Hartig GK, Ford CN. Morphological and functional changes of human vocal fold fibroblasts with hepatocyte growth factor. Ann Otol Rhinol Laryngol 2003;112:1026–1033
73. Hirano S, Bless DM, del Rio AM, Connor NP, Ford CN. Therapeutic potential of growth factors for aging voice. Laryngoscope 2004;114:2161–2167

Chapter 15

Vocal Fold Medialization, Arytenoid Adduction, and Reinnervation

Andrew Blitzer, Steven M. Zeitels, James L. Netterville, Tanya K. Meyer, and Marshall E. Smith

Restoration of vocal function with laryngeal framework surgery (laryngoplastic phonosurgery) was introduced at the beginning of the 20th century. Today, these procedures have emerged as the dominant surgical management approach for the treatment of the aerodynamic incompetence and acoustic deterioration associated with vocal fold paralysis/paresis. Other indications include cancer defects, vocal fold scar, sulcus vocalis, bowing associated with vocal fold atrophy, laryngeal trauma, and neuromuscular disorders including abductor spasmodic dysphonia and parkinsonism. Laryngeal framework surgery has also been employed to alter pitch for gender reassignment; however, this topic is not discussed here.

Although medialization of the musculomembranous vocal fold by means of rearranging the laryngeal cartilage framework was described by Payr[1] in 1915, and others in the mid–20th century,[2,3] Isshiki et al[4-6] championed the systematic analysis and laryngoplastic treatment of glottal incompetence in the 1970s. He designed his medialization procedure of the musculomembranous vocal fold with the use of a synthetic implant in 1974.

In 1978, Isshiki et al[5] designed the arytenoid adduction procedure to treat patients with large glottal gaps secondary to a malpositioned arytenoid. One of his outstanding contributions is that he taught surgeons that laryngeal framework procedures could be done with facility utilizing local anesthesia with sedation. The concept that the cricoarytenoid joint could be dissected and manipulated under local anesthesia to allow for phonatory feedback was revolutionary. Based on this seminal work, the adduction arytenopexy[2,7-9] and cricothyroid subluxation[7,8,10] procedures were introduced to further enhance phonatory reconstruction.

♦ Laryngeal Framework Surgery

Isshiki's Classification

Isshiki[6] described four basic surgical procedures that he termed thyroplasty types I to IV for altering the conformation of the thyroid cartilage and the arytenoid adduction, which attempts to close the posterior (cartilaginous) glottis.

Thyroplasty Type I

Thyroplasty type I (**Fig. 15.1**) is the most widely used of Isshiki's original thyroplasty techniques. It involves creating a rectangular cartilaginous window at the level of the true vocal fold and using cartilage, Silastic, Gore-Tex, or other implant material to medialize the true vocal fold. This procedure achieves closure of the musculomembranous vocal fold only; arytenoid position is not appreciably altered by the implant. Thyroplasty type I is a relatively simple and reversible procedure that is ideally performed with local anesthesia to facilitate fine-tuning of the voice with precise placement of the implant material. There have been a large number of manuscripts describing a multitude of variations of the original procedure, primarily introducing different implant materials and their placement. As thyroplasty type I does not primarily influence arytenoid position, this procedure is often coupled with an arytenoid adduction or arytenopexy to close both the anterior (musculomembranous) and posterior (cartilaginous) glottis.

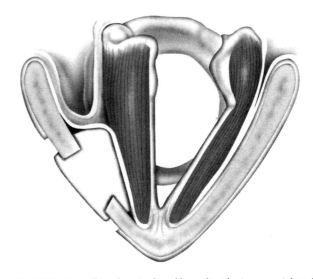

Fig. 15.1 A small implant is placed lateral to the inner perichondrium of the thyroid lamina.

Thryoplasty Types II to IV

Thyroplasty type II is a procedure in which the posterolateral thyroid lamina is lateralized; there are few indications for its use. Thyroplasty type III is used to lower the vocal pitch by shortening the anteroposterior (AP) dimension of the glottis. The primary function is to release vocal fold tension to lower pitch. Conversely, thyroplasty type IV increases the AP dimension of the glottis, thereby increasing the tension on the vocal folds and raising the vocal pitch. Thyroplasty types III and IV have been used in gender reassignment surgery to bring the fundamental frequency into the normal range for the newly assigned sex.

Arytenoid Adduction

Arytenoid adduction was described by Isshiki et al[5] as a way of mimicking the medializing effect of the lateral cricoarytenoid muscle on the vocal process. A paralyzed arytenoid tends to fall forward and laterally on the cricoid facet, shortening the AP length of the vocal fold and moving the arytenoid away from the midline. The classic arytenoid adduction procedure is performed under local anesthesia with sedation by exposing the posterior aspect of the thyroid lamina. The cricoarytenoid joint is identified, and a suture is placed through the muscular process of the arytenoid and passed anteriorly through the thyroid lamina, thereby rotating the vocal process medially to meet the opposite vocal process during phonation. Prior to the conclusion of the surgical procedure the position is visually verified by means of a flexible fiberoptic laryngoscope.

Principles and Theory of Laryngeal Framework Surgery

The ideal procedure(s) to treat aerodynamic glottal incompetence that is associated with paralytic/paretic dysphonia should attempt to simulate the normal vocal fold position during phonation with regard to the following interdependent parameters: (1) position of the musculomembranous region in the axial plane, (2) position of the arytenoid in the axial plane, (3) height of the vocal fold, (4) length of the vocal fold, (5) contour of the vocal fold edge in the musculomembranous region, (6) contour of the vocal fold edge in the arytenoid region, and (7) mass and viscoelasticity of the vocal fold.

Furthermore, the procedure(s) ideally should be easy to perform, associated with few complications, reliable, reversible, and not threatening to the airway.[11] The basic technique for medialization laryngoplasty is very similar for each of the implant materials. If one understands the fundamental principles behind placing the vocal cord into the physiologic phonating position, the choice of implant material is of secondary importance. One can achieve very good results with almost any implant, if the principles outlined below are adhered to. Some implants due to their size constraints may make it harder to place the vocal fold in the correct position. Other implants offer initial excellent voice results, but are not stable and may move from the initial location with delayed decrease in voice quality. Following the outlined steps in any described technique is secondary to a basic understanding of the physiologic phonating position of the vocal cord.

Unless contraindicated, some authors start patients on a Medrol DosePack the day before surgery, and patients are given 0.2 mg/kg of Decadron 1 hour prior to the procedure. This helps to minimize intraoperative swelling, which can interfere with determining the implant size, and reduces postoperative airway swelling.

The anesthetic preparation of the patient is extremely important. It is very easy to oversedate the patient, leading to slurred lethargic speech. With slight oversedation the muscle tone of the hypopharynx grows weak, making it very difficult to see the vocal folds on the monitor, or judge voice improvement in the lethargic patient. The majority of patients need only a few milligrams of Versed to undergo the entire procedure. It is critical to have an alert and oriented patient to obtain good results. Some anesthesiologists prefer to administer intravenous propofol, which can be quickly reversed when patient cooperation is necessary, and then the patient can be quickly sedated after implant placement.

Once the patient is mildly sedated, the patient's nose is anesthetized by instilling 4 cc of 5% cocaine into the nasal cavity. A flexible fiberoptic scope is introduced transnasally, suspended above the patient, and attached to the video monitor system so that the larynx can be visualized on the monitor during the entire procedure (**Fig. 15.2**). Other surgeons pass an endoscope at critical times during the procedure when visualization is important. This makes the patient more comfortable during the procedure.

Preoperative intramuscular Robinal is administered to decrease the pharyngeal secretions during the procedure. To increase the likelihood of success, one needs both auditory and visual feedback, to access the position of the vocal fold during testing. Intraoperative visualization of the vocal fold provides two distinct advantages: (1) The relative position of the vocal fold within the window can be identified early in the procedure. (2) Initial hyperfunctional, pressed, strained voice, can be very confusing to the surgeon unless he can observe the position of the vocal fold on the monitor. In this

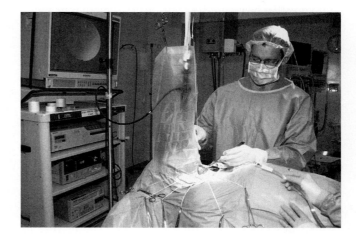

Fig. 15.2 The flexible nasolaryngoscope, suspended above the patient, and attached to the video monitor, is used to view the position of the vocal cord throughout the procedure.

setting, with the vocal fold displaced toward the midline, the hyperfunctional state of the larynx can be readily seen on the monitor. As outlined below, the patient is coached to relax his larynx during continued voice testing, until the hyperfunctional state is released. This slow, relaxation of the supraglottic larynx is seen on the monitor as the voice begins to improve. In the rare patient, where the hyperfunctional voice does not break, one can complete the operation, by observing the television monitor and placing the paralyzed vocal fold in the midline. Even though the perioperative voice continues to be strained, the majority of these patients will develop reasonable quality voice. Without the ability to visualize the glottis it would be very difficult to acquire good voice results in this subgroup of patients.

Local anesthesia is injected into the skin and subcutaneous tissues of the anterior neck. It is infiltrated along the thyroid cartilage extending deeply to the posterior border of this cartilage. This is usually sufficient to perform the entire procedure. Local anesthesia is never injected into the paraglottic space or the postcricoid region. As long as the mucosa of the endolarynx, and the piriform sinuses, are not violated, the patients will have very little sensation in these two regions.

Procedures

Netterville's Technique for Silastic Implants

An incision is created in a skin crease overlying the cricothyroid membrane. If an arytenoid adduction is planned, the incision should be at least 5 to 6 cm in length. Initial elevation is performed superficial to the strap muscle layer. If one anticipates atrophy of the thyroarytenoid muscle, then fat is carefully left approximated to the fascia overlying the strap muscles. If needed later in the procedure, this can be developed into a laterally based vascularized fat flap to use in reconstruction of the paraglottic space. After the strap mussels have been separated in the midline, the medial 2 cm of the sternohyoid muscle is divided 6 to 7 mm inferior to its attachment to the hyoid bone. The sternothyroid muscle is lifted up as the perichondrium is elevated off the thyroid cartilage. If the addition of an arytenoid adduction (AA) is anticipated, the perichondrium is elevated to the posterior border of the thyroid cartilage. The window is laid out on the lateral surface of the cartilage. There has been considerable debate over the location of this window. Many formulas have been described to accurately locate this window just lateral to the vocal fold. Most of these formulas result in a window that is too high. The implant, if placed in the center portion of these higher windows, leads to overmedialization of the false vocal fold and the ventricle, resulting in rough or diplophonic voice. The lower the window is, the easier it is to accomplish medialization in the appropriate plane. Therefore, the window is placed as low on the thyroid cartilage as possible, leaving a 2- to 3-mm inferior strip of cartilage below the edge of the window **(Fig. 15.3)**.

In other descriptions of the surgical technique, the cartilage island is left within the window and displaced into the paraglottic space as a biologic tissue implant. Leaving the island as a natural tissue barrier is not necessary, and in reality

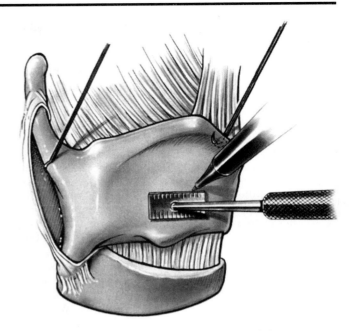

Fig. 15.3 The window is outlined as low as possible leaving a 2- to 3-mm strut of cartilage below the window. The anterior border of the window is placed back from the anterior commissure 5 mm in women and 7 mm in men.

the island impedes consistently good voice results. Early in our series we realized that the cartilage island was not stable. The island often shifted out of position, or atrophied, resulting in loss of the initial improvement in voice quality.

Also, if the cartilage island is left within the window, and used to displace the vocal fold, the window must be placed in exactly the right location to achieve optimal results. It is also common for the needed plane of medialization to be so discrete that medialization within the superior portion of a 6-mm-wide window results in poor strained voice, whereas medialization within the lower third results in normal voice. It is far more practical to use the window as an entry into the paraglottic space, using an implant system that allows one infinite variability in placing the vocal fold in the physiologic phonating position, no matter where the position of the vocal fold is in relation to the window. Another common mistake is creating a window that is too small. This makes it very difficult to test medialization in all aspects of the paraglottic space. It is also very difficult to place an appropriate-size implant through a small window. In view of this, we recommend creating a window that is it least 6 by 13 mm in size. The window is placed parallel to the imagined plane of the vocal fold as low as possible on the thyroid cartilage, as outlined above. The window is started back from the anterior commissure approximately 5 mm in the female and 7 mm in the male. The window may need to extend to 15 to 16 mm in length in large men to have access to the paraglottic space to appropriately test and medialize the posterior one third of the vocal fold. In a female of small stature, it may be necessary to extend the window toward the anterior commissure of the thyroid cartilage. These intraoperative window adjustments are usually easy to determine as one tests for the location of the vocal fold within the window.

A high-speed drill with a 3-mm cutting burr is used to remove the cartilage from the window. The inner perichondrium is carefully protected as the cartilage is removed, to prevent damage of the underlying muscle by the drill bit. The early descriptions of medialization laryngoplasty (ML) recommended preservation of the inner perichondrium as a biologic barrier to prevent implant extrusion. In 1987 we began to remove the entire cartilage island and carefully divide the inner perichondrium to consistently obtain discrete medialization at the level of the vocal fold. We recommend dividing the perichondrium at the edge of the window and removing it from within the window. This can be done carefully with a small sharp knife blade without injuring the underlying thyroarytenoid (TA) muscle fascia. As the perichondrium is divided, one can see the natural space between the perichondrium and the TA muscle fascia (**Fig. 15.4**). The vascular supply of the paraglottic space runs deep to the TA fascia; therefore, this potential space between the two layers can be quite dry and avascular. At this point one carefully elevates the paraglottic soft tissue away from the inner perichondrium, leaving the inner perichondrium still in place attached to the medial surface of the thyroid cartilage. The position of the vocal fold in relation to the window can now be ascertained by gently displacing the TA muscle with a blunt probe in all quadrants of the window while observing the soft tissue movement on the monitor. Displacement of the soft tissue in the superior half of the window often results in prolapse of the ventricle and or the false vocal fold. In most men, the maximum plane of medialization, necessary to obtain quality voice, is in the lower third of the window. Even in females, with the window placed near the lower border of the cartilage, the plane of medialization is usually in the middle to lower half of the window. Determination of the appropriate plane of maximum medialization (the level within the window) is critical in obtaining good voice. One of the major causes of poor voice results, leading to revision surgery, is an appropriately sized implant that is placed 2 to 3 mm too high. This results in rough raspy voice quality, with marked vocal fatigue.

To judge the size of the implant the voice is tested during medialization of the focal fold with the depth gauge. The size and shape of a depth gauge should simulate the medialization that will be obtained with the implant (**Fig. 15.5**). Due to the smaller size and more obtuse angle of the thyroid cartilage in females, a smaller depth gauge is needed for the female larynx. The voice is tested by moving the depth gauge in all aspects of the window with varying degrees of medialization. The medialization of the vocal fold is observed on the television monitor as this testing occurs.

The majority of patients who present with vocal cord paralysis have developed compensatory speech patterns with a hyperfunctional pressed voice quality. During the initial aspect of testing, as the paralyzed vocal fold is displaced toward the midline this hyperfunctional, pressed voice quality only becomes worse. Instead of the beautiful voice the surgeons hope to hear, it is very common for the patient to develop an extremely strained voice during the initial aspect of testing. When this occurs, the surgeon, while observing the position of the vocal fold on the monitor, depresses and holds it as near the midline as possible. The patient is then coached to relax and try to speak in a softer voice, releasing the strained quality. It may take anywhere from 2 to 20 minutes of continued coaching for this hyperfunctional speech pattern to break. With a persistent, stubborn, pressed voice, the patient is asked to start each word by humming, which relaxes the larynx. The patient is instructed to count to 10, starting each word with the humming sound. In the majority of patients this hyperfunctional speech breaks within 5 to 10 minutes. It takes patience on

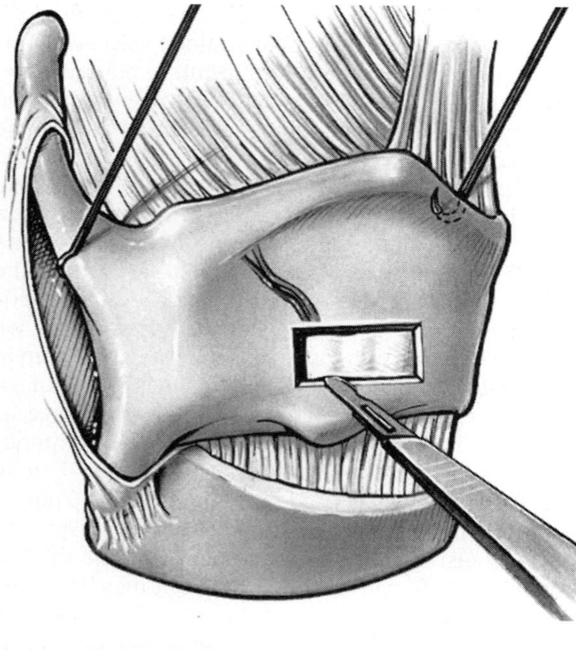

Fig. 15.4 To prepare for implant placement, the inner perichondrium is divided around the window edge. The plane of elevation is medial to the inner perichondrium, and superficial (lateral) to the thyroarytenoid muscle fascia.

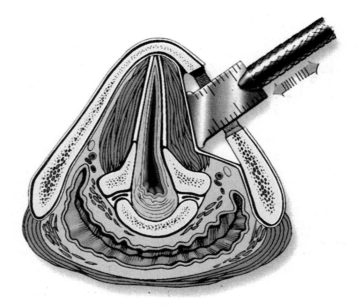

Fig. 15.5 The depth gauge is used within the window for intraoperative voice testing. The testing gauge should simulate the shape of the implant.

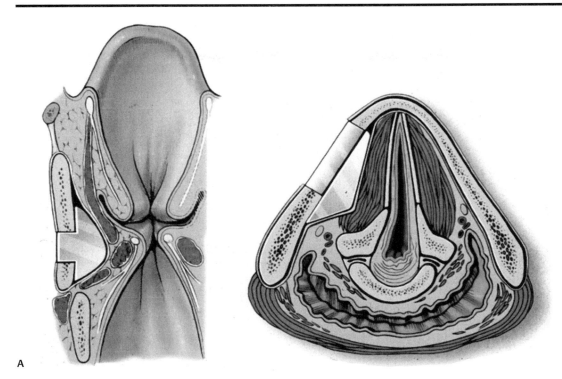

Fig. 15.6 The final implant is placed within the pocket just deep to the thyroid cartilage displacing the thyroarytenoid (TA) muscle toward the midline. The implant is carved with wide flanges to fit snugly against the inner surface of the thyroid cartilage, creating a stable implant that resists movement or migration.

the part of the surgeon to wait for a good voice to develop. After the pressed voice begins to break, and reasonable voice quality develops, one can then judge the size of the implant needed by the position of the depth gauge within the window. The average depth of medialization in most men and women is approximately 5 mm in the posterior aspect of the implant, with 1 mm or less medialization needed in the anterior aspect of the window.

An implant is fashioned matching the measurements that produced excellent voice during testing with the depth gauge. The lower flange is placed into the window first as the implant is rotated and compressed through the window. The flanges and lateral strut lock the implant into position (**Fig. 15.6**). A 4-0 Prolene suture placed through the implant around the lower strut of the window further stabilizes the implant. As one gains experience with this procedure, it is impressive how subtly different patients are. To achieve consistently good voice results, one must tailor the size of the implant and the level of medialization to each patient. As can be realized from the above discussion, starting with a limited selection of prefabricated implants can compromise the voice results in some patients.

Meyer and Blitzer's Rationale and Technique for Using the VoCoM (Nonporous Hydroxylapatite Ceramic) Prosthesis

Rationale The VoCoM thyroplasty method[12] is a self-contained system of implants and instruments to allow accurate vocal fold medialization. The implants come in five sizes and are secured with one of four shims, allowing placement of the implant in several different positions. Specifically, the implant can be secured in a horizontal or vertical position, at the superior or inferior boarder of the thyroplasty window, and at any position along the anterior to posterior position of the thyroplasty window (**Fig. 15.7**).

There are several advantages inherent in the design of this system, which streamlines the actual surgical procedure. This is critical to the success of the thyroplasty technique, as tissue edema, which develops from excessive operative time or manipulation, can make it difficult for the surgeon to judge the appropriate vocal endpoint. A specially designed surgical instrument set facilitates window placement, determination of implant size and optimal location, and insertion of the implant. The graduated prefabricated implants and shims obviate the need to hand carve implants on the back table during the procedure, saving valuable operative time. The implant is made of hydroxylapatite with proven biocompatibility that generates a thin fibrous encapsulation. In some individuals there may be osteogenesis in the region of the fenestra, creating lamellar bone bridging between the implant and the thyroid lamina.[13] For individuals with paresis and residual motion, this provides implant stability and minimizes the risk of migration or extrusion. Although the osteogenesis is localized and does not preclude implant removal, this system should not be used in individuals in whom removal is anticipated.

The main disadvantage of the system is that the firm nature of the implant does not allow for further carving, and additional modification of the shape must be done with a diamond drill. Additionally, osteointegration in the area of

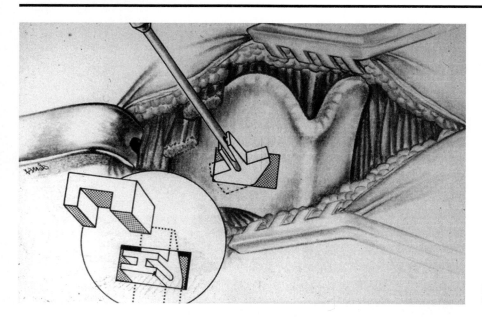

Fig. 15.7 The VoCoM implant and shim system for vocal cord medialization.

the thyroid lamina may make the procedure less easily reversible than other implants such as Silastic.

Technique A 4- to 5-cm horizontal incision is made over the lateral aspect of the thyroid lamina and extended 1 cm across the midline (**Fig. 15.8**). Subplatysmal flaps are elevated superiorly and inferiorly, and the strap muscles are separated in the midline and retracted laterally. Fibers of the thyrohyoid are divided with electrocautery to delineate the inferior boarder of the thyroid cartilage, and the thyroid lamina is exposed by retraction of the strap muscles laterally and by rotating the larynx to the contralateral side using a single hook placed at the thyroid notch.

To prevent coughing during implant manipulation, topical anesthetic can be injected into the subglottic airway or 50 to 100 mg of lidocaine can be given intravenously just prior to the entry through the thyroid lamina. Interestingly, no local anesthetic is needed in the paraglottic tissues during implant manipulation.

The position of the cartilage window is determined. The superior aspect of the window should be placed at the level of the true vocal fold. This position lies at the halfway vertical distance between the fundus of the thyroid notch and the anterior inferior edge of the thyroid cartilage. A line from this point extending posteriorly parallel to the inferior boarder of the thyroid cartilage will approximate the level of the true vocal fold (TVF). For females, the anterior aspect of the window is positioned 5 to 8 mm lateral to the midline and for males 8 to 10 mm. The window is carefully outlined using the template, and the outer perichondrium and cartilage are removed taking care to accurately maintain the dimensions of the window (this is important to ensure a snug fit of the prosthesis). The cartilage can be removed using a scalpel, a Kerrison punch, or a small otologic drill. If possible, the integrity of the inner perichondrium is preserved.

Some experts place the implant external to the inner perichondrium, and others feel that the perichondrium tethers the medialization and strip it away. Regardless, care should be taken to ensure hemostasis and to make sure that the airway is not violated. The paraglottic tissues are carefully freed from the inner table of the thyroid cartilage using the perichondrial elevator.

A series of trial implants are then placed ranging from 3 to 7 mm of displacement (**Fig. 15.9**). The implants can be rotated into four orientations and placed throughout the four quadrants of the window to determine the placement for optimal phonation (**Fig. 15.10**). We have found that the most common position is in the inferior posterior quadrant in the vertical position with the bevel facing inferiorly. To medialize the vocal process of the arytenoid, the implant can be rotated to the horizontal position and placed posteriorly. The patient is asked to vocalize to confirm optimal placement. The trial implant is then removed.

If inadequate voicing is obtained, and a persistent posterior glottic gap is evident on laryngoscopy, an arytenoid adduction procedure can be considered at this point, prior to placement of the final implant. Medialization thyroplasty does not affect the level of the vocal fold in the vertical plane. If there is significant discrepancy, it may be necessary to add an arytenoids repositioning procedure to the medialization.

It is important that once the window is created to proceed with implant placement with alacrity to minimize distortion of the voice from glottic edema. The appropriate implant and shim are chosen. Just before placement of the final prosthesis, the field is flooded with saline and the patient is asked to perform a Valsalva maneuver. Any appearance of air bubbles suggests violation of the airway, in which case the procedure should be terminated.

Assuming the integrity of the airway has been maintained, the implant is loaded onto the handle of the implant

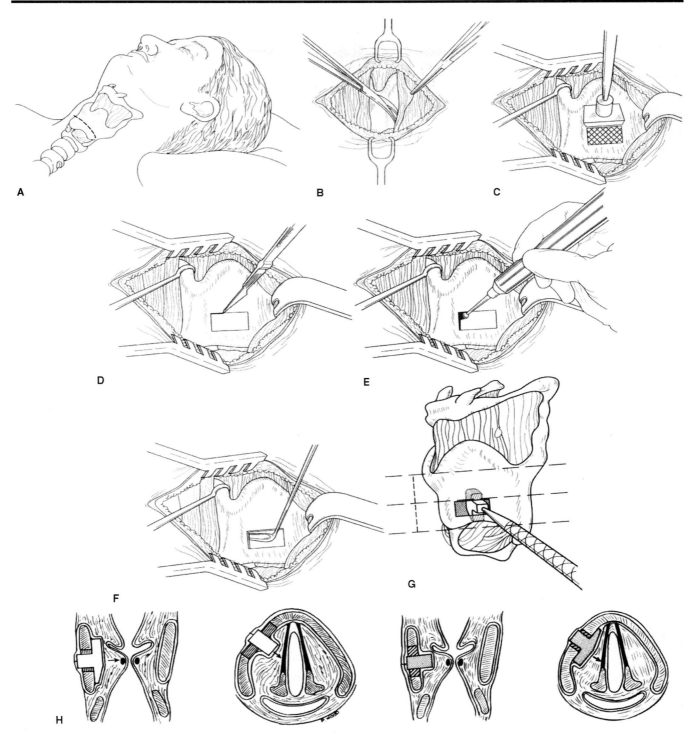

Fig. 15.8 Thyroplasty technique. **(A)** Skin incision. **(B)** After elevation of subplatysmal flaps, the strap muscles are divided and retracted laterally. **(C)** The larynx is rotated using a single hook, and the fenestra template tool is used to mark the location of the window. **(D,E)** The window can be fashioned using a scalpel, Kerrison punch, or drill. **(F)** The paraglottic tissues are freed from the inner table of the thyroid cartilage. **(G)** A series of trial inserts are placed to determine optimum implant size and position, after which the final implant will be placed and secured with the appropriate shim. The position of the vocal fold relative to external landmarks is shown. **(H)** The implants can be placed vertically or horizontally to achieve optimum phonation. (From Cummings CW, Haughey BH, Thomas JR, et al, eds. Otolaryngology: Head and Neck Surgery. 4th ed. St. Louis: Elsevier-Mosby, 2005:2194. Reprinted with permission of Elsevier. Copyright © 2005.)

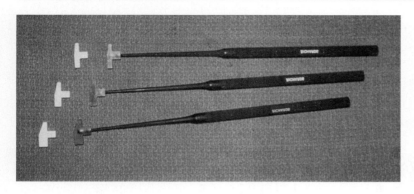

Fig. 15.9 Trial implant tools alongside the corresponding final implants.

inserter and placed in the proper position. The correct shim is then placed using a smooth dressing forceps, thus securing the implant in the desired position in the fenestra (**Fig. 15.11**). The wound is irrigated with antibiotic solution. A drain is placed deep to the strap muscles. The strap muscles and platysma are closed with an absorbable suture and the skin is closed as desired.

Postoperatively, the patient is monitored overnight in the hospital for possible hematoma formation and airway obstruction. The drain is removed on postoperative day 1. The patient is given a regular diet but encouraged to minimize aggressive vocal activity such as coughing, throat clearing, or yelling, although absolute voice rest is not necessary. Patients are told that the voice may deteriorate on

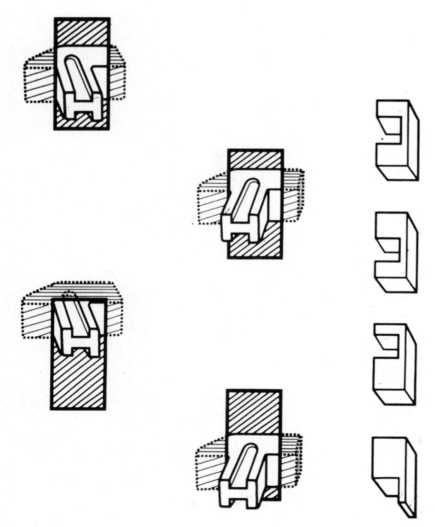

Fig. 15.10 Depending on the shim used, the implant can be variably positioned along the anterior/posterior and superior/inferior axis of the fenestra.

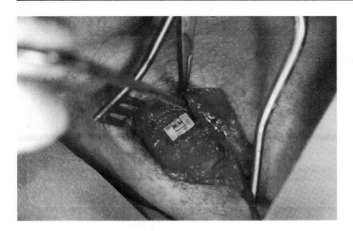

Fig. 15.11 An implant in situ just prior to closure.

the first postoperative day, but will reemerge between postoperative days 3 and 5. Prophylactic antibiotics are continued for 5 days.

Revision The surgical approach for revision is the same as for the primary surgery. After exposure of the implant, any osteogenesis is disrupted using a Freer elevator or a diamond drill. Closure and postoperative care are the same as in the original surgery.

Complications The most serious complication is postoperative airway compromise. In light of this, all patients are monitored in the hospital overnight. The performance of concomitant arytenoid adduction increases this risk and also the risk of hematoma formation. Other complications include penetration of the endolaryngeal mucosa, implant migration, infection, chondritis, and implant extrusion.

Results A study from Johns Hopkins evaluated 35 patients implanted for vocal fold paralysis and reported subjective improvement in 89%.[14] There were two complications including one implant extrusion and one case of airway obstruction. These results compare favorably with the results of other implant techniques in the literature.

Summary The VoCoM implant system is a simple, efficient, and flexible method to achieve accurate vocal fold medialization. It is compatible with concomitant arytenoid adduction, although in itself may provide modest medialization of the vocal process. The implant material is biocompatible with a clinical history of more than 10 years of use. The procedure is technically reversible, although it should be used in individuals who are candidates for a permanent implant.

Zeitel's Rationale and Technique for Gore-Tex Implants

Rationale Gore-Tex medialization has become Zeitel's implant of choice for medialization due to the unique qualities of the material.[7,8,15] The use of Gore-Tex as a medialization implant for the musculomembranous vocal fold was introduced by Hoffman and McCulloch[11] and has been employed by Zeitel for 7 years.[7,8,15] The primary advantages of Gore-Tex are its ease of handling, placement, and adjustability, all of which enhance the speed and precision with which the operation can be performed. The position of the Gore-Tex can even be adjusted and fine-tuned extensively while the implant remains within the patient rather than removing it for modification as is done with Silastic. This is unlike virtually all other implant approaches. Furthermore, precise positioning of the thyroid-lamina window is less critical since Gore-Tex can be placed into appropriate position despite a slightly malpositioned window.

Because of these characteristics, Gore-Tex is also well suited to restore aerodynamic glottal competence in scenarios in which there are complex anatomic defects such as those encountered with trauma and cancer resections. Even subtle contour changes from the loss of superficial lamina propria associated with sulcus vergeture can be reconformed to treat a small glottal gap. The versatility of Gore-Tex is evidenced by its ease of use in the treatment of these varied irregular tissue abnormalities. The clinical experience in part reported in a recent review entailed minimal complications in over 200 cases.[15]

Technique Zeitel's technique usually combines arytenopexy, laryngoplasty, and cricoid subluxation.

A horizontal incision is made in a natural neck crease overlying the region of the cricothyroid space. Subplatysmal flaps are raised to expose the infrahyoid strap musculature, and Gelpi retractors are placed to maintain the flaps. A transverse incision is made through the strap muscles to expose the thyroid lamina. A double-pronged skin hook is placed lateral to the edge of the thyroid lamina and it is rotated anteromedially. This defines the edge of the thyroid lamina and inferior cornu of the thyroid cartilage. A needle-tipped electrocautery knife is used to separate the inferior constrictor from the thyroid lamina (**Fig. 15.12**). The inferior cornu is identified and isolated so that the cricothyroid joint can be separated with Mayo scissors (**Fig. 15.13**). Separating the cricothyroid joint and associated inferior constrictor muscle from the thyroid cartilage allows for further anteromedial rotation of the thyroid lamina (**Fig. 15.14**). Blunt dissection is performed in a cephalad and slightly anterior direction from the cricothyroid facet along the cricoid cartilage until the superior rim of the cricoid is encountered (**Fig. 15.15**). In performing these maneuvers, the lateral aspect of the piriform mucosa has been bluntly dissected from the inner aspect of the thyroid lamina, and the medial aspect of the piriform mucosa has been separated from the posterolateral aspect of the cricoid (**Fig. 15.14**). Posterior superior dissection along the top of the cricoid results in separation of the lateral cricoarytenoid muscle from the muscular process and enables easy identification of the cricoarytenoid joint (**Fig. 15.15**). The dissection along the superior rim of the cricoid leads to the muscular process of the arytenoid. The lateral cricoarytenoid muscle is severed from its attachment to the arytenoid. The posterior cricoarytenoid muscle is then separated from the muscular process of the arytenoid (**Fig. 15.15**). The cricoarytenoid joint is opened widely with Stevens scissors, and the curved, glistening

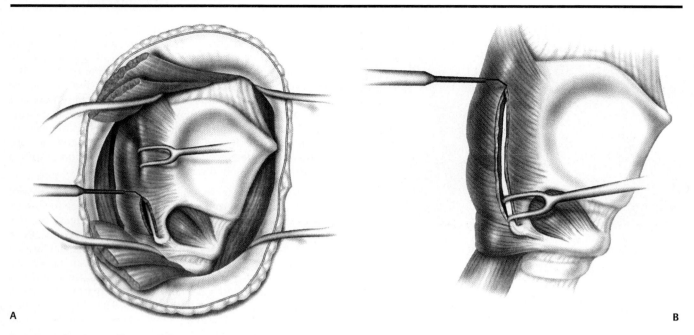

Fig. 15.12 (A,B) A needle-tipped electrocautery knife is used to separate the inferior constrictor from the thyroid lamina.

white surface of the cricoid facet is identified (**Fig. 15.16**). The posterior cricoarytenoid muscle is separated from the posterior plate of the cricoid so that the posterior aspect of the cricoarytenoid joint is well visualized and there is room to place a suture through this region (**Fig. 15.16**). A 4-0 Prolene suture on a cutting needle is placed through the posterior plate of the cricoid just medial to the facet, and the needle is brought out through the medial aspect of the cricoarytenoid joint (**Fig. 15.17**). The needle is then passed through the body of the arytenoid, followed by the inner aspect of

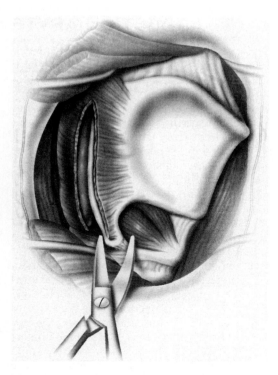

Fig. 15.13 The inferior cornu is identified and isolated so that the cricothyroid joint can be separated with Mayo scissors.

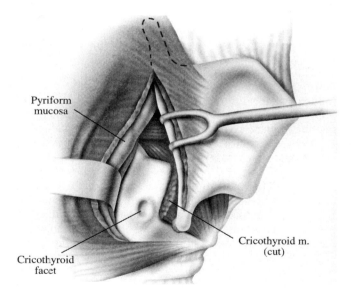

Fig. 15.14 Separating the cricothyroid joint and associating the inferior constrictor muscle from the thyroid cartilage allows for further anteromedial rotation of the thyroid lamina. Blunt dissection is performed in a cephalad and slightly anterior direction from the cricothyroid facet along the cricoid cartilage until the superior rim of the cricoid is encountered. The lateral aspect of the pyriform mucosa is bluntly dissected from the inner aspect of the thyroid lamina and the medial aspect of the pyriform mucosa is separated from the posterolateral aspect of the cricoid.

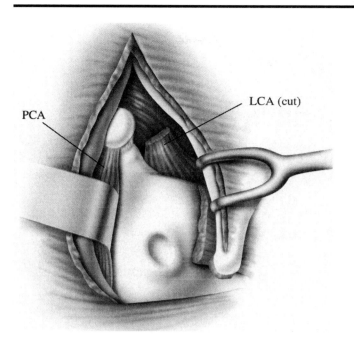

Fig. 15.15 Posterior superior dissection along the top of the cricoid results in separation of the lateral cricoarytenoid muscle from the muscular process and ensures that the cricoarytenoid joint will be identified easily. LCA, lateral cricoarytenoid; PCA, posterior cricoarytenoid.

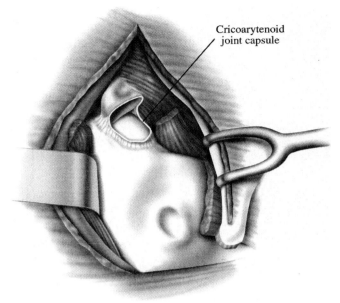

Fig. 15.16 The cricoarytenoid joint is opened widely with Stevens scissors and the curved glistening white surface of the cricoid facet is identified.

the cricoid. The needle is then advanced under the cricoid facet and through the posterior plate of the cricoid, where a slip knot is placed (**Fig. 15.17**). The arytenoid is positioned so that its body is subluxed medially, just off the facet, and so that it is rocked internally in the natural plane of the curved joint. The adduction arytenopexy procedure results in a slightly longer vocal fold, which is appropriately aligned in all three dimensions with a well-conformed medial edge of the glottal aperture. Once the arytenoid is secured, the thyroid lamina is replaced into its natural anatomic position. The arytenoid is visualized by means of a flexible fiberoptic laryngoscope to check its position during several phonatory tasks. If the arytenoid is in good position, the arytenoid suture is affixed permanently. The voice is typically still dysphonic until the implant is placed to support the paraglottic musculature.[2]

Subsequently, an inferiorly based thyroid perichondrial flap is developed and a standard window is made in the thyroid lamina lateral to the musculomembranous vocal fold as previously described by Isshiki (**Fig. 15.18**). The inner perichondrium of the thyroid lamina is preserved as is appropriate at the perimeter of the window. A small implant is then fashioned from a thin sheet of Gore-Tex so that it can be layered lateral to the inner perichondrium of the thyroid lamina. The Gore-Tex can be stabilized with a 4-0 Prolene suture and the thyroid-lamina window can be repositioned. The external perichondrium (**Fig. 15.19**) can be preserved and closed over the thyroid-lamina window. The primary goal of the implant with arytenopexy is to prevent the lateral excursion of the flaccid paraglottic tissue during oscillatory cycles, rather than to medialize the vocal edge, which is accomplished mostly by the arytenopexy.

Once the adduction arytenopexy and medialization laryngoplasty are completed, a cricothyroid subluxation is performed to further enhance vocal quality. Observations made from the vocal-outcome data in the patients who underwent adduction arytenopexy and medialization laryngoplasty revealed that fairly normal conversational level phonation was achieved.[2,7–9] However, there were remarkable limitations of maximal range capabilities, especially frequency variation and maximal phonation time. This was thought to be secondary to suboptimal viscoelastic tension in the denervated vocal fold soft tissues despite the aforementioned improvements in three-dimensional repositioning of the vocal edge. The need to increase viscoelastic tension in the denervated vocal fold and thereby improve aerodynamically efficient entrained oscillation, catalyzed the development of the cricothyroid (CT) subluxation procedure.[7,10]

The newly described CT subluxation is accomplished, by placing a 2-0 Prolene suture around the inferior cornu of the thyroid lamina. It is then passed in a submucosal fashion underneath the cricoid anteriorly (**Fig. 15.20**). The suture is pulled taut (**Fig. 15.21**), which increases the distance between the cricoid facet and the attachment of the anterior commissure ligament. This ultimately increases the tension and length of the musculomembranous vocal fold on the paralyzed side. The tension on this suture is adjusted by using a slip-knot while the patient performs several phonatory tasks. This includes maximal-range tasks such as the use of pulse register (vocal fry) through a falsetto register and glissando sliding scales.

This cricothyroid subluxation suture simulates CT muscle contraction for countertension on the thyroarytenoid muscle

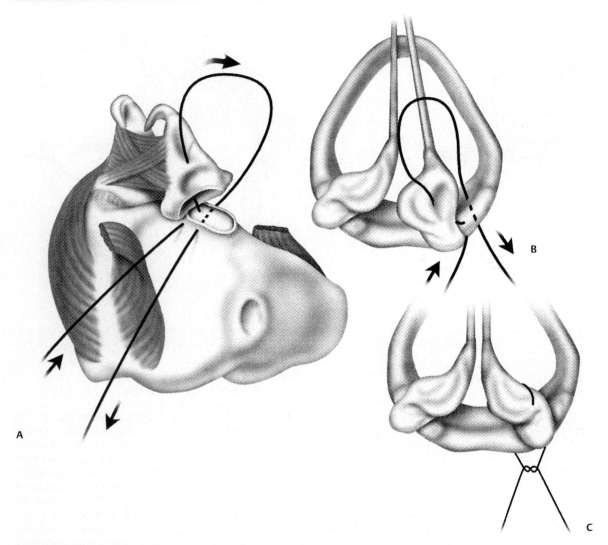

Fig. 15.17 (A) A 4-0 Prolene suture on a cutting needle is placed through the posterior plate of the cricoid just medial to the facet, and the needle is brought out through the medial aspect of the cricoarytenoid joint. **(B)** The needle is passed through the body of the arytenoid and then through the inner aspect of the cricoid. **(C)** The needle is advanced under the cricoid facet and through the posterior plate of the cricoid, where a slip knot is placed.

and for increasing the length of the musculomembranous vocal fold. The CT subluxation (CT sub) procedure has further enhanced postoperative vocal quality because it is an easily adjustable method of increasing and varying tension and length of the paralyzed and denervated musculomembranous vocal fold. This is unlike all prior operations, which were designed primarily to treat paralytic dysphonia by repositioning the vocal fold edge.[2,4–6,16] Those procedures that alter tension and length of the vocal fold were conceived to modify pitch rather than to treat paralytic dysphonia.[6] Once this is completed, the strap muscles are reattached with 3-0 Vicryl suture in a running fashion. The wound is irrigated and a Penrose drain is placed. The platysma is approximated in a running fashion with Vicryl suture as well, and then the skin is closed with 4-0 nylon suture. A pressure dressing is applied and the drain is removed 1 to 4 days later, based on surgeon preference and individualized by the wound characteristics. The patient is started on a liquid diet directly after the procedure and is advanced to a normal diet as tolerated. Fiberoptic laryngoscopy is performed prior to discharge to ensure that there is not an excessive amount of edema that would warrant further observation. Typically, patients can be discharged on the first postoperative day. The modified biomechanical properties of vocal fold vibration that occurred subsequent to CT sub resulted in improved vocal outcome in all patients[10] and was most remarkable in maximal range capabilities. CT sub enhanced the postoperative voice of patients, regardless of whether they required medialization laryngoplasty alone or with adduction arytenopexy. Unlike stretching/lengthening procedures associated with gender reassignment, voice results in denervated patients have not deteriorated, as

15 Vocal Fold Medialization, Arytenoid Adduction, and Reinnervation

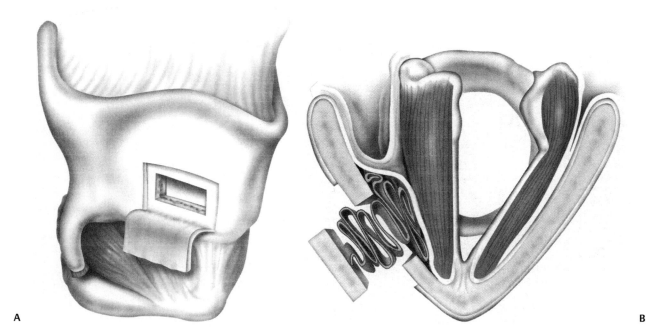

Fig. 15.18 **(A)** An inferiorly based thyroid perichondrial flap is developed, and a standard window is made in the thyroid lamina lateral to the musculomembranous vocal fold. **(B)** A thin sheet of Gore-Tex is used; it is layered in position and can be stabilized with a 4-0 Prolene suture.

evidenced by a follow-up exam after 1 year or longer. Due to the decreased elasticity of denervated vocal folds, the optimal length (for vibration) is longer than that of normal vocal folds. Denervated vocal fold tissue has a different resonant frequency than if it is innervated.

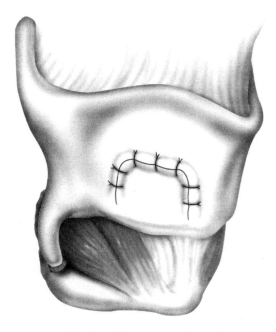

Fig. 15.19 The thyroid lamina external perichondrium is repositioned with 4-0 Vicryl suture.

Netterville's Arytenoid Adduction Technique

In spite of the significant advancements seen with medialization laryngoplasty, there are still a large number of patients who fail to achieve good results with medialization laryngeal surgery (MLS) alone. Thus we perform an AA in the majority of patients undergoing MLS.

In the first five patients in our series, prior to 1990, AA was performed in a similar manner to the original description by Isshiki et al.[5] In these patients, the muscular process of the arytenoid was exposed via a posterior approach in which the cricothyroid joint was disrupted, losing some of the laryngeal stability that this joint provides. In addition, the posterior cricoarytenoid (PCA) was divided off its attachment to the arytenoid and the cricoarytenoid joint capsule was opened. Long-term follow-up in these patients revealed that the disruption of the joint with loss of the posterior support often leads to prolapse of the arytenoid cartilage into the laryngeal lumen with overadduction of the posterior commissure. Over time the voice became very coarse and dysphonic.

Due to these observations, we modified the surgical technique to prevent this loss of support to either the thyroid or the arytenoid cartilage. Our approach now is completely anterior to the strap musculature, with elevation of the outer perichondrium until the posterior border of the thyroid cartilage can be visualized. Removal of the midportion of the posterior border of the thyroid cartilage provides excellent access to the arytenoid, without opening the cricothyroid joint. As outlined in detail below, the cricoarytenoid joint and the muscles inserting on the arytenoid are not disturbed. This approach allows both ML and AA to be completed in the same field of view, and obviates the need

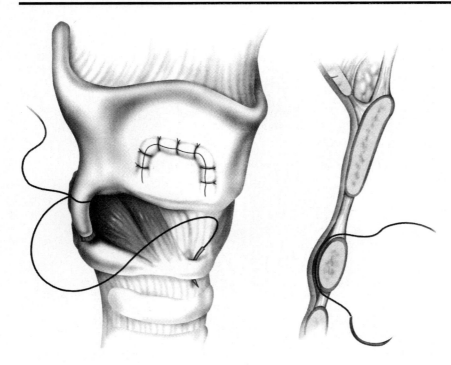

Fig. 15.20 The cricothyroid subluxation is accomplished by placing a 2-0 Prolene suture around the inferior cornu of the thyroid lamina. It is then passed in a submucosal fashion underneath the cricoid anteriorly.

to divide the inferior constrictor muscle to reach the posterior border of the thyroid cartilage. The ability to preserve the integrity of the inferior constrictor muscle, the cricothyroid joint, the cricoarytenoid joint, and the PCA and lateral cricoarytenoid (LCA) attachment on the arytenoid, along with the partial reinnervation that commonly occurs within the paralyzed TVC, adds further stability to the arytenoid cartilage and entire larynx.

We exposed the muscular process of the arytenoid in all patients irrespective of the preoperative position of the vocal process to access directly the benefit of the AA along with MLS. After one has become familiar with the procedure, this step does not dramatically lengthen the procedure. The opportunity to judge in all patients the added benefit of AA has significantly improved our ability to acquire the best voice results with one procedure.

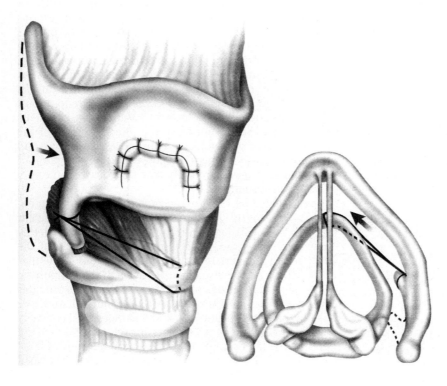

Fig. 15.21 The suture is pulled taut, which increases the distance between the cricoid facet and the attachment of the anterior commissure ligament.

The placement of an implant alone does not apply the vector of displacement on the arytenoid that replicates the anterior pull of the thyroarytenoid muscle, as it positions the arytenoid and vocal cord in the physiologic phonating position. The cricoarytenoid joint functions as a complex sliding joint that allows the arytenoid to rock into the lumen during adduction and rock out of the lumen during abduction. The thyroarytenoid muscle with its forward vector slides the arytenoid into the larynx with a slight rotation of the vocal process toward the midline. This rotation results in a small change in length with a slight increase in tension. The major benefit of AA is in stabilizing the arytenoid and therefore the TVC in the midline adducted position. Often if the TVC is in excellent position with the implant alone, the voice is only good at a lower volume. As the patient attempts to increase volume to communicate in a noisy setting, the voice drops off and becomes less audible. To increase vocal volume, there must be an increase in subglottic airflow, which effects an increase in subglottal pressure. With unilateral paralysis, as the pressure increases, the nonstabilized arytenoid "blows" laterally, creating an increase in air leak, with a drop in volume. The AA stitch increases the stability of the arytenoid, which prevents its lateral displacement during voice use with increasing subglottic pressure. This controls the mean airflow rate through the glottis, and leads to significant increase in volume.

However, patients with unilateral paralysis, who also present with either contralateral paresis or severe chronic obstructive pulmonary disease (COPD), present a relative contraindication to AA, as it may result in a loss of functional airway in this select group. The posterior one third of the glottis is the ventilating portion of the glottis. A decrease in the lumen in the posterior half produces significantly more laryngeal resistance than a comparable medialization in the anterior membranous larynx. It may be prudent in these two groups to limit surgical therapy to medialization alone.

Arytenoid adduction alone with no implant has been reported to produce quality voice results. In our series this is the exception not the rule. It appears that AA alone will aid only a very limited number of patients; however, if the implant is always placed first prior to testing the effects of the AA suture, one will not identify these rare patients.

During the initial approach for AA, the thyroid perichondrium, along with the thyrohyoid muscle, is elevated to the posterior border of the thyroid cartilage. Elevation of the thyroid perichondrium up to the superior process and down to the cricothyroid joint provides excellent exposure without further division of the muscles. Once the perichondrium has been widely elevated, a skin hook placed on the posterior border of the ala is used to rotate the thyroid ala and facilitate exposure posteriorly. The elevated perichondrium is divided at the posterior border of the thyroid cartilage by sweeping a sharp elevator along the posterior edge, or sharply dividing it with a knife, thus preventing elevation of the inner perichondrium. This elevation continues deep to the medial surface of the cartilage elevating the piriform sinus away from the inner perichondrium, which is purposely left attached to the inner surface of the cartilage. We completely elevate the paraglottic soft tissue away from the inner perichondrium, extending from the window to the posterior border of the thyroid cartilage. This exposure is created to ensure the AA suture can pass through this space without catching on the inner perichondrium or fascial bands that may act as slings to alter the vector of pull of the AA suture.

Although Isshiki described separation of the cricothyroid joint for better exposure, we purposely maintain the integrity of this joint. This preserves the stability of the laryngeal framework, and prevents injury to the recurrent laryngeal nerve as it passes adjacent to the posterior surface of the joint. A majority of paralyzed larynges undergo some degree of reinnervation, which helps to maintain muscle bulk and tone. Therefore, we strive in these procedures to avoid further injury to the recurrent laryngeal nerve (RLN).

At this point a 5-mm right-angle Kerrison rongeur is used to remove a window of cartilage at the posterior aspect of the cartilage, to visualize the paraglottic space lateral to the muscular process of the arytenoid. The cartilage is removed until one can palpate the muscular process of the arytenoid and see the anterior extension of the piriform sinus. The piriform sinus can be distended laterally, by asking the patient to blow out against pursed lips. The anterior extension of the piriform sinus is identified and elevated away from the muscular process of the arytenoid, with further elevation of the postcricoid mucosa off PCA muscle to near the midline. While the surgeon watches the television monitor, the arytenoid is slowly moved along its plane of adduction and abduction to access its mobility and demonstrate potential closure of the posterior glottis.

We rarely remove the posterior cricoarytenoid muscle from the arytenoid or open up the cricoarytenoid joint. These steps may produce an unstable arytenoid cartilage that can prolapse medially into the airway with very poor voice results. A normally mobile arytenoid can be positioned into the physiologic phonating position without removing any of the muscle attachments. In fact, these attachments provide stability for the adducted cartilage, allowing it to rotate into the physiologic phonating position.

To obtain a secure purchase on the muscular process, a 4-0 Prolene suture is passed through the lateral edge of the muscular process in a figure-of-eight fashion, passing through cartilage, the perichondrium, and the ligamentous attachments of the muscles **(Fig. 15.22)**. Both ends of the suture, with the needles still in place, are then passed through the dissected paraglottic space into the window. The needles are passed butt end first through the open space to ensure that the suture does not catch on any tissue still attached to the cartilage along its course. If the suture is caught on any lateral tissue, this entrapment acts as a pulley, which may change the vector of pull of the AA suture, making it difficult to position the arytenoid in the physiologic adducted position. We previously passed the AA suture through either the paraglottic soft tissue via an 18-gauge needle or passed it through the posterior edge of the implant. However, this altered the vector of pull on the arytenoid, which created difficulties in acquiring a true adduction of the arytenoid

One end of the suture is passed through the cartilage at the anterior border of the window. If this area is calcified, then a small hole is drilled with a 1-mm wire-pass bit. The second needle is passed below the window medial to the lower cartilage strut, then through the cricothyroid membrane soft

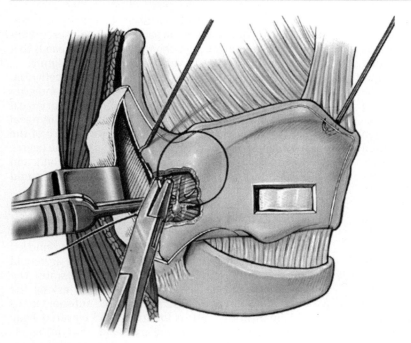

Fig. 15.22 After retraction of the piriform sinus, the suture is passed twice through the muscular process and its muscular ligamentous cover.

tissue in the midline (**Fig. 15.23**). The intent of this AA suture placement is to mimic the pull of the thyroarytenoid muscle. The larynx is then allowed to fall back into its anatomic position, and the arytenoid is slowly adducted and abducted to demonstrate the appropriate arytenoid movement as seen on the television monitor.

The depth gauge is used to palpate through the window to identify the position the vocal cord relative to the window. As the patient speaks during voice testing, the vocal cord is displaced medially with the depth gauge to assess voice change. When the maximum benefit from medialization has been identified with the depth gauge, the AA suture is then gently pulled to demonstrate any further improvement that may be derived (**Fig. 15.24**). By testing medialization and AA jointly and independently, one can decide whether one or both are needed to obtain maximum benefit. Based on the measurements obtained from the depth gauge, the implant is carved as previously described, and

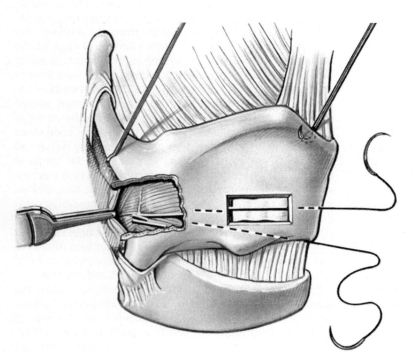

Fig. 15.23 The superior limb of the arytenoid adduction (AA) suture is brought out through the cartilage anterior to the window. The inferior limb of the suture is passed below the lower strut and brought out through the cricothyroid ligament.

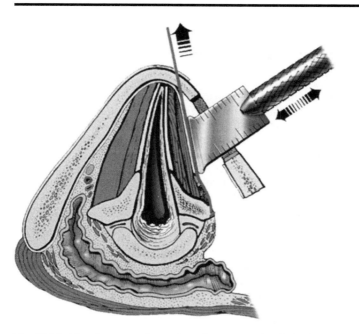

Fig. 15.24 After the maximal voice benefit is acquired with the depth gauge, slight tension is placed on the AA suture to assess its additional benefit.

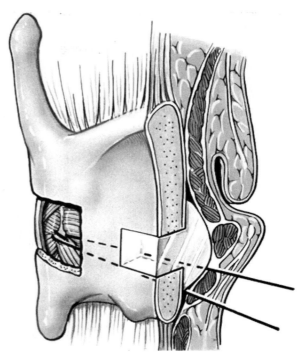

Fig. 15.25 After correct placement of the implant, both limbs of the AA suture are deep to the implant.

inserted through the window before the AA suture is tied. The untied strands of the AA suture are held medially, as the implant is inserted through the window, to prevent the AA sutures from slipping above or below the implant and being trapped between the implant flanges and the cartilage (**Fig. 15.25**). This entrapment would alter the vector of pull on the arytenoid. The two AA sutures should lie medial to the implant along the lateral fascia of the thyroarytenoid muscle. Almost no tension is needed to adduct the arytenoid when the suture has been placed in the manner described. In fact, it is very easy to overadduct the vocal process, with too much tension on the suture. As the AA suture is tied, to prevent slipping of the knot, a small hemostat is used to hold the knot after the first throw of the surgeon's knot is laid down. After multiple gentle pulls on the AA suture during voice testing, the arytenoid tends to stay close to its adducted position. In the majority of cases the AA suture is tied with no tension, with a small area of air under the knot. This is the just-loose technique. Once the arytenoid has been coaxed into the phonating position, the major benefit of the suture is to stabilize the arytenoid, preventing it from lateral displacement, during forceful phonation. A simple intraoperative test demonstrates the stabilizing function of the AA suture. During the patient's quiet respiration the surgeon can pull up on the tied knot at the anterior loop of an appropriately placed AA suture. The knot will stand up in the air, with space under the tied suture. But with the next phonation, the knot is drawn down against the cartilage, preventing the arytenoid from being displaced laterally by the pressure of the contralateral arytenoid, or increasing subglottic airflow.

In a very small subset of patients the voice only improves with forceful continued pull on the arytenoid. In this group the AA suture is tied with the indicated level of tension. It is very easy to place too much tension on the suture, causing the vocal process to cross the midline, resulting in decreased voice quality and compromise of the airway. The AA suture is tied only after the implant has been placed. If the suture is tied prior to placement of the implant, the implant can deflect the tied AA suture, resulting in a change in tension with overadduction of the vocal process.

Arytenoid adduction has been a significant addition to MLS in the treatment of patients with unilateral vocal cord paralysis. Whereas MLS may effect medialization of the membranous vocal fold, it cannot reproduce the vector of force that the thyroarytenoid muscle exerts in adducting the arytenoid cartilage. Only AA can mimic this vector, placing the arytenoid in the physiologic phonating position. The indications for the use of arytenoid adduction are probably broader than has been previously reported.

Dr. Smith's Rationale and Technique of Reinnervation

Rationale Vocal fold paralysis may be accompanied by a sensory deficit causing dysphagia and aspiration in addition to dysphonia. The goal of reestablishing physiologic movement and sensation to a paralyzed larynx is not consistently attainable by current techniques. But there are several laryngeal reinnervation procedures that have been sufficiently tested in this area to provide some recommendations and options for clinical management. This particularly applies to restoring phonatory function in unilateral laryngeal paralysis, and intraoperative management of the divided RLN.

Reinnervation of the paralyzed larynx has been an area of clinical and research interest for many years. Over 100 years ago, the successful repair of an injured RLN after a gun-shot wound was reported.[17] Success with reinnervation of the RLN with a branch of the ansa cervicalis was reported in 1924 and 1926.[18] Extensive reviews of research and clinical experience in laryngeal reinnervation have recently been published.[19,20] The reader is directed to these reports for further information and references.

Recurrent Laryngeal Nerve Anatomy Related to Laryngeal Reinnervation

The main trunk of the RLN contains roughly 1000 to 4000 myelinated axons, which carry efferent (motor), afferent, sympathetic, and parasympathetic secretomotor fibers. Of these, 500 to 1000 are motor fibers to the intrinsic laryngeal muscles.[21,22] This means that the fibers going to both adductor and abductor muscles are carried in the same bundle, until just before they branch into their target muscle. This was demonstrated in the human RLN by careful serial sectioning in 1952.[22] In their study, Sunderland and Swaney[22] found varying fascicle arrangements and plexus formation, with rearrangement and redistribution of nerve fibers along the length of the RLN. Muscle groups varied within these fascicles, and there was no consistent fascicular arrangement of adductor- or abductor-targeted muscle fibers. Significant variation in branching and bundling of these nerve fibers occurs individually, without an intraneural topographic organization.[23,24] The RLN branch to the PCA muscle can be seen to originate before, at, or after the nerve traverses behind the cricothyroid joint. As another example, 40% of human larynx specimens have demonstrated innervation of the thyroarytenoid (TA) muscles from fibers of the superior laryngeal nerve (SLN) which run through the CT muscle and under the thyroid lamina.[25] All these variations may affect vocal fold position in vocal fold paralysis, and thus influence outcomes in reinnervation procedures.

Nerve Injury and Repair The nerves that innervate the larynx are at risk for injury due to their long course through the neck and chest. They are in proximity to many vital structures and are vulnerable during a variety of surgical procedures. The degree and extent of injury can systematically vary.[26] Minor injuries result in conduction block through the axon (first degree). This is usually due to compression or ischemia. Axonal degeneration is termed second degree, and is caused by compression or crushing. The distal axon undergoes wallerian degeneration, and then gradually regenerates along a core of Schwann cells inside the intact endoneurial tubule. When axonal and endoneurial injury occurs, it is termed third degree. In this situation the endoneurial tubule continuity is disrupted. The same degeneration and regeneration process occurs, but the potential for aberrant regeneration of axonal sprouts exists, which will enter distal tubules that are different from the original neural pathways. Fourth-degree injury involves disruption of the perineurium. As in third-degree injury, the potential for disorganized regeneration exists because the regenerating axon not only can enter the incorrect nerve tubules but also can grow into adjacent nerve fascicles. The potential for scar tissue and neuroma formation also exists, which inhibits the ability of axons to regenerate. Complete transection of the nerve, including the epineurium, is termed fifth-degree injury. The hope for spontaneous recovery from this injury and the potential for nerve loss and misdirection of axonal sprouts is significant. Microsurgical repair of the transected nerve provides the best chance for at least some axonal regeneration to occur. If some regeneration occurs, then muscle atrophy may be avoided and the possibility of some recovery of function still exists.

Laryngeal nerves have a high capacity for regeneration when injured. This is seen by the moderate recovery rate from idiopathic vocal fold paralysis,[26] and even the high rate of symptom recurrence of spasmodic dysphonia in patients who underwent RLN transection.[27] Electromyography (EMG) studies on the transected RLN side of spasmodic dysphonia patients with recurrent symptoms often show muscle activation with phonation, demonstrating that some regeneration has occurred, even though one vocal fold is paralyzed (immobile).[28,29]

This leads to the concept of laryngeal synkinesis. This phenomenon was described in 1968 by Hiroto et al[30] using laryngeal EMG, and the concept was articulated by Crumley.[31] It is analogous to the synkinesis seen in facial paralysis.[32] This condition may occur in nerve injuries from the third degree through the fifth degree, which means that the nerve does not have to be entirely transected for vocal fold paralysis and laryngeal synkinesis to develop. Laryngeal synkinesis occurs when adductor and abductor nerves regenerate aberrantly to innervate the opposite muscles from their original function. This is highly likely in the case of RLN injury, because approximately 75% of motor axons go to the adductors and 25% to the abductor (PCA). When laryngeal synkinesis is present, laryngeal adductor muscles activate during abductor tasks and abductor muscles activate during adductor tasks. The vocal fold is usually immobile from the antagonistic cocontraction. Maronian et al[33] reported on 10 patients with EMG evidence of laryngeal synkinesis. They defined synkinesis with EMG criteria that compared motor unit recruitment amplitude on opposing tasks. They used this information in attempts to localize botulinum toxin injections to abnormally activating muscles to improve laryngeal function.

Blitzer et al[34] reported on 14 patients with immobile vocal folds. Seven with good voices were found to have EMG evidence of laryngeal synkinesis, and those with poor voices had reduced signs of laryngeal reinnervation and tipped arytenoid position. The authors postulated that the muscle tone positioned the arytenoid favorably for phonation, even though the vocal fold was immobile. In summary, laryngeal synkinesis may be a favorable state in recovery of capacity for phonation in unilateral vocal fold paralysis. Though the vocal fold is immobile, the motor units of the intrinsic laryngeal muscles are populated to some degree and are able to maintain vocal fold position and tone, which allow the paralyzed vocal fold to aid in glottal closure and mucosal wave entrainment necessary for phonation. A procedure such as ansa-RLN reinnervation accomplishes this through a nonselective regeneration of laryngeal motor units. Crumley[35] estimated that approximately 20% of intact axonal fibers may be all that are needed to create laryngeal muscle tone sufficient for phonation.

History of Laryngeal Reinnervation The first report of primary repair of the RLN was in 1909, when Horsley[17] reported on a 40-year-old woman who was shot in the neck with a pistol. The RLN was found to be transected and was repaired primarily, with purported complete recovery of vocal function. Frazier and Mosser[18] are credited with reporting the first cases of ansa cervicalis to RLN neurorrhaphy, an idea they claimed was given to them by Chevalier Jackson. They used this procedure to treat four patients with bilateral vocal fold paralysis, three with a mixed bilateral vocal fold paralysis, and three with unilateral vocal fold paralysis. Overall, they reported that six of ten had improvement in vocal fold movement and laryngeal function.

Laryngeal Reinnervation Techniques and Options The most useful donor nerve in laryngeal paralysis treatment is the ansa cervicalis nerve. It has a favorable size match with the RLN. There is little to no dysfunction from transection of the branch to the sternohyoid or omohyoid muscles. It can be obtained from either the ipsilateral or the contralateral side. Other donor nerves have been studied in animal experiments, including the hypoglossal,[36] phrenic,[35,37,38] superior laryngeal nerve,[39] and contralateral RLN.[40] Each of these carries more donor-site morbidity than the ansa cervicalis.

The donor nerve can be connected to the larynx in several ways, including direct neurorrhaphy, nerve-muscle-pedicle, and direct muscle implant. This section confines itself to the direct end-to-end neurorrhaphy technique. Zheng et al[41] performed a series of canine experiments with laryngeal adductor branch reinnervation and found that although all three techniques yielded successful reinnervation, the direct neurorrhaphy technique worked most effectively.

The technique of ansa-RLN reinnervation will be briefly described. The procedure is usually performed with the patient under general anesthesia. However, if there is the possibility that the nerves cannot be found and the patient thus may be a medialization laryngoplasty candidate, the procedure may commence under local anesthesia until the nerves are found, and then converted to general anesthesia or completed under monitored anesthesia care (MAC).[20] The neck is entered through an anterior incision at approximately the level of the inferior edge of the cricoid cartilage that extends laterally to the anterior border of the sternocleidomastoid muscle. The platysma muscle is divided, but care is taken to raise the subplatysmal flaps without trauma, as the ansa cervicalis branches may be fairly superficial. Either the ansa cervicalis or the RLN may be identified first. In cases where the RLN may have been injured from prior surgery, it is our preference to look for it first, because an inadequate length of distal RLN prevents the operation from successful completion. The superior thyroid pole vessels are identified and individually suture ligated as distally as possible to prevent injury to the external branch of the superior laryngeal nerve. The larynx is rotated with a hook placed on the lateral thyroid ala above the cricoid and the region of the cricothyroid joint identified. At this location the nerve is found entering the larynx. It is dissected for several centimeters inferiorly. The RLN may also be found by dissection inferior to the thyroid gland and followed superiorly toward the larynx.

The ansa cervicalis is next found by retracting the medial border of the sternocleidomastoid muscle and identifying the nerve running on top of the internal jugular vein. Dissection of the underside of the sternohyoid or omohyoid muscles will also reveal nerve branches entering these muscles. A portable nerve stimulator can be used to confirm identification of these branches. The nerve needs to be dissected for sufficient length to reach the RLN, and this can be measured with a vessel loop. The sternohyoid muscle branch is most frequently used due to its long length. If the ipsilateral ansa cervicalis is not available due to scarring and injury from prior neck surgery, the contralateral ansa cervicalis may be used. The neck incision then needs to be extended to the opposite side for the ansa dissection. Additionally, there must be sufficient length, especially on the RLN side, to bring the nerves together and sew them over the cricothyroid membrane. The ansa branch may bifurcate into several small branches and these can be used and incorporated into the neurorrhaphy if there is a size mismatch between the ansa and RLN. The ansa branch is cut sharply and then tunneled under the strap muscles to the RLN. The RLN is transected and the end sharply freshened with a razor knife. An end-to-end neurorrhaphy is performed with an operating microscope, using three to four 8-0 or 9-0 sutures placed in the epineurium circumferentially. Paniello[20] suggests protecting the nerve repair with a small vein graft that has been slid over the nerve prior to suturing. The wound is then closed and a surgical drain placed. The procedure usually takes approximately 2.5 hours, a little longer than a medialization procedure. The patient is generally observed overnight in the hospital, although we have performed the procedure on an outpatient basis.

The patient's voice following ansa-RLN neurorrhaphy may be unchanged or may be slightly more breathy, depending on the number of axons to laryngeal adductors that had previously been present. It is reasonable to tell patients that their voice may get a little worse before it gets better. The reinnervation process usually begins to improve the voice 3 to 4 months after the procedure, and continues for a year or more. Thus, patients may expect continued improvement in the voice for the first year. Improvement is noted in voice quality, volume, pitch range, and dynamic range of the voice. If the patient desires immediate temporary improvement in the voice while waiting for the reinnervation to take place, an augmentation injection of the vocal fold can be done at the same operation with a temporary filler material such as Cymetra®, collagen, or cross-linked hyaluronan gel.

It can be argued that the ansa-RLN laryngeal reinnervation procedure is technically easier to perform than medialization procedures.[19] There are no intraoperative assessments to make about voice quality and adjustments of implant position or arytenoid suture tension. The procedure can be done under general instead of local anesthesia. The operation has no learning curve, and is done in the same way each time. In current otolaryngology residency and head/neck fellowship training programs residents become well experienced in the relevant head and neck anatomy. The microsurgical skills are practiced, and the neurorrhaphy procedure is straightforward and easier than microvascular suturing.

Ansa–Recurrent Laryngeal Nerve Neurorrhaphy Results Beginning with Frazier and Mosser's[18] reports, there have been several case series of the ansa-RLN neurorrhaphy for vocal fold paralysis. In the 1980s and early 1990s Crumley et al[42,43] reported on their experience with this procedure in treatment of unilateral vocal fold paralysis. Though improvement was seen in 18 of 20 cases, the reports did not contain data with which to adequately assess the postoperative voice outcomes. Zheng et al[44] reported on eight patients with unilateral vocal fold paralysis who underwent ansa-RLN adductor branch reinnervation. They conducted postoperative voice analysis, laryngostroboscopy, and EMG studies. They found that on laryngostroboscopy the patients exhibited little to no movement of the paralyzed vocal fold, but synchronous mucosal waves were observed during phonation. This implies that vocal fold stiffness and viscoelastic properties between the two folds were favorable to sustain symmetric mucosal wave vibration. Olson et al[45] reported on 12 cases of unilateral vocal fold paralysis treated with ansa-RLN neurorrhaphy who underwent preoperative and postoperative acoustic and perceptual assessment. Significant improvements were measured in acoustic measures of breathiness and perceptual ratings of overall voice quality. Those with an isolated RLN paralysis without other associated morbidities obtained the best results. Maronian et al[46] reported on nine patients with unilateral vocal fold paralysis who underwent ansa-RLN neurorrhaphy. Four of these consented to undergo postoperative EMG studies. It was found that early EMG recordings of the reinnervated TA muscle showed activation with tasks that typically activate the strap muscle. However, late (more than 12 months) EMG recordings of the TA muscle showed activation with phonation, suggesting a relearning of the nerve innervating the TA muscle.

Chhetri et al[47] reported on comparison of two groups of patients with unilateral vocal paralysis (UVP). One group underwent ansa-RLN combined with an arytenoid adduction laryngoplasty, and the second group underwent arytenoid adduction alone. No difference was seen on perceptual, aerodynamic, and stroboscopic measures. This study did not have any group that underwent only ansa-RLN neurorrhaphy. The only study to date that directly compares ansa-RLN neurorrhaphy with medialization laryngoplasty techniques was submitted by Paniello.[48] He studied the voice outcomes in 12 patients who underwent each procedure. At 1-year follow-up, perceptual ratings of the overall quality of the speaking voice reading a standard passage were rated by blinded listeners on a 50-point visual analogue scale. The reinnervation group rating averaged 35, with a range of 22 to 47. The medialization group averaged 27.5, with a range of 13 to 35 ($p = .0046$). These patients were not prospectively randomized. The next step needed is a prospective randomized surgical trial that directly compares the outcomes of these procedures.

When to Consider Laryngeal Reinnervation The idea of replacing an injured or paralyzed nerve is conceptually appealing. Instead of repositioning the paralyzed vocal fold with a static implant or injectable material, the restoration of laryngeal muscle tone to improve the voice has been felt to have theoretical advantages by restoring viscoelastic symmetry and not just geometric symmetry.[49,50] Although the peripheral nervous system has the capacity to repair and regenerate when injured, in the larynx the functional outcome is less predictable. Studies to date indicate that reinnervation of the paralyzed larynx results in more capacity for improved laryngeal adduction and phonation but not abduction and enlargement of the glottic airway.

The following advantages of laryngeal reinnervation have been reported by Crumley et al[42,43]:

- It can restore normal or near-normal voice without synthetic materials placed inside the laryngeal framework.
- It does not alter the stiffness of the vocal folds, particularly the pliability of the layered vocal fold microstructure.
- It restores bulk to the thyroarytenoid muscle.
- It improves vocal fold positioning due to muscular contraction of the lateral cricoarytenoid, interarytenoid, and posterior cricoarytenoid muscles.
- It is reversible (by nerve section).
- It does not preclude static methods of laryngeal repositioning and medialization if needed.
- It eliminates dysphonia due to synkinesis if present (by section of the RLN).

The potential disadvantages of laryngeal reinnervation include the following:

- An intact donor nerve is needed.
- The distal stump of the RLN must be able to be dissected and available.
- There is a several-month delay before reinnervation becomes effective and the voice improves.

There are no published studies currently available that directly compare laryngeal reinnervation with other techniques of unilateral vocal fold paralysis treatment, such as static medialization or injection. At this time it is reasonable to suggest that laryngeal reinnervation be considered in the following situations:

- When the RLN is transected accidentally, a primary RLN-RLN repair is advised.[50,51]
- When the RLN is transected intentionally for extirpative cancer surgery, a primary ansa-RLN neurorrhaphy (if the ansa is available) is recommended.[52-54]
- In younger patients with unilateral vocal fold paralysis in whom there is concern about their ability to tolerate a procedure under local anesthesia and potential long-term complications of a foreign implant in the larynx.
- In professional vocalists with unilateral vocal fold paralysis who hope to regain some pitch and dynamic range to their voice.
- In patients with unilateral vocal fold paralysis and dysphonia who also have real or potential concerns for

airway obstruction, such as those with sleep apnea or athletes at risk for exertional dyspnea. A medialization or injection procedure may encroach on the glottic airway. Arytenoid adduction has a slight increased risk of postoperative airway complications.[55,56]

♦ Conclusion

Paralytic dysphonia is the most common indication for static reconstruction of the larynx. Prior procedures have addressed primarily the position of the vocal fold in the axial and vertical planes. Several different types of implant materials and techniques have been reviewed in this chapter. However, achieving wide dynamic pitch-range capabilities and vocal flexibility have been limited secondary to the flaccid, denervated vocal fold tissue. Novel procedures have been designed to address these issues by optimally positioning the arytenoid and restoring tension in the flaccid vocal fold. These procedures include the arytenoids adduction and arytenopexy procedures.

The future surgery should lie primarily in dynamic reconstruction (reinnervation and electrical pacing) of the intrinsic laryngeal musculature.

References

1. Payr E. Plastik am schildknorpel zur Behebung der Folgen einseitiger Stimmbandlahmung. Dtsch Med Wochenschr 1915;43:1265–1270
2. Zeitels SM, Hochman I, Hillman RE. Adduction arytenopexy: a new procedure for paralytic dysphonia and the implications for medialization laryngoplasty. Ann Otol Rhinol Laryngol 1998;107(Suppl 173):1–24
3. Zeitels SM. The evolution of the assessment and treatment of paralytic dysphonia. Otolaryngol Clin North Am 2000;33:803–816
4. Isshiki N, Morita H, Okamura H, Hiramoto M. Thyroplasty as a new phonosurgical technique. Acta Otolaryngol 1974;78:451–457
5. Isshiki N, Tanabe M, Sawada M. Arytenoid adduction for unilateral vocal cord paralysis. Arch Otolaryngol 1978;104:555–558
6. Isshiki N. Phonosurgery: Theory and Practice. Tokyo: Springer-Verlag; 1989
7. Zeitels SM. Adduction arytenopexy with medialization laryngoplasty and crico-thyroid subluxation: a new approach to paralytic dysphonia. Operative Tech Otolaryngol Head Neck Surg 1999;10:9–16
8. Zeitels SM, Jarboe J, Franco RA. Phonosurgical reconstruction of early glottic cancer. Laryngoscope 2001;111:1862–1865
9. Zeitels SM. Adduction arytenopexy for vocal fold paralysis: indications and technique. J Laryngol Otol 2004;118:508–516
10. Zeitels SM, Hillman RE, Desloge RB, Bunting GA. Cricothyroid subluxation: a new procedure for enhancing the voice with laryngoplastic phonosurgery. Ann Otol Rhinol Laryngol 1999;108:1126–1131
11. McCulloch TM, Hoffman HT. Medialization laryngoplasty with expanded polytetrafluoroethylene: surgical technique and preliminary results. Ann Otol Rhinol Laryngol 1998;107:427–432
12. http://www.gyrus-ent.com
13. Flint PW, Corio RL, Cummings CW. Comparison of soft tissue response in rabbits following laryngeal implantation with hydroxylapatite, silicone rubber, and Teflon. Ann Otol Rhinol Laryngol 1997;106:399–407
14. Cummings CW, Purcell LL, Flint PW. Hydroxylapatite laryngeal implants for medialization. Preliminary report. Ann Otol Rhinol Laryngol 1993;102:843–851
15. Zeitels SM, Mauri M, Dailey SH. Medialization laryngoplasty with Gore-Tex for voice restoration secondary to glottal incompetence: indications and observations. Ann Otol Rhinol Laryngol 2003;112:180–184
16. Neuman TR, Hengesteg A, Lepage MS, Kaufman KR, Woodson GE. Three-dimensional motion of the arytenoid adduction procedure in cadaver larynges. Ann Otol Rhinol Laryngol 1994;103:265–270
17. Horsley JS. Suture of the recurrent laryngeal nerve, with report of a case. Trans South Surg Gynecol Assoc 1909;22:161–167
18. Frazier CH, Mosser WB. Treatment of recurrent laryngeal nerve paralysis by nerve anastomosis. Surg Gynecol Obstet 1926;43:134–139
19. Goding GS. Laryngeal reinnervation. In: Cummings CW, Haughey BH, Thomas JR, et al, eds. Otolaryngology: Head and Neck Surgery. 4th ed. St. Louis: Elsevier-Mosby, 2005:2207–2221.
20. Paniello RC. Laryngeal reinnervation. In: Sulica L, Blitzer A, eds. Vocal Fold Paralysis. Berlin, Heidelberg, New York: Springer-Verlag, 2006: 189–202
21. Hayashi M, Isozaki E, Oda M, Tanabe H, Kimura J. Loss of large myelinated nerve fibres of the recurrent laryngeal nerve in patients with multiple system atrophy and vocal cord palsy. J Neurol Neurosurg Psychiatry 1997;62:234–238
22. Sunderland S, Swaney WE. The intraneural topography of the recurrent laryngeal nerve in man. Anat Rec 1952;114:411–426
23. Gacek RR, Malmgren LT, Lyon MJ. Localization of adductor and abductor motor nerve fibers to the larynx. Ann Otol Rhinol Laryngol 1977;86:771–776
24. Damrose EJ, Huang RY, Ye M, Berke GS, Sercarz JA. Surgical anatomy of the recurrent laryngeal nerve: implications for laryngeal reinnervation. Ann Otol Rhinol Laryngol 2003;112:434–438
25. Sanders I, Wu BL, Mu L, Li Y, Biller HF. The innervation of the human larynx. Arch Otolaryngol Head Neck Surg 1993;119:934–939
26. Sulica L, Cultrara A, Blitzer A. Vocal fold paralysis: causes, outcomes, and clinical aspects. In: Sulica L, Blitzer A, eds. Vocal Fold Paralysis. Berlin, Heidelberg, New York: Springer, 2006:33–54
27. Aronson AE, De Santo LW. Adductor spastic dysphonia: three years after recurrent laryngeal nerve section. Laryngoscope 1983;93:1–8
28. Sulica L, Blitzer A, Brin MF, Stewart CF. Botulinum toxin management of adductor spasmodic dysphonia after failed recurrent laryngeal nerve section. Ann Otol Rhinol Laryngol 2003;112:499–505
29. Ludlow CL, Naunton RF, Fujita M, Sedory SE. Spasmodic dysphonia: botulinum toxin injection after recurrent nerve surgery. Otolaryngol Head Neck Surg 1990;102:122–131
30. Iroto I, Hirano M, Tomita T. Electromyographic investigation of human vocal cord paralysis. Ann Otol Rhinol Laryngol 1968;77:296–304
31. Crumley RL. Laryngeal synkinesis: its significance to the laryngologist. Ann Otol Rhinol Laryngol 1989;98:87–92
32. Crumley RL. Mechanisms of synkinesis. Laryngoscope 1979;89:1847–1854
33. Maronian NC, Robinson L, Waugh P, Hillel AD. A new electromyographic definition of laryngeal synkinesis. Ann Otol Rhinol Laryngol 2004;113:877–886

34. Blitzer A, Jahn AF, Keidar A. Semon's law revisited: an electromyographic analysis of laryngeal synkinesis. Ann Otol Rhinol Laryngol 1996;105:764–769

35. Crumley RL. Experiments in laryngeal reinnervation. Laryngoscope 1982;92:1–27

36. Paniello RC, West SE, Lee P. Laryngeal reinnervation with the hypoglossal nerve. I. Physiology, histochemistry, electromyography, and retrograde labeling in a canine model. Ann Otol Rhinol Laryngol 2001;110:532–542

37. van Lith-Bijl JT, Stolk RJ, Tonnaer JA, Groenhout C, Konings PN, Mahieu HF. Laryngeal abductor reinnervation with a phrenic nerve transfer after a 9-month delay. Arch Otolaryngol Head Neck Surg 1998;124:393–398

38. Baldissera F, Tredici G, Marini G, et al. Innervation of the paralyzed laryngeal muscles by phrenic motoneurons. A quantitative study by light and electron microscopy. Laryngoscope 1992;102:907–916

39. Rice DH. Laryngeal reinnervation. Laryngoscope 1982;92:1049–1059

40. Sercarz JA, Nguyen L, Nasri S, Graves MC, Wenokur R, Berke GS. Physiologic motion after laryngeal nerve reinnervation: a new method. Otolaryngol Head Neck Surg 1997;116:466–474

41. Zheng H, Zhou S, Chen S, Li Z, Cuan Y. An experimental comparison of different kinds of laryngeal muscle reinnervation. Otolaryngol Head Neck Surg 1998;119:540–547

42. Crumley RL. Update: ansa cervicalis to recurrent laryngeal nerve anastomosis for unilateral laryngeal paralysis. Laryngoscope 1991;101:384–387 discussion 388

43. Crumley RL, Izdebski K, McMicken B. Nerve transfer versus Teflon injection for vocal cord paralysis: a comparison. Laryngoscope 1988;98:1200–1204

44. Zheng H, Li Z, Zhou S, Cuan Y, Wen W. Update: laryngeal reinnervation for unilateral vocal cord paralysis with the ansa cervicalis. Laryngoscope 1996;106:1522–1527

45. Olson DE, Goding GS, Michael DD. Acoustic and perceptual evaluation of laryngeal reinnervation by ansa cervicalis transfer. Laryngoscope 1998;108:1767–1772

46. Maronian N, Waugh P, Robinson L, Hillel A. Electromyographic findings in recurrent laryngeal nerve reinnervation. Ann Otol Rhinol Laryngol 2003;112:314–323

47. Chhetri DK, Gerratt BR, Kreiman J, Berke GS. Combined arytenoid adduction and laryngeal reinnervation in the treatment of vocal fold paralysis. Laryngoscope 1999;109:1928–1936

48. Paniello RC. Medialization vs. reinnervation for vocal cord paralysis. NIH Grant 2001;DC004681:56

49. Titze IR. Comments on the myoelastic-aerodynamic theory of phonation. J Speech Hear Res 1980;23:495–510

50. Green DC, Ward PH. The management of the divided recurrent laryngeal nerve. Laryngoscope 1990;100:779–782

51. Crumley RL. Repair of the recurrent laryngeal nerve. Otolaryngol Clin North Am 1990;23:553–563

52. Chou FF, Su CY, Jeng SF, Hsu KL, Lu KY. Neurorrhaphy of the recurrent laryngeal nerve. J Am Coll Surg 2003;197:52–57

53. Miyauchi A, Matsusaka K, Kihara M, et al. The role of ansa-to-recurrent-laryngeal nerve anastomosis in operations for thyroid cancer. Eur J Surg 1998;164:927–933

54. Miyauchi A, Yokozawa T, Kobayashi K, Hirai K, Matsuzuka F, Kuma K. Opposite ansa cervicalis to recurrent laryngeal nerve anastomosis to restore phonation in patients with advanced thyroid cancer. Eur J Surg 2001;167:540–541

55. Abraham MT, Gonen M, Kraus DH. Complications of type I thyroplasty and arytenoid adduction. Laryngoscope 2001;111:1322–1329

56. Weinman EC, Maragos NE. Airway compromise in thyroplasty surgery. Laryngoscope 2000;110:1082–1085

Chapter 16

Diagnostic-Based Treatment Approaches

JoAnne Robbins, Stephanie K. Daniels, and Soly Baredes

Swallowing is a highly complex balancing act that most people do not think about until a bit of food or a pill is caught in the throat or until more than an occasional sip of liquid is aspirated. Approximately 30 oral and pharyngeal muscles and multiple nerves must perform precisely on cue so that the upper aerodigestive tract is reconfigured from a mechanism that channels air for breathing and speaking (**Fig. 16.1**) to a food-propelling mechanism that safely accomplishes ingestion (**Fig. 16.2**).

The four morphologic regions serving these purposes are the oral cavity, pharynx, larynx, and esophagus. Of these, the first three collectively are termed the upper aerodigestive tract because they also serve the airway-dependent functions of respiration and speech production. In humans, with our upright posture, it is the adjacent position of the anatomy for breathing to the anatomy for food passage that unfortunately facilitates gravitational influences on food to flow into an unprotected airway.

The larynx is essential to safe swallowing and is neurologically wired to protect the airway from entry of food, liquid, medications, or secretions. However, a perspective of dysphagia that focuses on the presence or absence of aspiration, as it relates only to the larynx, ignoring the critical elements of the propulsive pump for bolus transfer and the opening of the upper esophageal sphincter (UES) for clearance, would result in limited and largely erroneous treatment plans that could prove fatal to the patient who aspirates in the presence of an intact larynx. Indeed, essential to normal swallow physiology, including three levels of airway protection, is normal clearance of food from the oropharynx so that when the larynx returns to an open inspiratory position, no residual foreign material is in oropharyngeal recesses to be inhaled and aspirated. Further, esophageal integrity is critical as well to minimize aspiration that may occur long after swallowing is completed due to material maintained in the esophagus (intraesophageal stasis and reflux)[1] or below, in the form of gastroesophageal reflux. These latter events may occur in the presence of an intact larynx.

Thus aspiration may occur at mealtime or at other times. When aspiration is *during* the meal, particularly early in the meal, then the biomechanics and anatomy of the oropharyngeal swallow or the esophagus must be carefully considered. If aspiration is reported to occur *after* the meal, and often seemingly not present during eating, then intraesophageal or gastroesophageal reflux is more likely the culprit and warrants evaluation. In the latter scenario, the larynx is often functionally intact but reacting to the refluxate that moves posteriorly/superiorly and may enter the airway, damaging the larynx and causing related sequelae.

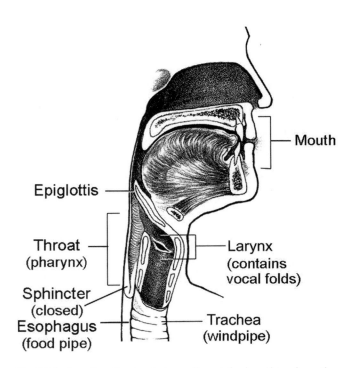

Fig. 16.1 Aerodigestive tract channeling air for breathing from the nose and mouth through the open larynx into the lungs and back up and out. For speaking, air is channeled similarly, but the vocal folds vibrate to produce voice.(From Weihofen D, Robbins J, Sullivan P. The Easy to Swallow, Easy to Chew Cookbook. New York: John Wiley; 2002. Adapted with permission.)

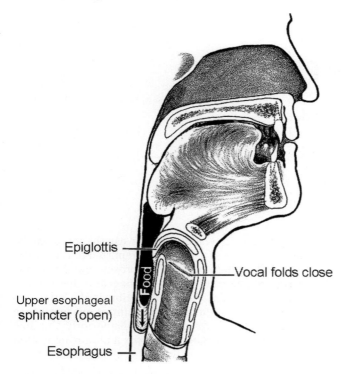

Fig. 16.2 Aerodigestive tract reconfigured from an air channel to a food-propelling mechanism. The tongue propels food into the throat; the epiglottis covers the larynx, which is the airway entrance; and the vocal folds close to protect the trachea and lungs from foreign material. (From Weihofen D, Robbins J, Sullivan P. The Easy to Swallow, Easy to Chew Cookbook. New York: John Wiley; 2002. Adapted with permission.)

♦ Neurologic Conditions Affecting Swallowing

Disease or damage to any region along the neural axis from the cerebral cortex to muscles of the oral cavity, pharynx, larynx, and esophagus may produce dysphagia (**Table 16.1**). The temporal relationship of dysphagia to neurologic disease is variable, with some disorders associated with the acute onset of dysphagia (e.g., stroke) and other, typically degenerative disorders (e.g., Parkinson disease [PD]) associated with a gradual onset of swallowing problems (**Table 16.2**). Stroke has been the most studied of the neurologic etiologies of dysphagia. Since the advent of neuroimaging techniques, it is well established that in addition to brainstem or bilateral hemispheric stroke, a single stroke involving either cerebral hemisphere may produce significant and protracted dysphagia.[2,3]

Neurologic disorders may affect the oropharyngeal or esophageal phases of swallowing. Although patterns of swallowing kinematics emerge from underlying etiologies, none has been shown with adequate statistical power to be identified as providing distinguishing hallmarks in swallowing characteristics that differentiate one neurologic disease from another.

Table 16.1 Medical and Surgical Treatments for Dysphagia

Medical
Botulinum toxin injection
Dilation
Nasogastric tube
Surgical
Cricopharyngeal myotomy
Laryngeal framework surgery with or without arytenoid adduction
Vocal fold augmentation—injection of medialization thyroplasty
Tracheostomy
Laryngotracheal separation
Hypopharyngoplasty
Stents
Cervical esophagostomy, gastrostomy, jejunostomy

Table 16.2 Neurologic Disorders Impacting Swallowing

Central nervous system
Nondegenerative
Stroke
Traumatic brain injury
Cerebral palsy
Neoplasms
Neck surgery
   Carotid endarterectomy
   Cervical fusion
Degenerative
Dementia
Movement disorders
   Parkinson disease
   Progressive supranuclear palsy
   Olivopontocerebellar atrophy
   Huntington's disease
   Wilson's disease
Multiple sclerosis
Peripheral nervous system
Amyotrophic lateral sclerosis
Postpolio syndrome
Myasthenia gravis
Guillain-Barré
Myopathy
   Myotonic dystrophy
   Oculopharyngeal muscular dystrophy
   Inclusion body myositis
   Polymyositis
   Dermatomyositis
   Hyper- and hypothroidism

Symptoms of neurogenic dysphagia may be obvious, characterized by coughing with swallowing or a patient's complaint of pharyngeal retention or a feeling of something "stuck." However, unlike dysphagia resulting from head and neck cancer in which the dysphagia symptoms are apparent, swallowing problems resulting from neurogenic disorders may not be as obvious because the disorder may more commonly affect the sensory system.[4] Thus, a cough reflex may not be evoked with aspiration, or a patient may not be aware of pharyngeal residue. Moreover, neurologic disorders may affect a person's cognition or language, which can limit a patient's awareness of, or ability to communicate about, a swallowing disturbance.

♦ Diagnosis and Treatment Evaluation

Evaluating the Swallow

Before determining the type of treatment to employ for neurogenic dysphagia, the specific biomechanic or physiologic disorder(s) of the dysphagia (e.g., decreased anterior laryngeal movement, delayed evocation of the pharyngeal swallow response) must be identified. To identify the exact nature of the swallowing disorder, an instrumental swallowing examination must be completed. The videofluoroscopic swallow study (VSS) is generally the method of choice in evaluating oropharyngeal dysphagia in that kinematic events comprising all stages of swallowing, from the oral cavity through the esophagus, can be visualized and examined while in motion, and the dynamics of bolus flow also are visualized.

Evaluating the Treatment

By employing an instrumental examination to determine the exact mechanism of dysphagia, one can use a specifically designed treatment to target the underlying biomechanical problem during the fluoroscopic examination. Certain compensatory strategies such as postures and food or fluid consistency modification as well as swallowing maneuvers should be attempted during the instrumental examination to determine their effectiveness. Other less immediate treatments, such as rehabilitative, medical, surgical, or prosthetic, should be employed to target the area of dysfunction identified on the instrumental examination.

♦ Treatment

Medical Treatment

As with direct swallowing rehabilitation, any medical or surgical intervention for swallowing should be performed to address the pathophysiology underlying specific swallowing biomechanical contributors to the dysphagia identified on the instrumental examination. No randomized, controlled clinical trials have been conducted to determine the effectiveness of medical or surgical interventions on the rehabilitation of neurogenic dysphagia.

Botulinum toxin (Botox) type A has been used in treating UES dysfunction. Studies generally report improved swallowing on the instrumental examination or by patient report,[5-10] with results lasting from 1 to 14 months postinjection.[7] However, these studies are limited in that they are retrospective, and completed in heterogeneous populations; no study has incorporated a placebo control.

Botox type A injection into the salivary glands (parotid, submandibular) also has been used to treat sialorrhea (hypersalivation) in neurogenic patients including those with PD and amyotrophic lateral sclerosis.[11,12] Double-blind, placebo-controlled studies have been completed in patients with PD using Botox type A[13] and type B.[14] Subjective improvement in drooling was identified in the patients receiving either type of Botox, whereas the placebo group in both studies reported no change.

Dilation, either pneumatic or bougienage, may be used to treat cricopharyngeal dysfunction; however, no study has specifically focused on this procedure in a group of patients with neurogenic dysphagia. Symptomatic response to cricopharyngeal disruption with either dilation or myotomy was studied in a heterogeneous group of subjects.[15] Results revealed 58% of subjects who underwent dilation had a subjective improvement in swallowing.

Surgical Treatment

Patients with severe swallowing disorders may require surgical intervention at some point in the course of their illness. Surgery in the patient with a swallowing disorder aims to (1) improve passage of the bolus, (2) prevent aspiration, or (3) facilitate non-oral feedings. Surgery is indicated in patients with neurogenic dysphagia when (1) there is clearly a surgical lesion, such as a tumor, stricture, or diverticulum, which is generally a coincidental finding with this population; (2) a deficit, such as a vocal cord paralysis or UES dysfunction, persists and is symptomatic despite a period of observation and appropriate nonsurgical management; (3) there are actual or imminent complications from chronic aspiration despite the cessation of oral feedings; (4) remaining without oral feedings to prevent aspiration is an unacceptable alternative to the patient; or (5) there is a need to establish a route for long-term non-oral feedings.[16,17]

Treatment of Laryngeal Incompetence

Laryngeal incompetence can result from vocal cord paralysis, a sensory deficit, or mechanical disruption and scarring. The most critical element of the sphincteric function of the larynx preventing aspiration is the closure of the true vocal cords during deglutition. A vocal cord paralysis can cause aspiration by producing incomplete glottic closure during swallowing, and an ineffective cough. Loss of laryngeal sphincteric function also decreases subglottic pressure during swallowing, which is felt to decrease efficiency of swallowing and increase aspiration.[18] Aspiration is more commonly seen when laryngeal paralysis causes a deficit in closure at the posterior aspect of the glottis.

The techniques devised primarily to improve phonation in patients with vocal cord paralysis also may aid in the management of aspiration. The details of these procedures are discussed elsewhere in this text, but essentially include laryngeal framework surgery with or without arytenoid adduction, and injection thyroplasty. Aspiration can be corrected by medialization of the immobile vocal cord, thus permitting the contralateral vocal cord to achieve glottic closure when it is adducted. Framework surgery in which medialization is achieved by inserting an implant lateral to the vocal cord (type I thyroplasty) has been demonstrated to decrease aspiration in a variety of disorders associated with vocal cord paralysis and dysphagia, and to facilitate elimination of the need for tracheostomy.[19] The addition of an arytenoid adduction procedure is necessary when the laryngeal deficit includes a significant posterior glottic gap. Despite positioning thyroplasty implants to extend to the level of the vocal process of the arytenoids, the arytenoid adduction procedure is more effective in closing posterior gaps. The procedure is performed by inserting a suture into the muscular process of the arytenoid. By applying anterior traction and fixing the suture to the lateral ala of the thyroid cartilage, the arytenoid is rotated, thus positioning the vocal process in a median position. The arytenoid adduction procedure is usually performed in combination with a thyroplasty medialization procedure, although it can be performed as the initial step, after which the need for thyroplasty is assessed.[20-22]

Medialization thyroplasty and arytenoid adduction procedures may be performed under general anesthesia, but they are usually performed under local anesthesia to allow intraoperative monitoring of the voice, airway, and adequacy of glottic closure. Thyroplasty procedures are reversible (i.e., the implant can be easily removed) and, therefore, can be performed even if return of function may occur at a future time. On the other hand, because of the dissection at the cricoarytenoid joint, arytenoid adduction should be considered a permanent alteration of laryngeal anatomy, and should be performed only when no return of function is anticipated (e.g., after transection of the vagus nerve during skull base surgery).

Injection thyroplasty accomplishes medialization of the immobile cord by injecting the cord directly to close an identified glottic gap. Many materials are currently used for injection including fat, fascia, gelatin powder, collagen, and acellular micronized human dermis.[23] The advantage of injection thyroplasty is that the procedure is less invasive and can sometimes be performed percutaneously as an office procedure. Also, resorbable material such as gelatin powder can be used for short-term trials. These injection procedures, however, do not afford the control and precision that surgical thyroplasty and arytenoids adduction provide. Resorption of injected materials can also make long-term results unpredictable. Injections can be used as an adjunct to surgical medialization.[24,25]

A recently introduced hypopharyngoplasty procedure may be a useful adjunct in the management of patients with laryngeal incompetence and pharyngeal paralysis.[26] The procedure is performed at the time of thyroplasty and arytenoid adduction. Insensate and redundant piriform sinus mucosa on the paralyzed side is resected to prevent dilation and pooling, and the inferior constrictor muscle is advanced anteriorly to increase tone. To date, the procedure has been performed only by its progenitors on eight patients who were reported to have good outcomes.

When glottic incompetence results from mechanical disruption or scarring (e.g., after trauma or partial laryngeal resection), one may not be able to improve competency with standard implants or injections. Procedures for specific situations need to be employed, such as the subperichondrial implantation of a portion of the superior thyroid cartilage to medialize the vocal cord in patients after laser treatment of glottic carcinoma.[27] Partial collapse of the cricoid cartilage has also been used to correct glottic incompetence after extended supraglottic laryngectomy.[28]

The appropriate application of procedures for laryngeal incompetence is dependent on a complete multidisciplinary evaluation of the causes of aspiration in an individual patient. The position of an immobile vocal cord, the status of posterior glottic closure, associated dysmotility of the tongue and pharynx, and general strength and mental status contribute to the likelihood of aspiration. The procedures discussed above are effective for localized, well-defined areas of laryngeal incompetence. The effectiveness of these procedures is diminished in situations where there is associated diffuse incoordination and sensory loss, as may occur in stroke patients or patients with advanced neuromuscular disorders.

Treatment of Cricopharyngeal Muscle Dysfunction

Failure of the cricopharyngeus muscle, the major component of the UES, to relax appropriately may cause dysphagia, pooling of secretions, and aspiration. There is much conflicting information in the literature regarding the incidence and management of cricopharyngeal dysfunction (spasm or incoordination during the pharyngeal phase of swallowing).[29,30] Evidence supporting the use of cricopharyngeal myotomy for neurogenic dysphagia is limited. No trial for cricopharyngeal myotomy for neurogenic dysphagia has been conducted. If one were performed, it would have to include those with a hyperactive cricopharyngeus muscle, and exclude the patients with more generalized dysfunction. Such a problem was noted in the study reviewing cricopharyngeal myotomy for dysphagia in head and neck cancer patients. In this study by Jacobs et al,[31] no significant differences were seen in swallowing between patients who had a myotomy and those who did not. Of course, the entire cohort included patients with multiple swallowing disabilities, which are not likely to be improved with myotomy alone. The studies to date for myotomy in the neurogenic dysphagia population have used subjective, rather than objective, measures, and had small sample sizes.[32-34] Dysfunction associated with a systemic disorder (e.g., parkinsonism, myasthenia gravis, or polymyositis) may improve with specific treatment of the disorder or specific swallowing rehabilitation. Persistent cricopharyngeal dysfunction may need to be addressed directly; however, before this can be undertaken, the exact nature of the disorder must be understood, as isolated cricopharyngeal dysfunction is rare in patients with neurogenic dysphagia. In this population, decreased anterior hyolaryngeal traction to open the UES is the etiology often related to reduced lingual pressure generation and therefore reduced intrabolus pressures to assist in optimizing UES opening, not failure of the muscle to relax[35]. In these cases, myotomy would not improve swallowing.

Cricopharyngeal myotomy is the most effective treatment for persistent, isolated cricopharyngeal dysfunction.[36,37] This has been shown to be effective in some patients who suffered lateral medullary brainstem stroke in which the relaxation of the UES is disinhibited. The procedure is most successful when combined with a behavioral opening maneuver such as the Mendelsohn,[38] because even after the surgical "relaxation" of the UES is accomplished, opening of the sphincter must occur and that is accomplished best with a voluntary mechanical maneuver. Lateral medullary stroke patients (particularly the unilateral patients who are the ones most likely to survive) are generally very cognitively intact. The operation can be performed endoscopically, usually using a CO_2 laser, but is still most often performed via an external approach. In the endoscopic approach, the muscle is transected submucosally in the midline posteriorly to the prevertebral fatty tissue.[39] In the external approach, the cricopharyngeus muscle is exposed via a lateral cervical incision. The lower fibers of the inferior constrictor muscle and 1 cm of adjacent circular esophageal muscle fibers are also transected because these participate in the UES. The operation weakens the UES, but does not eliminate it. The remaining pressure is sufficient to prevent significant reflux or air swallowing.[40–43] Cricopharyngeal myotomy has also been used successfully with arytenoid adduction to manage aspiration.[44]

A Zenker's or hypopharyngeal diverticulum is an outpouching of mucosa at the level of the UES, usually protruding posteriorly and to the left between the transverse fibers of the cricopharyngeus muscle and the inferior constrictor muscle. It may result in dysphagia, regurgitation of undigested food, and aspiration. Although its etiology is unclear, it is likely related to cricopharyngeus muscle dysfunction.[30] Thus identification of a Zenker's diverticulum in the neurogenic population may be a coincidental finding; however, patients with chronic neurogenic dysphagia involving UES dysfunction may develop a diverticulum over time. Treatment can be via an endoscopic approach or by open approach via a lateral cervical incision. Endoscopic approaches divide the diverticuloesophageal wall (including the cricopharyngeus muscle), permitting the bolus to pass unobstructed.[45–47] Such approaches that require the transmucosal division of the wall without closure never gained wide acceptance because of the fear of mediastinitis. The introduction of staple-assisted diverticulostomy, in which the wall is stapled when incised, diminished the risks and has made endoscopic management of Zenker's diverticulum the treatment of choice for many surgeons.[48,49] Open approach with resection of the diverticulum and cricopharyngeal myotomy is still necessary for small diverticula that cannot accommodate the surgical stapler or if anatomic factors make endoscopic access difficult. Open extramucosal diverticulopexy combined with cricopharyngeal myotomy has also been used successfully to eliminate dysphagia and aspiration. In this procedure the sac is not resected but is repositioned superiorly so the apex of the diverticulum can no longer act as a reservoir.

General Procedures for Managing Aspiration

The procedures described above are designed to address specific defects that hinder proper passage of the bolus or result in aspiration. When there is significant aspiration but no defect can be corrected, the aim is to provide a means of dealing with the aspiration even though the primary dysfunction cannot be improved. Procedures used in such instances are designed to separate, partially or totally, the airway from the digestive passages. It should be noted that these surgical approaches have either not been studied in the neurogenic population or have been limited to case reports.[50,51]

The most commonly used procedure to achieve this goal is the tracheostomy with a cuffed tube. To some degree the tracheostomy does protect the tracheobronchial tree from material that may pass through the laryngeal sphincter. It also provides easy access for suctioning aspirated material. However, its effectiveness diminishes as the volume of aspirated secretions and food increases, because these will eventually seep around the cuff or pass into the distal trachea when the cuff is temporarily deflated. Furthermore, the presence of the tracheostomy may itself promote some laryngeal dysfunction and aspiration.[18,52–54]

Because of the tracheostomy's limitations, other techniques for separating the air and digestive passages have been devised. Habal and Murray[55] described a supraglottic closure technique. Via a pharyngotomy, an incision is made around the perimeter of the epiglottis, aryepiglottic folds, arytenoids, and interarytenoid area. The epiglottis is then used as a flap that is sutured back to the arytenoids. The difficulty with this procedure is that there is a tendency for the epiglottic flap to separate from the posterior aspect of the larynx. Although such a separation has the advantage of restoring some phonation and can be intentionally created for this purpose, it obviously can result in recurrent aspiration. Modification of the technique to diminish the elasticity of the epiglottic cartilage has helped reduce posterior dehiscence.[56]

Biller et al[57] described a vertical supraglottic closure procedure for patients undergoing total glossectomy. After incising the margins of the epiglottis, aryepiglottic folds, arytenoids, and interarytenoid area, the epiglottis is vertically tubed, leaving a small opening at the tip. This procedure is more reliable in maintaining supraglottic closure than the horizontal epiglottic flap. The opening superiorly is sufficient to permit phonation in some patients. Both the horizontal and vertical supraglottic closures are potentially reversible, and have the advantage of leaving the vocal cords intact.[58]

Montgomery[59] described a glottic closure procedure. Via a thyrotomy, the glottis is denuded of epithelium circumferentially by resecting a strip of mucous membrane.

The de-epithelialized halves of the glottis are sutured to each other. The procedure is potentially reversible, although the degree of scarring that is created makes it difficult to restore normal laryngeal function.

Krespi et al[60] introduced the technique of partial cricoid resection for the management of aspiration in patients after head and neck cancer surgery. The posterior half of the cricoid lamina is removed via a submucosal dissection, and a cricopharyngeal and inferior constrictor myotomy is performed. This maneuver leaves a large hypopharyngeal portal for secretions and food and decreases anteroposterior diameter of the larynx, thus eliminating or reducing aspiration. The irreversibility of the subglottic collapse is a disadvantage of this procedure.

Lindeman[61] described a tracheoesophageal diversion technique that provides complete separation of the airway and digestive tract. The trachea is divided at the level of the third or fourth tracheal ring, and the proximal stump is anastomosed to the cervical esophagus. The distal portion of the trachea is brought out to the skin where a tracheostome is created. This procedure channels all aspirated material into the esophagus. The procedure is reversible with preservation of voice and laryngeal airway. When a high tracheostomy exists, a laryngotracheal separation can be performed without diversion into the esophagus.[62-65] The proximal portion of the trachea is closed on itself, creating a blind pouch. Pooling of secretions in this pouch does not seem to be problematic. Krespi et al[50] described a modification of the procedure that permits diversion into the esophagus when a high tracheostomy is present.

Laryngeal stents that occlude the laryngeal inlet above a tracheostomy have been used with some success. Because of difficulty in their use and care, they are infrequently used, but are still useful in selected short-term situations.[66,67]

Before the development of the multiple techniques available for managing chronic aspiration, total laryngectomy was used for cases of intractable aspiration. Although the role for laryngectomy for aspiration has diminished, it is still used in selected patients (such as patients with uncorrectable aspiration after partial laryngeal surgery for cancer).

Despite the effectiveness of the above techniques in controlling aspiration, all procedures that separate the airway from the digestive tract require the use of a tracheostomy, and most impair phonation. Preliminary work to restore dynamic laryngotracheal separation with implantable recurrent laryngeal nerve stimulators has the potential to control aspiration without airway disruption.[68]

Nonoral Feedings

If a stable situation can be achieved by simply withholding oral feedings from a patient, and if this is acceptable to the patient, more elaborate procedures for aspiration can be avoided. Nasogastric tube feedings and parenteral alimentation are usually not satisfactory for long-term nutritional support. Preferable techniques include the creation of a cervical esophagostomy, feeding gastrostomy, or feeding jejunostomy. A feeding gastrostomy is best in most situations. The percutaneous endoscopic approach has greatly simplified the creation of the gastrostomy.

Prosthetic Devices

A category of compensatory options to improve swallowing biomechanics is prosthetic devices. Neurologic patients with trigeminal (mandible), vagus (velopharynx), or hypoglossal (tongue) involvement may be candidates for this approach.

A palatal lift prosthesis lifts the soft palate into an elevated (closed) position in patients with velar paresis/paralysis. A palatal reshaping or augmentation prosthesis can be extremely effective in patients with bilateral lingual paralysis.[69,70] These prostheses recontour the hard palate to interact with the more intact portion of the tongue, enabling the patient to control and propel the bolus more efficiently. If a patient has generalized reduction in lingual elevation both anteriorly and posteriorly, the palate may be lowered uniformly. If the patient exhibits a hemiparesis the prosthesis would contain more material in the affected side. These intraoral prostheses are usually constructed by a maxillofacial prosthodontist in cooperation with the swallowing therapist.

A jaw sling has been described for mandibular elevation to effect closure of the mouth in patients with trigeminal damage. A buccinator apparatus[71] to remind the patient to keep the mouth closed until closure can be accomplished automatically also is described. The device consists of a flat-shaped 16-gauge wire cut to encircle the patient's lips. By contouring the wire around the buccinator muscle and by applying pressure at the base of the nose and at the base of the lower teeth, the device pulls the lips in and holds the teeth together.[71]

In some cases a guide plane prosthesis is helpful. Such a device comprises a vertical bar attached to a lower denture or partial plane. When the patient closes his or her mouth, the vertical bar guides the mandible into proper alignment and thus proper occlusion.

Behavioral Treatment

Behavioral treatment for dysphagia is usually categorized as either rehabilitative or compensatory in nature. *Rehabilitative* interventions have the capacity to directly improve the dysphagia at the biologic level. That is, neuromuscular anatomy (e.g., muscle) or neural circuitry is the target of therapy that may have direct influence on physiology, biomechanics, and bolus flow. On the other hand, *compensatory* interventions avoid or reduce the effects of the impaired structures or neuropathology and resultant disordered physiology and biomechanics on bolus flow. Examples are presented in the following sections.

Compensatory Interventions

Traditionally, interventions for dysphagia in neurologic patients, particularly the elderly, are most often compensatory in nature and are directed at modifying bolus flow by targeting neuromuscularly induced pathobiomechanics or by adapting the environment. Compensatory strategies are believed by clinicians to be less demanding of the patient in terms of effort, and many of the strategies can be imposed on a relatively frail or passive patient. A nonexclusive sampling of compensatory strategies includes postural adjustment,

16 Diagnostic-Based Treatment Approaches

slowing the rate of eating, limiting bolus size, adaptive equipment, and diet modification, which is the most commonly used environmental adaptation.

Postural Adjustments Postural adjustments are relatively simple to teach a patient, require little effort to employ and can eliminate misdirection of bolus flow through biomechanical adjustment. A general postural rule to facilitate safe swallowing is to eat in an upright posture in order for the vertical phase of the oropharyngeal swallow to capitalize on the gravitational forces when sitting with the torso and head and neck at a 90-degree angle to the horizon (**Fig. 16.3**). This posture also can assist in precluding early spillage of food or liquid from the horizontal oral phase into the vertical pharynx and a potentially open airway as well as diminishing the probability of nasal regurgitation.

A less obvious postural adjustment would be useful to patients with disease-specific hemiparesis resulting from unilateral stroke. For this group of patients, a common strategy is a head turn toward the hemiparetic side, effectively closing off that side to bolus entry and facilitating bolus transit through the nonparetic pharyngeal channel and successfully through the UES. On the other hand, if the pathophysiologic underpinning is the uncoupling of the oral from the pharyngeal phase of the swallow, a simple chin tuck (**Fig. 16.3B**) at approximately a 45-degree angle reduces the speed of bolus passage, thereby giving the neural system the time it needs to initiate the pharyngeal and airway protection events prior to bolus entry. Other postural adjustments are facilitative of safe swallowing and are designed to specifically compensate for pathophysiologic conditions that, upon referral for a swallowing assessment and treatment, are analyzed with videofluoroscopy and treated by the swallowing clinician.

Limiting Food and Liquid Eating Rate and Amounts In contrast to the "fast-food society" in which we live, individuals with neurogenic dysphagia, as a rule, take longer to eat. Eating an adequate amount of food becomes a challenge, not only because of the increased time required to do so, but also because fatigue frequently becomes an issue. Typically, smaller amounts per swallow are less likely to enter or block the airway, but in individuals who experience a sensory loss to the mouth or throat, larger amounts of food or liquid may be necessary to trigger a swallow response. To promote a safe and efficient swallow in most individuals with swallowing and chewing difficulty, the following recommendations to patients are useful:

- Eat slowly and allow enough time for a meal.
- Do not eat or drink while rushed or tired.
- Take small amounts of food or liquid into the mouth. Use a teaspoon rather than a tablespoon.
- Concentrate on swallowing. Eliminate distractions like television.
- Avoid mixing food and liquid in the same mouthful.
- Place the food on the stronger side of the mouth if there is unilateral weakness, and tilt the head or lean toward the stronger side, using gravity to facilitate flow by the more intact musculature.

Adaptive Equipment Eating and drinking aids can assist in placing, directing, and controlling the bolus of food or liquid and maintaining proper head posture while eating. For example, modified cups with cut-out rims (placed over the bridge of the nose) or straws will prevent a backward head

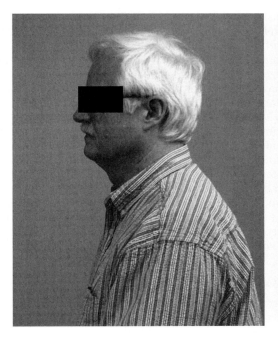
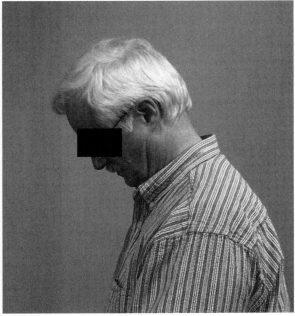

Fig. 16.3 (A,B) A compensatory chin tuck posture may facilitate increased airway protection when swallowing.

tilt and in fact facilitate a chin tuck, when drinking to the bottom of a cup. In contrast, a backward head tilt, which results in neck extension, should be avoided in most cases because when the head is tilted back, food and liquid are more likely misdirected into the airway. Spoons with narrow, shallow bowls or glossectomy feeding spoons (a spoon developed for moving food to the back of the tongue) are useful to individuals who require assistance in placing food in certain locations in the mouth. More importantly, these utensils and devices promote independence in eating and drinking. A speech pathologist/swallowing clinician can make suggestions regarding appropriate aids to optimize swallowing safety and satisfaction. Occupational therapists are experts in the area of adaptive equipment and can be helpful in obtaining products that are often available only commercially.

Diet Modification The most common compensatory intervention is diet modification, a totally passive environmental adaptation. Withholding thin liquids such as water, tea, or coffee, which are most easily aspirated by older adults, and restricting liquid intake to thickened liquids is almost routine in nursing homes in an attempt to minimize or eliminate thin liquid aspiration, presumably the long-term related outcome of which is pneumonia. Despite the huge impact these seemingly unappealing practices may have on quality of life, they are commonly implemented in the absence of efficacy data. In keeping with the current call for evidence-based practice in health care, a National Institutes of Health (NIH)-funded clinical trial recently was conducted to determine efficacy of the latter practice for patients with dementia or PD.[72–74] With the recent appearance on the clinical scene of the Swal-QOL[75–77] (a quality-of-life assessment for patients with swallowing difficulties), some of these ongoing practices can be evaluated from the patient's perspective as well as by the clinicians who are recommending them with good intent. Additional diet modifications include recommending a soft food diet in which the bolus maintains itself in a cohesive mass during transit. The use of sauces and gravies to minimize the formation of dry particles that may easily be misdirected into the airway is a common recommendation. Other strategies within this category of interventions are available, and the dietician should work closely with the team to ensure the safest diet is provided and effective in maintaining adequate nutrition and hydration for the patients.[78]

Knowing the Heimlich Maneuver Educating care providers and family members about the signs of choking and the standard first-aid technique to clear the airway, namely the Heimlich maneuver, is essential. Although the Heimlich maneuver in fact can be self-administered, it is recommended that individuals with dysphagia eat in the company of someone who knows this first-aid technique. Family members should be trained in emergency techniques for clearing the airway.

Rehabilitative Interventions

Rehabilitative exercises are, by nature, more active and rigorous than compensatory strategies. Often a rehabilitative approach to dysphagia intervention is withheld from the elderly population because such demanding activity is assumed to deplete any limited remaining swallowing reserve, thus potentially exacerbating dysphagia symptoms; however, sufficient treatment efficacy data are emerging to change assumption-based patterns of practice.[79,80]

Although progressive resistance training appears safe and effective for the limb musculature in older adults,[81,82] it has only begun to be systematically applied to the muscles of swallowing.[80] But there are two exercise regimens that are supported with efficacy data for improving swallowing-related function in neurogenic dysphagia. The first is a simple isotonic/isometric neck exercise performed over a 6-week period in which the patient simply lies flat on his back and lifts his head (keeping shoulders flat) for a specified number of repetitions.[83] The improved physiologic outcome of UES opening that effects swallowing is speculated as a result of strengthening the mylohyoid/geniohyoid muscle groups and possibly the anterior segment of the digastric muscle. The second is a lingual resistance exercise that has been used to strengthen the tongue,[80] which as mentioned earlier is a key to successful oropharyngeal swallowing.[79] Stroke patients have demonstrated increased lingual strength and improved timing of the biomechanics, and have broadened their dietary intake, in part, as a function of the exercise.[82]

Such findings suggest that older individuals and those with neurogenic dysphagia of specific etiologies are able to benefit from rehabilitative exercises focused on bulbar-innervated head and neck musculature. The methods not only hold promise for influencing safe, efficient bolus flow with significant functional gains but also may restore health and quality of life as well.

Combined Interventions

Optimal swallowing usually is the result of a combination of interventions each selected because it addresses a component of the pathobiomechanical pattern of the swallow. Not infrequently, the combination includes compensatory strategies early on post-insult and as a first step in a plan of dysphagia therapy, because simple interventions, like a chin tuck, are quickly learned. These may provide immediate safety while the strengthening of muscles takes practice over time and may be ongoing. Most importantly, clinicians must identify strategies that provide the safest swallow in the timeliest manner so that patients are nourished and hydrated as a result of the care provided. Although rehabilitation strategies appear to be associated with a sense of self-improvement in addition to improved bolus flow, they must be preceded or combined with the "quick fix" that compensatory interventions provide as a successful starting point with a combined intervention program.

Senescent Swallowing and Prevention

The term *presbyphagia*[84] refers to characteristic changes in the swallowing mechanism in otherwise healthy older adults. The progressive change that is normal with aging appears to put the elderly at increased risk for dysphagia, particularly when they are faced with stressors such as acute medical conditions (e.g., stroke) or perturbations such as medication or nasogastric tubes, which might not elicit dysphagia in a less vulnerable system.

Changes in the peripheral nervous system as well as central changes are documented with age and appear to be related to sarcopenia[85] in muscles of the head and neck. Structurally, sarcopenia is associated with reductions in muscle mass and cross-sectional area, a reduction in the number or size of muscle fibers, and a transformation or selective loss of specific muscle fiber types.[86-89] Reductions in tongue muscle fiber diameter are reported for the superior longitudinal muscle from 50 human tongues. Reductions in fiber diameters began at age 40 in males and age 30 in females.[90] In addition, an increase in fatty and connective tissue and increased amyloid deposits in the blood vessels of the tongue have also been reported.[91] In the larynx, changes in human laryngeal muscle specimens (thyroarytenoid) from autopsy or laryngectomy show a tendency for decreasing type II (fast) muscle fibers and increasing type I (slow) fiber composition with increasing age.[92] Accordingly, there are reports in our literature of sarcopenia-like changes in muscles of the upper aerodigestive tract. However, most of the work performed in the area of sarcopenia has been performed in the limb musculature, and further work is certainly indicated in cranial muscles.

The research in the area of exercise for elderly people has typically been applied to reducing falls in elderly persons,[93] rather than swallowing impairment. However, both clinical and animal studies examining this issue are beginning to emerge in the literature. In studies of progressive resistance exercise in the limbs, results demonstrated that elderly men and women can increase muscle size and strength with training, even subjects who were 90 years old or older.[94-97] According to Evans,[98] "There is no pharmacologic intervention that holds a greater promise of improving health and promoting independence in the elderly than does exercise."

There are compelling preliminary data to suggest that increased muscle activation or strength and effort training may play an important role in swallowing rehabilitation.[82,83,99-103] For example, reports in the clinical literature are suggestive of improvements in swallowing function following performance of tongue exercises in combination with other factors.[104] Thus, although there is substantial literature in limb systems to date, some preliminary data in head and neck systems are pointing to the potential benefits of strength training as a useful intervention for swallowing disorders. Exercise targeting sarcopenia with or without additional impairment warrants further clinical study, because such an approach holds the promise of prevention of age-related dysphagia for individuals who employ exercise regimes focusing on head and neck musculature.

♦ Conclusion

As the population ages, strategies for treating persons with neurogenic dysphagia will be of crucial importance. Research into the underlying pathophysiology of age-related swallowing disorders is of primary importance to allow development of interventions with sound scientific bases to encourage prevention, slowing, or reversal of these conditions. Certainly the state of the evidence calls for more research with a need for randomized clinical trials in this area. Contributions by all team members involved in the care of these patients are valuable in the challenging decision-making process, with the patient's family or care provider's point of view perhaps the most critical contribution.

References

1. Waite BK, Palmer R, Nicosia M, et al. Intraesophageal reflux and intraesophageal stasis are distinct from gastroesophageal reflux as seen radiographically. Gastrointest Endosc 2002;122:283
2. Robbins J, Levine RL. Swallowing after unilateral stroke of the cerebral cortex: Preliminary experience. Dysphagia 1988;3:11–17
3. Robbins J, Levine RL, Maser A. Swallowing after unilateral stroke of the cerebral cortex. Arch Phys Med Rehabil 1993;74:1295–1300
4. Rosenbek JC, Robbins JA, Roecker EB, Coyle JL, Wood JLA. Penetration-Aspiration Scale. Dysphagia 1996;11:93–98
5. Haapaniemi JJ, Laurikainen EA, Pulkkinen J, Marttila RJ. Botulinum toxin in the treatment of cricopharyngeal dysphagia. Dysphagia 2001;16:171–175
6. Alberty J, Oelerich M, Ludwig K, Hartmann S, Stroll W. Efficacy of botulinum toxin A for treatment of upper esophageal sphincter dysfunction. Laryngoscope 2000;110:1151–1156
7. Shaw GY, Searl JP. Botulinum toxin treatment for cricopharyngeal dysfunction. Dysphagia 2001;16:161–167
8. Parameswaran MS, Soliman AMS. Endoscopic botulinum toxin injection for cricopharyngeal dysphagia. Ann Otol Rhinol Laryngol 2002;111:871–874
9. Ahsan SF, Meleca RJ, Dworkin JP. Botulinum toxin injection of the cricopharyngeal muscle for the treatment of dysphagia. Otolaryngol Head Neck Surg 2000;122:691–695
10. Liu LWC, Tarnopolsky M, Armstrong D. Injection of bolulinum toxin A to the upper esophageal sphincter for oropharyngeal dysphagia in two patients with inclusion body myositis. Can J Gastroenterol 2004;18:397–399
11. Pal PK, Calne DB, Calne S, Tsui JKC. Botulinum toxin A as treatment for drooling saliva in PD. Neurology 2000;54:244–247
12. Giess R, Naumann M, Werner E, et al. Injections of botulinum toxin A into the salivary glands improve sialorrhoea in amyotrophic lateral sclerosis. J Neurol Neurosurg Psychiatry 2000;69:121–123
13. Mancini F, Zangaglia R, Cristina S, et al. Double-blind, placebo-controlled study to evaluate the efficacy and safety of botulinum toxin type A in the treatment of drooling in Parkinsonism. Mov Disord 2003;18:685–688
14. Ondo WG, Hunter C, Moore W. A double-blind placebo-controlled trial of botulinum toxin B for sialorrhea in Parkinson's disease. Neurology 2004;62:37–40
15. Ali GN, Wallace KL, Laundl TM, Hunt DR, deCarle DJ, Cook IJ. Predictors of outcome following cricopharyngeal disruption for pharyngeal dysphagia. Dysphagia 1997;12:133–139

16. Baredes S. Surgical management of swallowing disorders. Otolaryngol Clin North Am 1988;21:711–720
17. Blitzer A, Krespi YP, Oppenheimer RW, et al. Surgical management of aspiration. Otolaryngol Clin North Am 1988;21:743–750
18. Eibling DE, Gross RD. Subglottic air pressure: a key component of swallowing efficiency. Ann Otol Rhinol Laryngol 1996;105:253–258
19. Carrau RL, Pou A, Eibling DE, et al. Laryngeal framework surgery for the management of aspiration. Head Neck 1999;21:139–145
20. Woodson GE, Murry T. Glottic configuration after arytenoid adduction. Laryngoscope 1994;104:965–969
21. Kraus DH, Orlikoff RF, Rizk SS, et al. Arytenoid adduction as an adjunct to type I thyroplasty for unilateral vocal cord paralysis. Head Neck 1999;21:52–59
22. Bielamowicz S, Gupta A, Sekhar LN. Early arytenoid adduction for vagal paralysis after skull base surgery. Laryngoscope 2000;110:346–351
23. Damrose EJ, Berke GS. Advances in the management of glottic insufficiency. Curr Opin Otolaryngol Head Neck Surg 2003;11:480–484
24. Hoffman H, McCabe D, McCulloch T, et al. Laryngeal collagen injection as an adjunct to medialization laryngoplasty. Laryngoscope 2002;112:1407–1413
25. Bhattacharyya N, Kotz T, Shapiro J. Dysphagia and aspiration with unilateral vocal cord immobility: incidence, characterization, and response to surgical treatment. Ann Otol Rhinol Laryngol 2002;111:672–679
26. Mok P, Woo P, Schaefer-Mojica J. Hypopharyngeal pharyngoplasty in the management of pharyngeal paralysis: new procedure. Ann Otol Rhinol Laryngol 2003;112:844–852
27. Sittel C, Friedrich G, Zorowka P, et al. Surgical voice rehabilitation after laser surgery for glottic carcinoma. Ann Otol Rhinol Laryngol 2002;111:493–499
28. Sacks S, Lawson W, Biller HF. Correction of late glottic insufficiency. Otolaryngol Clin North Am 1988;21:761–769
29. Baredes S, Shah SS, Kaufman R. The frequency of cricopharyngeal dysfunction on videofluoroscopic swallowing studies in patients with dysphagia. Am J Otolaryngol 1997;18:185–189
30. Veenker EA, Andersen PE, Cohen JI. Cricopharyngeal spasm and Zenker's diverticulum. Head Neck 2003;25:681–694
31. Jacobs JR, Logemann J, Pajak T, et al. Failure of cricopharyngeal myotomy to improve dysphagia following head and neck cancer surgery. Arch Otolaryngol Head Neck Surg 1999;125:942–946
32. Poirier NC, Bonavina L, Taillefer R, Nosadini A, Peracchia A, Duranceau A. Cricopharyngeal myotomy for neurogenic oropharyngeal dysphagia. J Thorac Cardiovasc Surg 1997;113:233–241
33. St Guily JL, Perie S, Thiebaut-Noel W, Chaussade S, Eymard B, Angelard B. Swallowing disorders in muscular diseases: functional assessment and indications of cricopharyngeal myotomy. Ear Nose Throat J 1994;73:34–40
34. Born LJ, Harned RH, Rikkers LF, Pfeiffer RF, Quigley EM. Cricopharyngeal dysfunction in Parkinson's disease: role in dysphagia and response to myotomy. Mov Disord 1996;11:53–58
35. Songman JA. Evaluation and treatment of swallowing disorders (2nd ed) 1998 Austin, TX: Pro-Ed.
36. Takes RP, van den Hoogaen FJA, Marres HAM. Endoscopic myotomy of the cricopharyngeal muscle with CO2 laser surgery. Head Neck 2005;27:703–709
37. Ross ER, Green R, Auslander MO, et al. Cricopharyngeal myotomy: management of cervical dysphagia. Otolaryngol Head Neck Surg 1982;90:434–441
38. Robbins J, Levine RL. Swallowing after lateral medullary stroke syndrome plus. Clin Commun Disord 1993;3:45–55
39. Takes RP, van den Hoogaen FJA, Marres HAM. Endoscopic myotomy of the cricopharyngeal muscle with CO2 laser surgery. Head Neck 2005;27:703–709
40. Seaman WB. Cineroentgenographic observations of the cricopharyngeus. Am J Roentgenol Radium Ther Nucl Med 1966;96:922–931
41. Hurwitz AL, Duranceau A. Upper-esophageal sphincter dysfunction-pathogenesis and treatment. Am J Dig Dis 1978;23:275–281
42. Redmond P, Berliner L, Ambos M, et al. Radiological assessment of pharyngoesophageal dysfunction with emphasis on cricopharyngeal myotomy. Am J Gastroenterol 1982;77:85–92
43. Ellis FH Jr, Crozier RE. Cervical esophageal dysphagia. Ann Surg 1981;194:279–289
44. Woodson G. Cricopharyngeal myotomy and arytenoid adduction in the management of combined laryngeal and pharyngeal paralysis. Otolaryngol Head Neck Surg 1997;116:339–343
45. Dohlman F, Mattson O. The endoscopic operation for hypopharyngeal diverticula. AMA Arch Otolaryngol 1960;71:744–752
46. Kuhn FA, Bent JP. Zenker's diverticulotomy using the KTP/532 laser. Laryngoscope 1992;102:946–950
47. Bradwell RA, Bieger AK, Strachan DR, et al. Endoscopic laser myotomy in the treatment of pharyngeal diverticula. J Laryngol Otol 1997;111:627–630
48. Scher RL, Richtsmeier WJ. Long-term experience with endoscopic staple-asssisted esophagodiverticulostomy for Zenker's diverticulum. Laryngoscope 1998;108:200–205
49. Smith SR, Genden EM, Urken ML. Endoscopic stapling technique for the treatment of Senker diverticulum vs standard open-neck technique. Arch Otolaryngol Head Neck Surg 2002;128:141–144
50. Krespi YP, Quatela VC, Sisson GA, et al. Modified tracheoesophageal diversion for chronic aspiration. Laryngoscope 1984;94:1298–1301
51. Butcher RB. Treatment of chronic aspiration as a complication of cerebrovascular accident. Laryngoscope 1982;92:681–685
52. Cameron JL, Reynolds J, Zuidema GD. Aspirations in patients with tracheostomies. Surg Gynecol Obstet 1973;136:68–70
53. Bonanno PC. Swallowing dysfunction after tracheotomy. Ann Surg 1971;174:29–33
54. Ding R, Logemann JA. Swallow physiology in patients with trach cuff inflated or deflated: a retrospective study. Head Neck 2005;27:809–813
55. Habal MB, Murray JE. Surgical treatment of life-endagering chronic aspiration pneumonia. Plast Reconstr Surg 1972;49:305–311
56. Strome M, Fried MP. Rehabilitative surgery for aspiration. Arch Otolaryngol 1983;109:809–811
57. Biller HF, Lawson W, Baek SM. Total glossectomy: a technique of reconstruction eliminating laryngectomy. Arch Otolaryngol 1983;109:69–73
58. Harcourt JP, Brookes GB. Epiglottic placation for intractable aspiration. Clin Otolaryngol Allied Sci 1996;21:360–365
59. Montgomery WW. Surgery to prevent aspiration. Arch Otolaryngol 1975;101:679–682
60. Krespi YP, Pelzer HJ, Sisson GA. Management of chronic aspiration by subtotal and submucosal cricoid resection. Ann Otol Rhinol Laryngol 1985;94:580–583
61. Lindeman RC. Diverting the paralyzed larynx: a reversible procedure for intractable aspiration. Laryngoscope 1975;85:157–180
62. Baron BC, Dedo HH. Separation of the larynx and trachea for intractable aspiration. Laryngoscope 1980;90:1927–1932
63. Eisele DW, Yarington CT, Lindeman RC, et al. The tracheoesophageal diversion and laryngotracheal separation procedures for treatment of intractable aspiration. Am J Surg 1989;157:230–236
64. Eibling DE, Snyderman CH, Eibling C. Laryngotracheal separation for intractable aspiration: a retrospective review of 34 patients. Laryngoscope 1995;105:83–85
65. Yamana T, Kitano H, Hanamitsu M, et al. Clinical outcome of laryngotracheal separation for intractable aspiration pneumonia. ORL J Otorhinolaryngol Relat Spec 2001;63:321–324
66. Eliachar I, Robert JK, Hayes JD, et al. A vented laryngeal stent with phonatory and pressure relief capability. Laryngoscope 1987;97:1264–1269

67. Eliachar I, Nguyen D. Laryngotracheal stent for internal support and control of aspiration without loss of phonation. Otolaryngol Head Neck Surg 1990;103:837–840
68. Broniatowski M, Grundfest-Broniatowski S, Tyler DJ, et al. Dynamic laryngotracheal closure for aspiration: a preliminary report. Laryngoscope 2001;111:2032–2040
69. Logemann JA, Kahrilas P, Hurst P, Davis J, Krugler C. Effects of intraoral prosthetics on swallowing in oral cancer patients. Dysphagia 1989;4:118–120
70. Davis JW, Lazarus C, Logemann J, Hurst P. Effect of a maxillary glossectomy prosthesis on articulation and swallowing. J Prosthet Dent 1987;57:715–719
71. Mitchell P. Buccinator apparatus to improve swallowing. Phys Ther 1967;47:1135
72. Robbins J, Hind JA, Logemann J. An ongoing randomized clinical trial in dysphagia. J Commun Disord 2004;37:425–435
73. Logemann JA, Gensler G, Robbins J, et al. A randomized study of three interventions for aspiration of thin liquids in patients with dementia or Parkinson's disease. J Speech Lang Hear Res 2008;51:173–183
74. Robbins JA, Gensler G, Hind JA, et al. Comparison of two interventions for liquid aspiration on pneumonia incidence: a randomized controlled trial. Ann Intern Med 2008;148:509–518
75. McHorney CA, Bricker DE, Kramer AE, et al. The SWAL-QOL outcomes tool for oropharyngeal dysphagia in adults: I. Conceptual foundation and item development. Dysphagia 2000;15:115–121
76. McHorney CA, Bricker DE, Robbins JA, Kramer AE, Rosenbek JC, Chignell KA. The SWAL-QOL outcomes tool for oropharyngeal dysphagia in adults: II. Item reduction and preliminary scaling. Dysphagia 2000;15:122–133
77. McHorney CA, Robbins JA, Lomax K, et al. The SWAL-QOL outcomes tool for oropharyngeal dysphagia in adults: III. Extensive evidence of reliability and validity. Dysphagia 2002;17:97–114
78. Weihofen D, Robbins J, Sullivan P. The Easy to Swallow, Easy to Chew Cookbook. New York: John Wiley; 2002
79. Robbins J, Gangnon R, Theis S, Kays SA, Hind J. The effects of lingual exercise on swallowing in older adults. J Am Geriatr Soc 2005;53:1483–1489
80. Robbins JA, Carnes M, Hind JA, et al. Lingual isometric and swallowing strength in the elderly: Is intervention warranted? Gerontology 1998;38:6
81. Fiatarone MA, O'Neill EF, Ryan ND, et al. Exercise training and nutritional supplementation for physical frailty in very elderly people. N Engl J Med 1994;330:1769–1775
82. Robbins J, Kays SA, Gangnon R, Hewitt A, Hind J. The effects of lingual exercise in stroke patients with dysphagia. Arch Phys Med Rehabil 2007;88:150–158
83. Shaker R, Kern M, Bardan E, et al. Augmentation of deglutitive upper esophageal sphincter opening in the elderly by exercise. Am J Physiol 1997;272:G1518–G1522
84. Robbins JA. Old swallowing and dysphagia: thoughts on intervention and prevention. Nutr Clin Pract 1999;14:S21–S26
85. Evans WJ. What is sarcopenia? J Gerontol A Biol Sci Med Sci 1995;50A:5–8
86. Brown M, Hasser EM. Differential effects of reduced muscle use (hindlimb unweighting) on skeletal muscle with aging. Aging (Milano) 1996;8:99–105
87. Carlson BM. Factors influencing the repair and adaptation of muscles in aged individuals: satellite cells and innervation. J Gerontol A Biol Sci Med Sci 1995;50:96–100
88. Lexell J. Human aging, muscle mass, and fiber type composition. J Gerontol A Biol Sci Med Sci 1995;50:11–16
89. Lexell J, Taylor CC, Sjostrom M. What is the cause of ageing atrophy? Total number, size and proportion of different fiber types studied in whole vastus lateralis muscle from 15 to 83-year old men. J Neurol Sci 1988;84:275–294
90. Nakayama M. Histological study on aging changes in the human tongue. Nippon Jibiinkoka Gakkai Kaiho 1991;94:541–555
91. Yamaguchi A, Nasu M, Esali Y, et al. Amyloid deposits in the aged tongue. A post mortem study of 107 individuals over 67 years of age. J Oral Pathol 1982;11:237–244
92. Rodeno MT, Sanchez-Fernandez JM, Rivera-Pomar JM. Histochemical and morphometrical ageing changes in human vocal cord muscles. Acta Otolaryngol (Stockholm) 1993;113:445–449
93. Fiatarone MA, Evans WJ. The etiology and reversibility of muscle dysfunction in the aged. J Gerontol 1993;48(Spec. No):77–83
94. Fiatarone MA, Marks EC, Ryan ND, Meredith CN, Lipsitz LA, Evans WJ. High intensity strength training in non-agenarians. Effects on skeletal muscle. JAMA 1990;263:3029–3034
95. Frontera WR, Meredith CN, O'Reilly KP, et al. Strength conditioning in older men: skeletal muscle hypertrophy and improved function. J Appl Physiol 1988;64:1038–1044
96. Grimby G, Aniansson A, Hedberg M, et al. Training can improve muscle strength and endurance in 78–84 year old men. J Appl Physiol 1992;73:2517–2523
97. Tracy BL, Ivey FM, Hurlbut D, et al. Muscle quality. II. Effects of strength training in 65- to 75-year old men and women. J Appl Physiol 1999;86:195–201
98. Evans WJ. Exercise, nutrition, and aging. Clin Geriatr Med 1995;11:725–734
99. Burnett TA, Mann EA, Cornell SA, Ludlow CL. Laryngeal elevation achieved by neuromuscular stimulation at rest. J Appl Physiol 2003;94:128–134
100. El Sharkawi A, Ramig LO, Logemann JA, et al. Swallowing and voice effects of Lee Silverman Voice Treatment (LSVT[R]): a pilot study. J Neurol Neurosurg Psychiatry 2002;72:31–36
101. Hind J. The effects of lingual exercises on swallowing. Paper presented at the American Speech Language Hearing Association annual convention, Washington, DC, 2000
102. Lazarus C, Logemann J, Huang C, Rademaker A. Effects of two types of tongue strengthening exercises in young normals. Folia Phoniatr Logop 2003;55:199–205
103. Sullivan P, Hind J, Robbins J. Lingual exercise protocol for head and neck cancer. Poster presentation at the 9th Annual Meeting of Dysphagia Research Society, Savannah, GA, 2000
104. Neumann S, Bartolome G, Buchholz D, Prosiegel M. Swallowing therapy of neurologic patients: correlation of outcome with pretreatment variables and therapeutic methods. Dysphagia 1995;10:1–5

Chapter 17

Movement Disorders of the Larynx

Mitchell F. Brin, Andrew Blitzer, and Miodrag Velickovic

Phonation and the production of sound require precise coordination of muscles and consequent airflow and are nearly always perturbed in patients with neuromuscular disorders affecting movement. The neurologic subspecialty of movement disorders has played an increasingly important role in clinical care. Since the last edition of this volume, there has been an explosion of information about genetics, protein chemistry, neurophysiology, and neuropathology. However, with the exception of the major advances in the neurosurgical management of many of these disorders, and in particular the application of high-frequency deep brain stimulation, in addition to the growth in the use of local injections of botulinum toxin as a focal therapy for hyperkinetic disorders, there has been a paucity of specific new pharmacologic interventions. This chapter discusses the fundamental clinical and physiologic characteristics of the more common movement disorders, with special emphasis on the relevant neurolaryngologic aspects. There are several excellent sources for a more detailed general review of movement disorders[1,2] in addition to the official journal of the Movement Disorder Society, *Movement Disorders*.

Patients are classified as having a movement disorder if they have a disorder of motor programming resulting in either a paucity of movement (akinesia or bradykinesia), excessive movement (hyperkinesia), or a combination thereof (**Table 17.1**). In general, for each disorder we classify the disorder as a primary or secondary condition. When the condition is primary, there is no identifiable cause or etiology for the symptoms, which are highlighted when each disorder is discussed.

Proper diagnosis and treatment of these disorders typically requires a team approach including an otolaryngologist, neurologist, and speech-language pathologist. It is helpful to have consultative assistance from a speech-language scientist, psychiatrist, and radiologist. The treating team should be committed to managing these disorders. Once a diagnosis is established, appropriate steps should be taken to appropriately classify symptoms and design a treatment program. Often a treatment program includes treatment of the underlying condition, which may include social support (psychotherapy, family therapy), physical therapies,[3] and pharmacotherapy.

For most movement disorders, patients are classified as either idiopathic, that is, without a known etiology or the presence of any other disorder that can present with the phenotype, or symptomatic, that is, with an underlying disorder causing the phenotype. Since the first edition of this book, numerous genetic loci and associated mutations have been identified for cases that historically have been classified as idiopathic or symptomatic, which makes it difficult to classify a patient with genetic underpinnings as "idiopathic"; thus, many authors are classifying patients as "primary" when there is no other underlying neurologic disorder for a disease. It is notable that classifications are typically descriptive of physical signs and have evolved over time as molecular and genetic biology evolve and etiologies become known.[4]

♦ Parkinson Disease

Definition

Parkinsonism is a neurologic syndrome manifested by any combination of tremor at rest, rigidity, bradykinesia, and loss of postural reflexes.[5] At least two of these four cardinal features should be present for the diagnosis of parkinsonism. There are many causes of parkinsonism, and they can be divided into three major categories: idiopathic, symptomatic, and parkinsonism-plus disorders (**Table 17.2**). The specific diagnosis depends on details of the clinical history, the neurologic examination, and laboratory tests.

Table 17.1 Movement Disorders

Movement Disorder	Bradykinetic	Hyperkinetic
Parkinsonism	X	
Chorea	X	X
Essential tremor		X
Dystonia		X
Stuttering		X
Myoclonus		X
Tics (Tourette syndrome)		X

Table 17.2 Classification of Parkinsonism

I. Idiopathic (primary)
   A. Parkinson disease
II. Symptomatic (secondary)
   A. Drugs—neuroleptics
   B. Postencephalitic
   C. Toxins—Mn, CO, MPTP, cyanide
   D. Vascular
   E. Brain tumor
   F. Head trauma
III. Parkinsonism-plus syndromes
   A. Progressive supranuclear palsy
   B. Multiple system atrophy
      1. Pyramid type (formerly known as striatonigral degeneration)
      2. Cerebellar type (formerly known as olivopontocerebellar atrophy [OPCA] degeneration)
   C. Dementia syndromes
      1. Alzheimer's disease
      2. Normal pressure hydrocephalus
   D. Hereditary disorders
      1. Wilson disease
      2. Huntington disease
      3. Pantothenate kinase–associated neurodegeneration (formerly known as Hallervorden-Spatz disease)

Abbreviations: Mn, manganese; CO, carbon monoxide; MPTP, 1-methyl-4-phenyl-1,2,3,6-tetrahydropyridine.

Table 17.3 Criteria for the Diagnosis of Parkinson Disease

A. *Inclusions*
   1. At least two of the following:
      a. Rest tremor
      b. Rigidity
      c. Bradykinesia
      d. Loss of postural reflexes
B. *Exclusions*
   1. History of:
      a. Encephalitis
      b. Exposure to carbon monoxide, manganese, MPTP, or other toxins
      c. Recent exposure to neuroleptic medication
   2. Onset of parkinsonian symptoms following:
      a. Head trauma
      b. Stroke
   3. Presence on examination of:
      a. Cerebellar ataxia
      b. Loss of downward ocular movements
      c. Pronounced postural hypotension not due to concurrent medication
      d. Vocal cord paralysis
   4. Magnetic resonance imaging or computed tomography of the head revealing:
      a. Lacunar infarcts
      b. Capacious cerebral ventricles
      c. Cerebellar atrophy
      d. Atrophy of the midbrain or other parts of the brainstem
   5. Failure to respond to levodopa therapy

Source: Fahn S. Disorders with parkinsonism features. In: Hurst JW, ed. Medicine for the Practicing Physician. 2nd ed. Boston: Butterworths; 1988:1522–1525. Adapted with permission.

Idiopathic parkinsonism, also known as Parkinson disease (PD), is the most common type of parkinsonism encountered by the neurologist. It is a progressive disorder of unknown etiology, and the diagnosis is usually made by excluding known causes of parkinsonism; however, many patients who present with a classical phenotype have a genetic etiology. The major exclusion criteria, which if present indicate another cause of parkinsonism, are presented in **Table 17.3**.

Clinical Features

Parkinson disease begins insidiously. Tremor is usually the first symptom recognized by the patient; however, the disorder can begin with hypophonia, slowness in movement, or shuffling gait. In the early stages, the symptoms and signs tend to remain on one side of the body, but with time the other side slowly becomes involved as well. Nevertheless, most patients have asymmetric symptoms throughout the course of their disease.

Tremor, approximately 3 Hz, is present in the distal parts of the extremities and the lips while the involved body part is at rest. "Pill-rolling" tremor of the hands is the most typical. The tremor ceases upon active movement of the limb. Resting tremor must be differentiated from postural and kinetic tremors, in which tremor appears only when the arm is being used. These tremors are typically caused by other disorders, namely essential tremor and cerebellar disorders. However, after maintaining outstretched hands for a few seconds, some patients have a reemergence of the rest tremor with the classical approximately 3-Hz frequency.

Bradykinesia is manifested by masked facies; decreased blinking; drooling of saliva due to decreased spontaneous swallowing; loss of spontaneous movement such as gesturing; smallness and slowness of handwriting (micrographia); difficulty with hand dexterity for shaving, brushing teeth, and putting on makeup; short-stepped, shuffling gait with decreased arm swing; and difficulty arising from a chair, getting out of automobiles, and turning in bed. Bradykinesia thus encompasses a loss of automatic movements as well as slowness in initiating movement on command and reduction in amplitude of the voluntary movement. The latter can be observed as decrementing amplitude with repetitive finger tapping or foot tapping.

Rigidity is an increased resistance to passive movement, is equal in all directions, and usually is manifested by a ratchety "give" in the range of motion, so-called cogwheel rigidity. Eventually the patient assumes a stooped posture and begins to lose balance, with a tendency to fall due to loss of postural reflexes. Loss of postural reflexes with stooped posture leads to festination, whereby the patient walks faster and faster.

In addition to these motor signs, most patients with PD have behavioral signs as well. The patient slowly becomes more dependent, fearful, indecisive, and passive. The spouse gradually makes more of the decisions and becomes the dominant decision-maker. Eventually, the patient sits much of the day unless encouraged to exercise. Passivity also expresses itself by the patient not desiring to attend social events. Depression is a frequent feature in patients with PD. Dementia occurs in approximately 30% of patients with PD and is nearly universal in the bed-bound patient. More common is bradyphrenia, in which the patient is slow in responding to questions, but cognitive function appears to be intact.

Onset is usually above the age of 50, but younger patients can be affected, particularly in genetic cases. Onset before age 30 does not preclude a diagnosis of PD, but juvenile parkinsonism raises questions of other etiologies, such as Wilson disease and the Westphal variant of Huntington disease. The disease is more common in men, with a male/female ratio of 3:2. The incidence in the United States is 20 new cases per 100,000 population per year, with a prevalence of 187 cases per 100,000 population.[6] With modern medications the mortality rate is close to normal for age.

Pathology and Biochemistry

The pigmented nuclei of the brainstem, namely the pars compacta of the substantia nigra, the locus coeruleus, and the dorsal motor nucleus of the vagus, are affected in PD. There is loss of nerve cells and increased gliosis in these nuclei. The cytoplasm of intact neurons often shows eosinophilic inclusions called Lewy bodies.[7]

The substantia nigra neurons contain dopamine; the locus coeruleus, norepinephrine; and other pigmented neurons, serotonin. Thus the loss of these neurons results in a loss of these monoamine neurotransmitters in their nerve terminals. The most consistent biochemical alteration in PD is a marked depletion of dopamine in the neostriatum. Most of the symptoms of PD can be directly related to the loss of striatal dopamine. However, some of the motor (e.g., postural instability) and nonmotor (e.g., dementia, depression) features are either incompletely responsive or unresponsive to dopamine replacement therapy, nor is there a halt in the progression of the disease, suggesting that other neurotransmitter systems are involved.[8]

Historically, environmental factors were deemed to be the primary cause of the condition. Twenty years ago, there was a sparse literature suggesting that PD could have genetic underpinnings,[9] and the role of genetics in this condition was hotly debated with the primary example in twin studies. Subsequently, with advances in molecular biology and genetic enabling technologies, including population epidemiology and genetics techniques, nearly a dozen loci have been identified that segregate with the phenotype of idiopathic PD, with additional loci associated with other forms of parkinsonism.[10] The current thinking is similar to that recognized by Barbeau[11] for which environmental and other factors play upon the neurobiology of appropriately genetically primed individuals and the symptoms of PD emerge. In individual cases, it may be difficult to tease out the relative contributions of nature and nurture. However, the current hypothesis is that the condition is a complex multifactorial neurodegenerative disease whereby the cellular molecular machinery becomes clogged, associated with protein misfolding and subsequent protein aggregation.[12] These insights have led to new strategies for both symptom relief and neuroprotection with the hope for more effective therapies in the future.

Speech

In PD, speech production is compromised due to hypokinetic dysarthria with lack of vocal fold closure[13] and possibly poor presentation of air to the vocal apparatus (sound generator) due to decreased flow associated with a bradykinetic bellows mechanism. Family members may be first to recognize a change, with patients being unaware. Ultimately, patients complain of hypophonia with a high self-reported voice handicap on formal rating scales such as the Voice Handicap Index.[14] The dysphonia, which is often the first speech symptom, is characterized by a decreased loudness with monopitch, monoloudness, and prosodic insufficiency. Voice is decreased in loudness and tends to fade out at the end of breath groups, often with a harsh breathy voice quality. Breath groups are shortened and pauses for breaths may occur at inappropriate times. Speech may be produced in short rushes with inappropriate silences between words and syllables. Tremor may be present (discussed later in the chapter). Articulation is produced with reduced range of articulation for both lingual and labial sounds.[15,16] Laryngoscopy often reveals bowing of the vocal cords, present to some degree in 87% of patients in one study[14] with a midcord opening of the glottis on phonation. The vocal cord motion is often slowed or associated with tremulous movements[17] in 53% in one study.[14] There may be pooling of secretions in the hypopharynx and difficulties in swallowing. The abnormal movements can be complicated by dyskinesias associated with symptomatic therapy.

Speech is almost invariably affected in multiple system atrophy (MSA), one of the parkinsonism-plus syndromes.[18] Autonomic dysfunction is the hallmark of the disease. In parkinsonian type of MSA (MSA-p), formerly known as striatonigral degeneration, the vocal cords may be paralyzed. Ataxic dysarthria is present in cerebellar type of MSA (MSA-c), formerly known as olivopontocerebellar atrophy. There may also be a sensory aberration causing a diminished or absent cough reflex and intermittent aspiration. The respiratory laryngeal function may deteriorate during sleep with stridor and obstructive events, at times life-threatening and result in unanticipated death.[19,20] Consequently, a sleep study and appropriate consultations are recommended for all patients who have signs or symptoms of stridor, sleep disturbance, or pulmonary dysfunction. When appropriate, tracheostomy may be required. Surgery may be hazardous and requires close monitoring because of the potential for severe blood pressure fluctuations in MSA patients.

Treatment

A multidimensional approach to treating PD is generally recommended.[21] During the past decade, there have been significant advances in the management of PD, including new options for pharmacotherapy, surgical intervention, and speech therapy.

Speech therapy is a primary therapy for PD patients with vocal dysfunction.[22] The primary goal is to increase loudness, typically accompanied by increasing the subglottal air pressure, which results in improved vocal fold vibration.[23,24] Clinical efficacy has been demonstrated using the Lee Silverman Voice Treatment (LSVT), which has been shown to improve speech and voice measures and vocal fold closure facial expression,[25] and lead to changes in neural correlates as seen on neuroimaging.[26] However, other treatments are under investigation.[27] Speech therapy for PD is discussed in more detail in Chapter 12.

Pharmacotherapy

Patients with idiopathic PD (IPD) typically experience amelioration of symptoms with dopamine precursors (levodopa with carbidopa) either alone or in combination with a catechol-o-methyltransferase inhibitor (entacapone, tolcapone) or dopamine agonists (bromocriptine, pergolide mesylate, ropinirol, pramipexole); however, cases of secondary parkinsonism are typically resistant to medication. Propargylamines[28] including selegiline[29] and rasagiline,[30] have been reported, although not confirmed, to slow progression of IPD if added early in the course of the disease. Their symptomatic effect is mediated through inhibition of monoamine oxidase type B enzyme. Select dopamine agonists have been suggested to slow progression of IPD. However, because of the methodologic challenges in distinguishing symptomatic benefit from delayed neurodegeneration, conclusive data are not yet available.[31,32]

Long-term levodopa therapy often leads to late complications, including response oscillations, dyskinesias, and drug-induced psychiatric effects. Early in therapy, most patients have continuous benefit from three or four doses per day; subsequent response oscillations typically develop within 5 years of treatment. Even more troubling, some patients develop unpredictable oscillations with no apparent relation to their dosing regimen. Response oscillations may be accompanied by dyskinesias; chorea, with or without dystonia, is common, especially at the time of peak levels. Although dose reduction may be effective for peak-dose dyskinesias, many patients have a very narrow therapeutic window, and titrating an effective dose versus reduction of the dyskinesia may be difficult. Strategies include sustained-release preparations, coadministration of dopamine agonists, liquid preparations, metabolic inhibitors such as catechol-o-methyltransferase inhibitors, or subcutaneous apomorphine. Delayed gastric emptying may be responsible in some cases. Cisapride[33] had been used in select patients in the past to improve gastric motility but was withdrawn from the U.S. market due to its cardiac side effects. Psychiatric effects of chronic levodopa therapy include vivid dreams and hallucinations, and an exacerbation of memory loss, confusion, and anxiety. Although some of these effects may be treated symptomatically[8] with other medications, a reduction in levodopa may be necessary.

Oral therapies that result in enhanced stimulation of dopamine receptors (e.g., levodopa, dopamine agonists, dopamine releasers) and an overall improvement in motor function have been clearly demonstrated to improve speech production in general.[34] Although paradoxical, many of the characteristics of speech, including respiration, phonation, and articulation may be perturbed by levodopa-related fluctuations. In addition, pharmacologic treatment can sometimes worsen speech by making it more rapid, less distinct, with some "freezing of speech," that is, repetition of a syllable or phrases. Vocal cord augmentation[35] has been used to correct the open glottis on phonation, but the results may be poor if there is a significant reduction in air presented to the larynx. Therefore, pulmonary function studies are important before augmentation.

Neurosurgery

In the early 20th century, lesions of the motor cortex were performed in an effort to ameliorate hyperkinetic movements, including tremor associated with PD.[36] However, these excisional procedures in addition to incising the pyramidal tracts in the upper cervical cord often resulted in a spastic hemiparesis as a substitute for the dyskinesia. In 1940, Meyers[37] described pallidotomy for PD, later demonstrating that dyskinesias can be improved with his procedure without pyramidal tract damage.[38] During a surgical procedure in a postencephalitic PD patient, Cooper[39] accidentally severed the anterior choroidal artery, which feeds the medial globus pallidus and lateral ventral thalamus, and discovered marked improvement in tremor and rigidity. Cooper[40] later reported that dystonic posturing in parkinsonian patients improved with anterior choroidal artery ligation, and he began to operate on primary dystonia patients. Cooper performed lesions in the pallidum and thalamus with improved tremor control.[41] With bilateral procedures, there was a significant morbidity due to dysarthria and dysphagia. Once levodopa became available in the late 1960s, surgical interventions were rarely performed until recent decades.

During the past two decades, there has been a resurgence of interest in surgical interventions for PD prompted by several factors. Chronic levodopa therapy typically results in motor fluctuations, which emerge within the first 3 to 5 years of therapy. Strategies have been developed to attempt to delay the onset of motor fluctuations, but for most patients these complications ultimately emerge. Technical advancements in neuroimaging, stereotactic neurosurgery, and microelectrode intraoperative recording have permitted improved localization of surgical targets and placement of either lesions or implants. Finally, our understanding of the organization of the basal ganglia and those pathways important to the pathophysiology of PD has led to a more rational approach to target selection.[42]

Neurosurgical procedures for PD can be broadly classified into (1) ablative procedures, (2) stimulation procedures, and (3) potentially restorative procedures. Detailed reviews are available.[43]

Ablative procedures have been performed in the thalamus and internal segment of the pallidum. Thalamotomy can be performed with modest morbidity, and has demonstrated improvement in contralateral tremor and, to a lesser extent, in rigidity, in up to 90% of patients.[44] In most cases, thalamotomy does not result in improvement for bradykinesia, postural instability, or ipsilateral tremor. Currently, mortality is less than 1%[44]; complications include contralateral hemiparesis, seizures, paresthesias, ataxia, apraxia, hypotonia, abulia, and gait disturbances. Pallidotomy gained attention[45] because when the lesion is placed in the posteroventral portion of the internal segment of the globus pallidus (GPi), there can be long-lasting improvement in tremor, rigidity, hypokinesia, speech, gait, dystonia, and, importantly, levodopa-induced dyskinesias. Utilizing microelectrode recordings for target localization, many groups have reported impressive and dramatic improvements in dyskinesias with more modest improvements in the cardinal signs of PD.[46]

Deep brain stimulation (DBS) for the management of PD was introduced by Benabid and colleagues.[47] They showed that high-frequency (>100 Hz), low-voltage (<5 V) electrical stimulation of the ventro-intermediate (V_{im}) nucleus of the thalamus improved tremor in PD and essential tremor. Based on a growing understanding of the neural networks controlling basal ganglia function in PD and other disorders, attention shifted to stimulating the GPi, and subthalamic nucleus (STN) in patients with intractable PD. Early trials[48] demonstrated that in addition to improvement in tremor, the other cardinal features of PD, namely bradykinesia, gait disturbance, rigidity, and balance, may be improved by DBS of the GPi or STN. This has translated into an improvement in activities of daily living (ADL) scores and motor function.[49,50]

Transplantation is an experimental procedure whereby dopamine-containing cells are transplanted into the nigral targets of patients with intractable PD. The foundation for this therapy is based on our understanding that PD is associated with specific degeneration of the dopaminergic nigrostriatal neurons, and dopaminergic replacement strategies result in improvement of the motor signs and symptoms of PD. There are numerous factors to consider when considering transplantation therapy, including choice of tissue to be transplanted (adrenal, fetal nigral, retinal pigment epithelial, stem cells, etc.), density and quantity of tissue to be transplanted, location of transplant, and the role of immunosuppressive therapy. Transplantation of adrenal medullary cells into the caudate nucleus was initially reported by Madrazo et al[51] to have dramatic results, but the results were not reproduced by other investigators[52,53]; the procedure has been abandoned. Early open-label studies of fetal nigral cell transplantation into the posterior putamen demonstrated feasibility, improvement in symptoms, and improved striatal uptake in levodopa.[54,55] Postmortem studies demonstrate that with at least some transplant protocols, implanted cells can survive in large numbers and reinnervate the striatum in an organotypic fashion.[56] In grafted regions, there is normal-appearing staining for dopamine transporter and cytochrome oxidase, normal tyrosine hydroxylase (TH) messenger RNA (mRNA) expression, and normal-appearing synaptic connections between grafted and host neurons without evidence of host-derived sprouting.[57] Two double-blind studies of fetal nigral transplantation, supported by the National Institutes of Health, have been reported. The first study, reported by Freed et al[58] in 2001 demonstrated modest benefit in the younger patients (under age 60). No improvement was derived from the implant despite neuron-imaging evidence that the graft survived and produced dopamine. However, there was a marked placebo effect and some patients developed unanticipated severe dyskinesias when not on medication that could not be ameliorated by decreasing dopamine therapy.[59] The second study performed under a different transplantation protocol showed no overall treatment effect, but milder patients did show significant improvement.[60] Neuroimaging demonstrated transplant survival, and postmortem examination showed robust survival of dopamine neurons. Although neuroimaging and immunohistochemistry supports the potential role of neurotransplantation, the technology is not considered accepted at this time.

Recently, investigators have reported speech and intelligibility benefits of DBS of the subthalamic nucleus when used to treat PD. One study reported mild improvement, particularly for modulation in loudness and pitch, at the expense of intelligibility.[61] Others have reported improvement in perceptual speech as documented on global PD rating scales and quantitative acoustic and force analyses.[62] However, not all authors have reported benefits from DBS at this site.[63–67] The benefits from DBS are dependent on an anatomic substrate of speech dysfunction in PD, the pharmacologic status of the patient, and stimulation location and parameters. Pinto et al[68] examined four patients under a variety of conditions and concluded that motor speech subcomponents can be improved similar to limb motor function, but that the complex coordination of all speech anatomic substrates are not uniformly responsive to subthalamic nucleus stimulation. It should also be noted that brain surgery can contribute to speech disorders by impacting the motor and language circuits, and this must be taken into consideration when evaluating a patient who has had central nervous system (CNS) surgery.[69]

♦ Dystonia

Dystonia is a syndrome dominated by sustained muscle contractions frequently causing twisting and repetitive movements or abnormal postures that may be sustained or intermittent. Dystonia can involve any voluntary muscle. Because the movements and resulting postures are often unusual and the condition is rare, it is one of the most frequently misdiagnosed neurologic conditions.[70] The prevalence estimates of dystonia suggest approximately 50,000 to 200,000 cases of idiopathic dystonia in the United States.[71] Additional epidemiologic studies have shown the following: a service-based prevalence of primary focal dystonia of 13.7/100,000 in the Tottori Prefecture of Japan[72] and a crude prevalence for all types of primary dystonia of 37.1/100,000 and laryngeal dystonia of 5.9/100,000 in Iceland.[73] During the past decade, major advances have occurred in the understanding of the genetics and biology of the condition, in addition to providing further support for therapeutic management with botulinum toxin and DBS.

As a clinical syndrome, patients can be classified according to clinical symptomatology, age at onset, and etiology. Classification may be important as it can give us clues about prognosis and also an approach to management. The classification scheme is outlined in **Table 17.4**.

Dystonia may begin at any age. We have seen presenting signs as early as 9 months and as late as 85 years. In general, there is a bimodal age-at-onset distribution with peaks

Table 17.4 Classification of Dystonia

I. Age at onset
   A. Infantile (<2 year)
   B. Childhood (2–26 year)
   C. Adult (>26 year)

II. Etiology
   A. Primary
      1. With hereditary pattern
         a. Autosomal dominant
            i. Classical types
- Childhood-onset dystonia
- Focal dystonia

            ii. Variant types
- Dopa-responsive dystonia
- Myoclonic dystonia

         b. X-linked recessive
      2. Sporadic (without a documented hereditary pattern)
         a. Classical types
         b. Variant types

   B. Symptomatic
      1. Associated with hereditary neurologic syndromes and with known enzyme defect (Wilson disease, GM1 gangliosidosis, GM2 gangliosidosis, hexosaminidase A and B deficiency, metachromatic leukodystrophy, Lesch-Nyhan syndrome, homocystinuria, glutaric acidemia, triosephosphate isomerase deficiency, methylmalonic aciduria)
      2. Associated with probable hereditary neurologic syndromes, without known enzyme defect, but with a chemical marker (Leigh disease, familial basal ganglia calcifications, Hallervorden-Spatz disease, dystonic lipidosis (sea-blue histiocytosis), juvenile neuronal ceroid-lipofuscinosis, ataxia-telangiectasia, chorea-acanthocytosis, Hartnup disease, intraneuronal inclusion disease, hereditary bilateral optic atrophy with dystonia [mitochondrial])
      3. Associated with hereditary neurologic syndromes, without known enzyme defect or chemical marker (Huntington disease, hereditary juvenile dystonia-parkinsonism, Pelizaeus-Merzbacher disease, progressive pallidal degeneration, Joseph disease, Rett syndrome, spinocerebellar degenerations, olivopontocerebellar atrophies, hereditary spastic paraplegia with dystonia)
      4. Due to known environmental cause (perinatal cerebral injury, athetoid cerebral palsy, delayed onset dystonia, encephalitis and postinfectious [a. Reye syndrome, subacute sclerosing leukoencephalopathy, wasp sting Creutzfeldt-Jakob disease], head trauma, thalamotomy, brainstem lesion (including pontine myelinolysis), focal cerebral vascular injury, arteriovenous malformation, brain tumor, multiple sclerosis, cervical cord injury, peripheral injury, drugs [D2 receptor antagonists, levodopa, ergotism, anticonvulsants], toxins: Mn, CO, carbon disulfide, cyanide, methanol, disulfiram, metabolic [hypoparathyroidism])
      5. Dystonia associated with presumed sporadic disorder, of unknown etiology (parkinsonism)
      6. Psychogenic dystonia
      7. Pseudodystonia (Sandifer syndrome, stiff-person syndrome, rotational atlantoaxial subluxation, soft tissue nuchal mass, bone disease, ligamentous absence, laxity or damage, congenital muscular torticollis, congenital postural torticollis, congenital Klippel-Feil syndrome, posterior fossa tumor, syringomyelia, Arnold-Chiari malformation, trochlear nerve palsy, vestibular torticollis)

III. Distribution
   A. Focal
      1. Blepharospasm (forced, involuntary eye-closure)
      2. Oromandibular dystonia (face, jaw, or tongue)
      3. Torticollis (neck)
      4. Writer's cramp (action-induced dystonic contraction of hand muscles)
      5. Spasmodic dysphonia (vocal cords)
   B. Segmental (cranial/axial/crural)
   C. Multisegmental
   D. Generalized (ambulatory, non-ambulatory)

Source: Data from Fahn,[501] Calne,[502] and Bressman.[503] Those reviews should be consulted for references regarding the literature citations for these etiologies.

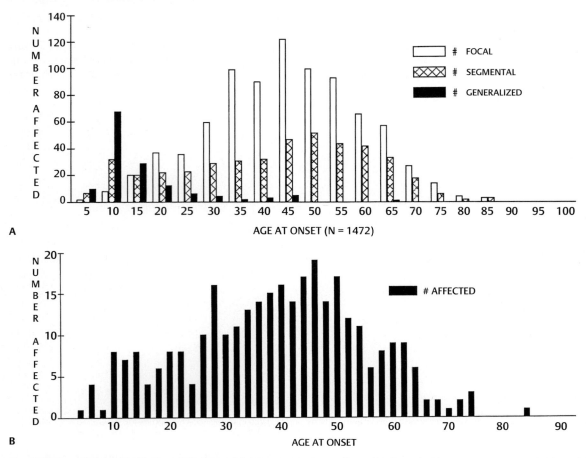

Fig. 17.1 Age at onset distribution of patients with primary dystonia evaluated at the Columbia University Dystonia Clinical Research Center as of 1990. **(A)** All patients with primary dystonia. **(B)** All patients with primary laryngeal dystonia.

at ages 8 and 42 **(Fig. 17.1)**. Therefore, we classify patients as early onset when the presenting signs are before age 26, and as late onset at older ages. Alternatively, we can classify patients as infantile onset when the presenting signs are before age 2, childhood onset between ages 2 and 12, adolescent onset between ages 13 and 20, and adult onset at older ages. The significance of this distinction is discussed below.

According to the etiologic classification, patients with idiopathic disease have no evidence by history, examination, or laboratory studies of any identifiable cause for the dystonic symptoms. Therefore, there must be a normal perinatal and early developmental history; no prior history of neurologic illness or exposure to drugs known to cause acquired dystonia (e.g., phenothiazines); normal intellectual, pyramidal, cerebellar, and sensory examinations; and normal diagnostic studies. Patients who have abnormalities noted above are classified as having secondary dystonia. The clinical phenomenology will often be a clue as to etiology. Primary dystonia is typically action-induced; symptoms are enhanced with use of the affected body part, and the region may appear normal at rest. Secondary dystonia frequently results in fixed dystonic postures. The presence of extensive dystonia limited to one side of the body (hemidystonia) suggests a secondary etiology.

When classified by the distribution, patients are categorized as having focal, segmental, or generalized symptoms. Focal dystonia symptoms involve one small group of muscles in one body part, segmental disease involves a contiguous group of muscles, and generalized dystonia is widespread. Dystonia may involve muscles of the oral cavity, larynx, pharynx, tongue, and jaw. Common examples of focal dystonia **(Table 17.4)** include blepharospasm (forced, involuntary eye closure), oromandibular dystonia (face, jaw, or tongue), torticollis (neck), writer's cramp (action-induced dystonic contraction of hand muscles), and spasmodic dysphonia (vocal cords).

Idiopathic and hereditary generalized dystonia almost always begins as a focal dystonia before spreading to involve other parts of the body. Spread may not take place or may be limited and then plateau as a focal or segmental dystonia. Age at onset, genetic predisposition, or other factors likely contribute to the phenotypic expression in any particular individual. The coexistence of dystonic symptoms affecting the vocal cords and other body parts further supports the notion that the laryngeal symptoms are dystonic, as discussed below **(Table 17.5)**.

Table 17.5 Dystonia at the Columbia University Neurological Institute

	All Dystonia N = 2556		Laryngeal Dystonia N = 562	
	Primary Dystonia	Secondary Dystonia	Primary Dystonia	Secondary Dystonia
N	1828 (72%)	728 (28%)	464 (83%)	98 (17%)
F	1097 (60%)	416 (57%)	273 (59%)	58 (59%)
M	730 (40%)	306 (43%)	191 (41%)	40 (41%)
F:M	1.5	1.4	1.4	1.4
Jewish	407 (22%)	141 (19%)	92 (20%)	18 (18%)
Non-Jewish	1421 (78%)	587 (81%)	372 (80%)	80 (82%)
Positive family history	366 (20%)	63 (9%)	95 (20%)	10 (10%)
Focal	1053 (58%)	235 (32%)	296 (64%)	37 (38%)
Seg cran	271 (15%)	80 (11%)	81 (17%)	18 (18%)
All seg	596 (33%)	264 (36%)	141 (29%)	35 (36%)
Gnlized	162 (9%)	161 (22%)	26 (6%)	26 (27%)

Abbreviations: N, number of patients; M, male; F, female; F:M, female to male ratio; Seg cran, segmental cranial; All seg, all segmentals and hemidystonia; Gnlized, generalized.
Data as of July 1991.

Spasmodic Dysphonia (Laryngeal Dystonia)

Idiopathic spasmodic dysphonia (SD) and laryngeal dystonia (LD) are clinical terms used to describe an action-induced, laryngeal motion disorder. Most cases represent manifestations of primary dystonia, but many are secondary to other neurologic entities (**Table 17.4**).

In 1871, Traube[74] coined the term *spastic dysphonia* when describing a patient with nervous hoarseness. Schnitzler et al[75] used the terms *spastic aphonia* and *phonic laryngeal spasm* to describe such patients. Gerhardt[76] called the condition "coordinated laryngeal spasm." Fraenkel[77,78] uses the word *mogiphonia* for a slowly developing disorder of the voice characterized by increasing vocal fatigue, spasmodic constriction of throat muscles, and pain around the larynx. Of note, he compared the laryngeal disorder to "mogigraphia" or occupational writer's cramp, or dystonic cramping of the arm when writing. In 1899, Gowers[79] described functional laryngeal spasm whereby the cords were brought together too forcibly while speaking (currently classified as adductor type). He contrasted this to phonic paralysis, whereby the vocal cords could not be brought together while speaking (currently classified as abductor type). Gowers wrote, "The affection has been compared to writer's cramp... a case reported by Gerhardt, in which the patient had actually suffered from writers' cramp, and, at the age of 50, learned to play the flute. The act of blowing the flute brought on laryngeal spasm and an unintended voice sound, accompanied by muscular contractions in the arm and angle of the mouth." Here again, the focal dystonia of LD is being compared with dystonia involving other segments of the body (mouth, arm). Critchley[80] described the voice pattern as a condition in which the patient sounds as though he were "trying to talk whilst being choked." Bellussi[81] described the condition as "stuttering with the vocal cords."

Aronson drew specific attention to this disorder in the laryngeal literature. At the time of his 1968 review,[82] there were approximately 122 cases in the literature, including 34 of his own cases. Minnesota Multiphasic Personality Inventory (MMPI) testing and psychiatric interviews did not discriminate between patients with LD and those in the normal population, distinguishing those affected with LD from patients with psychogenic dysphonias, thus helping to establish SD as an organic, or nonpsychiatric, condition. Nevertheless, many patients are referred to psychiatrists for treatment because the correct diagnosis is not made when the patient initially presents for treatment.

Aronson[83] later formally distinguished and reviewed two types of spasmodic dysphonia: adductor, due to irregular hyperadduction of the vocal folds; and abductor, due to intermittent abduction of the vocal folds. Patients with adductor LD exhibit a choked, strained-strangled voice quality with abrupt initiation and termination of voicing, resulting in short breaks in phonation. The voice is generally reduced in loudness and monotonal. Vocal tremor is frequently observed along with a slow speech rate and decreased smoothness of speech. Speech intelligibility is generally decreased. Occasionally patients with adductor LD exhibit compensatory pseudo-abductor spasmodic dysphonia, compensating for severe adductor laryngeal spasms by abducting their vocal cords and whispering. Patients with abductor LD exhibit a breathy, effortful, voice quality with abrupt termination of voicing, resulting in aphonic whispered segments of speech. The voice is reduced in loudness and vocal tremor is frequently observed. Speech intelligibility is generally reduced. Some patients display a combination of adductor and abductor signs and have been classified as mixed.

Aronson and Hartman[84] later noted that LD has tremor characteristics similar to those found in essential tremor (ET). The differential diagnosis between LD due to ET and that due to a dystonic tremor can be difficult. We noted that spasmodic dysphonia is not a spastic disorder[85]; electromyographic characteristics were inconsistent with those seen in pyramidal disorders. We found an irregular tremor in 25% of patients as opposed to the regular tremor of essential tremor (discussed below). The findings were comparable to those of patients who had generalized dystonia with laryngeal involvement. Schaefer et al[86] used electromyography to establish further that LD is a disorder of vocal motor control. Because the condition is not a spastic disorder, we had favored the term *spasmodic dysphonia* rather than *spastic dysphonia*.

Several lines of evidence further supported the notion that spasmodic dysphonia is a form of dystonia. Fraenkel[77,78] and Gowers[79] compared the involuntary movements in spasmodic dysphonia to those of other dystonias. However, in the earlier works, a psychogenic etiology was proposed.[87] Jacome and Yanez[88] associated spasmodic dysphonia with Meige disease, or segmental-cranial dystonia (**Table 17.4**); other authors subsequently have concurred.[89–92] Many of the clinical and electrophysiologic phenomenologic and genetic features of patients with focal spasmodic dysphonia are similar to those with more generalized disease (see below), and we have recommended that the condition be properly called "laryngeal dystonia."

Furthermore, dystonia is characterized by abnormal involuntary movements that are typically action induced. In LD, the *action* is that of speaking. The vocal apparatus is usually normal at rest, but functions abnormally with speaking. Adductor LD is characterized by abnormal involuntary cocontraction of the vocalis muscle complex muscles resulting in inappropriate adduction of the vocal folds. As an action-induced, task-specific, or functional movement disorder, the muscles and anatomic structures are typically normal at rest but move inappropriately with action. Conversely, abductor LD is characterized by action-induced inappropriate cocontraction of the posterior cricoarytenoid muscles during the action of speaking, resulting in inappropriate abduction of the vocal cords. Patients with mixed adductor and abductor dysphonia have both prominent adductor and abductor spasms.[93]

We have reported patients with respiratory adductor laryngeal dystonia.[94-97] These patients have abnormal involuntary adduction of the vocal cords on respiration, but may have grossly normal function with speech. In this case, the specific action is the movements of the vocal cords during respiration. Patients may be idiopathic or have a tardive etiology. Symptoms may be laryngeal at onset or begin in other cranial regions (upper face as blepharospasm) and progress to involve the larynx and other cranially innervated structures (e.g., jaw, diaphragm). Laryngeal stridor was relieved with local injections of botulinum toxin in some of our cases whereby the respiratory dysrhythmia persisted. Furthermore, we have also reported cases whereby the laryngeal hyperkinesias were induced by the action of singing,[98] with normal vocal cord function and connected speech at initial presentation. It is notable that whereas singing provoked dystonic symptoms in these patients, we have also treated cases of cervical dystonia (CD) and blepharospasm whereby singing was a trick used to temporarily improve dystonic symptoms.

Dystonic movements can be rapid and repetitive and tremor may be seen in dystonia affecting any segment of the body. Dystonic tremors are typically irregular and have a directional preponderance; symptoms are increased when the patient's posture places the affected body part in a position opposed to the primary dystonic contractions. For instance, patients with torticollis often have a head tremor that can be damped by placing the head into the preferred posture. Many patients with SD have an irregular vocal tremor that is both audible and can be recorded electromyographically.[86] Similar to the dystonic tremor seen in individuals with arm or neck dystonia, the irregular dystonic tremor of SD may be due to posturing of dystonic muscles in a position where the agonist contractions do not fully neutralize those of the antagonists. This tremor may be differentiated from the regular tremor seen in benign essential voice tremor (see Tremor, later in this chapter). The clinical distinction may be difficult in many cases, particularly when a patient presents with symptoms of essential tremor in other body parts. In many cases, the clinical distinction cannot be made.

Sensory System and Dystonia

Sensory tricks often ameliorate dystonic movements and postures, and this maneuver can be effective in different parts of the body. These sensory tricks are also known as a *geste antagonistique* or *gegendruckphanomen*. The patients with CD often find that gently touching the chin, back of head, or top of head relieves the symptoms; blepharospasm patients may relieve symptoms by gently touching the lateral canthus. The use of the sensory tricks to keep the head in the body midline position was reported by 88.9% of patients in one series.[99] The physiology of sensory tricks remains unknown. In a recent study, 13 of 25 patients with idiopathic CD had markedly reduced electromyography (EMG) activity (50% or more) even during arm movement, but before the arm touched the skin, while performing a sensory trick.[100] Some patients have been reported to have reduced dystonia while thinking about a sensory trick.[101] Patients with SD have reported that symptoms momentarily improve by pinching the nares, pressing the hand against the back of the head,[102] pressing the hand into the abdomen, pulling on an ear, or touching the clavicular notch (personal experience). Many patients observe that they speak better after a yawn or sneeze, or when they sing or yell; these are common experiences in patients with other craniocervical dystonias and were reported in early descriptions of dystonia.[103,104]

Botulinum toxin type A (BONTA) may also modify the sensory feedback loop to the CNS, and this mechanism may be partially responsible for its beneficial effect in treating dystonia. Ludlow et al[105] and Zwirner et al[106] proposed that reduced muscle activity and therefore feedback to laryngeal motoneuron pools may be a primary mechanism of action of BONTA. We offered the possibility that toxin might have a direct effect on sensory afferents by blocking intrafusal fibers, resulting in decreased activation of muscle spindles.[107] This would effectively change the sensory afferent system by reducing the Ia traffic. Filippi et al[108] supported this hypothesis by establishing that local injections of BONTA directly reduce afferent Ia fiber traffic, and therefore exert a modulatory effect on sensory feedback. This may also account for the clinical observation that injections of BONTA have an effect on regional noninjected muscles, which is most striking in spastic limbs.[109]

Support for this mechanism derives from the cumulative work of Ryuji Kaji and colleagues,[110-115] who showed that the increase in severity of dystonic writer's cramp associated with enhancing Ia muscle spindle activity with the tonic vibration maneuver can be decreased by intramuscular injections of dilute lidocaine, which preferentially affects the afferent innervation of the muscle spindle. Both ethanol and lidocaine block sodium channels; however, the former blocks the channels for a longer duration than the anesthetic. Kaji et al called the treatment of lidocaine plus ethanol the "muscle afferent block" (MAB), and it has shown an effect in neck, jaw,[114] and limb dystonia[110,111] and spasticity.[113,115] The benefit for each treatment lasts only a few weeks, and therefore is of limited use in most dystonic and spastic situations. However, this model of blocking Ia afferents supports the proposed mechanism of action with BONTA on conditions associated with excessive muscle contraction. These studies support the importance of the afferents system in the clinical manifestations of dystonia.[116]

Also notable is the growing appreciation of the importance of the integrative sensory function of the basal ganglia as reviewed by Kaji's group[117,118] and recently DeLong and Wichmann.[42] In addition to the observations described above in patients with dystonia who can respond to a sensory or tactile stimulus, PD patients have demonstrated a remarkable ability to have enhanced motor function as a consequence of specific sensory cues, the phenomenon of *kinesie paradoxale*[119] (as discussed by Riess and Weghorst[120]). For instance, PD patients in the "off" state may be able to run out of a room in response to an emergency, such as someone yelling "fire," or walk more effectively on a sandy beach rather than on a floor. Sensory cues, such as stepping over lines on a floor, have been used to facilitate gait in PD patients. These observations, coupled with the remarkable understanding of the basal ganglia stimulated by advances in cellular recording during DBS surgery, have supported the notion that the basal ganglia are an important relay for the gating of both sensory and motor circuits whereby sensory inputs have the ability to control motor output.

In patients with cranial dystonia, involuntary hissing or humming may be present. It is difficult to know if it is primarily associated with the disorder or is a secondary trick to relieve the patient of symptoms.[121] We have observed numerous patients with laryngeal dystonia who hum before speaking, as if to initiate vibration of the vocal cords to prepare them for vocalization.

Trauma has become generally accepted as a factor that may trigger dystonic symptoms,[122-124] although this matter is debated by some.[125] Head/neck trauma has been reported in 5 to 21% of cervical dystonia cases.[126-129] Patients with spasmodic dysphonia may report the onset of symptoms immediately after a laryngeal/pharyngeal trauma, most often following a viral infection[130,131]; this observation has been borne out in our series of patients. Whereas up to approximately 30% of our patients with dystonia have a clear family history of dystonia, and therefore a genetic predisposition to the development of symptoms, some of the sporadic cases may be genetically susceptible or "primed," and after exposure to the appropriate environmental factors ("trigger factors") such as exposure to infections or trauma, symptoms manifest. Limb dystonia[132,133] and jaw dystonia[134] may occur after peripheral traumas. Similar models have been proposed for other movement disorders.[11] There is a growing body of experimental evidence that the appropriately predisposed may develop dystonia,[135,136] including with overuse/overactivity.[137] In our practice, we accepted trauma as a trigger for dystonia when the onset of the dystonia is within 6 to 12 months of the identified trauma. In many cases, the peripheral injury that preceded the dystonia was acute, brief, and well defined. In some of our patients, the injury was relatively mild or chronic or repetitive, as had been noted by Schott.[138] The dystonia typically occurs in the traumatized body part or region, and in many cases is associated with pain. Sometimes the dystonic posture evolves as the pain improves.

Psychogenic Dystonia

We consider psychogenic dystonia to be a form of secondary dystonia because the phenomenology is dystonic and the etiology is psychiatric. Suspicious findings on neurologic examination suggestive of a psychiatric etiology include false weakness, false sensory complaints, multiple somatizations, obvious psychiatric disturbances such as self-inflicted injuries, incongruous and inconsistent movements and postures, and distractability. Some patients have improvement with suggestion, or unusual and nonphysiologic intervention. Psychogenic dystonia can be severe enough to lead to fixed contractures. Fahn and Williams[139] proposed a classification scheme, stating that the clinical diagnosis is made with certainty only after symptoms improve without pharmacotherapy in the setting of a history and examination that are inconsistent or incongruous with an organic movement disorder.[140-142] Improvement with a *gestes antagoniste* is uncommon but has been reported.[143,144]

However, many patients with unusual movement disorders are misdiagnosed as psychogenic because of the unusual nature of their symptoms and signs. Stanley Fahn and the late David Marsden stated, "Just because it is unusual does not mean it is psychogenic" (personal communication; also see Shale et al[145]), emphasizing that the diagnosis of a psychogenic movement disorder is complicated because the symptomatology often mimics that of other neurologic disorders.[146] These patients can be extraordinarily difficult to diagnose. For instance, the diagnosis of psychogenic dystonia was made in a patient with the classical DYT1 gene mutation in a family with dystonia.[147,148] Some patients may present with fixed dystonic postures[144,149]; neurophysiologic abnormalities, consistent with organic dystonia, have been observed in psychogenic dystonia.[142,150] However, the consequences of misdiagnosis, whereby psychogenic patients are classified with an organic movement disorder, and vice versa, can be significant. The patient with organic disease can be subjected to years of demoralization and psychotherapy associated with a diagnosis of an unreal disorder, whereas patients with psychogenic disease can undergo unnecessary treatments, including neurosurgical procedures,[142,151] with all good intentions, when they are diagnosed as having an organic etiology for their symptoms. A rating scale has recently been developed for understanding the phenomenology of patients with psychogenic movement disorders.[152] Although many patients remain chronic, a multidisciplinary approach including a focus on psychiatric intervention, can be successful.

In patients with LD, clinical features, such as improvement with alcohol, sedatives, and tranquilizers, and worsening under stress or when talking on the telephone, had been used as evidence that patients presenting with symptoms of LD have a psychogenic basis for their condition. However, these are common clinical features among the dystonias. Similar to torticollis,[153,154] remissions may occur in patients with LD, and some relapse.

We suspect that psychogenic LD is very rare, but the true incidence is not known. Speech language pathologists have described cases to us, and we suspect that we have not seen these patients because they are treated by speech-language pathologists and are not referred for evaluation. One of our patients had a very bizarre speech pattern that was thought to be psychogenic. With speech therapy, the bizarre speech resolved, and she was left with pure abductor LD. In retrospect, the bizarre speech was a manifestation of futile attempts to develop a compensatory strategy.

Laryngeal tension-fatigue syndrome and *muscle tension dysphonia* are terms used to describe secondary muscle tension disorders. The laryngeal, perilaryngeal, suprahyoid, neck, and jaw muscles may be involved.[155,156] Increased muscular tension in the neck and larynx has been found to be associated with palpable increased muscle tension in the suprahyoid and perilaryngeal muscles during phonation, elevation of the larynx with increased pitch, open posterior glottic chink on phonation, and associated vocal fold abnormalities such as nodules or chronic laryngitis.[157-159] Under mild conditions, alterations in pitch and easy fatigue may be present, and chronic intermittent dysphonia may occur. With more significant musculotension dysfunction, the voice may become breathy and harsh to variable degrees.[160] These vocal presentations are sometimes difficult to differentiate from spasmodic dysphonia.[161-163] Such muscular tension-related disorders are often noted in professional speakers. Relaxation techniques, appropriate neck and shoulder positioning, and instruction for efficient voice use is recommended. Nonsteroidal antiinflammatory drugs (NSAIDs), physical therapy, warm compresses, and massage may also help.[164] Forced whispering can result in muscle tension dysphonia (MTD).

Genetics

Idiopathic torsion dystonia (ITD) is thought to be etiologically heterogeneous and clinical and ethnic subtypes of ITD have been identified during the past three decades of focus. When the Dystonia Clinical Research Center in New York was funded in the early 1980s, the primary objective was to identify the causes of dystonia and develop effective therapies. At that time, based on our observations,[165] we thought that the age at onset of dystonia might provide some clues to the underlying pathobiology of the condition. The age-at-onset histogram with its bimodal distribution did indeed provide a window into the genetics, predicting that most patients with childhood-onset dystonia would have a different genetic etiology than those with adult-onset dystonia.[165] We also knew from the analysis of pedigrees that even in families that had a clear autosomal dominant pattern of inheritance, there was reduced penetrance whereby not all gene carriers manifested symptoms. Family studies suggested that different phenotypes likely indicated a different genetic basis for the observed clinical heterogeneity.

The initial focus of our research was to understand the genetics of one of the most severe forms of inherited dystonia, childhood-onset idiopathic dystonia, also known as primary generalized torsion dystonia (PTD), dystonia musculorum deformans, or Oppenheim's dystonia.[166] It is inherited as an autosomal dominant disease with a 30 to 40% penetrance.[166] The symptoms usually start in an arm or leg in childhood, and generalize by adulthood. Occasionally onset is in later life, with the symptoms typically presenting in the cranial structures (e.g., neck, larynx, and upper face), and tending to stay more localized.[167] The cause for this variation in distribution with different age of onset is not known, but likely reflects the underlying neurobiology of the condition[168] caused by the *DYT1* gene deletion mutation, which was identified in 1997. Although the deletion mutation is most prevalent in Ashkenazi Jews due to a founder mutation,[166] it can appear in most ethnic populations, including African-Americans and Asians. In some cases the deletion appears as a spontaneous mutation.[169,170]

Extensive work on *DYT1* dystonia led to the identification of torsinA, the protein product of the *DYT1* gene, and its localization to chromosome 9q34.1.[171-174] In most pedigrees with the clinical syndrome of childhood-onset PTD, there is a single amino acid (glutamic acid) deletion at residue 303.[174] This alteration in the amino acid sequence of the protein is necessary, but not sufficient, for the production of the clinical symptomatology, as not all gene carriers develop symptoms of dystonia. The reason for the lack of complete penetrance remains to be elucidated, but may be attributable to some property of the abnormal torsinA in dystonia, for example, the precipitation of neuronal dysfunction by an environmental factor(s) or by other modifier genes, small interfering RNAs or other transcriptional factors, resulting in alterations of gene-protein interactions.

The role of torsinA in cellular function has not yet been fully elucidated. Based on the amino acid sequence, torsinA has an adenosine triphosphate (ATP) binding domain, and has a sequence that is similar to that of the heat shock proteins (HSPs). HSPs have ATP and adenosine triphosphatase (ATPase) activity, and they have chaperone functions. Mutations in the carboxy region of these proteins can block binding to companion proteins. Therefore, if native torsinA functions in a multimer, then a mutation could result in disassociation, which is characteristic of dominant-negative disorders and manifest as a dominant disorder. Studies have demonstrated that the mutant torsinA that is normally localized in the endoplasmic reticulum relocates to the nuclear envelope, and potentially brings the wild-type torsinA with it, thus disrupting normal cellular function.[175-178]

Although the initial focus had been on *DYT1* dystonia, additional genetic subtypes, distinguished by phenotype, molecular biology, or genotype, have been identified and are summarized elsewhere.[179] Hereditary autosomal dominant myoclonus dystonia is a movement disorder characterized by involuntary lightning myoclonic jerks of the axial and appendicular structures, and mild dystonic movements and postures are typically alleviated by alcohol. We reported a family with eight members with myoclonus dystonia[180]; the index case presented with a diagnosis of laryngeal dystonia. Using a positional cloning approach, Zimprich et al[181] identified five different heterozygous loss-of-function mutations in the gene for varepsilon-sarcoglycan *(SGCE)*, in patients with myoclonus dystonia. Pedigree analysis showed a marked difference in penetrance depending on the parental origin of the disease allele, indicative of a maternal imprinting mechanism, similar to that which has been demonstrated in the mouse varepsilon-sarcoglycan gene. It is interesting that many of these patients have associated

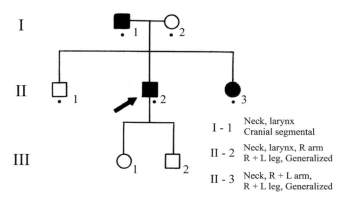

Fig. 17.2 Family C. The proband has generalized dystonia with vocal cord involvement. His sister has generalized dystonia with prominent torticollis. Their father has involvement of his neck and vocal cords.

obsessive-compulsive disorder (OCD) and alcohol dependence.[182] This is reflected in the neuropsychiatric manifestations and alterations in dopaminergic and serotonergic metabolites in an animal model of this condition.[183]

Mutations in the mitochrondrial genome can also result in dystonic signs. In addition to dystonia, these patients typically display additional features associated with mitochondrial dysfunction, such as optic atrophy, hearing loss, peripheral and neuropathy. In some cases abnormal neuroimaging provides diagnostic clues.[184]

In most families with dystonia, various members may have different presentations. For instance, in *DYT1* dystonia, individuals may present with generalized, segmental, or focal dystonia, suggesting that those with milder manifestations are related to the more generalized cases. This observation supports the concept that the less involved individuals are *formes frustes* of generalized dystonia. Across all forms of dystonia with laryngeal involvement, the presence of dystonic symptoms in other family members supports the concept that the laryngeal involvement is dystonic and genetic in these cases (**Fig. 17.2**). For instance in our series of patients, 11 to 31% of patients presenting for evaluation and treatment of laryngeal dystonia had other family members with dystonic symptoms involving the larynx or some other segment of the body.[185] Those with a family history of dystonia in general had a younger age at onset.

Laboratory Evaluation

Routine laboratory investigations are typically normal in patients with idiopathic dystonia, including idiopathic SD. Patients with secondary dystonia have laboratory findings consistent with the underlying disorder. Neuroimaging studies with positron emission tomography (PET) have suggested abnormalities in the basal ganglia and associated outflow pathways as reflected in the sensory[186,187] or motor[188] cortex in classical idiopathic disease, and motor cortex[189] in X-linked dystonia-parkinsonism ("Lubag"[190,191]). Eidelberg et al[192] has studied clinically nonmanifesting and manifesting *DYT1* carriers and found that they express a specific metabolic topography with increases in the posterior putamen, globus pallidus, cerebellum, and supplementary motor cortex.[193] Additional metabolic findings have been reported in other genetic and nongenetic forms of dystonia[194,195]; however, there are no consistent findings across all forms of dystonia.

There are no consistent brain pathologic findings in patients with idiopathic dystonia. Among the various reviews[196-200] of primarily idiopathic dystonia, the most frequently cited lesions are in the basal ganglia, including the putamen, the head of the caudate, and the upper brainstem. Hedreen et al[201] proposed that the putamen and the striatopallido-thalamo-cortical circuit appear to be the most likely sites in which to search for the unknown defect in primary dystonia.

In a review of the behavioral and motor consequences of focal lesions of the basal ganglia, Bhatia and Marsden[202] found that putaminal and globus pallidus (lentiform nuclei) lesions were frequent causes of dystonia. This observation has been confirmed with more recent publications and our own.[203] There are several reports of metabolic disorders, particularly those affecting mitochondrial function, causing dystonic symptoms,[204] including patients with Leber's[205] or related phenotype,[206] partial cytochrome b deficiency,[207] ragged-red fibers with complex III and IV deficiency,[208] complex I deficiency,[209] or other mitochondrial mutation.[210] These findings support the concept that disturbed basal ganglia function, including that caused by molecular defects, may be important in the genesis of the dystonia phenotype.

McNaught et al[211] recently reported perinuclear inclusion bodies in the midbrain reticular formation and periaqueductal gray in four cases of *DYT1* dystonia, suggesting that impaired protein handling may be a part of the molecular pathology of idiopathic dystonia, and brainstem nuclei may be important in the clinical manifestations. However, detailed histories were not available for all patients to assess whether there were other factors that may have contributed to the observations.

There is also little known about the precise biochemistry of dystonia. Some patients derive benefit from pharmacotherapy with anticholinergics, benzodiazepines, baclofen, dopamine depletors, or dopamine blocking agents. However, from the few autopsies,[212] there is normal choline acetyltransferase in the cortex and striatum. In examples of secondary dystonia,[213] there is a marked and consistent elevation of norepinephrine in several regions of brainstem. In our case of primary putamenal degeneration, the substantia nigra pars compacta contained a normal number of neurons but decreased tyrosine hydroxylase immunoreactivity.[203]

Treatment

Various options are available for treating patients with dystonia.[214] Aside from the case of levodopa-responsive dystonia, which responds exquisitely to levodopa/carbidopa therapy,[215,216] no drug has emerged as uniformly effective, and the surgical approaches are not uniformly beneficial or without risk. One must choose a treatment strategy keeping the risk to a minimum. To avoid potential harm when searching for an effective therapy, surgical therapies and drugs that may cause irreversible harm should be avoided. Very few systematic drug trials have been conducted in dystonia[217,218]; much of what we know about pharmacotherapy has resulted from empiric observations.[219,220] Indeed, in the past two decades, no new oral agent has emerged as specifically effective for patients with idiopathic dystonia, including the focal dystonias.

As genetic and molecular biologic research advances, there is growing concern about the use of ablative CNS surgery. The primary goal of research is to find out more about the etiologic pathophysiology with the intent to develop specific pharmacotherapeutic intervention. With that goal in mind, ablative brain therapy is generally avoided as one might ablate regions of the brain that may hold important receptors to future interventional pharmacotherapy. However, deep brain stimulation of the pallidum and other basal ganglia targets has emerged as an effective therapy for patients with more generalized or focal dystonia that is resistant to other therapies including local injections of botulinum toxin.[221-225]

Specific pharmacotherapy directed at the underlying identified biochemical defect is available for only a limited number of symptomatic dystonias.[226] The most notable is Wilson disease. For tardive dystonia, the best treatment is avoidance of offending medications when possible, and providing the patient with a list of these medications to avoid.

Physical methods temporize symptoms but, in our clinical experience, help very few. Systemic pharmacotherapy provides little relief of symptoms. However, many patients report mild symptom relief with muscle-relaxing agents and anxiolytics such as baclofen and benzodiazepines. Dedo and Izdebski[227] described dramatic relief of symptoms by sectioning the recurrent laryngeal nerve. However, the results were not long lasting, due to either reinnervation or central reorganization. The initial favorable reports were temporized by Aronson and De Santo's[228,229] review of 33 patients treated with surgery. By 3 years, only 36% of patients had some persistent improvement and only one of 33 achieved a persistent normal voice. Adverse effects included breathiness, hoarseness, diplophonia, and falsetto. Of the 64% with failed voices at 3 years, 48% were worse than before surgery. Failures were more common among women (77%) than among men (36%). Since that time, other surgical procedures have been reported with limited success. These include a laryngoplastic procedure where there is either an anterior commissure pushback, widening of the anterior commissure, or a vocal fold medialization (for abductor SD).[230,231] Myectomy[232] and myoplasty[233] of the thyroarytenoid (TA), lateral cricoarytenoid (LCA), and posterior cricoarytenoid (PCA) have also been reported to reduce the breaks, but produce unpredictable results. The denervation/reinnervation procedure[234] cuts the adductor branch of the recurrent laryngeal nerve (RLN) bilaterally, which is then anastomosed to the ansa cervicalis bilaterally. An LCA myotomy was also added in some patients. The results to date may be promising, but there are not enough long-term vocal results available.

Long-term treatment focal dystonia, and in particular LD, was unrewarding until the advent of local injections of botulinum toxin type A. We began using botulinum toxin type A for the treatment of focal and segmental dystonias in April 1984.[235] Improvement in symptoms of LD with local injections of botulinum toxin type A is remarkable and reviewed elsewhere in this volume and supported by consensus statements. The American Academy of Neurology,[236] the American Academy of Otolaryngology,[237] the National Institutes of Health Consensus Panel,[238] and other organizations[107,236-242] have reviewed the clinical usefulness of botulinum toxin therapy; the expert panels found this modality of treatment safe and effective for most focal dystonias.

Patients with more than focal dystonia (segmental, multifocal, generalized) are usually treated with pharmacotherapy. However, many patients have benefited from botulinum toxin type A therapy directed toward one or many discrete regions of the body. Pharmacotherapy is usually initiated with an anticholinergic, benzodiazepine, or baclofen. The choice of drug to initiate usually depends on the age of the patient, prior exposure to medications, and other concurrent medications or medical problems. Drug dosage is low initially, and gradually increased as tolerated. If the medication is of no benefit at a dose necessary to cause adverse effects, then it is gradually tapered and discontinued. If a medication is documented to be helpful, then it can be continued, and the next medication is added. In difficult cases, dopamine depleting (e.g., tetrabenazine[243,244]) and receptor blocking agents[245-247] may be added.

Intrathecal baclofen, which has been approved by the Food and Drug Administration (FDA) for patients with spasticity of spinal and cerebral origin, has been used in a limited number of studies and has helped many patients with dystonia. Patients are considered candidates for intrathecal baclofen after they have failed pharmacotherapy, or other conservative treatment. Because of the complexities of patient management, it is recommended that intrathecal baclofen be administered by a team of specialists, including a neurologist and neurosurgeon, familiar with the treatment program, and equipped to manage side effects.[248-252]

As noted elsewhere, the effectiveness of DBS for the treatment of drug-induced dyskinesias in PD has revitalized interest in the surgical treatment of dystonia. The globus pallidus internus (GPi) appears to be the optimal target for intractable dystonia.[253,254] The most dramatic improvement occurs in patients with primary dystonia and those with the DYT1 gene mutation. A lesser degree of improvement may be seen in patients with secondary dystonia.[221,222,225,255,256] DBS of the pallidal nucleus recently received a Humanitarian Use Device designation by the FDA.[257]

Other Cranial Neurolaryngeal Dystonias

Dystonia may affect the soft palate, pharynx, mandible, and other nearby regions. The principles of classification and therapy are similar to those for laryngeal dystonia. It should be emphasized that, associated with their rarity, we have cared for patients who have been misdiagnosed as having glossopharyngeal neuralgia or psychogenic disorders, typically "globus hystericus," who, on further careful examination, have involuntary muscular contractions of the oropharyngeal, lingual, or mandibular musculature. If dystonia is suspected, then appropriate referral to a team with expertise in laryngeal movement disorders is indicated.

♦ Tremor

The appearance of tremor is that of a rhythmical movement of a part of the body. The appearance implies that the movement has a relatively fixed periodicity and possesses an amplitude and waveform that are to some extent invariable over reasonable amounts of time. If these characteristics do not hold, then movements have an irregular appearance and historically have been classified as different phenomena.[258] Tremor has been defined as "a series of involuntary, relatively rhythmic, purposeless, oscillatory movements"[259] that have been observed in axial, distal, or proximal musculature, or any combination thereof. Tremors have been classified by their etiology or clinical appearance and are characterized by their frequency, amplitude, distribution over the body, and exacerbating and relieving factors.[260] The classifications terms are for the most part descriptive or associative and may describe a purported neuroanatomic etiology, such as rubral, basal ganglia; some other causative factor, such as drug-induced, anxiety, or thyroid tremor; frequency; or provoking position/action, such as action-induced or rest tremor **(Table 17.6)**. All individuals have normal physiologic tremor, which occurs with a frequency of approximately 6 to 12 Hz. Abnormal (pathologic) tremor, on the other hand, has been reported to range from 3 to 7 Hz and is considered a sign of neurologic disorder.[261] Rest tremor occurs in relaxed, unsupported limbs, and action tremors occur during muscle contraction. Action tremors have been classified further as postural tremors (when holding a position against gravity), contraction tremor (produced by isometric voluntary contraction independent of gravity, such as making a fist), and kinetic or intention tremor (during goal-directed movement such as touching a finger to the nose). Few of these descriptive classifications precisely identify the cause of the tremor and are confounded by overlap. Nevertheless, the descriptive terms may be used as a context from which to consider therapeutic intervention. Pathologic tremor is frequently observed in the limb, hand, and foot musculature of these patients, and vocal tremor may accompany these diseases as well.[83,262] The proposed underlying neural bases for tremor include a central mechanism, as in essential tremor and that associated with parkinsonism and dystonia, or a peripheral mechanism, such as the tremor associated with a polyneuropathy.[263] This section discusses predominantly those associated with central causes.

Voice Analysis and Characteristics Accompanying Tremulous Diseases

The involuntary, rhythmic, oscillatory movements that affect the distal musculature in patients with tremulous diseases may also affect the muscles of the speech production mechanism and generate rhythmic alterations in pitch and loudness, called "vocal tremor." Vocal tremor may result in rapid decreases and increases in loudness and pitch or in complete phonation stoppages. Intelligibility and rate of speech may be decreased. Vocal tremor has been described perceptually as "tremulous voice,"[262] "wavy voice,"[264] or "tremulous, quavering speech,"[265] and has been associated with neurologic disorders such as essential tremor, PD, cerebellar ataxia, and flaccid dysarthria.[83]

Various sites have been documented as anatomic bases of vocal tremor within the speech mechanism. Oscillations in musculature of the respiratory, laryngeal, or articulatory systems or elsewhere in the body have been associated with vocal tremor. Critchley[266] suggested that "tremor of muscles of the larynx, lips, tongue and diaphragm may be responsible for quavering speech." Vocal tremor has been reported to result from changes in subglottal air pressure induced by an action tremor of the respiratory muscles,[267] rhythmic activity in the rectus abdominus respiratory muscle,[268] and rhythmic fluctuations in contraction of expiratory chest muscles.[269] Vertical movement of the larynx[262] and rhythmic abduction[270] and adduction of the vocal folds and rhythmic reduction of tension of the vocal folds due to cricothyroid action[270] have been associated with vocal tremor and the accompanying vocal arrests and breaks. Lips, tongue, soft palate, and jaw movements have been reported to contribute to vocal tremor as well.[269,270] It has also been suggested that passive vibration from gross tremor elsewhere in the body may be reflected in secondary vocal tremor.[16,271]

We recommend a careful neurologic and laryngologic examination to define to anatomic substrate for tremor in patients presenting with vocal tremulousness, as vocal tremor may be the first symptom or the only symptom of a neurologic disease. Clinicians may require special training to differentiate vocal tremor from other conditions such as spasmodic dysphonia.[272] Furthermore, the frequency, amplitude, and regularity of vocal tremor may differ among diseases of different neural subsystems.[83,269,273] Therefore, analysis of vocal tremor may make important contributions to early and differential diagnosis of neurologic diseases and consequently to treatment decisions.

Teams of researchers and clinicians from speech pathology, otolaryngology, and neurology have contributed to our knowledge about vocal tremor. The primary quantification of vocal tremor has been through acoustic analysis and, more recently, laryngeal electromyography. Most of the acoustic data on vocal tremor have been obtained from visual inspection of oscillographic displays of waveform

Table 17.6 Different Adjectives Used to Describe Tremor

Action	Kinetic	Postural
Cerebellar	Midbrain	Primary writing
Drug-induced	Multiple sclerosis	Psychogenic
Dystonic	Orthostatic	Reemergent
Enhanced physiologic	Palatal myoclonic	Rubral
Essential	Parkinsonian	Toxin induced
Head	Peripheral neuropathy	Vocal
Hyperthyroid	Physiologic	Wing beating
Intention	Posttraumatic	

Source: Data from Louis ED. Tremor disorders: identification and treatment. Med Update Psych 1997;2:172–178.

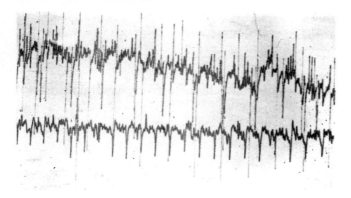

Fig. 17.3 This patient presented for the evaluation of laryngeal dystonia and had a tremulous voice on examination. Laryngeal electromyography revealed myotonic discharges consistent with a primary muscle disorder.

data or graphic level recorder displays of amplitude contours of sustained vowel phonation. Vocal tremor may involve oscillations in frequency in addition to the amplitude oscillations previously reported,[273,274] and tremor is a complex waveform comprising several components[275–277] rather than the single frequency usually measured from oscillographic data.

Laryngeal electromyography has been useful in directly assessing muscle status and the interaction among muscles in patients who present with tremor.[85,91,278–280] The electromyographic patterns, including those that occur during phonation tasks, can often differentiate essential tremor from spasmodic dysphonia and other neurologic conditions, such as Tourette's and vocal tics,[278] associated with laryngeal movement disorders. For instance, we evaluated a patient referred for laryngeal dystonia who presented with a tremulous voice and was found to have myotonic discharges in the laryngeal muscles (**Fig. 17.3**). Furthermore, multichannel studies permit an assessment of the association of the laryngeal muscles with each other and with nearby muscles such as the strap and pharyngeal muscles. By obtaining quantitative data on the frequency, amplitude, and regularity of vocal tremor, researchers have proposed various hypotheses about the physiologic basis within the speech mechanism (respiratory, laryngeal, or articulatory muscle oscillation). Commonly, the frequency of vocal tremor accompanying neurologic diseases has been reported to range from 4 to 11 Hz[274,278] with amplitudes of oscillation ranging widely. In PD, a tremor with rhythmic bursts of 5 to 6 Hz has been reported, whereas in spasmodic dysphonia, increased thyroarytenoid muscle activity has been observed with bursts with phonation, or asymmetric activity, but typically without a tremor signature.[278] Some vocal tremors may be constant throughout sustained phonation, others may crescendo in amplitude and slow in frequency toward the end of the phonation, and still others may be too variable for analysis. Reports of normal physiologic vocal tremor have most often been in the 8- to 20-Hz range[273] with amplitudes of oscillation of approximately 25%.[262] Whereas these more precise analyses may facilitate distinctions among tremors accompanying different neurologic diseases, the studies contribute to our understanding about underlying physiologic bases of vocal tremor within the speech mechanism.

Essential Tremor

Essential tremor (ET) is the most common presentation of tremor. The tremor of ET is a rhythmic oscillatory movement of 4- to 12-Hz frequency, with variable amplitude,[281–283] most commonly due to reciprocal activation of antagonistic muscles, although periods of cocontraction may be observed.[284] The frequency of tremor affecting different individuals is quite variable, and there is overlap with the characteristic frequencies of physiologic and parkinsonian tremors. Therefore, frequency cannot be the sole criterion by which essential tremor may be distinguished.[285] Clinical criteria for the diagnosis of ET have been recommended.[69,286] ET is characterized by a progressive kinetic tremor of the upper limbs, sometimes accompanied by voice or head tremor, and is not due to some other identifiable condition, that is, not "symptomatic." ET is typically absent at rest, maximal during maintenance of a posture, attenuated but still present during movement, and often accentuated at the termination of movement. It is present at rest only in the occasional patient; differentiation from parkinsonism can be difficult in these individuals. The upper extremities, head, and voice are commonly affected, often with asymmetrical limb involvement. Although originally coined "benign essential tremor," the condition is disabling for many.[287]

An important clinical distinction is between ET and the tremor of classical parkinsonism. ET has classically been considered to be a monosymptomatic disorder, with rigidity, bradykinesia, and postural instability typically being absent; however, mild rigidity may be present in some patients.[284] The tremor of ET is present with posture and action, varying between 4 and 12 Hz, faster than the rest tremor of PD at 3 to 5 Hz. Additional clinically significant signs of parkinsonism suggests that the patient may have a neurodegenerative condition, either as the cause of the tremor or coincidental.[287]

The fundamental pathogenesis of ET is unknown. Affecting 1 to 6% of the population[288] and reported to be familial (autosomal dominant) in 17 to 100% of those affected,[289] ET is genetically heterogeneous and has been associated with two genetic loci, 3q13.3 (FET1, Online Mendelian Inheritance in Man [OMIM] Project number 190300)[184,290] and 2p25-p22 (ETM2, OMIM 602134)[291]; however, until recently, identification of a gene and consequently a gene product has failed, and more complex genetics or an interaction among genetics, environmental factors, and other susceptibility factors may be etiologic.[292,293] However, recently, FET1 has been associated with a specific polymorphism in the *DRD3* gene[294] in 23 of 30 unrelated French families.

No anatomic or neurochemical correlates have been identified in the brain or body fluids of essential tremor patients.[287] Current theories have derived from knowledge of the anatomic basis of other tremors, physiologic investigations of essential tremor, response of essential tremor to various pharmacologic agents, animal models of tremor,[295] and neurocognitive testing.[296,297] For instance, various β-adrenergic antagonist agents may attenuate the symptoms of essential tremor, with most evidence suggesting an effect on peripheral $β_2$-adrenoceptors in skeletal muscle,[295] similar to the effect of β-adrenergic antagonists on physiologic tremor. The effect of botulinum toxin on the symptoms of ET[298-301] supports the role of peripheral influences. Intravenous and intraarterial epinephrine enhance the amplitude of physiologic tremor, mediated by peripheral β-adrenoceptors in the forearm. This tremorgenic effect is attenuated by propranolol. $β_2$-receptors are located on both intrafusal and extrafusal muscle fibers.

However, there is also evidence that β-adrenergic antagonists may exert an effect on central pathways important in the attenuation of essential tremor, and the therapeutic effects of ethanol, primidone, phenobarbital, alprazolam, and topiramate[302] on essential tremor are most probably exerted via central pathways, as is obvious for the therapeutic effect of brain surgical approaches (ablative and stimulation of the thalamus, pallidum, and subthalamic nucleus). These observations have collectively led to a model of three interconnected oscillatory loops in the nervous system important in the genesis of tremor, with essential tremor partially due to oscillations occurring in the olivocerebellorubral loop system, which releases normal damping influences to allow oscillations to occur within the spinal reflex loop.[303,304] Furthermore, peripheral inputs, possibly mediated by adrenoreceptors, further modulate these central oscillators. Studies with PET have supported the contention that the olivocerebellar tracts are abnormal in this condition.[305] As discussed earlier in this chapter, CNS ablation of lesions of the thalamus and DBS has emerged as an effective therapy for tremor. Interestingly, DBS of the thalamus,[306] pallidum, and subthalamic region[307] is effective in treating essential tremor, reducing functional disability and in some cases vocal symptoms. Benefit is seen with stimulation/modulation in these nuclear regions, suggesting that either common fibers traverse the region of all three nuclei, or the propagation and maintenance of the oscillatory outflow depends on intact interconnections among these three key regions of the basal ganglia. For instance, benefit by stimulation in the subthalamic region is reported to be attributed to disruption of the ascending dentate- and interpositus-thalamic fibers within a small region in the subthalamic region as compared with the relatively large wedge-shaped volume of the Vim nucleus of the thalamus, the latter being the target of thalamic ablative lesions or stimulation.[307]

Vocal tremor occurs in approximately 10 to 20% of patients with essential tremor.[269] It may be the first or only sign of the disease, or it may accompany tremors in other body parts. Vocal tremor may parallel the onset of other symptoms or have a sudden onset and cause rapid deterioration in speech intelligibility. Vocal tremor may be modulated with emotional stress or fatigue.[83] Pitch breaks (octave breaks to a lower frequency) and phonation arrests have been reported in certain cases of essential tremor[269,308] and have been associated with visible vertical oscillations of the larynx.[15] Aronson's group[15] stated, "When organic voice tremor becomes sufficiently severe, the range or amplitude of the adductor phases of most or all of the vocal fold tremor cycles is so extensive that the folds momentarily meet in the midline and seal the glottis, producing a strained or staccato voice arrest." These characteristics have been misdiagnosed as the voice arrests and adductory laryngeal spasms accompanying adductor spasmodic dysphonia.[80] Vocal tremor has been observed in 30% of a group of patients with adductor spasmodic dysphonia[131] **(Fig. 17.4)**. A comparison between these patient groups suggests that essential tremor patients have greater regularity in vocal arrests[84] and vocal tremor than spasmodic dysphonia patients.[273,309] Furthermore, it has been reported that in essential tremor patients, frequency oscillations were more predominant than amplitude oscillations,[273] whereas in spasmodic dysphonia patients only amplitude oscillations, or bursts with phonation, were observed.[278]

Reductions in vocal tremor have been reported with administration of propranolol,[277,305] primidone,[310] and benzodiazepines (lorazepam, clonazepam, diazepam), either alone or in combination.[268] In practice, we and others have found limited clinically significant changes in vocal tremor with administration of propranolol[265] and primidone[311]; benzodiazepines such as clonazepam or lorazepam may result in mild amelioration of symptoms. Local injections of botulinum toxin into the vocal folds have been reported, sometimes with dramatic

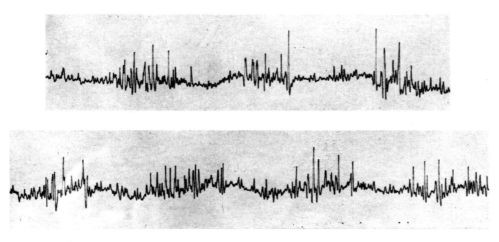

Fig. 17.4 Laryngeal electromyography recording from the vocalis muscle in a patient with spasmodic dysphonia and tremor.

results.[300,312–317] Furthermore, some patients who have DBS for the management of their somatic tremor experience improvement in vocal tremor.[318–321] Clinicians unfamiliar with these voice disorders can be taught to identify predominant speech symptoms leading to improved accuracy in diagnosis.[272] However, presumably because of the complexity of the muscle movements and the limitation in clinical diagnosis-by-symptom, a clinical pathophysiologic differentiation between a voice disorder caused by tremor and a dystonia disorder can be elusive.

Vocal Tremor in Other Disorders

In addition to the other voice disturbances seen in PD (above), Logemann et al[16] reported that 13.5% of a group of patients with PD had tremulousness of speech. The frequency of vocal tremor in patients with PD has been reported in the range of 5 to 7 Hz[322] and 4 to 6 Hz.[277] This is similar to the tremor frequencies reported in the lip and jaw musculature of parkinsonian patients.[275] Vocal tremor in PD patients has been reported to include both frequency and amplitude oscillations[322] and mainly frequency oscillations.[277] It has been suggested that patients with postencephalitic parkinsonism have the greatest degree of tremor in the laryngeal muscles. Quivering of the interarytenoid muscles and the false folds has been associated with the quivering voice quality observed in these patients.[323]

"Coarse voice tremor"[83] or irregular vocal tremor[261] has been reported in patients with cerebellar ataxia. Zemlin et al[324] reported "galloping" in the phonation of a study of patients with ataxic involvement associated with multiple sclerosis. The authors associated this with tremors or ataxia of the cricothyroid, vocalis, or thyroarytenoid muscles.

Aronson[83] has reported tremor and "flutter" (rapid tremor) on vowel prolongation of flaccid patients with unilateral vocal fold paralysis and myasthenia gravis. He has also reported this rapid tremor flutter in voices of patients with the flaccid-spastic mixed dysarthria of amyotrophic lateral sclerosis. A 5- to 6-Hz vocal tremor was quantified in a patient with amytrophic lateral sclerosis and associated with respiratory muscle oscillation.[324]

◆ Stuttering

Stuttering is the oldest known, most researched, and possibly the least understood communication disorder. Stuttering was first described around 2000 B.C. during the Middle Egyptian Dynasty in hieroglyphics that refer to a speech disorder as "to walk haltingly with a tongue that is sad."[325] Since then, there has been considerable debate about whether the etiology of this condition is psychological, learned, or organic. Since the first edition of this book, there has been increasing evidence that stuttering is a neurologic disorder and indeed a movement disorder of cranially innervated muscles. Since the phenomenology includes abnormal, involuntary, and inappropriate use of the muscles of speech production resulting in dysfluency, it might best be considered a movement disorder. Classifying stuttering from this vantage point can give us a new perspective on the motor derangement of stuttering. We can also draw upon the proposed models of motor control, as applied to stuttering, to further understand the dysfluencies and motor derangements associated with the more classical movement disorders discussed in this chapter.

As a CNS disorder characterized by involuntary and inappropriate use of the muscles of speech production resulting in dysfluency, stuttering is properly classified as an involuntary movement disorder. Phenomenologically, stuttering has been described as "the involuntary (done contrary to or without choice... not subject to control of the will) disruption of a continuing attempt to produce a spoken utterance"[326] and an "involuntary disruption of a word the speaker is otherwise attempting to utter."[327] Because stuttering is involuntary and the affected individual experiences a loss of control, it is associated with frustration and consequently associated with apprehension, struggle, and avoidance, ultimately becoming integrally associated with neuropsycholinguistic impact.[328]

Patients typically present in childhood with repetitions of words or parts of words, syllables, prolongations of sound, and speech interruptions (blocks). Structures involved include the lips, jaw, tongue, and vocal folds. Stuttering is found in all age levels beginning with the onset of speech. It is almost always reported to begin before adolescence, most commonly in the early years. Dysfluencies may be normal during early speech development, such as through the age of 4; however, for some children, these dysfluencies continue. Bloodstein[329] reported that the estimates of lifetime incidence of stuttering average 10%, which is much higher than the 1% prevalence previously assumed. Others have stated that approximately 5% of the population has experienced stuttering for at least 6 months, with approximately 1% of the pediatric population stuttering,[329,331] with males more commonly affected.[333] In addition, fewer previously fluent children develop stuttering as their age advances. Throughout childhood there is much fluidity in the prevalence of stuttering because occurrences of new cases are balanced by the remission of old ones. There is a marked tendency for children to recover spontaneously after periods of stuttering of different lengths. Bloodstein stated that estimates of spontaneous recovery range from 36 to 79% of children who stutter; this range is supported by other researchers.[333,334] Recovery occurs at any age, but the younger the person the better the chance of a persistent recovery. Seider et al[335] reported that spontaneous recovery occurs at ages ranging from 3 to 38 years. Their data also demonstrated a decreased probability of recovery with increased age. Andrews et al[336] estimated that 75% of those who stutter at age 4, 50% of those who stutter at age 6, and 25% of those who stutter at age 10 will recover. Adult-onset stuttering suggests an underlying neurologic disorder such as brain injury or a parkinsonism syndrome.[337,338]

Competing stimuli such as emotional arousal or sensory stimuli, motor actions such as walking, and using rhythmical patterns such as those provided by a metronome, increase fluency. Novel modes of speaking, such as singing, speaking in a singsong, using a monotone, shouting, using a foreign accent, and using clear or slurred articulation, also increase fluency for a period of time. Communicative pressures such as audience size, listener reactions, concern about social approval, time pressure, and the degree to which the stutterer is responsible for conveying a meaningful message to a listener are found to increase stuttering. Eisenson and Horowitz[339] reported that stutterers stuttered more frequently on meaningful stimuli than on lists of words. Burke[340] noted that stutterers can repeat sentences fluently from dictation. Choral reading[341] is described as another situation that increased fluency. Talking to animals or infants are some of the easiest situations for stutterers and therefore some of the most fluent. Although these observations had been interpreted as supporting a psychological etiology, they indeed support a neurologic basis of the brain circuit interactions in the neurobiology of stuttering and may represent de-automatization (see below) occurring in the basal ganglia. Psychological factors likely influence the disorder and in particular the patient's response to the physical manifestations of CNS dysregulation.

Over the years many theories about the cause of stuttering have emerged. From the 1930s to the 1940s, most of the dominant theories came from a medical model that focused on the organic cause of stuttering. These theories are shaped by research in perseveration,[342] blood sugars,[343] cerebral dominance,[344] and delayed myelination of the nerve fibers.[345] Ingham[346] described how, in the 1940s, Freud and Carl Rogers changed the favored perspective from a medical to a psychological approach. Ingham also stated that B. F. Skinner's theories on learning helped to change the orientation back toward a medical model. The behaviorist approach became popular, experimental methods were used, and programmed therapy became popular. Webster and Lubker[347,348] theorized that impaired auditory feedback causes stuttering. Aberrant interaction of air-conduction and bone-conduction components of the feedback system were believed to distort the feedback signal from speech and cause the stutterer to compensate for the speech perception distortion by stuttering.

With the availability of new technology, organic theories became increasingly popular in the 1970s and 1980s. Using electromyography, Freeman and Ushijima[349] measured muscle activity during fluent and nonfluent utterances. Analysis revealed that stuttering is accompanied by high levels of laryngeal muscle activity and disruption of normal reciprocity between abductor and adductor muscle groups. Results have been interpreted to demonstrate a strong correlation between abnormal laryngeal muscle activity and stuttering. Neuroimaging techniques[350,351] further supported dysfunction in cortical-subcortical-cerebellar processing in stuttering subjects.

Continuing with the medical model, investigators at Yale University[352,353] formulated a hypothesis about the genetic and environmental interactions that produce the family patterns seen in stuttering. Studies among stuttering relatives revealed a pattern indicating transmission of a susceptibility to the disorder with sex-modified expression; girls were more resistant to the expression of the disorder, suggesting why fewer women than men stutter. Ambrose et al[333] performed a segregation analysis based on relatives of childhood stutterers and concluded that there is a single major locus that is responsible for the transmission of stuttering in relatives of preschool children who stuttered. They suggested that the failure of the Yale investigators to identify the mendelian inheritance was due to their bias associated with their studying adults with chronic stuttering, rather than the population of children who have ever stuttered and may have recovered. In addition, enrolling school-aged children permits a broader sample of living family members to interview and study. Further segregation studies support a model of autosomal dominant major gene effect, further influenced by the two covariates—sex and affected status of parents.[354] Recovery from stuttering was more frequent in females as opposed to males, supporting the change in male/female sex ratio from approximately 2:1 in childhood to approximately 4–5:1 in subjects that persisted into adulthood. Persistence of developmental stuttering into adulthood, as opposed to recovery, is potentially due to additional genetic factors, suggesting that there may be a polygenic component in patients who continue to stutter into adulthood.[332]

Alm[355] and Ludlow and Loucks[356] reviewed evidence that stuttering is a dynamic motor control disorder with features similar to dystonia and chronic motor tics and, consistent with other movement disorders, likely involves perturbations in the basal ganglia circuits as they broadly influence and modify motor control output from other regions of the brain. They note that the basal ganglia and connections subserve important integrative functions for sensory input and motor output, including timing of motor output. Furthermore, during the past two decades, neurobiologists have recognized that brain connection and receptor density is dynamic and changes in utero and throughout life, often with dramatic changes in the neonate and young child.[357,358] For instance, dopamine subtype density and ratios (D1/D2) change during early development,[359,360] with the time course of D2 receptor density falling by age 5, which is similar to the onset of developmental stuttering and the onset of chronic motor tics and childhood-onset dystonia. Furthermore, development and learning are associated with dynamic synaptic changes throughout many critical brain regions.[361,362]

As a disorder of speech production, similar to dystonia, stuttering is action induced. Stuttering and abnormal timing events occur in three subsystems of speech: respiratory, phonatory, and articulatory. The abnormal involuntary movements are task specific, and the movements may be repetitive and stereotyped. Stuttering has the phenomenology of increased muscle tension or lack of appropriate smooth motor control in those three subsystems that causes the muscles to move too quickly or too far.[363] Electromyographic studies have shown that the normal reciprocal behavior of the laryngeal muscles is perturbed in stuttering[349]; this type of phenomenology is seen in dystonia. The postures may be sustained for longer than expected or in quick repetitive movements of the same posture. Patients may have primarily focal systems (phonatory, respiratory, articulatory) or have segmental symptomatology involving two or three regions. In addition, other cranial musculature may inappropriately contract during stuttering, including the eyelids and other muscles of facial expression.[364] One report that specifically examined the abnormal involuntary movements that are associated with stuttering[364] described the phenomenology into two categories: involuntary abnormal movements associated with stuttering, and voluntary abnormal movements performed to assist with alleviation of the stuttering. These motor abnormal movements extended beyond the face, and included muscles not associated with articulation, including the upper and lower extremities, including a *geste antagonistique*, which is characteristic of dystonia. Subclinical limb tremor may be observed in stutterers,[365] also supporting an extrapyramidal etiology for the dysfluency disorder. Studies also report slower manual reaction times in unaffected limbs of patients with dystonia[366-368] and stuttering with greater voice onset times in the latter.[369]

Further support for the association between stuttering and dystonia includes the response to sensory feedback seen in both disorders, such as the *geste antagonistique* in dystonia (see above), whereas in stuttering, masking of auditory feedback,[370] shifting the frequency of auditory feedback,[371] and delaying auditory feedback[372] have been used as tools to improve fluency. In explaining these latter observations, Alm[355] notes that the basal ganglia are important in executing automatic behaviors based on the anticipated, usual, or habituated environment. Changing the aural inputs alters the environment and results in "de-automatization" of sensory processing resulting in modified basal ganglia processing strategies that result in temporary improved fluency. This can compare with the striking improvement in the ability to run when a PD patient has an emergency to attend to. In addition, the putamen and globus pallidus, two critical nuclei of the basal ganglia, are commonly implicated in acquired dystonia,[202] and the thalamus and striatum are commonly implicated in stuttering.[373] It is intriguing to note that lesions that result in stuttering rarely involve the speech and language regions, and when patients recover from lesions in the primary speech areas of the brain they rarely stutter.[356] Furthermore, dopamine-receptor blocking agents have been reported to benefit patients with dystonia[244] and stuttering.[375] Aggravation of symptoms under stress is common in both conditions, suggesting that the sensorimotor integration systems are more vulnerable in these disorders.

Abwender et al[375] examined the phenotype of stuttering, and identified an increased incidence of tic-like associated movements and obsessive-compulsive disorder, suggesting a common neurobiology in developmental stuttering and Tourette's syndrome. Mulligan et al[376] suggested that the cranial and other somatic movements associated with stuttering are phenomenologically more tic-like than dystonic. They reported tic-like involuntary movements of the face, oral structures, and limbs in stutterers. Furthermore, a genetic study of patients with Gilles de la Tourette syndrome (GTS) found an increased incidence of a history of stuttering in the patients as opposed to controls without GTS.[377] GTS patients and the associated behavioral comorbidities (including stuttering) demonstrated an association with genes involved in dopamine neurobiology (dopamine D2 receptor, dopamine β-hydroxylase, and dopamine transporter). However, inconsistent with this association are the following findings: patients with stuttering do not report the typical premonitory sensory "urge" that is so characteristic of chronic motor tics; and the movements associated with stuttering are task-specific, unlike the purposeless movements associated with tics. In addition, an EMG study[378] of intrinsic laryngeal muscle contraction in four patients with stuttering, including those with severe disease, did not demonstrate an increase in thyroarytenoid muscle activation as compared with normally fluent individuals. Although the sample size was small, these findings would not be consistent with dystonic contraction of the laryngeal musculature, and suggest that local muscle weakening with botulinum toxin may not demonstrate efficacy in this population. It would be interesting to perform these studies in patients who displayed the phenomenology of adductor laryngeal blocks.

Regardless of whether one deems stuttering to be a form of dystonia or a unique manifestation of another primary movement disorder, it is clear that further work is needed to clarify the complex neurobiology and genetics of the condition.

Primary therapy for stuttering, and the cornerstone of care, has been speech therapy with the goal of increasing fluency.[379] As noted above, many patients recover. Intensive treatment has been reported to have a more favorable result,[380] but treated patients are at a significant risk of relapse.[381] However, for those who continue with dysfluency, other options are considered. Although a variety of medications have been reported to either induce or improve stuttering, no consistent therapeutic picture has emerged. Brady[382] reviewed 16 case reports of 22 patients with stuttering symptoms after introduction of specific medications. In all instances the dysfluency resolved upon discontinuation of the offending agent. The evidence that the drugs were causally related was the recurrence of symptoms upon rechallenge or a double-blind assessment. It was notable that there was an overrepresentation of females among the cases supporting a secondary etiology. Some reported to improve stuttering also caused stuttering in this series, such as phenothiazines, tricyclic antidepressants, and serotonin reuptake inhibitors.

Haloperidol, a dopamine receptor antagonist has been the most effective medication for stuttering.[374,383] However, in practice, intolerable side effects of sedation and extrapyramidal symptoms preclude broad use in this population. A double-blind study of clomipramine and desipramine[384] demonstrated statistically significant improvement in the former group for both fluency and associated obsessive-compulsive behavioral comorbidities such as the preoccupation with stuttering, in addition to the amount of energy reportedly spent resisting stuttering. A subsequent study that included a placebo confirmed the modest benefits afforded by clomipramine.[385] The serotonin reuptake inhibitors sertraline[386] and paroxetine (mentioned by Costa and Kroll[386]) have demonstrated fluency and comorbidity benefits in case reports, the former also being implicated in causing stuttering also.[387] Although the strength of the evidence to support pharmacotherapy has been questioned,[389] in clinical practice medications have been considered predominantly for patients with significant disability.

Botulinum toxin has been tried in patients with disabling stuttering[389,390] with benefit modest at best, and very few patients continue on therapy.

◆ Myoclonus

Myoclonus refers to sudden, brief, shocklike involuntary movements caused by muscular contractions (positive myoclonus) or inhibitions (negative myoclonus, "asterixis") arising from the CNS.[391,392] The muscle twitches of fasciculations due to lesions of the lower motor neuron are excluded from this definition. Phenomenologically, similar muscle jerks may be produced by peripheral nerve or plexus lesions[393]; some have classified hemifacial spasm as a myoclonic syndrome.[394] Myoclonus may be classified according to etiology, phenomenology (**Table 17.7**), physiology, or pharmacology.[394] In the past decade there has been increasing attention to progressive neurologic conditions, which are often genetic, either with prominent myoclonus or myoclonic features such as the myoclonic dystonias, epilepsies, and ataxias. Recent reviews are available.[392,395]

Laryngeal involvement can become problematic in patients with myoclonic involvement of the primary laryngeal structures or muscles of respiration. Because of the irregular and often unpredictable nature of the myoclonic movements, aspiration can occur.[396] Singulus (hiccup) and palatal myoclonus are of particular importance to the otolaryngologist, and these will be discussed in additional detail below.

Table 17.7 Classification of Myoclonus

Etiologic classification of myoclonus

I. Physiologic myoclonus in normal subjects: sleep jerks (hypnic jerks), anxiety-induced, exercise-induced, hiccough (singultus), benign infantile myoclonus with feeding

II. Essential myoclonus (no known cause and no other gross neurologic deficit): hereditary (autosomal dominant), sporadic

III. Epileptic myoclonus (seizures dominate and no encephalopathy initially): with fragments of epilepsy, childhood myoclonic epilepsies, benign familial myoclonic epilepsy, progressive myoclonus epilepsy

IV. Symptomatic myoclonus (progressive or static encephalopathy dominates): storage disease, spinocerebellar degenerations, basal ganglia degenerations, dementias, viral encephalopathies, metabolic, toxic encephalopathies, physical encephalopathies, focal CNS damage

Phenomenologic classification of myoclonus

I. Distribution: focal, segmental, multifocal, generalized

II. Regularity: arrhythmic, rhythmic, oscillatory

III. Synchronization: synchronous, asynchronous

IV. Relation to motor activity: at rest, with action, intention

V. Positive versus negative (asterixis)

Source: From Fahn S, Marsden CD, Van Woert MH. Definition and classification of myoclonus. Adv Neurol 1986;43:1–5. Reprinted with permission.

Singulus Myoclonus

A common form of myoclonus is singulus or hiccup. Hiccup is an intermittent, abrupt, involuntary contraction of the diaphragm that results in sudden inspiration, which is opposed by a closed glottis. It is a segmental, rhythmical myoclonus, typically stimulated by peripheral irritation of the diaphragm, more often on the left side. Like other forms of myoclonus, the etiologies may be cortical (neurodegenerative, brain tumor, meningitis, encephalitis), spinal (tumor, abscess), metabolic (uremia), or peripheral (gastric irritation, pulmonic and thoracic cavity disorders).[397] Experimental electrophysiologic studies[398] have demonstrated sudden inspiratory muscle contractions of diaphragm and external intercostal muscles associated with inhibition of expiratory muscle activity. Glottic closure occurs within 35 milliseconds of the diaphragmatic stimulation. Hiccup frequency decreased with a rise in arterial PCO_2, and increased with its decline. Treatment has included physical maneuvers such as breath-holding, rapidly drinking liquids, breathing into a bag, and pharmacotherapies such as baclofen,[399] amyl nitrite, atropine, narcotics, barbiturates, chlorpromazine, and gabapentin,[400,401] in addition to pharyngeal stimulation[402] and phrenic nerve stimulation[403] in intractable cases.

Palatal Myoclonus

Branchial or oculopalatal myoclonus refers to myoclonic symptoms affecting cranial structures, and is therefore of interest to the laryngologist.[404,405] Spencer, in 1886, used the term *nystagmus* for a case of rhythmic synchronous pharyngeal, laryngeal, and ocular movements in a young girl with a presumed tumor. Because of the association of the term *nystagmus* with physiologically and phenomenolocally different eye movements, the term *myoclonus* was later proposed by Guillain et al[406] for the syndrome affecting the branchial musculature. When peering into the oral cavity, the movements are characterized by involuntary, usually unconscious, movements of the soft palate and pharynx.[407] Further exploration often documents synchronous jerks affecting the eyes, face, palate, larynx (**Fig. 17.5**), diaphragm, neck, shoulder, and arm, giving rise to the syndrome of "myoclonies velo-pharyngo-laryngo-oculo-diaphragmatiques."[408]

Palatal myoclonus has been classified as "essential" (EPM) when there are no signs of other neurologic dysfunction, and "symptomatic" when there are other symptoms, signs, or evidence of structural neurologic disease.[409] EPT has been considered to be a relatively homogeneous and distinct idiopathic condition with a widening clinical spectrum of features.[410,411] Similar to other idiopathic conditions, such as dystonia, as more becomes known about the condition, further pathophysiologic and molecular classification will be possible.

The pharyngeal movements are most commonly bilateral and symmetric, but can be unilateral, with the palate and uvula being drawn to one side. The rhythmicity nearly always persists in sleep, usually between 1.5 and 3 Hz, with a range of 0.3 and 100 Hz[407]; variation with respiration has been documented.[412] Myoclonic jerks can be briefly suppressed in

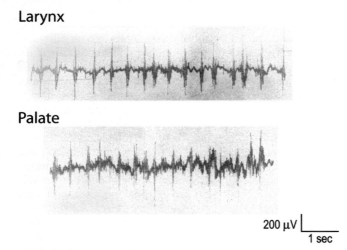

Fig. 17.5 Laryngeal electromyographic recording from the vocalis muscle complex and soft palate from a patient with branchial myoclonus showing rhythmical bursts.

some patients. Once symptoms begin, they are usually lifelong, but may rarely disappear.[413]

The patient's complaint of clicking in the ears or tinnitus,[414–416] thought to be due to involvement of the eustachian tube and tensor veli palatini muscle, was noted in the 19th century by Muller and then by Politzer.[417] The clicking can often be heard by family members and by clinicians. Laryngeal involvement may produce a broken speech pattern, simulating that heard in laryngeal dystonia or tremor (personal observation). Examination of the vocal cords often shows slow rhythmical adduction and abduction of the vocal cords at the same timing and frequency as the palatal, pharyngeal, and occasional diaphragmatic contractions. This causes the broken speech pattern and a respiratory dysrhythmia. Ventilatory dysfunction has been documented.[418]

An anatomic network abnormality has been identified in cases of branchial myoclonus. There is enlargement of the inferior olivary nucleus (ION) in the medulla (reviewed elsewhere[407,412]); these may be seen on magnetic resonance imaging (MRI) scans[419] and must be differentiated from a brainstem tumor.[420] There is gross hypertrophy of the olives with microscopic evidence of enlarged, vacuolated, bizarrely shaped neurons and enlarged astrocytes with prominent thick processes. Associated findings include fibrillary gliosis and demyelination of white matter. Functional imaging studies have demonstrated increased regional cerebral blood flow in the olivocerebellar circuits in patients with palatal myoclonus,[421] supporting the contention that these brainstem connections are important in the pathophysiology of palatal myoclonus.

Through anatomic and later histopathologic analysis, a specific pathway has been proposed to be involved. The ipsilateral central pontine tegmental tract and contralateral cerebellar dentate nucleus appear to be invariably involved. Guillain and Molleret et al[406] proposed a triangular pathway to relate hypertrophic ION degeneration to cerebellar lesions. However, it later became apparent that lesions of the olivodentate fibers have not been symptomatic. Trelles[422,423] proposed a pathway from the dentate nucleus to the contralateral ION, later substantiated by Ben Hamida[424] and Lapresle.[409] ION hypertrophy is thought to be due to a unique effect of transsynaptic degeneration.[425]

Focal palatal myoclonus is usually a minor annoyance; the syndrome is problematic when associated with spread to other muscles and in particular those involving the ear, or socially disabling when involving facial and platysmal muscles.[426] Although usually unresponsive to pharmacotherapy (therapies for all forms of myoclonus are reviewed elsewhere[392]), there have been isolated cases reported to have responded to the serotonin precursor 5-hydroxytryptophan (5-HTP), carbamazepine, clonazepam, tetrabenazine, trihexyphenidyl, sumatriptan, baclofen, and botulinum toxin type A.[427] Treatment with tenotomy of the tensor veli palatini, stapedius, or tensor tympani muscles and myringotomy may have a varying degree of success.[428]

More widespread myoclonus may be a clue to an underlying neural or metabolic disorder[392,395] (**Table 17.7**). For instance, opsoclonus-myoclonus, which is most often associated with viral conditions[429] and is present, often with ataxia, in more than 50% of children with neuroblastoma,[430,431] may present as a paraneoplastic condition.[433] It is believed to have an immunologic basis.

Other myoclonic-like conditions warrant additional note. In the first edition of this chapter, we described the following case, which we coined "laryngeal flutter": J.R. developed a clicking sound in his right nostril at age 31. The sound was intermittent and did not interfere with function. At age 39, he developed right chest and abdominal pain and a sensation of tightness in the right pharynx and palate. There was an intermittent twitching of the right nasolabial fold and a trembling sensation at the right costal margin. He subsequently developed marked sensory discomfort in the mouth, right chest, and right abdomen. Neurologic and complete gastrointestinal examinations were normal and he was referred to a psychiatrist. He continued to have feelings of poorly coordinated chest and abdominal muscles, and episodes of abdominal distention, nausea, and vomiting. Occasionally, he had interruptions in his speech, requiring a cough to clear his throat. He began to note a throat tremor and described "reverse peristalsis making me want to vomit." His wife reported that the clicking sound was audible during sleep. Examination at age 40 revealed an audible clicking coming from the mouth generally at 6 Hz, but occasionally irregular. It was associated with a palatal tremor and sometimes sustained contraction of the right palate and involuntary contraction of the intrinsic muscles of the right tongue with depression and twisting of the tongue to the right. The pharyngeal wall also moved, and there was a rare twitch of the right nasolabial fold. There were no involuntary movements of the extraocular muscles or abdomen. An esophagogram revealed fluttering involving the muscles of the pharynx and larynx; the diaphragm was normal. The larynx appeared to have fluttering movements like the "warble" of a sparrow. Phonation and swallowing suppressed the fluttering motion, only to return 30 to 60 seconds later. EMG showed irregular motion of the electrode and irregular bursts of motor unit potentials of the cricothyroid, geniohyoid, vocalis, and palatal muscles; there was no myoclonus or tremor. Spinal fluid, MRI of the brain and cervical cord, computed tomography (CT) of the brain, evoked potentials, and serologic studies were normal. We coined this condition as "laryngeal flutter" because the disorder appeared on cine-esophagography like the fluttering of a sparrow's larynx when singing. His symptoms have responded to treatment with lorazepam. The condition was presented by one of the authors (M.F.B.) to the late C. David Marsden at the Unusual Movement Disorders Dinner at the American Academy of Neurology, and was compared with other skeletal muscle perivisceral movement disorders.[434]

Recently Andrew Larner reviewed a condition described by Antony Van Leeuwenhoek in 1723 as "diaphragmatic flutter"[434-437] or "respiratory myoclonus."[439] This condition was characterized by sudden and violent movements involving the upper abdomen. The symptoms were not persistent and were attributed to shock-like movements of the diaphragm. Patients may present with respiratory stridor. Neurologically, most cases are idiopathic or primary, but have been associated with viral conditions and postencephalitis. Recently, a case of recurrent belching was described in a patient with the neurodegenerative choreic condition neuroacanthocytosis.[438,439,441] In our experience, respiratory dysrhythmias and diaphragmatic dyskinesias (nonmyoclonic and myoclonic) may be more common than appreciated if the diagnosis is entertained and may be associated with idiopathic or symptomatic dystonia[96,97] or in tardive conditions,[442] and we have found that respiratory modified barium swallowing studies are helpful in establishing the diagnosis.

♦ Tic Disorder

The word *tic* refers to a brief, usually rapid, purposeless, stereotyped, often repetitive movement involving multiple muscle groups.[441,442] Tics belong to a spectrum of movements **(Table 17.8)** that may be simple (either motor or phonic) or complex (either motor or vocal). One of the key characteristics is that the movements or vocalizations can be voluntarily suppressed by the patient for minutes or hours, often followed by a flurry of movements afterward. In addition to their suppressibility, tics tend to wax and wane over the lifetime of the individual, and may change in characteristics and distribution over time. Tic disorder typically begins in childhood; however, onset in adulthood occurs.

Similar to other movement disorders, tics can be primary or idiopathic, or associated with other conditions[443] such as developmental conditions (Asperger syndrome, autism), brain injuries, drug therapies, and neurodegenerative disease (Huntington disease, chorea-acanthocytosis.[444-446]

Gilles de la Tourette syndrome (GTS) is the most severe form of the tic disorder spectrum; involuntary vocalizations are the hallmark of the disease. However, for the majority of patients with a tic disorder, the vocalizations can be subtle, manifesting as a sniff or throat clearing. Additional features include onset in childhood or adolescence, multiple tics of several body parts, variations in the intensity of the symptoms over weeks or months, suppressibility, and presence for more than one year. Obsessive-compulsive behavior is a commonly associated comorbidity that further impacts the patient's quality of life.[447] There is no meaningful cutoff point to distinguish GTS from a less severe form of tic disorder.

It is notable that an expert in stuttering, J. M. Itard,[448] was the first to describe GTS in 1825. As described by Borsel et al,[449] "Itard reported tics, barking sounds, uncontrollable utterances of obscenities in a French noblewoman, the marquise de Dampierre." Subsequently, in 1885, another French physician, George Gilles de la Tourette[450] published additional cases and the condition was named after him.

Vocal tics, which includes phonic tics, laryngeal tics, or coughing, may occur intermixed with speech rather than associated with periods of silence, and at times when a normal speaker would use hesitation phenomena,[451] or at rest such as in coughing or throat-clearing tics. Vocalizations can be either articulate words or inarticulate sounds. Patients with GTS frequently present to the otolaryngologist for evaluation of laryngeal tics manifesting as inappropriate coughing, barking, throat clearing, hooting, and grunting, lingual tics as hisses or clicks, or nasal tics as sniffs and snorts. In one case of severe, persistent tic involving retching and coughing, we observed mastoid process tenderness due to local muscle abuse. After obvious pathology is treated or ruled out, a detailed history of associated signs of a tic disorder in addition to a family history often clarifies the diagnosis. Many patients are reluctant to accept the diagnosis, and referral to a neurologist is frequently indicated.

One can often elicit a family history of tics among family members of affected individuals, and current evidence supports an autosomal dominant mode of inheritance in most cases; however, the pattern of inheritance for all cases remains to be clarified.[452,454] Genetic studies[456] have identified families in which the full spectrum of simple and complex tics with vocalizations coexist in the same pedigree; this broad phenotype has plagued attempts to identify the molecular genetic basis for this condition. However, recent linkage and association studies in two independent family populations have implicated chromosome 17q25 as a region for further investigation.[455] In a separate report, a candidate locus for the phenotypic spectrum of GTS, OCD, and chronic motor tics was identified on chromosome 18q22.[456]

Table 17.8 Classification of Tics

A. Simple motor tics: eye blinks, eye rolls, neck stretch, limb jerks, grimacing, toe curls
B. Simple phonic tics: sniffing, grunting, throat clearing, yelping, barking, squealing, coughing, hissing, humming
C. Complex motor tics: head shaking, wrist shaking, finger cracking, touching, hitting, squatting, smelling hands/objects, rubbing, echopraxia, copropraxia
D. Complex vocal tics: coprolalia, unintelligible words, belching, hiccough, stuttering, echolalia, palilalia, "Bronx cheer"

Source: From Weiner WJ, Lang AE. Movement disorders: a comprehensive survey. Mount Kisco, NY: Futura; 1989. Adapted with permission

Tic patients may have additional often disabling comorbidities (for review, see Singer[444]), including an increased incidence of migraines, sleep disorders, attention-deficit hyperactivity disorder, and OCD. It has been postulated that these conditions are genetically associated with the genes contributing to the tic spectrum. Furthermore, it has been proposed that a subset of tic patients has either the onset of their condition or an abrupt worsening of symptoms associated with a streptococcal infection. This condition has been called pediatric autoimmune neuropsychiatric disorders associated with streptococcal infection (PANDAS).[459] The theory is unproven, and there is significant debate about the existence of the poststreptococcal condition.[460]

Pharmacologic intervention is symptomatic (reviewed elsewhere[461,462]). Because of the waxing and waning nature of the disorder, assessing the efficacy of interventional pharmacology is difficult. Although phenothiazines, such as haloperidol, appear to offer the greatest relief, both tardive dyskinesia and tardive dystonia, severely disabling movement disorders, may occur as secondary effects of phenothiazine administration, and this form of therapy is reserved for resistant cases. The monoamine depleting agent tetrabenazine has been used to manage tics without the tardive complications.[243,244] Clonidine, an α2-adrenergic agonist, and clonazepam, a benzodiazepine, have been helpful in treating the movement disorder in many patients, whereas selective serotonin reuptake inhibitors are often initiated to treat the obsessive comorbidities.[463] One must consider the treatment of comorbid conditions when treating a tic/Tourette disorder, as many of these patients have associated disabling obsessive or attention-deficit conditions.[464,465]

Local injections of botulinum toxin have been used to treat rapid facial, vocal, and dystonic tics.[466–469] The benefits vary, likely due to the complex nature of the involuntary movements. This form of therapy may be appropriate for selected patients with severe, persistent tics involving one group of muscles, such as those of the larynx or eyelids. Interestingly, some patients report a decrease in the typical "urge" to make the movement, suggesting an effect on the sensory component of the disorder. Deep brain stimulation has recently been tested with encouraging results[470,471]; however, at the time of this writing, this approach is considered experimental.

♦ Choreic Disorders

Choreic movements refer to involuntary, irregular, purposeless, nonrhythmic, abrupt, rapid, unsustained movements that flow from one body part to another (reviewed elsewhere[472,473]). Rhythmical movements with the speed and duration of hours are seen in classical tardive dyskinesia. Because of the rhythmicity, tardive dyskinesia has also been called "rhythmic chorea."

The prototypical choreic movements are those seen in Huntington disease, in which the brief and rapid movements are irregular and occur randomly as a function of time. Choreic movements can be partially suppressed, and the patient with chorea can "hide" some of the movements by incorporating them into semipurposeful movements, known as parakinesia. Chorea is usually accompanied by "motor impersistence," the inability to maintain a sustained contraction. A common symptom of motor impersistence is the dropping of objects. Motor impersistence is detected by determining if the patient is unable to keep the tongue protruded and by the presence of "milk-maid" grips due to an inability to keep the fist in a sustained tight grip. The phenomenology of chorea in Huntington disease can be duplicated by the chorea or induced by levodopa, whereas the chorea of Sydenham's appears somewhat differently, being more of a restless and somewhat writhing quality, like choreoathetosis.

The primary laryngeal-associated disorder in chorea is dysphagia and aspiration, which may result in death from aspiration pneumonia; these are common as Huntington disease progresses. Patients typically are unable to control the quantity of food and the rate of eating. The gag reflex and coughing is often impaired; dysarthria is common. Dysphagia is usually greatest for liquids. Patients also display airway compromise during swallowing due to neck hyperextension in poor respiratory control. Speech is often abnormal as they typically display tic-like coarse irregular inspiratory spurts, grunts, or other vocalizations. Although not studied extensively, decreased verbal fluency is not uncommon.[474] Barium swallow studies demonstrate poor bolus formation, pharyngeal stasis, poor cricopharyngeal function, dysmotility of the esophagus, and irregular diaphragmatic movements. Pulmonary function evaluation often shows irregular respiratory movements. Laryngoscopy reveals abnormal irregular vocal cord motion during respiration.

Choreic disorders are usually classified by etiology (**Table 17.9**). They are divided into primary and secondary choreas, based on whether the disorder is idiopathic or hereditary (the primary choreas) or due to some degenerative disease or environmental insult (secondary choreas). A few choreas are discussed in the following subsections.

Table 17.9 Major Causes of Chorea

I. Primary
  A. Hereditary
    1. Chorea is dominant feature
      a. Huntington disease
      b. Hereditary nonprogressive chorea
      c. Familial inverted chorea
    2. Chorea is not dominant feature
      a. Neuroacanthocytosis
      b. Ataxia-telangiectasia
      c. Lesch-Nyhan syndrome
      d. Glutaric acidemia
      e. Cerebral lipidoses
      f. Familial chorea and myoclonus epilepsy
      g. Dentato-rubro-pallido-luysian atrophy
      h. Wilson disease
      i. Pyruvate decarboxylase deficiency

Table 17.9 Continued

  B. Idiopathic
  1. Essential chorea
  2. Senile chorea
  3. Spontaneous oral dyskinesia
  C. Paroxysmal
  1. Paroxysmal kinesigenic choreoathetosis
II. Secondary
  A. Vascular
  1. Hemichorea/hemiballism secondary to stroke
  2. Vasculitis: lupus erythematosus
  3. Polycythemia vera
  4. Henoch-Schönlein purpura
  5. Internal cerebral vein thrombosis
  6. Subdural hematoma
  B. Infectious
  1. Sydenham's chorea
  2. Encephalitides
    a. Epidemic, subacute sclerosing panencephalitis (SSPE), arthropod-borne
    b. Syphilis, measles, varicella
    c. Pertussis, typhoid
  3. Subacute bacterial endocarditis
  4. Creutzfeldt-Jakob disease
  C. Chemicals/toxins
  1. Drugs
    a. Levodopa, neuroleptics, anticholinergics
    b. Antihistamines, oral contraceptives
    c. Phenytoin, ethosuximide, imipramine
    d. α-Methyldopa, methylphenidate,
    e. Pemoline, methadone
  2. Chemicals: CO, Hg, Li, azide
  3. Kernicterus
  4. Alcoholism (hepatic?)
  D. Metabolic disorders
  1. Chorea gravidarum
  2. Idiopathic hypoparathyroidism
  3. Hypomagnesemia
  4. Addison disease
  5. Hypernatremia
  6. Thyrotoxicosis
  7. Hypoglycemia
  8. Nonketotic hyperglycemia
  9. Chronic hepatocerebral degeneration
  E. Tumors including metastases
  F. Tuberous sclerosis
  G. Degeneration of centrum medianum

Huntington Disease

Huntington disease (HD)[473] is the most common cause of idiopathic chorea. Its prevalence in the United States and in Western Europe is approximately 4 to 8/100,000[470] population. The diagnosis depends on a positive family history of this autosomal dominant inherited disorder with confirmatory genetic testing. The cardinal features of HD, aside from the presence of chorea, are other motor signs and symptoms (clumsiness, motor impersistence, abnormal gait, and loss of postural reflexes), personality change (inappropriate behavior, such as getting too close to people when talking to them, impetuousness, irritability with loss of social inhibitions, striking out at people due to a low threshold to frustration), emotional disorder (especially depression), lack of motivation (e.g., apathy, constantly needing to be reminded to perform daily chores, decreased conversation), cognitive decline (especially subtractions, number recall, serial sevens, handling money), caudate atrophy on CT scan, decreased glucose metabolism in striatum on PET scan, and a progressive course.

The average age at onset is around 38 years; approximately 10% of cases begin before the age of 20. When the disease begins in childhood, 90% of such cases inherit the HD gene from the father. Childhood-onset HD is expressed with a more rapid course and with a propensity toward rigidity and akinesia rather than chorea.

Molecular genetic studies, using restriction fragment length polymorphism of DNA, led to the discovery that the HD gene is located near the tip of the short arm of chromosome 4. The abnormality is an expanded unstable CAG trinucleotide repeat sequence in exon 1 of the *huntingtin* gene; the protein product has an uncertain function.[474] A few homozygote cases were discovered in a large Venezuelan pedigree, the offspring of a marriage between two affected individuals. The onset in such cases was in childhood, but otherwise looked phenotypically like heterozygotes. HD is fully penetrant when there are 40 or greater CAG repeats.[475] The age at onset in patients correlates with the number of CAG repeats and accounts for approximately 50% of the variation in age of onset.[476] The disease is incompletely penetrant when there are 36 to 39 CAG repeats; when there are 30 to 35 repeats, the carrier will typically not develop the disease. However, for CAG repeats between 30 and 39, a longer repeat length may be transmitted to the members of the next generation, who may consequently develop disease.

Unfortunately, no agent has emerged as markedly effective in managing the motor, cognitive, or neurodegenerative consequences of HD.[477-479] Supportive social and psychotherapy are considered primary in this population. Many patients with chorea, and in particular HD, develop severe depression, psychosis, and dementia. Depression is at least twice that of the general population; a minimum estimate is 10% attempting suicide.[480,481] These are addressed with supportive and therapeutic medications. In view of the propensity for disabling and often life-threatening dysphagia, speech and swallowing therapy are important.

If chorea interferes with daily activities, specific treatment may be indicated; the FDA has approved tetrabenazine for treatment of Huntington disease.[482] Antidopaminergic agents can suppress the movements. Because antipsychotic drugs may induce tardive dyskinesia on top of chorea, it is preferable to prescribe tetrabenazine in countries where it is available.[483,485] Tetrabenazine is also preferred to the antipsychotic drugs because they block dopamine receptors. Non-antidopaminergic drugs have been used to partially suppress choreic movements. Clonazepam, valproate, and baclofen may be somewhat effective.

Sydenham's Chorea

The most common secondary chorea associated with infection is Sydenham's chorea,[471,485] due to the β-hemolytic streptococcus. The incidence of Sydenham's chorea has fallen dramatically with the introduction of antibiotics. Neurologic manifestations other than chorea may also be present; the most common is speech impairment, but encephalopathy, reflex changes, weakness, gait disturbance, headache, seizures, and cranial neuropathy also occur. The age at onset is predominantly between 5 and 15 years, but chorea can also occur in adults. Chorea is generalized in 81% and unilateral in 19% of cases. Duration ranges from 1 to 22 weeks, with a median of 12 weeks. Recurrence of chorea occurs in 20%. A rare patient may have chorea persisting lifelong. Residual behavioral and electroencephalograph (EEG) changes are not uncommon in Sydenham's chorea. Susceptibility to chorea gravidarum and chorea from oral contraceptives are sequelae of Sydenham's chorea.

The clinical features of the chorea in Sydenham's chorea differs from that of HD.[486] In Sydenham's the movements are usually more flowing, with a restless quality. In HD the movements tend to be more individualistic and jerky. Physiologic recordings in Sydenham's reveal the bursts of EMG activity to last more than 100 milliseconds and to occur asynchronously in antagonistic muscles.[487] This contrasts to HD, in which more frequent bursts of 10 to 30 milliseconds and 50 to 100 milliseconds occur.

Although Sydenham's chorea is classified under infectious etiologies (**Table 17.9**), it may have been more reasonable to list it in the category of an immunologic disorder. Immunoglobulin G (IgG) antibodies in sera from children with rheumatic fever reacted with neuronal cytoplasmic antigens of caudate and subthalamic nuclei. Antibodies to cardiolipin, which have been found in chorea associated with lupus erythematosus, have not been found in Sydenham's chorea.

Antidopaminergic drugs have been used successfully to suppress choreic movements in Sydenham's chorea, but it seems more prudent not to administer an agent that could potentially produce tardive dyskinesia or tardive dystonia. If treatment is necessary, a benzodiazepine or valproate may suffice. A brief course of corticosteroids may also provide some benefit in patients with Sydenham's chorea.

Systemic Lupus Erythematosus

Systemic lupus erythematosus (SLE) is a cause of secondary chorea, of immunologic etiology. Cardiolipin antibodies and antiphospholipid antibodies (lupus anticoagulant) have been found in SLE chorea. Chorea is intermittent in SLE. PET scans have not found caudate hypometabolism in contrast to other choreas. Treatment with antidopaminergics has been successful.

Vascular Chorea

The most common cause of secondary hemichorea is vascular, with infarction or hemorrhage in the contralateral subthalamic nucleus or multimicroinfarcts in the contralateral caudate nucleus. In rare instances it occurs bilaterally due to bilateral lacunae in the basal ganglia. Often these lesions produce very large amplitude choreic movements, which are referred to as ballism. These large-amplitude excursions are expressed by flinging and flailing movements with their involvement of proximal musculature. Because vascular hemiballism is usually self-limited, long-term treatment with an antichoreic drug is seldom necessary, and a course of 4 to 6 weeks is usually satisfactory. Because of the relatively rapid onset and safety profile when used in a controlled setting, tetrabenazine would be preferred to a dopamine receptor blocking agent that can induce tardive dyskinesia.

Drug-, Chemical-, and Toxin-Induced Chorea

A large number of drugs and chemicals can induce chorea. The most obvious are the monoaminergic agents, including levodopa, tricyclics and cerebral stimulants. The anticholinergics and antihistaminics are also widely reported to induce chorea. Toxins affecting the basal ganglia in particular, such as those that interfere with oxygenation like carbon monoxide, are also chemicals known for their ability to produce movement disorders such as chorea. Less well known is that lithium, anticonvulsants, mercury, methadone, and alcohol can induce chorea.

Metabolic-Disorder– and Endocrine-Disorder– Induced Chorea

Chorea gravidarum and chorea induced by birth control pills occur in those who previously had Sydenham's chorea. The end of the pregnancy and discontinuation of the oral contraceptives typically provide relief of the involuntary movements. Antichoreic drugs can also provide relief. A postmortem examination of a case of chorea gravidarum revealed neuronal loss and astrocytosis in the striatum.[490] Thyrotoxicosis and other metabolic diseases listed in **Table 17.9** can induce chorea.

Acanthocytosis

Acanthocytes (*acanthos* is Greek for thorny or spiny) are mature red cells with multiple[5-10] irregularly arranged thorn- or spur-like, spiny or blunt protrusions; they are not seen in bone marrow preparations.[441] This characteristic morphology is seen associated with a heterogeneous spectrum of disorders including neurodegenerative, or other medical conditions such as advanced hepatic disease, anorexia nervosa, postsplenectomy, advanced malnutrition, myxedema, panhypopituitarism, hypothyroidism, Wolman's disease, or spur cell anemia. Acanthocytes differ from echinocytes because the spicules are less numerous and less regular in size and orientation or distribution.[489] The distinction between acanthocytes and echinocytes may be obscured in dried blood smears, but is facilitated in wet smears or scanning electron microscopy.

Excluding those conditions associated with a deficiency of lipoproteins and associated with fat malabsorption,[490,492] neuroacanthocytosis (NA, also known as Vogt-Hopf syndrome, Levine syndrome, or chorea-acanthocytosis) was initially called Levine-Critchley syndrome after the initial report in Levine's abstract in 1960.[439,446,492] Early descriptions emphasized the hyperkinetic movement disorder including the presence of oral self-mutilation, lingual dystonia, and vocal and nonvocal tics; however, some cases have prominent symptoms of parkinsonism or amytrophy. Although generalized bradykinesia is uncommon in most reported cases, masked facies, dysarthria, dysphagia, and postural instability are common and characteristic, as in Huntington's chorea. Seizures, tics, and mild chorea may be presenting features, with epilepsy present in 40 to 73% of patients reported. Subtle personality changes, depression, and overt dementia may be present in up to 64% of patients.[446] Most authors accept >10% acanthocytes as necessary on peripheral blood smear; an occasional case has over 50% acanthocytes.[493] Serum creatinine kinase is commonly elevated. Although a modest elevation may be present (usually <100 U/L), some cases have levels as high as 1900 U/L or greater; elevations in lactate dehydrogenase and hepatic enzymes are frequently observed but are not invariable features. Electromyographic studies may be abnormal, consistent with peripheral axonal pathology. Neuroimaging demonstrates caudate atrophy, similar to that seen in HD. Recent advances in molecular genetics have helped to clarify the different etiologies and modes of inheritance of this genetic condition and include classical chorea-acanthocytosis (ChAc) due to mutation of the chorein protein,[494] X-linked McLeod syndrome (MLS) due to mutation of the *XK* gene on the X chromosome,[495] pantothenate kinase-associated neurodegeneration (PKAN, previously called Hallervorden-Spatz syndrome),[496] and Huntington disease-like 2 (HDL2).[446,497–499]

Treatment is symptomatic. Affected individuals, depending on genotype and phenotypic presentation, variably suffer from seizures, tics, chorea, dystonia, parkinsonism, oral self-mutilation, and dysphagia. Speech, occupational, and physical therapy should be individualized to maintain independence. Depression is important to treat when possible. Seizures are usually easy to control with monotherapy including diphenylhydantoin, carbamazepine, valproate, or phenobarbitol; carbamazepine may worsen involuntary movements. Hypokinesia is usually not as disabling as hyperkinesia. Hyperkinetic movements may respond to benzodiazepines (diazepam, clonazepam), phenothiazines (pimozide, haloperidol), and dopamine depletors (reserpine, tetrabenazine), although the latter may aggravate depression. Brenes et al[500] reported complete remission of one patient taking the calcium channel blocker verapamil; these results have not been replicated. Dysphagia may require a feeding gastrostomy; aspiration may cause death.

Laboratory Evaluation

When one encounters a patient with chorea, one must direct the workup considering the causes of chorea listed in **Table 17.9**. The *huntingtin* gene test is performed in most cases of insidious onset. The workup is directed to the symptoms and clinical course and may typically also include when appropriate a complete blood count (CBC), Sequential Multiple Analyzer Computer (SMAC-20) test, uric acid, erythrocyte sedimentation rate (ESR), serology, fresh blood smear search for acanthocytes, serum ceruloplasmin, slit-lamp examination for Kayser-Fleischer rings, urinalysis, triiodothyronine resin uptake (T3RU)/thyroxine (T4), antinuclear antibody (ANA), latex fixation, immunoglobulins, chorein, CT, MRI, glucose PET scan, thyroid studies, tests for pregnancy, antistreptolysin titer, neurophysiology (EEG, EMG, nerve conduction, evoked potentials), lysosomal enzymes on peripheral blood, α-fetoprotein, arterial blood gases, cerebrospinal fluid (CSF) lactate and pyruvate, electron microscopy of leukocytes and skin and conjuctival biopsy, and urine for quantitative organic acids and amino acids.

References

1. Movement Disorders. Neurologic Principles & Practice. 2nd ed. New York: McGraw-Hill; 2004
2. Parkinson's Disease and Movement Disorders. 4th ed. Baltimore: Lippincott Williams & Wilkins; 2002
3. Bogey RA, Elovic EP, Bryant PR, Geis CC, Moroz A, O'Neill BJ. Rehabilitation of movement disorders. Arch Phys Med Rehabil 2004;85(3, Suppl 1)S41–S45
4. Klein C. Movement disorders: classifications. J Inherit Metab Dis 2005;28:425–439
5. Fahn S. Parkinson's disease and other basal ganglion disorders. In: Asbury AK, McKhann GM, McDonald WI, eds. Diseases of the Nervous System: Clinical Neurobiology. Philadelphia: Ardmore Medical Books; 1986:1217–1228
6. Schoenberg BS. Epidemiology of Movement Disorders. London: Butterworths; 1987
7. Forno LS. Pathology of Parkinson's disease. In: Marsden CD, Fahn S, eds. Movement Disorders. London: Butterworth Scientific; 1982: 25–40
8. Chaudhuri KR, Healy DG, Schapira AH. Non-motor symptoms of Parkinson's disease: diagnosis and management. Lancet Neurol 2006; 5:235–245
9. Barbeau A, Roy M. Familial subsets in idiopathic Parkinson's disease. Can J Neurol Sci 1984;11:144–150
10. Klein C. Implications of genetics on the diagnosis and care of patients with Parkinson disease. Arch Neurol 2006;63:328–334
11. Barbeau A. Etiology of Parkinson's disease: a research strategy. Can J Neurol Sci 1984;11:24–28
12. Gsponer J, Vendruscolo M. Theoretical approaches to protein aggregation. Protein Pept Lett 2006;13:287–293
13. Smith ME, Ramig LO, Dromey C, Perez KS, Samandari R. Intensive voice treatment in Parkinson disease: laryngostroboscopic findings. J Voice 1995;9:453–459
14. Blumin JH, Pcolinsky DE, Atkins JP. Laryngeal findings in advanced Parkinson's disease. Ann Otol Rhinol Laryngol 2004;113:253–258
15. Darley FL, Aronson AE, Brown JR. Motor Speech Disorders. Philadelphia: WB Saunders; 1975

16. Logemann JA, Fisher H, Boshes B, Blonsky E. Frequency and cooccurrence of vocal tract dysfunctions in the speech of a large sample of Parkinson's patients. J Speech Hear Disord 1978;43:47–57

17. Perez KS, Ramig LO, Smith ME, Dromey C. The Parkinson larynx: tremor and videostroboscopic findings. J Voice 1996;10:354–361

18. Geser F, Wenning GK. The diagnosis of multiple system atrophy. J Neurol 2006;253(Suppl 3):iii2–iii15

19. Nagashima T, Oda M, Tanabe H, et al. Sleep apnea and sudden death in multiple system atrophy—polysomnographic studies and brain stem neuropathology. In: Togawa K, Katayama S, Hishikawa Y, Ohta Y, Horie T, eds. Sleep Apnea and Rhonchopathy. Basel: Karger; 1993:128–131

20. Silber MH, Levine S. Stridor and death in multiple system atrophy. Mov Disord 2000;15:699–704

21. Rajput A, Rajput AH. Parkinson's disease management strategies. Expert Rev Neurother 2006;6:91–99

22. Suchowersky O, Gronseth G, Perlmutter J, Reich S, Zesiewicz T, Weiner WJ. Practice parameter: neuroprotective strategies and alternative therapies for Parkinson disease (an evidence-based review): report of the Quality Standards Subcommittee of the American Academy of Neurology. Neurology 2006;66:976–982

23. Ramig LO, Sapir S, Countryman S, et al. Intensive voice treatment (LSVT) for patients with Parkinson's disease: a 2 year follow up. J Neurol Neurosurg Psychiatry 2001;71:493–498

24. Ramig LO, Sapir S, Fox C, Countryman S. Changes in vocal loudness following intensive voice treatment (LSVT) in individuals with Parkinson's disease: a comparison with untreated patients and normal age-matched controls. Mov Disord 2001;16:79–83

25. Ramig LO, Fox C, Sapir S. Parkinson's disease: speech and voice disorders and their treatment with the Lee Silverman Voice Treatment. Semin Speech Lang 2004;25:169–180

26. Liotti M, Ramig LO, Vogel D, et al. Hypophonia in Parkinson's disease: neural correlates of voice treatment revealed by PET. Neurology 2003;60:432–440

27. de Swart BJ, Willemse SC, Maassen BA, Horstink MW. Improvement of voicing in patients with Parkinson's disease by speech therapy. Neurology 2003;60:498–500

28. Boulton AA. Symptomatic and neuroprotective properties of the aliphatic propargylamines. Mech Ageing Dev 1999;111:201–209

29. Effect of deprenyl on the progression of disability in early Parkinson's disease. N Engl J Med 1989;321:1364–1371

30. Parkinson Study Group. A controlled, randomized, delayed-start study of rasagiline in early Parkinson disease. Arch Neurol 2004;61:561–566

31. Schapira AH. Disease modification in Parkinson's disease. Lancet Neurol 2004;3:362–368

32. Schapira AH, Olanow CW. Neuroprotection in Parkinson disease: mysteries, myths, and misconceptions. JAMA 2004;291:358–364

33. Djaldetti R, Koren M, Ziv I, Achiron A, Melamed E. Effect of cisapride on response fluctuations in Parkinson's disease. Mov Disord 1995;10:81–84

34. Goberman AM, Coelho C. Acoustic analysis of parkinsonian speech II: L-Dopa related fluctuations and methodological issues. NeuroRehabilitation 2002;17:247–254

35. Berke GS, Gerratt B, Kreiman J, Jackson K. Treatment of Parkinson hypophonia with percutaneous collagen augmentation. Laryngoscope 1999;109:1295–1299

36. Horsley V. The functions of the so-called motor areas of the brain. BMJ 1909;124:5–28

37. Meyers R. Surgical procedure for postencephalitic tremor, with notes on the physiology of premotor fibres. Arch Neurol Psychiatry 1940;44:455–457

38. Meyers R. Surgical experiments in therapy of certain 'extrapyramidal' diseases: current evaluation. Acta Psychiatr Neurol Suppl 1951;67:1–42

39. Cooper IS. Ligation of the anterior choroidal artery for involuntary movements of parkinsonism. Psychiatr Q 1953;27:317–319

40. Cooper IS. Dystonia musculorum deformans: natural history and neurosurgical alleviation. J Pediatr 1969;74:585–592

41. Cooper IS, Bravo G, Riklan M, Davidson N, Gorek E. Chemopallidectomy and chemothalamectomy for parkinsonism. Geriatrics 1958;13:127–147

42. DeLong MR, Wichmann T. Circuits and circuit disorders of the basal ganglia. Arch Neurol 2007;64:20–24

43. Abosch A, Lozano A. Stereotactic neurosurgery for movement disorders. Can J Neurol Sci 2003;30(Suppl 1):S72–S82

44. Tasker RR. Thalamotomy. Neurosurg Clin N Am 1990;1:841–864

45. Laitinen LV, Bergenheim AT, Hariz MI. Leksell's posteroventral pallidotomy in the treatment of Parkinson's disease. J Neurosurg 1992;76:53–61

46. Lozano AM, Lang AE, Galvez-Jimenez N, et al. Effect of gpi pallidotomy on motor function in Parkinson's disease. Lancet 1995;346:1383–1387

47. Benabid AL, Pollak P, Gervason C, et al. Long-term suppression of tremor by chronic stimulation of the ventral intermediate thalamic nucleus. Lancet 1991;337:403–406

48. Limousin P, Pollak P, Benazzouz A, et al. Bilateral subthalamic nucleus stimulation for severe Parkinson's disease. Mov Disord 1995;10:672–674

49. Kleiner-Fisman G, Herzog J, Fisman DN, et al. Subthalamic nucleus deep brain stimulation: summary and meta-analysis of outcomes. Mov Disord 2006;21(Suppl 14):S290–S304

50. Pahwa R, Factor SA, Lyons KE, et al. Practice Parameter: treatment of Parkinson disease with motor fluctuations and dyskinesia (an evidence-based review): report of the Quality Standards Subcommittee of the American Academy of Neurology. Neurology 2006;66:983–995

51. Madrazo I, Drucker-Colin R, Diaz V, Martinez-Mata J, Torres C, Becerril JJ. Open microsurgical autograft of adrenal medulla to the right caudate nucleus in two patients with intractable Parkinson's disease. N Engl J Med 1987;316:831–834

52. Goetz CG, Olanow CW, Koller WC, et al. Multicenter study of autologous adrenal medullary transplantation to the corpus striatum in patients with advanced Parkinson's disease. [see comments] N Engl J Med 1989;320:337–341

53. Olanow CW, Koller W, Goetz CG, et al. Autologous transplantation of adrenal medulla in Parkinson's disease. 18-month results. Arch Neurol 1990;47:1286–1289

54. Lindvall B, Olsson JE. Monoamine metabolites and neuropeptides in patients with Parkinson's disease, Huntington's chorea, Shy-Drager syndrome, and torsion dystonia. Adv Neurol 1990;53:117–122

55. Hauser RA, Freeman TB, Snow BJ, et al. Long-term evaluation of bilateral fetal nigral transplantation in Parkinson disease. Arch Neurol 1999;56:179–187

56. Kordower JH, Freeman TB, Snow BJ, et al. Neuropathological evidence of graft survival and striatal reinnervation after the transplantation of fetal mesencephalic tissue in a patient with Parkinson's disease. [see comments] N Engl J Med 1995;332:1118–1124

57. Kordower JH, Rosenstein JM, Collier TJ, et al. Functional fetal nigral grafts in a patient with Parkinson's disease: chemoanatomic, ultrastructural, and metabolic studies. J Comp Neurol 1996;370:203–230

58. Freed CR, Greene PE, Breeze RE, et al. Transplantation of embryonic dopamine neurons for severe Parkinson's disease. N Engl J Med 2001;344:710–719

59. Greene PE, Fahn S. Status of fetal tissue transplantation for the treatment of advanced Parkinson disease. Neurosurg Focus 2002;13:e3

60. Olanow CW, Goetz CG, Kordower JH, et al. A double-blind controlled trial of bilateral fetal nigral transplantation in Parkinson's disease. Ann Neurol 2003;54:403–414

61. Rousseaux M, Krystkowiak P, Kozlowski O, Ozsancak C, Blond S, Destee A. Effects of subthalamic nucleus stimulation on parkinsonian dysarthria and speech intelligibility. J Neurol 2004;251:327–334

62. Hardy J, Cookson MR, Singleton A. Genes and parkinsonism. Lancet Neurol 2003;2:221–228

63. Krack P, Batir A, Van BN, et al. Five-year follow-up of bilateral stimulation of the subthalamic nucleus in advanced Parkinson's disease. N Engl J Med 2003;349:1925–1934
64. Wang E, Verhagen ML, Bakay R, Arzbaecher J, Bernard B. The effect of unilateral electrostimulation of the subthalamic nucleus on respiratory/phonatory subsystems of speech production in Parkinson's disease–a preliminary report. Clin Linguist Phon 2003;17:283–289
65. Moretti R, Torre P, Antonello RM, et al. 'Speech initiation hesitation' following subthalamic nucleus stimulation in a patient with Parkinson's disease. Eur Neurol 2003;49:251–253
66. Farrell A, Theodoros D, Ward E, Hall B, Silburn P. Effects of neurosurgical management of Parkinson's disease on speech characteristics and oromotor function. J Speech Lang Hear Res 2005;48:5–20
67. Alvarez L, Macias R, Lopez G, et al. Bilateral subthalamotomy in Parkinson's disease: initial and long-term response. Brain 2005;128(Pt 3):570–583
68. Pinto S, Gentil M, Krack P, et al. Changes induced by levodopa and subthalamic nucleus stimulation on parkinsonian speech. Mov Disord 2005;20:1507–1515
69. Bruce BB, Foote KD, Rosenbek J, et al. Aphasia and thalamotomy: important issues. Stereotact Funct Neurosurg 2004;82:186–190
70. Fahn S. The varied clinical expressions of dystonia. Neurol Clin 1984;2:541–554
71. Nutt JG, Muenter MD, Aronson A, Kurland LT, Melton LJ III. Epidemiology of focal and generalized dystonia in Rochester, Minnesota. Mov Disord 1988;3:188–194
72. Fukuda H, Kusumi M, Nakashima K. Epidemiology of primary focal dystonias in the western area of tottori prefecture in Japan: comparison with prevalence evaluated in 1993. Mov Disord 2006;21:1503–1506
73. Asgeirsson H, Jakobsson F, Hjaltason H, Jonsdottir H, Sveinbjornsdottir S. Prevalence study of primary dystonia in Iceland. Mov Disord 2006;21:293–298
74. Traube L. Gesammelte Beitrage zur Pathologie und Physiologie. 2nd ed. Berlin: Verlag von August Hirschwald; 1871
75. Schnitzler J, Hajek M, Schnitzler A. Klinischer Atlas der Laryngologie. Nebst Anleitung zur Diagnose und Therapie der Krankheiten des Kehlkopfes und der Luftrohre. Wien und Leipzig: Wilhelm Braumuller; 1895
76. Gerhardt P. Bewegungsstoerungen der stimmbaender. Nothnagels Spezielle Pathologie Und Therapie. 1896;13:307
77. Fraenkel B. Ueber Beschaeftigungsneurosen der Stimme. Leipzig: G Thieme; 1887
78. Fraenkel B. Ueber die beschaeftigungsschwaeche der stimme: mogiphonie. Dtsch Med Wochenschr 1887;13:121–123
79. Gowers WR. Manual of Diseases of the Nervous System. 3rd ed. London: Churchill; 1899
80. Critchley M. Spastic dysphonia ("inspiratory speech"). Brain 1939;62:96–103
81. Bellussi G. Le disfonie impercinetiche. Atti Labor Fonet Univ Padova 1952;3:1
82. Aronson AE, Brown JR, Litin EM, Pearson JS. Spastic dysphonia. II. Comparison with essential (voice) tremor and other neurologic and psychogenic dysphonias. J Speech Hear Disord 1968;33:219–231
83. Aronson AE. Clinical Voice Disorders. New York: Thieme; 1985
84. Aronson AE, Hartman DE. Adductor spastic dysphonia as a sign of essential (voice) tremor. J Speech Hear Disord 1981;46:52–58
85. Blitzer A, Lovelace RE, Brin MF, Fahn S, Fink ME. Electromyographic findings in focal laryngeal dystonia (spastic dysphonia). Ann Otol Rhinol Laryngol 1985;94:591–594
86. Schaefer S, Watson B, Freeman F, et al. Vocal tract electromyographic abnormalities in spasmodic dysphonia preliminary report. Trans Am Laryngol Assoc 1987;108:187–196
87. Bloch P, Rio J. Neuro-psychiatric aspects of spastic dysphonia. Folia Phoniatr (Basel) 1965;17:301–364
88. Jacome DE, Yanez GF. Spastic dysphonia and Meigs disease. [letter] Neurology 1980;30:349
89. Marsden CD, Sheehy MP. Spastic dysphonia, Meige disease, and torsion dystonia. [letter] Neurology 1982;32:1202–1203
90. Golper LAC, Nutt JG, Rau MT, Coleman RO. Focal cranial dystonia. J Speech Hear Disord 1983;48:128–134
91. Blitzer A, Brin MF, Fahn S, Lovelace RE. Clinical and laboratory characteristics of focal laryngeal dystonia: study of 110 cases. Laryngoscope 1988;98:636–640
92. Chhetri DK, Blumin JH, Vinters HV, Berke GS. Histology of nerves and muscles in adductor spasmodic dysphonia. Ann Otol Rhinol Laryngol 2003;112:334–341
93. Blitzer A, Brin MF, Stewart CF. Botulinum toxin management of spasmodic dysphonia (laryngeal dystonia): a 12-year experience in more than 900 patients. Laryngoscope 1998;108:1435–1441
94. Grillone GA, Blitzer A, Brin MF, Annino DJ Jr, Saint-Hilaire MH. Treatment of adductor laryngeal breathing dystonia with botulinum toxin type A. Laryngoscope 1994;104:30–32
95. Brin MF, Blitzer A, Braun N, Stewart C, Fahn S. Respiratory and obstructive laryngeal dystonia treatment with botulinum toxin (Botox). Neurology 1991;41(Suppl 1):293
96. Baer JW, Braun N, Brin MF, Stewart C, Austin J, Blitzer A. Disordered diaphragmatic motion in patients with cranial dystonia: a fluoroscopic study. Neurology 1992;42(Suppl 3):240
97. Braun N, Abd A, Baer J, Blitzer A, Stewart C, Brin M. Dyspnea in dystonia. A functional evaluation. Chest 1995;107:1309–1316
98. Chitkara A, Meyer T, Keidar A, Blitzer A. Singer's dystonia: first report of a variant of spasmodic dysphonia. Ann Otol Rhinol Laryngol 2006;115:89–92
99. Jahanshahi M. Factors that ameliorate or aggravate spasmodic torticollis. J Neurol Neurosurg Psychiatry 2000;68:227–229
100. Wissel J, Muller J, Ebersbach G, Poewe W. Trick maneuvers in cervical dystonia: investigation of movement- and touch-related changes in polymyographic activity. Mov Disord 1999;14:994–999
101. Greene PE, Bressman S. Exteroceptive and interoceptive stimuli in dystonia. Mov Disord 1998;13:549–551
102. Aronson AE, Peterson HW, Litin EM. Voice symptomatology in functional dysphonia and aphonia. J Speech Hear Disord 1964;29:367–380
103. Meige H. Les convulsions de la face: une forme clinique de convulsions faciales, bilaterale et mediane. Rev Neurol (Paris) 1910;21:437–443
104. Tolosa E, Marti MJ. Blepharospasm-oromandibular dystonia syndrome (Meige's syndrome): clinical aspects. Adv Neurol 1988;49:73–84
105. Ludlow CL, Hallett M, Sedory SE, Fujita M, Naunton RF. The pathophysiology of spasmodic dysphonia and its modification by botulinum toxin. In: Berardelli A, Benecke R, Manfredi M, Marsden CM, eds. Motor Disturbances II. New York: Academic Press; 1990:273–288
106. Zwirner P, Murry T, Swenson M, Wooodson G. Effects of botulinum toxin therapy in patients with adductor spasmodic dysphonia: acoustic, aerodynamic, and videoendoscopic findings. Laryngoscope 1992;102:400–406
107. Brin MF, Blitzer A, Stewart C, Fahn S. Treatment of spasmodic dysphonia (laryngeal dystonia) with local injections of botulinum toxin: review and technical aspects. In: Blitzer A, Brin MF, Sasaki CT, Fahn S, Harris KS, eds. Neurological Disorders of the Larynx. New York: Thieme; 1992:214–228
108. Filippi GM, Errico P, Santarelli R, Bagolini B, Manni E. Botulinum-A toxin effects on rat jaw muscle spindles. Acta Otolaryngol 1993;113:400–404
109. Borg-Stein J, Pine ZM, Miller JR, Brin MF. Botulinum toxin for the treatment of spasticity in multiple sclerosis. New observations. Am J Phys Med Rehabil 1993;72:364–368
110. Kaji R, Rothwell JC, Katayama M, et al. Tonic vibration reflex and muscle afferent block in writer's cramp. Ann Neurol 1995;38:155–162
111. Kaji R, Kohara N, Katayama M, et al. Muscle afferent block by intramuscular injection of lidocaine for the treatment of writer's cramp. Muscle Nerve 1995;18:234–235

112. Kaji R, Shibasaki H, Kimura J. Writer's cramp: a disorder of motor subroutine? [editorial; comment] Ann Neurol 1995;38:837–838
113. Kaji R, Mezaki T, Kubori T, Murase N, Kimura J. Treatment of spasticity with botulinum toxin and muscle afferent block. Rinsho Shinkeigaku 1996;36:1334–1335
114. Yoshida K, Kaji R, Kubori T, Kohara N, Iizuka T, Kimura J. Muscle afferent block for the treatment of oromandibular dystonia. Mov Disord 1998;13:699–705
115. Mezaki T, Kaji R, Hirota N, Kohara N, Kimura J. Treatment of spasticity with muscle afferent block. Neurology 1999;53:1156–1157
116. Hallett M. Physiology of dystonia. Adv Neurol 1998;78:11–18
117. Murase N, Shimadu H, Urushihara R, Kaji R. Abnormal sensorimotor integration in hand dystonia. Suppl Clin Neurophysiol 2006;59:283–287
118. Kaji R, Urushihara R, Murase N, Shimazu H, Goto S. Abnormal sensory gating in basal ganglia disorders. J Neurol 2005;252(Suppl 4):IV13–IV16
119. Martin JP. The Basal Ganglia and Posture. London: Pitman Medical (& JP Lippincott); 1967
120. Riess T, Weghorst S. Augmented reality in the treatment of Parkinson's disease. In: Morgan K, Satava RM, Sieburg HB, Mattheus R, Christensen JP, eds. In: Proceedings of Medicine Meets Virtual Reality 95: Interactive Technology and the New Paradigm for Health Care. Amsterdam: IOS Press; 1995:298–302
121. Tolosa ES. Clinical features of Meige's disease (idiopathic orofacial dystonia). A report of 17 cases. Arch Neurol 1981;38:147–151
122. Brin MF, Fahn S, Bressman SB, Burke RE. Dystonia precipitated by peripheral trauma. Neurology 1986;36(Suppl 1):119
123. Jankovic J. Can peripheral trauma induce dystonia and other movement disorders? Yes! Mov Disord 2001;16:7–12
124. O'Riordan S, Hutchinson M. Cervical dystonia following peripheral trauma—a case-control study. J Neurol 2004;251:150–155
125. Weiner WJ. Can peripheral trauma induce dystonia? No! Mov Disord 2001;16:13–22
126. Chan J, Brin M, Fahn S. Idiopathic cervical dystonia: clinical characteristics. Mov Disord 1991;6:119–126
127. Jankovic J, Leder S, Warner D, Schwartz K. Cervical dystonia: clinical findings and associated movement disorders. Neurology 1991;41:1088–1091
128. Samii A, Pal PK, Schulzer M, Mak E, Tsui JK. Post-traumatic cervical dystonia: a distinct entity? Can J Neurol Sci 2000;27:55–59
129. Sa DS, Mailis-Gagnon A, Nicholson K, Lang AE. Posttraumatic painful torticollis. Mov Disord 2003;18:1482–1491
130. Teoh KH, Christakis GT, Weisel RD, et al. Dipyridamole preserved platelets and reduced blood loss after cardiopulmonary bypass. J Thorac Cardiovasc Surg 1988;96:332–341
131. Schaefer SD. Neuropathology of spasmodic dysphonia. Laryngoscope 1983;93:1183–1204
132. Frucht S, Fahn S, Ford B. Focal task-specific dystonia induced by peripheral trauma. Mov Disord 2000;15:348–350
133. Hollinger P, Burgunder J. Posttraumatic focal dystonia of the shoulder. Eur Neurol 2000;44:153–155
134. Sankhla C, Lai EC, Jankovic J. Peripherally induced oromandibular dystonia. J Neurol Neurosurg Psychiatry 1998;65:722–728
135. Schicatano EJ, Basso MA, Evinger C. Animal model explains the origins of the cranial dystonia benign essential blepharospasm. J Neurophysiol 1997;77:2842–2846
136. Evinger C. Animal models of focal dystonia. NeuroRx 2005;2:513–524
137. Byl N, Wilson F, Merzenich M, et al. Sensory dysfunction associated with repetitive strain injuries of tendinitis and focal hand dystonia: a comparative study. J Orthop Sports Phys Ther 1996;23:234–244
138. Schott GD. The relationship of peripheral trauma and pain to dystonia. J Neurol Neurosurg Psychiatry 1985;48:698–701
139. Fahn S, Williams DT. Psychogenic dystonia. Adv Neurol 1988;50:431–455
140. Fahn S. Psychogenic movement disorders. In: Marsden CD, Fahn S, eds. Movement Disorders 3. Oxford: Butterworth-Heinemann; 1994:359–372
141. Reich SG. Psychogenic movement disorders. Semin Neurol 2006;26:289–296
142. Leventon G, Man A, Floru S. Isolated psychogenic palatal myoclonus as a cause of objective tinnitus. Acta Otolaryngol 1968;65:391–396
143. Munhoz RP, Lang AE. Gestes antagonistes in psychogenic dystonia. Mov Disord 2004;19:331–332
144. Pearce J. Palatal myoclonus. Proc R Soc Med 1969;62:267
145. Shale H, Fahn S, Koller WC, Lang AE. What is it? Case 1, 1987: unusual tremors, bradykinesia, and cerebral lucencies. Mov Disord 1987;2:321–338
146. Krem MM. Motor conversion disorders reviewed from a neuropsychiatric perspective. J Clin Psychiatry 2004;65:783–790
147. Bentivoglio AR, Loi M, Valente EM, Ialongo T, Tonali P, Albanese A. Phenotypic variability of DYT1-PTD: does the clinical spectrum include psychogenic dystonia? Mov Disord 2002;17:1058–1063
148. Rao DB, Kataria MS. A case of "palato-pharyngeal myoclonus". Gerontol Clin (Basel) 1969;11:165–168
149. Schrag A, Trimble M, Quinn N, Bhatia K. The syndrome of fixed dystonia: an evaluation of 103 patients. Brain 2004;127(Pt 10):2360–2372
150. Espay AJ, Morgante F, Purzner J, Gunraj CA, Lang AE, Chen R. Cortical and spinal abnormalities in psychogenic dystonia. Ann Neurol 2006;59:825–834
151. Bramstedt KA, Ford PJ. Protecting human subjects in neurosurgical trials: the challenge of psychogenic dystonia. Contemp Clin Trials 2006;27:161–164
152. Hinson VK, Cubo E, Comella CL, Goetz CG, Leurgans S. Rating scale for psychogenic movement disorders: scale development and clinimetric testing. Mov Disord 2005;20:1592–1597
153. Friedman A, Fahn S. Spontaneous remissions in spasmodic torticollis. Neurology 1986;36:398–400
154. Jayne D, Lees AJ, Stern GM. Remission in spasmodic torticollis. J Neurol Neurosurg Psychiatry 1984;47:1236–1237
155. Koufman JA, Blalock PD. Functional voice disorders. Otolaryngol Clin North Am 1991;24:1059–1073
156. Morrison MD, Nichol H, Rammage LA. Diagnostic criteria in functional dysphonia. Laryngoscope 1986;96:1–8
157. Altman KW, Atkinson C, Lazarus C. Current and emerging concepts in muscle tension dysphonia: a 30-month review. J Voice 2005;19:261–267
158. Angsuwarangsee T, Morrison M. Extrinsic laryngeal muscular tension in patients with voice disorders. J Voice 2002;16:333–343
159. Sama A, Carding PN, Price S, Kelly P, Wilson JA. The clinical features of functional dysphonia. Laryngoscope 2001;111:458–463
160. Belafsky PC, Postma GN, Reulbach TR, Holland BW, Koufman JA. Muscle tension dysphonia as a sign of underlying glottal insufficiency. Otolaryngol Head Neck Surg 2002;127:448–451
161. Roy N, Smith ME, Allen B, Merrill RM. Adductor spasmodic dysphonia versus muscle tension dysphonia: examining the diagnostic value of recurrent laryngeal nerve lidocaine block. Ann Otol Rhinol Laryngol 2007;116:161–168
162. Roy N, Gouse M, Mauszycki SC, Merrill RM, Smith ME. Task specificity in adductor spasmodic dysphonia versus muscle tension dysphonia. Laryngoscope 2005;115:311–316
163. Sapienza CM, Walton S, Murry T. Adductor spasmodic dysphonia and muscular tension dysphonia: acoustic analysis of sustained phonation and reading. J Voice 2000;14:502–520

164. Bhalla RK, Wallis J, Kaushik V, Carpentier JP. How we do it: adjunctive intravenous midazolam: diagnosis and treatment of therapy-resistant muscle tension dysphonia. Clin Otolaryngol 2005;30:367–369

165. Fahn S. Generalized dystonia: concept and treatment. Clin Neuropharmacol 1986;9(Suppl 2):S37–S48

166. Ozelius L, Kramer PL, Moskowitz CB, et al. Human gene for torsion dystonia located on chromosome 9q32-q34. Neuron 1989;2:1427–1434

167. Bressman SB, de Leon D, Kramer PL, et al. Dystonia in Ashkenazi Jews: clinical characterization of a founder mutation. Ann Neurol 1994;36:771–777

168. Ozelius LJ, Hewett JW, Page CE, et al. The gene (DYT1) for early-onset torsion dystonia encodes a novel protein related to the Clp protease/heat shock family. Adv Neurol 1998;78:93–105

169. Risch NJ, Bressman SB, deLeon D, et al. Segregation analysis of idiopathic torsion dystonia in Ashkenazi Jews suggests autosomal dominant inheritance. Am J Hum Genet 1990;46:533–538

170. Klein C, Brin MF, de Leon D, et al. De novo mutations (GAG deletion) in the DYT1 gene in two non-Jewish patients with early-onset dystonia. Hum Mol Genet 1998;7:1133–1136

171. Kramer PL, de Leon D, Ozelius L, et al. Dystonia gene in Ashkenazi Jewish population is located on chromosome 9q32–34. [see comments] Ann Neurol 1990;27:114–120

172. Ozelius LJ, Kramer PL, de Leon D, et al. Strong allelic association between the torsion dystonia gene (DYT1) and loci on chromosome 9q34 in Ashkenazi Jews. Am J Hum Genet 1992;50:619–628

173. Rostasy K, Augood SJ, Hewett JW, et al. TorsinA protein and neuropathology in early onset generalized dystonia with GAG deletion. Neurobiol Dis 2003;12:11–24

174. Ozelius LJ, Hewett JW, Page CE, et al. The early-onset torsion dystonia gene (DYT1) encodes an ATP-binding protein. Nat Genet 1997;17:40–48

175. Goodchild RE, Kim CE, Dauer WT. Loss of the dystonia-associated protein torsinA selectively disrupts the neuronal nuclear envelope. Neuron 2005;48:923–932

176. Hewett JW, Kamm C, Boston H, et al. TorsinB-perinuclear location and association with torsinA. J Neurochem 2004;89:1186–1194

177. Naismith TV, Heuser JE, Breakefield XO, Hanson PI. TorsinA in the nuclear envelope. Proc Natl Acad Sci U S A 2004;101:7612–7617

178. Gonzalez-Alegre P, Paulson HL. Aberrant cellular behavior of mutant torsinA implicates nuclear envelope dysfunction in DYT1 dystonia. J Neurosci 2004;24:2593–2601

179. Bressman S. Genetics of dystonia. J Neural Transm Suppl 2006;70: 489–495

180. Klein C, Brin MF, Kramer P, et al. Association of a missense change in the D2 dopamine receptor with myoclonus dystonia. Proc Natl Acad Sci U S A 1999;96:5173–5176

181. Zimprich A, Grabowski M, Asmus F, et al. Mutations in the gene encoding varepsilon-sarcoglycan cause myoclonus-dystonia syndrome. Nat Genet 2001;29:66–69

182. Hess CW, Raymond D, Aguiar PC, et al. Myoclonus-dystonia, obsessive-compulsive disorder, and alcohol dependence in SGCE mutation carriers. Neurology 2007;68:522–524

183. Yokoi F, Dang MT, Li J, Li Y. Myoclonus, motor deficits, alterations in emotional responses and monoamine metabolism in epsilon-sarcoglycan deficient mice. J Biochem 2006;140:141–146

184. McKusick VA. Online Mendelian Inheritance in Man (OMIM). http://www ncbi nlm nih gov/sites/entrez?db=omim 2008; http://www.ncbi.nlm.nih.gov/sites/entrez?db=omim

185. de Leon D, Brin MF, Blitzer A, Heiman G, Fahn S. Genetic factors in spastic dysphonia. Neurology 1990;40(Suppl 1):142

186. Tempel LW, Perlmutter JS. Abnormal vibration-induced cerebral blood flow responses in idiopathic dystonia. Brain 1990;113:691–707

187. Perlmutter JS, Raichle ME. Pure hemidystonia with basal ganglion abnormalities on positron emission tomography. Ann Neurol 1984; 15:228–233

188. Playford ED, Rassingham RE, Marsden CD, Brooks DJ. Abnormal activation of striatum and dorsolateral prefontal cortex in dystonia. Neurology 1992;42(Suppl 3):377 Ref Type

189. Takahashi H, Snow B, Waters C, et al. Evidence for nigrostriatal lesions in Lubag (X-linked dystonia- parkinsonism in the Philippines). Neurology 1992;42(Suppl 3):441

190. Fahn S, Moskowitz C. X-Linked recessive dystonia and parkinsonism in Filipino males. Ann Neurol 1988;24:179

191. Wilhelmsen KC, Weeks DE, Nygaard TG, et al. Genetic mapping of the "Lubag" (X-linked dystonia-parkinsonism) in a Filipino kindred to the pericentromeric region of the X chromosome. Ann Neurol 1991;29:124–131

192. Eidelberg D, Moeller JR, Ishikawa T, et al. The metabolic topography of idiopathic torsion dystonia. Brain 1995;118(Pt 6):1473–1484

193. Trost M, Carbon M, Edwards C, et al. Primary dystonia: is abnormal functional brain architecture linked to genotype? Ann Neurol 2002;52:853–856

194. Asanuma K, Ma Y, Huang C, et al. The metabolic pathology of dopa-responsive dystonia. Ann Neurol 2005;57:596–600

195. Asanuma K, Carbon-Correll M, Eidelberg D. Neuroimaging in human dystonia. J Med Invest 2005;52(Suppl):272–279

196. Obeso JA, Gimenez Roldan S. Clinicopathological correlation in symptomatic dystonia. Adv Neurol 1988;50:113–122

197. Marsden CD, Obeso JA, Zarranz JJ, Lang AE. The anatomical basis of symptomatic hemidystonia. Brain 1985;108:463–483

198. Narbona J, Obeso JA, Tunon T, Martinez Lage JM, Marsden CD. Hemidystonia secondary to localized basal ganglia tumour. J Neurol Neurosurg Psychiatry 1984;47:704–709

199. Jankovic J, Patel SC. Blepharospasm associated with brainstem lesions. Neurology 1983;33:1237–1240

200. Zweig RM, Hedreen JC. Brain stem pathology in cranial dystonia. Adv Neurol 1988;49:395–407

201. Hedreen JC, Zweig RM, DeLong MR, Whitehouse PJ, Price DL. Primary dystonias: a review of the pathology and suggestions for new directions of study. Adv Neurol 1988;50:123–132

202. Bhatia KP, Marsden CD. The behavioural and motor consequences of focal lesions of the basal ganglia in man. Brain 1994;117:859–876

203. Walker RH, Purohit DP, Good PF, Perl DP, Brin MF. Severe generalized dystonia due to primary putaminal degeneration: case report and review of the literature. Mov Disord 2002;17:576–584

204. Berkovic SF, Karpati G, Carpenter S, Lang AE. Progressive dystonia with bilateral putaminal hypodensities. Arch Neurol 1987;44: 1184–1187

205. Novotny EJ Jr, Singh G, Wallace DC, et al. Leber's disease and dystonia: a mitochondrial disease. Neurology 1986;36:1053–1060

206. Bruyn GW, Vielvoye GJ, Went LN. Hereditary spastic dystonia: a new mitochondrial encephalopathy? Putaminal necrosis as a diagnostic sign. J Neurol Sci 1991;103:195–202

207. Nigro MA, Martens ME, Awerbuch GI, Peterson PL, Lee CP. Partial cytochrome b deficiency and generalized dystonia. Pediatr Neurol 1990;6:407–410

208. Donnet A, Guinot H, Pellissier JF, et al. Segmental dystonia and mitochondrial encephalomyopathy. Rev Neurol (Paris) 1992;148:51–53

209. Benecke R, Strumper P, Weiss H. Electron transfer complex I defect in idiopathic dystonia. Ann Neurol 1992;32:683–686

210. Jun AS, Brown MD, Wallace DC. A mitochondrial DNA mutation at np 14459 of the ND6 gene associated with maternally inherited Leber's Hereditary Optic Neuropathy and dystonia. Proc Natl Acad Sci U S A 1994;91:6206–6210

211. McNaught KS, Kapustin A, Jackson T, et al. Brainstem pathology in DYT1 primary torsion dystonia. Ann Neurol 2004;56:540–547

212. Jankovic J, Svendsen CN, Bird ED. Brain neurotransmitters in dystonia. N Engl J Med 1987;316:278–279

213. de Yebenes JG, Brin MF, Mena MA, et al. Neurochemical findings in neuroacanthocytosis. Mov Disord 1988;3:300–312
214. Brin MF. Treatment of dystonia. In: Jankovic J, Tolosa E, eds. Parkinson's Disease and Movement Disorders. New York: Williams & Wilkins; 1998:553–578
215. Nygaard TG, Trugman JM, de Yebenes JG, Fahn S. Dopa-responsive dystonia: the spectrum of clinical manifestations in a large North American family. Neurology 1990;40:66–69
216. Fletcher NA, Holt IJ, Harding AE, Nygaard TG, Mallet J, Marsden CD. Tyrosine hydroxylase and levodopa responsive dystonia. J Neurol Neurosurg Psychiatry 1989;52:112–114
217. Burke RE, Fahn S, Marsden CD. Torsion dystonia: a double-blind, prospective trial of high-dosage trihexyphenidyl. Neurology 1986;36:160–164
218. Costa J, Espirito-Santo C, Borges A, Ferreira J, Coelho M, Sampaio C. Botulinum toxin type A versus anticholinergics for cervical dystonia. Cochrane Database Syst Rev 2005; :CD004312
219. Greene P, Shale H, Fahn S. Analysis of open-label trials in torsion dystonia using high dosages of anticholinergics and other drugs. Mov Disord 1988;3:46–60
220. Adler CH. Strategies for controlling dystonia. Overview of therapies that may alleviate symptoms. Postgrad Med 2000;108:151–159
221. Starr PA, Turner RS, Rau G, et al. Microelectrode-guided implantation of deep brain stimulators into the globus pallidus internus for dystonia: techniques, electrode locations, and outcomes. J Neurosurg 2006;104:488–501
222. Bittar RG, Yianni J, Wang S, et al. Deep brain stimulation for generalised dystonia and spasmodic torticollis. J Clin Neurosci 2005;12:12–16
223. Chou KL, Hurtig HI, Jaggi JL, Baltuch GH. Bilateral subthalamic nucleus deep brain stimulation in a patient with cervical dystonia and essential tremor. Mov Disord 2005;20:377–380
224. Halbig TD, Gruber D, Kopp UA, Schneider GH, Trottenberg T, Kupsch A. Pallidal stimulation in dystonia: effects on cognition, mood, and quality of life. J Neurol Neurosurg Psychiatry 2005;76:1713–1716
225. Vidailhet M, Vercueil L, Houeto JL, et al. Bilateral deep-brain stimulation of the globus pallidus in primary generalized dystonia. N Engl J Med 2005;352:459–467
226. Bressman SB, Greene PE. Treatment of hyperkinetic movement disorders. Neurol Clin 1990;8:51–75
227. Dedo HH, Izdebski K. Intermediate results of 306 recurrent laryngeal nerve sections for spastic dysphonia. Laryngoscope 1983;93:9–16
228. Aronson AE, DeSanto LW. Adductor spastic dysphonia: 1 1/2 years after recurrent laryngeal nerve resection. Ann Otol Rhinol Laryngol 1981;90:2–6
229. Aronson AE, De Santo LW. Adductor spastic dysphonia: three years after recurrent laryngeal nerve resection. Laryngoscope 1983;93:1–8
230. Isshiki N, Tsuji DH, Yamamoto Y, Iizuka Y. Midline lateralization thyroplasty for adductor spasmodic dysphonia. Ann Otol Rhinol Laryngol 2000;109:187–193
231. Chan SW, Baxter M, Oates J, Yorston A. Long-term results of type II thyroplasty for adductor spasmodic dysphonia. Laryngoscope 2004;114:1604–1608
232. Koufman JA, Rees CJ, Halum SL, Blalock D. Treatment of adductor-type spasmodic dysphonia by surgical myectomy: a preliminary report. Ann Otol Rhinol Laryngol 2006;115:97–102
233. Shaw GY, Sechtem PR, Rideout B. Posterior cricoarytenoid myoplasty with medialization thyroplasty in the management of refractory abductor spasmodic dysphonia. Ann Otol Rhinol Laryngol 2003;112:303–306
234. Berke GS, Blackwell KE, Gerratt BR, Verneil A, Jackson KS, Sercarz JA. Selective laryngeal adductor denervation-reinnervation: a new surgical treatment for adductor spasmodic dysphonia. Ann Otol Rhinol Laryngol 1999;108:227–231
235. Brin MF, Fahn S, Moskowitz C, et al. Localized injections of botulinum toxin for the treatment of focal dystonia and hemifacial spasm. Mov Disord 1987;2:237–254
236. American Academy of Neurology. Assessment: the clinical usefulness of botulinum toxin-A in treating neurologic disorders. Report of the Therapeutics and Technology Assessment Subcommittee of the American Academy of Neurology. Neurology 1990;40:1332–1336
237. AAO-HNS. American Academy of Otolaryngology–Head and Neck Surgery Policy Statement: Botox for spasmodic dysphonia. AAO-HNS Bull 1990;9:8
238. National Institutes of Health Concensus Development Conference. Clinical use of botulinum toxin. National Institutes of Health Consensus Development Statement, November 12–14, 1990. Arch Neurol 1991;48:1294–1298
239. Botulinum-A toxin for ocular muscle disorders. Lancet 1986;1:76–77
240. American Academy of Ophthalmology. Botulinum toxin therapy of eye muscle disorders: safety and effectiveness. Ophthalmology 1989;96(part 2):37–41
241. Jankovic J, Brin M. Therapeutic uses of botulinum toxin. N Engl J Med 1991;324:1186–1194
242. Brin MF. Interventional neurology: treatment of neurological conditions with local injection of botulinum toxin. Arch Neurobiol (Madr) 1991;54:173–189
243. Kenney C, Jankovic J. Tetrabenazine in the treatment of hyperkinetic movement disorders. Expert Rev Neurother 2006;6:7–17
244. Paleacu D, Giladi N, Moore O, Stern A, Honigman S, Badarny S. Tetrabenazine treatment in movement disorders. Clin Neuropharmacol 2004;27:230–233
245. Jankovic J. Dystonia: medical therapy and botulinum toxin. Adv Neurol 2004;94:275–286
246. Fahn S. Systemic therapy of dystonia. Can J Neurol Sci 1987;14:528–532
247. Brin MF. Pharmacological treatment of movement disorders. In: Germano I, ed. Neurosurgical Treatment of Movement Disorders. Lebanon: American Associaton of Neurological Surgeons; 1998:83–104
248. Albright AL, Turner M, Pattisapu JV. Best-practice surgical techniques for intrathecal baclofen therapy. J Neurosurg 2006; 104(4, Suppl) 233–239
249. Dykstra DD, Mendez A, Chappuis D, Baxter T, DesLauriers L, Stuckey M. Treatment of cervical dystonia and focal hand dystonia by high cervical continuously infused intrathecal baclofen: a report of 2 cases. Arch Phys Med Rehabil 2005;86:830–833
250. Dachy B, Dan B. Electrophysiological assessment of the effect of intrathecal baclofen in dystonic children. Clin Neurophysiol 2004;115:774–778
251. Albright AL, Barry MJ, Shafton DH, Ferson SS. Intrathecal baclofen for generalized dystonia. Dev Med Child Neurol 2001;43:652–657
252. Walker RH, Swope D, Danisi FO, Germano IM, Goodman RR, Brin MF. Intrathecal baclofen therapy for dystonia. Neurology 1999;52 (Suppl 2):A521
253. Kumar R, Dagher A, Hutchison WD, Lang AE, Lozano AM. Globus pallidus deep brain stimulation for generalized dystonia: clinical and PET investigation. Neurology 1999;53:871–874
254. Yoshor D, Hamilton WJ, Ondo W, Jankovic J, Grossman RG. Comparison of thalamotomy and pallidotomy for the treatment of dystonia. Neurosurgery 2001;48:818–824
255. Marks WJ. Deep brain stimulation for dystonia. Curr Treat Options Neurol 2005;7:237–243
256. Tagliati M, Shils J, Sun C, Alterman R. Deep brain stimulation for dystonia. Expert Rev Med Devices 2004;1:33–41
257. FDA. Medtronic Activa Dystonia Therapy–H020007, 2003
258. Gresty MA, Findley LJ. Definition, analysis and genesis of tremor. In: Findley LJ, Capildeo R, eds. Movement Disorders: Tremor. New York: Oxford University Press; 1984:15–26
259. DeJong RN. The Neurologic Examination. 3rd ed. New York: Hueber; 1967
260. Jankovic J. Tremors: pathophysiology, differential diagnosis and pharmacology. Neuro Cons 1984;2:1–8

261. Marsden CD, Obeso JA, Rothwell JC. Benign essential tremor is not a single entity. In: Yahr MD, ed. Current Concepts in Parkinson's Disease. Amsterdam: Excerpta Medica; 1983

262. Brown JR, Simonson J. Organic voice tremor: a tremor of phonation. Neurology 1963;13:520–525

263. Marsden CD. Origins of normal and pathological tremor. In: Findley LJ, Capildeo R, eds. Movement Disorders: Tremor. New York: Oxford University Press; 1984:37–84

264. Hartman DE, Overholt SL, Vishwanat B. A case of vocal cord nodules masking essential (voice) tremor. Arch Otolaryngol 1982; 108:52–53

265. Koller W, Graner D, Mlcoch A. Essential voice tremor: treatment with propranolol. Neurology 1985;35:106–108

266. Critchley M. Observations on essential (heredo-familial) tremor. Brain 1949;72:113–139

267. Hachinski VC, Thomsen IV, Buch NH. The nature of primary vocal tremor. Can J Neurol Sci 1975;2:195–197

268. Tomoda H, Shibasaki H, Huroda Y, Shin T. Voice tremor: dysregulation of voluntary expiratory muscles. Neurology 1987;37:117–122

269. Lebrun Y, Devreux F, Rousseau JJ, Darimont P. Tremulous speech. A case report. Folia Phoniatr (Basel) 1982;34:134–142

270. Ardran G, Kinsbourne M, Rushworth G. Dysphonia due to tremor. J Neurol Neurosurg Psychiatry 1966;29:219–223

271. Findley LJ, Gresty M. Head facial and voice tremor. Adv Neurol 1988; 49:239–253

272. Barkmeier JM, Case JL, Ludlow CL. Identification of symptoms for spasmodic dysphonia and vocal tremor: a comparison of expert and nonexpert judges. J Commun Disord 2001;34:21–37

273. Ludlow CL, Bassich C, Connor N, Coulter D. Phonatory characteristics of vocal fold tremor. J Phon 1986;14:509–515

274. Ramig LA, Shipp T. Comparative measures of vocal tremor and vocal vibrato. J Voice 1987;1:162–167

275. Hunker C, Abbs J. Physiological analysis of parkinsonian tremors in the oral facial system. In: The Dysarthrias. San Diego: College Hill Press; 1984:69–100

276. Freund HJ, Dietz V. The relationship between physiological and pathological tremor in physiological tremor, pathological tremor and clonus. In: Desmedt J, ed. Progress in Clinical Neurophysiology. Basel: S. Karger; 1978:66–89

277. Philippbar SA, Robin DA, Luschei ES. Limb, jaw and vocal tremor in Parkinson's patients. In: Yorkston K, Beukelman D, eds. Recent Advances in Clinical Dysarthria. San Diego: College Hill Press; 1991

278. Kimaid PA, Quagliato EM, Crespo AN, Wolf A, Viana MA, Resende LA. Laryngeal electromyography in movement disorders: preliminary data. Arq Neuropsiquiatr 2004;62:741–744

279. Maronian NC, Robinson L, Waugh P, Hillel AD. A new electromyographic definition of laryngeal synkinesis. Ann Otol Rhinol Laryngol 2004;113:877–886

280. Maronian NC, Waugh PF, Robinson L, Hillel AD. Tremor laryngeal dystonia: treatment of the lateral cricoarytenoid muscle. Ann Otol Rhinol Laryngol 2004;113:349–355

281. Critchley E. Clinical manifestations of essential tremor. J Neurol Neurosurg Psychiatry 1972;35:365–372

282. Davis CH, Kunkle CE, Durham NC. Benign essential (heredofamilial) tremor. Trans Am Neurol Assoc 1951;56:87–89

283. Marshall J. Pathology of tremor. In: Findley LJ, Capildeo R, eds. Movement Disorders: Tremor. New York: Oxford University Press; 1984: 95–123

284. Marshall J. Observations on essential tremor. J Neurol Neurosurg Psychiatry 1962;25:122–125

285. Findley LJ. Essential tremor: introductory remarks. In: Findley LJ, Capildeo R, eds. Movement Disorders: Tremor. New York: Oxford University Press; 1984:207–209

286. Deuschl G, Bain P, Brin M. Consensus statement of the Movement Disorder Society on Tremor. Ad Hoc Scientific Committee. Mov Disord 1998;13(Suppl 3):2–23

287. Rajput A, Robinson CA, Rajput AH. Essential tremor course and disability: a clinicopathologic study of 20 cases. Neurology 2004;62:932–936

288. Louis ED, Ottman R, Hauser WA. How common is the most common adult movement disorder? Estimates of the prevalence of essential tremor throughout the world. Mov Disord 1998;13:5–10

289. Kovach MJ, Ruiz J, Kimonis K, et al. Genetic heterogeneity in autosomal dominant essential tremor. Genet Med 2001;3:197–199

290. Gulcher JR, Jonsson P, Kong A, et al. Mapping of a familial essential tremor gene, FET1, to chromosome 3q13. Nat Genet 1997;17:84–87

291. Higgins JJ, Pho LT, Nee LE. A gene (ETM) for essential tremor maps to chromosome 2p22-p25. Mov Disord 1997;12:859–864

292. Ma S, Davis TL, Blair MA, et al. Familial essential tremor with apparent autosomal dominant inheritance: Should we also consider other inheritance modes? Mov Disord 2006;21:1368–1374

293. Louis ED. Etiology of essential tremor: Should we be searching for environmental causes? Mov Disord 2001;16:822–829

294. Lucotte G, Lagarde JP, Funalot B, Sokoloff P. Linkage with the Ser9Gly DRD3 polymorphism in essential tremor families. Clin Genet 2006; 69:437–440

295. Lee RG. The pathophysiology of essential tremor. In: Marsden CD, Fahn S, eds. Movement Disorders 2. London: Butterworths; 1987:423–437

296. Troster AI, Woods SP, Fields JA, et al. Neuropsychological deficits in essential tremor: an expression of cerebello-thalamo-cortical pathophysiology? Eur J Neurol 2002;9:143–151

297. Gasparini M, Bonifati V, Fabrizio E, et al. Frontal lobe dysfunction in essential tremor: a preliminary study. J Neurol 2001;248:399–402

298. Trosch RM, Pullman SL. Botulinum toxin A injections for the treatment of hand tremors. Mov Disord 1994;9:601–609

299. Jankovic J, Schwartz K, Clemence W, Aswad A, Mordaunt J. A randomized, double-blind, placebo-controlled study to evaluate botulinum toxin type A in essential hand tremor. Mov Disord 1996;11:250–256

300. Brin MF, Lyons KE, Doucette J, et al. A randomized, double masked, controlled trial of botulinum toxin type A in essential hand tremor. Neurology 2001;56:1523–1528

301. Ferreira J, Sampaio C. Essential tremor. Clin Evid 2004;11:1674–1686

302. Connor GS. A double-blind placebo-controlled trial of topiramate treatment for essential tremor. Neurology 2002;59:132–134

303. Deuschl G, Elble RJ. The pathophysiology of essential tremor. Neurology 2000;54(11, Suppl 4)S14–S20

304. McIntyre CC, Savasta M, Walter BL, Vitek JL. How does deep brain stimulation work? Present understanding and future questions. J Clin Neurophysiol 2004;21:40–50

305. Massey EW, Paulson GW. Essential vocal tremor: clinical characteristics and response to therapy. South Med J 1985;78:316–317

306. Schuurman PR, Bosch DA, Bossuyt PM, et al. A comparison of continuous thalamic stimulation and thalamotomy for suppression of severe tremor. N Engl J Med 2000;342:461–468

307. Plaha P, Patel NK, Gill SS. Stimulation of the subthalamic region for essential tremor. J Neurosurg 2004;101:48–54

308. Meeuwis CA, Baarsma EA. Essential (voice) tremor. Clin Otolaryngol 1985;10:54

309. Hartman DE, Abbs JH, Vishwanat B. Clinical investigations of adductor spastic dysphonia. Ann Otol Rhinol Laryngol 1988;97(3 Pt 1):247–252

310. Koller WC, Royse VL. Efficacy of primidone in essential tremor. Neurology 1986;36:121–124

311. Hartman DE. Neurogenic dysphonia. Ann Otol Rhinol Laryngol 1984;93:57–64

312. Pacchetti C, Mancini F, Bulgheroni M, et al. Botulinum toxin treatment for functional disability induced by essential tremor. Neurol Sci 2000;21:349–353

313. Warrick P, Dromey C, Irish J, Durkin L. The treatment of essential voice tremor with botulinum toxin A: a longitudinal case report. J Voice 2000;14:410–421

314. Warrick P, Dromey C, Irish JC, Durkin L, Pakiam A, Lang A. Botulinum toxin for essential tremor of the voice with multiple anatomical sites of tremor: a crossover design study of unilateral versus bilateral injection. Laryngoscope 2000;110:1366–1374

315. Hertegard S, Granqvist S, Lindestad PA. Botulinum toxin injections for essential voice tremor. Ann Otol Rhinol Laryngol 2000;109:204–209

316. Adler CH, Bansberg SF, Hentz JG, et al. Botulinum toxin type A for treating voice tremor. Arch Neurol 2004;61:1416–1420

317. Nishida H, Sahashi K. Penicillamine-induced myasthenia gravis. Ryoikibetsu Shokogun Shirizu 2001;36:351–353

318. Moringlane JR, Putzer M, Barry WJ. Bilateral high-frequency electrical impulses to the thalamus reduce voice tremor: acoustic and electroglottographic analysis. A case report. Eur Arch Otorhinolaryngol 2004;261:334–336

319. Lyons KE, Pahwa R. Deep brain stimulation and essential tremor. J Clin Neurophysiol 2004;21:2–5

320. Putzke JD, Uitti RJ, Obwegeser AA, Wszolek ZK, Wharen RE. Bilateral thalamic deep brain stimulation: midline tremor control. J Neurol Neurosurg Psychiatry 2005;76:684–690

321. Taha JM, Janszen MA, Favre J. Thalamic deep brain stimulation for the treatment of head, voice, and bilateral limb tremor. J Neurosurg 1999;91:68–72

322. Ramig LA, Scherer RC, Titze IR, Ringel SP. Acoustic analysis of voices of patients with neurologic disease: rationale and preliminary data. Ann Otol Rhinol Laryngol 1988;97:164–172

323. Zemlin WR, Daniloff RG, Shriner TH. The difficulty of listening to time-compressed speech. J Speech Hear Res 1968;11:875–881

324. Ramig LO, Scherer RC, Klasner ER, Titze IR, Horii Y. Acoustic analysis of voice in amyotrophic lateral sclerosis: a longitudinal case study. J Speech Hear Disord 1990;55:2–14

325. Eldridge M. A History of the Treatment of Speech Disorders. London: Livingston; 1968

326. Webster RL, Dorman MF. Changes in reliance on auditory feedback cues as a function of oral practice. J Speech Hear Res 1971;14:307–311

327. Perkins WH. What is stuttering? J Speech Hear Disord 1990;55:370–382 discus.

328. Perkins WH, Kent RD, Curlee RF. A theory of neuropsycholinguistic function in stuttering. J Speech Hear Res 1991;34:734–752

329. Guitar B. Stuttering: An Integrated Approach to Its Nature and Treatment. Philadelphia: Lippincott Williams & Wilkins; 1998

330. Bloodstein O. A Handbook on Stuttering. Chicago: National Easter Seal Society; 1987

331. Gordon N. Stuttering: incidence and causes. Dev Med Child Neurol 2002;44:278–281

332. Ambrose NG, Cox NJ, Yairi E. The genetic basis of persistence and recovery in stuttering. J Speech Lang Hear Res 1997;40:567–580

333. Ingham RJ, Bothe AK. Recovery from early stuttering: additional issues within the Onslow & Packman-Yairi & Ambrose (1999) exchange. J Speech Lang Hear Res 2001;44:862–867

334. Kim SS, Rosenfield RL. Hyperhidrosis as the only manifestation of hyperandrogenism in an adolescent girl. Arch Dermatol 2000;136:430–431

335. Seider RA, Gladstien KL, Kidd KK. Recovery and persistence of stuttering among relatives of stutterers. J Speech Hear Disord 1983;48:402–409

336. Andrews G, Craig A, Feyer AM, Hoddinott S, Howie P, Neilson M. Stuttering: a review of research findings and theories circa 1982. J Speech Hear Disord 1983;48:226–246

337. Baumgartner C, Sapir S, Ramig L. Perceptual voice quality changes following phonatory-respiratory effort treatment (LSVT) vs. respiratory effort treatment for individuals with Parkinson disease. N C V S Status Prog Rep 1999;14:123–130

338. Helm-Estabrooks N, Hotz G. Sudden onset of "stuttering" in an adult: neurogenic or psychogenic? Semin Speech Lang 1998;19:23–29

339. Eisenson J, Horowitz E. The influence of propositionality on stuttering. J Speech Hear Disord 1945;10:193–197

340. Burke BD. Variables affecting stutterers' initial reactions to delayed auditory feedback. J Commun Disord 1975;8:141–155

341. Johnson W, Rosen L. Studies in the psychology of stuttering: VI. The effect of certain changes in speech pattern upon fluency of stuttering. J Speech Hear Disord 1937;2:105–109

342. Schuell H. Sex differences in relation to stuttering: part 1. J Speech Hear Disord 1946;11:297–298

343. Kopp GA. Metabolic studies of stutterers: I. Biochemical study of blood composition. Speech Monogr 1934;1:117–132

344. Orton S, Travis LE. Studies in stuttering: IV. Studies of action currents in stutterers. Arch Neurol 1929;21:61–68

345. Karlin IW, Strazzulla M. Speech and language problems of mentally deficient children. J Speech Hear Disord 1952;17:286–294

346. Ingham R. Stuttering and Behavior Therapy: Current Status and Experimental Foundations. San Diego: College Hill Press; 1984

347. Webster RL, Lubker BB. Interrelationships among fluency producing variables in stuttered speech. J Speech Hear Res 1968;11:754–766

348. Webster RL, Lubker BB. Masking of auditory feedback in stutterers' speech. J Speech Hear Res 1968;11:221–223

349. Freeman FJ, Ushijima T. Laryngeal muscle activity during stuttering. J Speech Hear Res 1978;21:538–562

350. Ingham RJ, Ingham JC, Finn P, Fox PT. Towards a functional neural systems model of developmental stuttering. J Fluency Disord 2003;28:297–317

351. Fox PT. Brain imaging in stuttering: where next? J Fluency Disord 2003;28:265–272

352. Kidd KK, Heimbuch RC, Records MA. Vertical transmission of susceptibility to stuttering with sex-modified expression. Proc Natl Acad Sci U S A 1981;78:606–610

353. Cox NJ, Seider RA, Kidd KK. Some environmental factors and hypotheses for stuttering in families with several stutterers. J Speech Hear Res 1984;27:543–548

354. Viswanath N, Lee HS, Chakraborty R. Evidence for a major gene influence on persistent developmental stuttering. Hum Biol 2004;76:401–412

355. Alm PA. Stuttering and the basal ganglia circuits: a critical review of possible relations. J Commun Disord 2004;37:325–369

356. Ludlow CL, Loucks T. Stuttering: a dynamic motor control disorder. J Fluency Disord 2003;28:273–295

357. Webb SJ, Monk CS, Nelson CA. Mechanisms of postnatal neurobiological development: implications for human development. Dev Neuropsychol 2001;19:147–171

358. Chugani DC, Muzik O, Behen M, et al. Developmental changes in brain serotonin synthesis capacity in autistic and nonautistic children. Ann Neurol 1999;45:287–295

359. El Awar M, Freedman M, Seeman P, Goldenberg L, Little J, Solomon P. Response of tardive and L-dopa-induced dyskinesias to antidepressants. Can J Neurol Sci 1987;14:629–631

360. Teicher MH, Andersen SL, Hostetter JC Jr. Evidence for dopamine receptor pruning between adolescence and adulthood in striatum but not nucleus accumbens. Brain Res Dev Brain Res 1995;89:167–172

361. Mink JW. The basal ganglia: focused selection and inhibition of competing motor programs. Prog Neurobiol 1996;50:381–425

362. Reynolds JN, Hyland BI, Wickens JR. A cellular mechanism of reward-related learning. Nature 2001;413:67–70

363. Webster RL. Empirical considerations regarding stuttering therapy. In: Gregory HH, ed. Controversies About Stuttering Therapy. Baltimore: University Park Press; 1979

364. Kiziltan G, Akalin MA. Stuttering may be a type of action dystonia. Mov Disord 1996;11:278–282
365. Lastovka M. Tremor in stutterers. Folia Phoniatr Logop 1995;47:318–323
366. Buccolieri A, Avanzino L, Marinelli L, Trompetto C, Marchese R, Abbruzzese G. Muscle relaxation is impaired in dystonia: a reaction time study. Mov Disord 2004;19:681–687
367. Curra A, Berardelli A, Agostino R, Giovannelli M, Koch G, Manfredi M. Movement cueing and motor execution in patients with dystonia: a kinematic study. Mov Disord 2000;15:103–112
368. Gilio F, Curra A, Inghilleri M, et al. Abnormalities of motor cortex excitability preceding movement in patients with dystonia. Brain 2003;126(Pt 8):1745–1754
369. Hand CR, Haynes WO. Linguistic processing and reaction time differences in stutterers and nonstutterers. J Speech Hear Res 1983;26:181–185
370. Mena I, Horiuchi K, Burke K, Cotzias GC. Chronic manganese poisoning. Individual susceptibility and absorption of iron. Neurology 1969;19:1000–1006
371. Hargrave S, Kalinowski J, Stuart A, Armson J, Jones K. Effect of frequency-altered feedback on stuttering frequency at normal and fast speech rates. J Speech Hear Res 1994;37:1313–1319
372. Van Riper C. The Nature of Stuttering. 1st ed. Prentice Hall; 1982
373. Carluer L, Marie RM, Lambert J, Defer GL, Coskun O, Rossa Y. Acquired and persistent stuttering as the main symptom of striatal infarction. Mov Disord 2000;15:343–346
374. Brady JP. The pharmacology of stuttering: a critical review. Am J Psychiatry 1991;148:1309–1316
375. Abwender DA, Trinidad KS, Jones KR, Como PG, Hymes E, Kurlan R. Features resembling Tourette's syndrome in developmental stutterers. Brain Lang 1998;62:455–464
376. Mulligan HF, Anderson TJ, Jones RD, Williams MJ, Donaldson IM. Tics and developmental stuttering. Parkinsonism Relat Disord 2003;9:281–289
377. Comings DE, Wu S, Chiu C, et al. Polygenic inheritance of Tourette syndrome, stuttering, attention deficit hyperactivity, conduct, and oppositional defiant disorder: the additive and subtractive effect of the three dopaminergic genes—DRD2, D beta H, and DAT1. Am J Med Genet 1996;67:264–288
378. Smith A, Denny M, Shaffer LA, Kelly EM, Hirano M. Activity of intrinsic laryngeal muscles in fluent and disfluent speech. J Speech Hear Res 1996;39:329–348
379. Bothe AK, Davidow JH, Bramlett RE, Ingham RJ. Stuttering treatment research 1970–2005: I. Systematic review incorporating trial quality assessment of behavioral, cognitive, and related approaches. Am J Speech Lang Pathol 2006;15:321–341
380. Andrews G, Guitar B, Howie P. Meta-analysis of the effects of stuttering treatment. J Speech Hear Disord 1980;45:287–307
381. Craig AR, Calver P. Following up on treated stutterers: studies of perceptions of fluency and job status. J Speech Hear Res 1991;34:279–284
382. Brady JP. Drug-induced stuttering: a review of the literature. J Clin Psychopharmacol 1998;18:50–54
383. Ludlow CL, Braun A. Research evaluating the use of neuropharmacological agents for treating stuttering: possibilities and problems. J Fluency Disord 1993;18:169–182
384. Gordon CT, Cotelingam GM, Stager S, Ludlow CL, Hamburger SD, Rapoport JL. A double-blind comparison of clomipramine and desipramine in the treatment of developmental stuttering. J Clin Psychiatry 1995;56:238–242
385. Stager SV, Ludlow CL, Gordon CT, Cotelingam M, Rapoport JL. Fluency changes in persons who stutter following a double blind trial of clomipramine and desipramine. J Speech Hear Res 1995;38:516–525
386. Costa AD, Kroll RM. Sertraline in stuttering. [letter] J Clin Psychopharmacol 1995;15:443–444
387. McCall WV. Sertraline-induced stuttering. J Clin Psychiatry 1994;55:316
388. Bothe AK, Davidow JH, Bramlett RE, Franic DM, Ingham RJ. Stuttering treatment research 1970–2005: II. Systematic review incorporating trial quality assessment of pharmacological approaches. Am J Speech Lang Pathol 2006;15:342–352
389. Brin MF, Stewart C, Blitzer A, Diamond B. Laryngeal botulinum toxin injections for disabling stuttering in adults. Neurology 1994;44:2262–2266
390. Ludlow CL. Treatment of speech and voice disorders with botulinum toxin. [clinical conference] JAMA 1990;264:2671–2675
391. Marsden CD, Hallett M, Fahn S. The nosology and pathophysiology of myoclonus. In: Marsden CD, Fahn S, eds. Movement Disorders. London: Butterworth Scientific; 1982:196–248
392. Nirenberg MJ, Frucht SJ. Myoclonus. Curr Treat Options Neurol 2005;7:221–230
393. Marsden CD, Obeso JA, Traub MM, Rothwell JC, Kranz H, La Cruz F. Muscle spasms associated with Sudek's atrophy after injury. Br Med J (Clin Res Ed) 1984;288:173–176
394. Weiner WJ, Lang AE. Movement Disorders: A Comprehensive Survey. Mount Kisco, NY: Futura; 1989
395. Caviness JN, Brown P. Myoclonus: current concepts and recent advances. Lancet Neurol 2004;3:598–607
396. Brin MF, Younger D. Neurologic disorders and aspiration. Otolaryngol Clin North Am 1988;21:691–699
397. Shim C. Motor disturbances of the diaphragm. Clin Chest Med 1980;1:125–129
398. Davis JN. An experimental study of hiccup. Brain 1970;93:851–872
399. Guelaud C, Similowski T, Bizec JL, Cabane J, Whitelaw WA, Derenne JP. Baclofen therapy for chronic hiccup. Eur Respir J 1995;8:235–237
400. Hernandez JL, Pajaron M, Garcia-Regata O, Jimenez V, Gonzalez-Macias J, Ramos-Estebanez C. Gabapentin for intractable hiccup. Am J Med 2004;117:279–281
401. Smith HS, Busracamwongs A. Management of hiccups in the palliative care population. Am J Hosp Palliat Care 2003;20:149–154
402. Rohr H, Lenz H. Diaphragm paralysis after traumatic injury to cervical spine nerve roots. Acta Neurochir (Wien) 1960;8:44–69
403. Aravot DJ, Wright G, Rees A, Maiwand OM, Garland MH. Non-invasive phrenic nerve stimulation for intractable hiccups. Lancet 1989;2:1047
404. Deuschl G, Wilms H. Palatal tremor: the clinical spectrum and physiology of a rhythmic movement disorder. Adv Neurol 2002;89:115–130
405. Deuschl G, Wilms H. Clinical spectrum and physiology of palatal tremor. Mov Disord 2002;17(Suppl 2):S63–S66
406. Guillain G, Mollaret P, Rees A, Maiwand OH, Garland MH. Duex cas de myoclonies synchrones et rythmees velo-pharyngo-laryngo-oculo-diaphragmatiques. Le probleme anatomizue et physiopathologiqque de ce syndrome. Rev Neurol 1931;II:545–566
407. Lapresle J, Ben Hamida M. The dentato-olivary pathway. Somatotopic relationship between the dentate nucleus and the contralateral inferior olive. Arch Neurol 1970;22:135–143
408. Guillain G. The syndrome of synchronous and rhythmic palato-pharyngo-laryngo-oculo-diaphragmatic myoclonus. Proc R Soc Med 1938;31:1031–1038
409. Deuschl G, Mischke G, Schenck E, Schulte Monting J, Lucking CH. Symptomatic and essential rhythmic palatal myoclonus. Brain 1990;113:1645–1672
410. Samuel M, Kleiner-Fisman G, Lang AE. Voluntary control and a wider clinical spectrum of essential palatal tremor. Mov Disord 2004;19:717–719
411. Abbasi S, Danisi FO, Blitzer A, Sulica A, Brin M. Palatal myoclonus (PM). Phenotype of 15 patients. Mov Disord 2000;15(Suppl 3):106
412. Dubinsky RM, Hallett M. Palatal myoclonus and facial involvement in other types of myoclonus. Adv Neurol 1988;49:263–278

413. Jacobs L, Newman RP, Bozian D. Disappearing palatal myoclonus. Neurology 1981;31:748–751
414. Seidman MD, Arenberg JG, Shirwany NA. Palatal myoclonus as a cause of objective tinnitus: a report of six cases and a review of the literature. Ear Nose Throat J 1999;78:292–297
415. Abdul-Baqi KJ. Objective high-frequency tinnitus of middle-ear myoclonus. J Laryngol Otol 2004;118:231–233
416. Howsam GD, Sharma A, Lambden SP, Fitzgerald J, Prinsley PR. Bilateral objective tinnitus secondary to congenital middle-ear myoclonus. J Laryngol Otol 2005;119:489–491
417. Rondot P, Ben Hamida M. Myoclonies du voille et myoclonies squelettiques. Etude clinique et anatomique. Rev Neurol (Paris) 1968;119:59–83
418. Sumer M. Symptomatic palatal myoclonus: an unusual cause of respiratory difficulty. Acta Neurol Belg 2001;101:113–115
419. Shepherd GMG, Tauboll E, Bakke SJ, Nyberg-Hansen R. Midbrain tremor and hypertrophic olivary degeneration after pontine hemorrhage. Mov Disord 1997;12:432–437
420. Hommet CD, de Toffol B, Cottier JP, Autret A. Bilateral olivary hypertrophy and palatal myoclonus. Surg Neurol 1998;49:215–216
421. Nitschke MF, Kruger G, Bruhn H, et al. Voluntary palatal tremor is associated with hyperactivation of the inferior olive: a functional magnetic resonance imaging study. Mov Disord 2001;16:1193–1195
422. Trelles JO. Les ramollissements protuberantiels. These de Medicine, Paris, 1935
423. Trelles JO. La oliva bulbar. Su estructure, funcion, y patologia. Rev Neuropsiquiatr 1943;6:433–521
424. Ben Hamida M. Contribution a l'etude anatomique de couple olivo-dentele. A propos de 13 observations de degenerescence hypertrophique des olives. These de Medicine Paris, 1965
425. Barron KD, Dentinger MP, Koeppen AH. Fine structure of neurons of the hypertrophied human inferior olive. J Neuropathol Exp Neurol 1982;41:186–203
426. Teoh HL, Lim EC. Platysmal myoclonus in subclinical hyperthyroidism. Mov Disord 2005;20:1064–1065
427. Chitkara A, Cultrara A, Blitzer A. Palatal myoclonus: treatment with botulinum toxin. Operative Techniques in Otolaryngology Head and Neck Surgery 2004;15:114–117
428. Hanson B, Ficara A, McQuade M. Bilateral palatal myoclonus. Pathophysiology and report of a case. Oral Surg Oral Med Oral Pathol 1985;59:479–481
429. Dale RC, Heyman I, Surtees RA, et al. Dyskinesias and associated psychiatric disorders following streptococcal infections. Arch Dis Child 2004;89:604–610
430. Matthay KK, Blaes F, Hero B, et al. Opsoclonus myoclonus syndrome in neuroblastoma a report from a workshop on the dancing eyes syndrome at the advances in neuroblastoma meeting in Genoa, Italy, 2004. Cancer Lett 2005;228:275–282
431. Armstrong MB, Robertson PL, Castle VP. Delayed, recurrent opsoclonus-myoclonus syndrome responding to plasmapheresis. Pediatr Neurol 2005;33:365–367
432. Kumar A, Lajara-Nanson WA, Neilson RW Jr. Paraneoplastic opsoclonus-myoclonus syndrome: initial presentation of non-Hodgkin's lymphoma. J Neurooncol 2005;73:43–45
433. Iliceto G, Thompson PD, Day BL, Rothwell JC, Lees AJ, Marsden CD. Diaphragmatic flutter, the moving umbilicus syndrome, and "belly dancer's" dyskinesia. Mov Disord 1990;5:15–22
434. Vantrappen G, Decramer M, Harlet R. High-frequency diaphragmatic flutter: symptoms and treatment by carbamazepine. Lancet 1992;339:265–267
435. Porter WB. Diaphragmatic flutter with symptoms of angina pectoris. JAMA 1936;106:992–994
436. Kobayashi I, Tazaki G, Hayama N, Kondo T. A case of the diaphragmatic flutter with an electromyographic study of the respiratory muscles. Tokai J Exp Clin Med 2004;29:151–154
437. Cvietusa PJ, Nimmagadda SR, Wood R, Liu AH. Diaphragmatic flutter presenting as inspiratory stridor. [see comments] Chest 1995;107:872–875
438. Sibon I, Ghorayeb I, Arne P, Tison F. Distressing belching and neuroacanthocytosis. Mov Disord 2004;19:856–859
439. Brin MF. Acanthocytosis. In: Vinken PJ, Bruyn GW, Klawans HL, eds. Handbook of Clinical Neurology: Systemic Diseases, Part I (Goetz CG, Tanner CM, Aminoff MJ, volume eds.). Amsterdam: Elsevier; 1993:271–299
440. Burn DJ, Coulthard A, Connolly S, Cartlidge NEF. Tardive diaphragmatic flutter. Mov Disord 1998;13:190–192
441. Jankovic J. Differential diagnosis and etiology of tics. Adv Neurol 2001;85:15–29
442. Singer HS. Tourette's syndrome: from behaviour to biology. Lancet Neurol 2005;4:149–159
443. Mejia NI, Jankovic J. Secondary tics and tourettism. Rev Bras Psiquiatr 2005;27:11–17
444. Saiki S, Hirose G, Sakai K, et al. Chorea-acanthocytosis associated with Tourettism. Mov Disord 2004;19:833–836
445. Danek A, Walker RH. Neuroacanthocytosis. Curr Opin Neurol 2005;18:386–392
446. Walker RH, Jung HH, Dobson-Stone C, et al. Neurologic phenotypes associated with acanthocytosis. Neurology 2007;68:92–98
447. Peterson BS, Pine DS, Cohen P, Brook JS. Prospective, longitudinal study of tic, obsessive-compulsive, and attention-deficit/hyperactivity disorders in an epidemiological sample. J Am Acad Child Adolesc Psychiatry 2001;40:685–695
448. Itard J. Memoire sur quelques fonctions involuntaires des appareils de la locomotion, de la prehension et de la voix. Arch Gen Med 1825;3:387–407
449. Van Borsel J, Goethals L, Vanryckeghem M. Disfluency in Tourette syndrome: observational study in three cases. Folia Phoniatr Logop 2004;56:358–366
450. De la Tourette G. Etude sur une affection nerveuse caracterise par de l'incoordination motrice accompagnee d'echolalaie et de coprolalie. Arch Neurol 1885;9:19–42
451. Ludlow CL, Polinsky RJ, Caine ED, Bassich CJ, Ebert MH. Language and speech abnormalities in Tourette syndrome. Adv Neurol 1982;35:351–362
452. Pauls DL. A genome-wide scan and fine mapping in Tourette syndrome families. Adv Neurol 2006;99:130–135
453. Keen-Kim D, Freimer NB. Genetics and epidemiology of Tourette syndrome. J Child Neurol 2006;21:665–671
454. Kurlan R, Behr J, Medved L, et al. Familial Tourette's syndrome: report of a large pedigree and potential for linkage analysis. Neurology 1986;36:772–776
455. Paschou P, Feng Y, Pakstis AJ, et al. Indications of linkage and association of Gilles de la Tourette syndrome in two independent family samples: 17q25 is a putative susceptibility region. Am J Hum Genet 2004;75:545–560
456. Cuker A, State MW, King RA, Davis N, Ward DC. Candidate locus for Gilles de la Tourette syndrome/obsessive compulsive disorder/chronic tic disorder at 18q22. Am J Med Genet A 2004;130A:37–39
457. Swedo SE, Leonard HL, Rapoport JL. The pediatric autoimmune neuropsychiatric disorders associated with streptococcal infection (PANDAS) subgroup: separating fact from fiction. Pediatrics 2004;113:907–911
458. Kurlan R. The PANDAS hypothesis: losing its bite? Mov Disord 2004;19:371–374
459. Jankovic J. Tourette's syndrome. N Engl J Med 2001;345:1184–1192
460. Muller N. Tourette's syndrome: clinical features, pathophysiology, and therapeutic approaches. Dialogues Clin Neurosci 2007;9:161–171
461. Silay YS, Jankovic J. Emerging drugs in Tourette syndrome. Expert Opin Emerg Drugs 2005;10:365–380

462. Allen AJ, Kurlan RM, Gilbert DL, et al. Atomoxetine treatment in children and adolescents with ADHD and comorbid tic disorders. Neurology 2005;65:1941–1949

463. The Tourette's Syndrome Study Group. Treatment of ADHD in children with tics: A randomized controlled trial. Neurology 2002; 58:527–536

464. Salloway S, Stewart CF, Israeli L, et al. Botulinum toxin for refractory vocal tics. Mov Disord 1996;11:746–748

465. Kwak CH, Hanna PA, Jankovic J. Botulinum toxin in the treatment of tics. Arch Neurol 2000;57:1190–1193

466. Porta M, Maggioni G, Ottaviani F, Schindler A. Treatment of phonic tics in patients with Tourette's syndrome using botulinum toxin type A. Neurol Sci 2004;24:420–423

467. Marras C, Andrews D, Sime E, Lang AE. Botulinum toxin for simple motor tics: a randomized, double-blind, controlled clinical trial. Neurology 2001;56:605–610

468. Houeto JL, Karachi C, Mallet L, et al. Tourette's syndrome and deep brain stimulation. J Neurol Neurosurg Psychiatry 2005;76:992–995

469. Limousin-Dowsey P, Tisch S. Surgery for movement disorders: new applications? J Neurol Neurosurg Psychiatry 2005;76:904

470. Fahn S. Article on chorea, 1991, unpublished

471. Cardoso F. Chorea: non-genetic causes. Curr Opin Neurol 2004;17: 433–436

472. Cunningham MC, Maia DP, Teixeira AL Jr, Cardoso F. Sydenham's chorea is associated with decreased verbal fluency. Parkinsonism Relat Disord 2006;12:165–167

473. Walker FO. Huntington's disease. Lancet 2007;369:218–228

474. Bates G, Lehrach H. The Huntington disease gene—still a needle in a haystack. Hum Mol Genet 1993;2:343–347

475. A novel gene containing a trinucleotide repeat that is expanded and unstable on huntington's disease chromosomes. Cell 1993;72:971–983

476. Andrew SE, Goldberg YP, Kremer B, et al. The relationship between trinucleotide (CAG) repeat length and clinical features of Huntington's disease. Nat Genet 1993;4:398–403

477. Bonelli RM, Hofmann P. A review of the treatment options for Huntington's disease. Expert Opin Pharmacother 2004;5:767–776

478. Slaughter JR, Martens MP, Slaughter KA. Depression and Huntington's disease: prevalence, clinical manifestations, etiology, and treatment. CNS Spectr 2001;6:306–326

479. Baliko L, Csala B, Czopf J. Suicide in Hungarian Huntington's disease patients. Neuroepidemiology 2004;23:258–260

480. Paulsen JS, Nehl C, Hoth KF, et al. Depression and stages of Huntington's disease. J Neuropsychiatry Clin Neurosci 2005;17:496–502

481. Paulsen JS, Hoth KF, Nehl C, Stierman L. Critical periods of suicide risk in Huntington's disease. Am J Psychiatry 2005;162:725–731

482. Bonelli RM, Hofmann P. A systematic review of the treatment studies in Huntington's disease since 1990. Expert Opin Pharmacother 2007;8:141–153

483. Ondo WG, Tintner R, Thomas M, Jankovic J. Tetrabenazine treatment for Huntington's disease-associated chorea. Clin Neuropharmacol 2002;25:300–302

484. Savani AA, Login IS. Tetrabenazine as antichorea therapy in Huntington disease: a randomized controlled trial. Neurology 2007; 68:797

485. Demiroren K, Yavuz H, Cam L, Oran B, Karaaslan S, Demiroren S. Sydenham's chorea: a clinical follow-up of 65 patients. J Child Neurol 2007;22:550–554

486. Cardoso F, Eduardo C, Silva AP, Mota CCC. Chorea in fifty consecutive patients with rheumatic fever. Mov Disord 1997;12:701–703

487. Hallett M, Kaufman C. Physiological observations in Sydenham's chorea. J Neurol Neurosurg Psychiatry 1981;44:829–832

488. Ichikawa K, Kim RC, Givelber H, Collins GH. Chorea gravidarum. Report of a fatal case with neuropathological observations. Arch Neurol 1980;37:429–432

489. Lessin LS, Klug PP, Jensen WN. Clinical implications of red cell shape. Adv Intern Med 1976;21:451–500

490. Brin MF, Pedley TA, Lovelace RE, et al. Electrophysiologic features of abetalipoproteinemia: functional consequences of vitamin E deficiency. Neurology 1986;36:669–673

491. Triantafillidis JK, Kottaras G, Sgourous S, et al. A-beta-lipoproteinemia: clinical and laboratory features, therapeutic manipulations, and follow-up study of three members of a Greek family. J Clin Gastroenterol 1998;26:207–211

492. Levine IM, Yettra M, Stefanini M. A hereditary neurological disorder with acanthrocytosis. Neurology 1960;10:425

493. Hardie RJ, Pullon HW, Harding AE, et al. Neuroacanthocytosis. A clinical, haematological and pathological study of 19 cases. Brain 1991; 114:13–49

494. Ueno S, Maruki Y, Nakamura M, et al. The gene encoding a newly discovered protein, chorein, is mutated in chorea-acanthocytosis. Nat Genet 2001;28:121–122

495. Ho M, Chelly J, Carter N, Danek A, Crocker P, Monaco AP. Isolation of the gene for McLeod syndrome that encodes a novel membrane transport protein. Cell 1994;77:869–880

496. Hayflick SJ, Westaway SK, Levinson B, et al. Genetic, clinical, and radiographic delineation of Hallervorden-Spatz syndrome. N Engl J Med 2003;348:33–40

497. Walker RH, Rasmussen A, Rudnicki D, et al. Huntington's disease-like 2 can present as chorea-acanthocytosis. Neurology 2003;61: 1002–1004

498. Saiki S, Sakai K, Saiki M, Hirose G. Huntington's disease-like 2 can present as chorea-acanthocytosis. Neurology 2004;63:939–940

499. Danek A, Jung HH, Melone MA, Rampoldi L, Broccoli V, Walker RH. Neuroacanthocytosis: new developments in a neglected group of dementing disorders. J Neurol Sci 2005;229–230:171–186

500. Brenes LG, Sanchez MI, Antillon A. Verapamil induces complete remission of the clinical and laboratory findings in a patient with chorea-acanthocytosis. Clin Res 1990;38:93A

501. Fahn S, Marsden CD, Calne DB. Classification and investigation of dystonia. In: Marsden CD, Fahn S, eds. Movement Disorders 2. London: Butterworths; 1987:332–358

502. Calne DB, Lang AE. Secondary dystonia. Adv Neurol 1988;50:9–33

503. Bressman SB. Dystonia genotypes, phenotypes, and classification. Adv Neurol 2004;94:101–107

Chapter 18

Botulinum Toxin Treatment of Spasmodic Dysphonia and Other Laryngeal Disorders

Lucian Sulica and Andrew Blitzer

[Note to readers: Botulinum toxin is available in three commercial preparations: two of botulinum toxin type A (Botox®; Allergan, Irvine, CA; and Dysport®; Ipsen, Slough, UK) and one of type B (Myobloc®; Solstice Neurosciences, Inc., Malvern, PA). Dosages discussed in this chapter refer specifically Botox, and the reader should note that these are not equivalent to those of either of the two other preparations.]

Botulinum toxin is a naturally occurring neurotoxin that causes systemic muscle weakening by reversible blockade of acetylcholine release at the synaptic junction. In therapeutic applications, it is administered by intramuscular injection, and its effects are limited by dose and toxin distribution. The superficial location of the larynx makes its muscles accessible, and the clear anatomic division between adductors and abductors of the vocal fold, separated by the lamina of the cricoid cartilage, allows selective treatment of each functional group. As a result, botulinum toxin has proved useful in a variety of laryngeal disorders of inappropriate or hyperfunctional muscle activity, spasmodic dysphonia most prominent among them.

♦ Pharmacology of Botulinum Toxin

Botulinum neurotoxins are produced by *Clostridium botulinum* bacteria as protein complexes consisting of a 150-kd neurotoxin molecule and several associated nontoxin hemagglutinating and nonhemagglutinating proteins.[1] The protein complex sizes formed are approximately 300 kd, 600 kd, and 900 kd (previously called M, L, and LL) depending on the strain of the organism.[1] The nontoxin complex proteins appear to protect the neurotoxin from degradation and may influence the migration properties of therapeutic preparations.[2-5] Seven different botulinum neurotoxin serotypes have been identified (A, B, C_1, D, E, F, G),[6] although only types A and B are routinely used clinically. For all serotypes, the 150 kd neurotoxin molecule is produced as a single-stranded molecule that must be cleaved or nicked by proteases into a di-chain molecule consisting of a heavy chain and light chain.[7]

When injected into muscles, botulinum neurotoxins inhibit the release of acetylcholine from motor neurons, resulting in a reduction in muscle contractions.[6] This inhibition occurs via a multistep process that begins with the binding of the heavy chain of botulinum neurotoxin to nerve terminal receptors.[8] These receptors have recently been identified as synaptic vesicle (SV) proteins—SV2 for botulinum toxin type A[9,10] and synaptotagmins I and II in association with gangliosides for botulinum toxin type B.[11,12] Once bound, the neurotoxin protein is internalized into nerve cells along with the synaptic vesicles.[9,10]

After internalization, the neurotoxin light chain is translocated across the vesicular membrane into the cytosol via a process involving the heavy chain.[13] The light chain functions as a zinc-dependent endopeptidase that cleaves one or more proteins necessary for vesicular neurotransmitter release.[14] Each botulinum toxin serotype cleaves at least one peptide bond on a SNARE protein (soluble *N*-ethylmaleimide-sensitive factor attachment protein receptor),[15] which makes up the vesicle docking and fusion apparatus required for neurotransmitter exocytosis. Botulinum toxin types A, C_1, and E cleave SNAP-25 (synaptosomal membrane-associated protein, 25 kd), whereas types B, D, F, and G cleave one or more of the vesicle associated membrane proteins (VAMPs; synaptobrevins).[16] Serotype C1 also cleaves syntaxin.[17]

The clinical effects of botulinum neurotoxins appear approximately 24 to 72 hours following injection. As acetylcholine release is decreased, neuronal sprouts develop at the neuromuscular junction and begin to release neurotransmitter.[18,19] Eventually, these sprouts retract, and exocytosis is reestablished in the original nerve terminal.[19] The clinical effects of botulinum neurotoxins last on the order of months, and reinjection is typically required to maintain clinical benefits.

Botulinum neurotoxins not only inhibit acetylcholine release from α-motor neuron terminals, but also from γ-motor neurons.[20,21] This action has been found to reduce the muscle spindle inflow to α-motoneurons, which may alter reflex muscular tone.[20] Similarly, botulinum neurotoxins inhibit acetylcholine release from cholinergic autonomic fibers,[22] which makes them useful for the treatment of certain conditions characterized by localized autonomic overactivity (e.g., hyperhidrosis).

Botulinum neurotoxin has been found to inhibit the release of some noncholinergic transmitters in the central nervous system under experimental conditions.[23] However, unlike tetanus toxin, botulinum neurotoxins are not retrogradely transported to the central nervous system following peripheral administration and therefore do not directly influence central neurotransmitter release.[24] In contrast, botulinum toxin type A appears to inhibit the evoked release of several peripheral neuropeptides that are involved in the transmission of pain. Specifically, botulinum toxin type A has been found to inhibit the depolarization-induced release of substance P from primary culture of embryonic rat dorsal root ganglia neurons,[25] as well as the stimulated release of calcitonin gene-related peptide (CGRP) from cultured trigeminal ganglia neurons.[26] A preclinical study of bladder pain found that botulinum toxin type A inhibited CGRP release from afferent nerve terminals and reduced pain responses.[27] Botulinum toxin type A has also been found to inhibit the formalin-evoked release of glutamate from primary afferent terminals.[28] It is possible that some of these nonclassical mechanisms of action contribute to the clinical effects of botulinum toxin type A in a variety of indications.

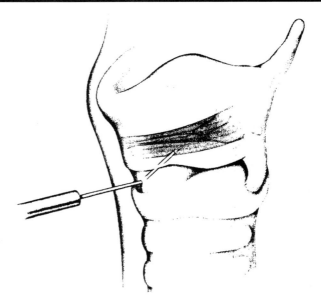

Fig. 18.1 Thyroarytenoid muscle injection for adductor spasmodic dysphonia. (From Sulica L, Blitzer A. Botulinum toxin treatment of spasmodic dysphonia. Op Tech Otolaryngol Head Neck Surg 2004;15: 76–80. Reprinted with permission.)

♦ Techniques for Laryngeal Injection

The small size and proximity of the laryngeal muscles to one another place a premium on accuracy in botulinum toxin injection. Electromyographic (EMG) guidance enables the clinician to locate deep, small muscles that are impossible to palpate, and enables localization of the most electrically active areas of target muscles. EMG can help to minimize unwanted effects on neighboring muscles, as well as to maximize the benefit of each treatment by placing toxin close to its site of action at the motor end plates, allowing a smaller dose and volume to be used. We inject botulinum toxin though a 27-gauge insulated needle attached to an EMG, functioning like a monopolar electrode, in virtually all laryngeal applications.

To treat the thyroarytenoid muscle, the patient is placed in a reclining position with the neck extended. A shoulder roll may be used. We find that local or intratracheal anesthesia is unnecessary in most cases, and may interfere with the EMG signal.[29] It is helpful to bend the needle upward some 30 to 45 degrees, especially when injecting women, as the shorter anterior-posterior distance of the female larynx requires a more acute angle of entry under the inferior border of the thyroid cartilage (**Fig. 18.1**). The needle is inserted through the skin at or just off of the midline at the level of the cricothyroid membrane and advanced superiorly and laterally toward the side of the target thyroarytenoid muscle. Often, the needle enters the air column in the laryngeal lumen after traversing the cricothyroid membrane, producing a characteristic "buzz" on EMG. This tells the injector that the needle lies medial to the vocal fold, and must be directed more laterally. Crossing the endolaryngeal mucosa is irritating to the patient, however, and may provoke a cough or a swallow. By piercing the cricothyroid membrane a few millimeters to the side of the midline, the experienced injector may enter the thyroarytenoid muscle directly without first entering the airway, significantly decreasing patient discomfort. Once the needle is in an area that demonstrates crisp motor unit potentials, the patient is asked to phonate. Brisk recruitment and a full interference pattern in EMG confirms placement, and the botulinum toxin is injected. With experience, the clinician becomes able to identify the characteristic acoustic signature of the motor unit end plates, making it unnecessary to refer to the visual signal.

The posterior cricoarytenoid muscle may be reached in two ways. Most commonly, the injector places his or her thumb at the posterior edge of the thyroid cartilage on the side to be injected and, using counterpressure from the other four fingers on the opposite thyroid lamina, rotates the entire larynx to expose its posterior aspect (**Fig. 18.2**). The needle is inserted along the lower half of the posterior edge of the thyroid cartilage, traversing the inferior constrictor, and it is advanced until it stops against the cricoid. The needle is then pulled back slightly and the patient is asked to sniff to activate the posterior cricoarytenoid to check placement. Alternately, the needle may be inserted through the cricothyroid membrane in the midline, guided across the lumen of the subglottic space (again identified by the characteristic airway "buzz") and through the posterior lamina of the cricoid cartilage to one side or the other of midline (**Fig. 18.3**).[30–32] An intratracheal injection of plain lidocaine helps to prevent coughing and does not affect the EMG signal, as the target muscle lies on the opposite side of the cricoid lamina. Once through the cricoid cartilage, the first electrical signal

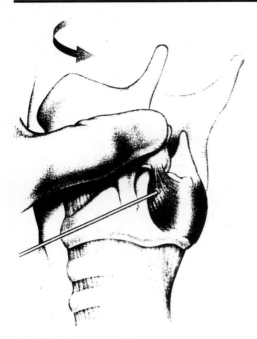

Fig. 18.2 Posterior cricoarytenoid muscle injection for abductor spasmodic dysphonia via the retrocricoid approach. (From Sulica L, Blitzer A. Botulinum toxin treatment of spasmodic dysphonia, Op Tech Otolaryngol Head Neck Surg 2004;15:76–80. Reprinted with permission.)

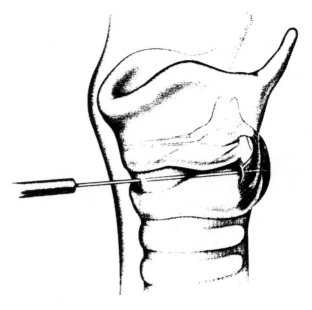

Fig. 18.3 Transcricoid injection of the posterior cricoarytenoid muscle for abductor spasmodic dysphonia. (From Sulica L, Blitzer A. Botulinum toxin treatment of spasmodic dysphonia, Op Tech Otolaryngol Head Neck Surg 2004;15:76–80. Reprinted with permission.)

encountered on the far side represents the posterior cricoarytenoid muscle. Placement is confirmed by muscle activation during sniffing, and the botulinum toxin is injected. In our experience, this approach is most useful in younger patients in whom the cartilage has not undergone extensive calcification. Even so, fragments of cartilage often plug the needle as it crosses the cricoid, and expelling them to begin injection may require considerable force on the plunger of the syringe.

Alternatives to EMG-guided injection include a variety of visually guided techniques. Botulinum toxin may be administered transcutaneously, as described above, under flexible fiberoptic laryngoscopic observation.[33] It may be injected transorally via a curved needle under endoscopic or mirror control,[34] or via the instrument channel of a flexible fiberoptic endoscope so equipped.[35] Probably only the last of these is suitable for reaching the posterior cricoarytenoid muscle. In any case, any method that enables the physician to achieve reliable and repeatable chemodenervation can be used to deliver the toxin. Subjecting the patient to a general anesthetic, as in the early days of the procedure, is no longer warranted.

♦ Clinical Applications

Spasmodic Dysphonia

Rationale for Use

Spasmodic dysphonia is a type of dystonia, a chronic disorder of central motor processing characterized by task-specific, action-induced muscle spasms. Initial use of botulinum toxin for this disorder was intended to relieve this involuntary muscle activity, based on encouraging treatment results in blepharospasm and torticollis, dystonias affecting the periocular and cervical muscles, respectively.

In his original description of recurrent nerve section, Dedo[36] proposed that the abnormality in spasmodic dysphonia was not solely a matter of abnormal neural signal to laryngeal muscles, but also involved abnormal feedback from the larynx to the central nervous system. The well-known action-induced, task-specific nature of dystonia suggests that afferent feedback may indeed play a role in the pathophysiology of spasmodic dysphonia. Further, the phenomenon of the sensory trick—a tactile or proprioceptive maneuver that can be used to improve symptoms—suggests that the alteration of afferent signals may be therapeutically useful. Over time, the sensory trick generally loses its effectiveness. The reason for this is not known, but it appears that the central nervous system tends to eventually overcome this change in input and return to sending inappropriate signals to involved muscles. This may explain why permanent interventions have been largely unable to control symptoms permanently in various dystonias. In the case of spasmodic dysphonia, although recurrent nerve section, anterior commissure release, and other surgical measures have all produced encouraging short-term results, long-term benefit has proved difficult to achieve.

The broad success of botulinum toxin as a treatment for focal dystonias, spasmodic dysphonia among them, may be due to the specificity, repeatability, and reversibility of the chemodenervation. Nerve terminal recovery from poisoning is a continuous, multiphase process, beginning practically as soon as acetylcholine release is blocked.[19]

The cycle of recovery and reinjection with botulinum toxin may make it impossible for the central nervous system to defeat the denervation, because it never reaches a stable plateau. That voice benefit from injection sometimes extends beyond that expected from the observed in vitro activity of botulinum toxin suggests that its clinical effect may be due to more than simple acetylcholine blockade at the neuromuscular junction. Some authors have hypothesized that botulinum toxin may affect neurotransmission in the afferent system as well. In fact, there is evidence that in dystonia, botulinum toxin transiently changes mapping of muscle representation areas in the motor cortex, and reorganizes inhibitory and excitatory intracortical pathways, probably through peripheral mechanisms.[37,38] In spasmodic dysphonia, changes in muscle activation are observed in both injected *and* noninjected muscles, further suggesting a central effect.[39]

Although the treatment cycle of recovery and reinjection translates clinically into some fluctuation of voice quality, results are generally satisfactory, as seen in posttreatment voice function ratings by clinicians and, more importantly, by the patients themselves.[40-44] Nowadays the American Academy of Otolaryngology–Head and Neck Surgery endorses botulinum toxin as primary therapy for this disorder (Policy Statement: Botulinum Toxin; reaffirmed March 1, 1999).

Injection Strategies

Approximately eight of 10 affected individuals have adductor spasmodic dysphonia, in which inappropriate glottal closure causes characteristic harshness, strain, and strangled beaks in connected speech. Abductor spasmodic dysphonia, in contrast, causes inappropriate glottal opening, which produces hypophonia and breathy breaks. Because of compensatory maneuvers or mixed dystonic features, voice patterns encountered clinically may not always be typical or easy to identify. Nevertheless, the division into adductor and abductor forms of the disorder is central to botulinum toxin treatment.

The standard treatment for adductor spasmodic dysphonia at our center is bilateral EMG-guided transcutaneous injections of the thyroarytenoid muscle, using equal amounts of botulinum toxin, based on our observation that the motor control disorder appears to be bilateral and symmetric in most patients. In patients with abductor spasmodic dysphonia, we inject both posterior cricoarytenoid muscles, although injections are not performed simultaneously for reasons of airway safety. Based on the response to initial treatment, we adjust dose and reassess the value of bilateral versus unilateral treatment. Rather than reinject after a predetermined interval, we instruct the patient to await the recurrence of symptoms. After a few cycles of treatment, the patient is often able to anticipate the return of spasms before they become audible to others.

A regimen of alternating unilateral injections is another means of controlling symptoms of glottic insufficiency, such as breathy dysphonia or dysphagia to liquids, in patients with adductor spasmodic dysphonia. In fact, at some centers, unilateral injection is standard treatment, as some have found that it appears to provide essentially equivalent symptomatic relief with less adverse effects.[45-49] That unilateral treatment is effective in a motor disorder usually observed to be bilateral again suggests that botulinum toxin has an effect on afferent neural systems.

Dosing

We use a standard dilution of 4.0 mL of preservative-free saline/100 U vial of botulinum toxin (Botox) for the larynx, diluting the solution further in the syringe as needed for each patient. The effective dose is not proportional to body mass or dysphonia severity, and varies considerably. Because injecting a large quantity of fluid into the vocal folds can cause dyspnea, we aim to limit the volume of each injection to 0.1 mL. For adductor spasmodic dysphonia, our initial dose is approximately 1 or 1.25 U per side, which represents a low average dose for our patient population. We may add a small dose a few weeks after the initial one if the voice does not become fluent. In the great majority of patients, dysphonia is well controlled for 3 months or more with injections of 0.625 to 2.5 U to each side. For abductor spasmodic dysphonia, we initially inject one posterior cricoarytenoid muscle with 3.75 U of botulinum toxin, and estimate the contralateral dose after evaluating vocal fold mobility 2 weeks later. A vocal fold that is completely unable to abduct requires that the other side be treated with a small dose, whereas a more mobile one permits a larger dose to be used. Asymmetric dosing is the rule in abductor spasmodic dysphonia. Fluctuations in disease severity in spasmodic dysphonia occasionally may require small adjustments in dose.

Adverse Effects

Botulinum toxin treatment results in an initial period of marked muscle weakness lasting several days, followed by a months-long plateau of somewhat milder weakening that constitutes the principal therapeutic effect. The reason for this is not known, but likely has to do with the two-stage mechanism of neural recovery from poisoning.[19] It is also hypothesized that partially cleaved SNAP-25 is repaired early, allowing for partial recovery. The completely cleaved SNAP-25, on the other hand, takes 3 months or longer to undergo full repair or replacement. The breathy dysphonia that usually follows thyroarytenoid injection in adductor spasmodic dysphonia is a clinical manifestation of this pattern; the initial effect of the toxin causes some glottic insufficiency. Inasmuch as it is to an extent inevitable, it is not truly a complication, but efforts must be made to minimize it. In general, the two phases of botulinum toxin effect are proportional. In the case of adductor spasmodic dysphonia, for example, the duration of breathiness can usually be shortened by sacrificing the duration of the therapeutic effect. Naturally, patients want to minimize the frequency of injections, but each patient has a different tolerance for a breathy voice. A person for whom voice is crucial, such as a performer or a teacher, may opt for smaller doses at more frequent intervals.

Dyspnea is the equivalent early effect in abductor spasmodic dysphonia, because the posterior cricoarytenoid is being weakened. As this is potentially life threatening, we treat only one side at a time, as detailed above. Even so, the potential for dyspnea imposes an important limitation in botulinum toxin treatment of abductor spasmodic dysphonia, and probably for this reason, results are less satisfactory than for adductor spasmodic dysphonia.[30] Thus, approximately 30% of our patients take small doses of systemic therapy in addition to botulinum toxin. The combination of toxin and systemic therapy seems to offer better symptom control than either therapy alone in these individuals.

Clinical features of dystonia vary between patients, as do functional requirements for voice; the physician must individualize the treatment of each patient, which entails selecting the muscles to be injected, adjusting doses, and varying the frequency of injections. There is often a balance between decreased spasms and loss of function, and the physician and the patient must arrive at an acceptable and flexible treatment plan together.

Essential Tremor

Essential tremor is an age-related disease of involuntary movement. Although generally acknowledged to be the most common adult-onset movement disorder, it is difficult to fix a precise incidence because essential tremor may be mild enough to go unnoticed in 50% or more of affected people.[50,51] In many cases, the disease is familial, and it can be inherited in an autosomal dominant fashion; the rest of the cases appear to be sporadic.[50-53] Voice tremor may be the only manifestation of essential tremor, and the phonatory apparatus may be affected in as many as 25 to 30% of cases.[52,54]

Essential tremor, when it affects the voice, is not usually restricted to the intrinsic muscles of the larynx. Other muscles of the phonatory tract that may be involved include extrinsic laryngeal muscles, pharyngeal and palatal muscles, the muscles of articulatory structures, as well as muscles of the diaphragm, chest wall, and abdomen, which affect phonatory expiration.[55-57] The term *essential voice tremor* thus describes the clinical situation better and is more apt than *essential laryngeal tremor*. Typically, laryngeal examination reveals rhythmic oscillatory motion of the vocal folds, palate, and pharynx. Vocal fold tremor is bilateral and grossly symmetric.

First-line treatment of essential tremor is pharmacologic. Propranolol and primidone are mainstays of treatment, with proven efficacy in controlled clinical trials. Their utility in treating voice tremor is less well established; neither primidone[58] nor propranolol[59] has been shown to improve voice tremor in studies of small numbers of patients. Promising early results using methazolamide, a carbonic-anhydrase inhibitor, have not been supported by subsequent blinded investigation.[60] A single case of effective treatment with gabapentin[61] awaits further study.

Botulinum toxin treatment of essential voice tremor is predicated on the assumption that vocal fold tremor and resulting inappropriate glottal aperture account for the greater part of the symptoms of essential tremor of the phonatory tract. Generally, botulinum toxin is injected into one[62] or both[62-66] thyroarytenoid muscles in the manner of treatment of adductor spasmodic dysphonia and in comparable doses. According to patient self-perception of vocal quality, botulinum toxin injections were useful in 67 to 80% of cases (**Table 18.1**). Acoustic measures documented benefit less often, leading investigators to hypothesize that much of the perceived improvement resulted from decreased phonatory effort.

Table 18.1 Botulinum Toxin Treatment of Essential Voice Tremor: Summary of Studies

Study	Type of Study	Number of Subjects	Muscles Injected	Dose Used	Outcome Patient Subjective Evaluation	Blinded Perceptual Evaluation	Acoustic Analysis
Hertegard and Adler[64]	Open trial	15	Bilateral TA, occasionally thyrohyoid and cricothyroid	0.6–5 U per side (TA)	10 of 15 (67%) reported benefit	Significant mean improvement on VAS	Significant decrease of F_0 and F_0 variation
Warrick et al[62,65]	Open trial with crossover (unilateral versus bilateral injection)	10	Bilateral TA Unilateral TA	2.5 U per side 15 U	8 of 10 (80%) wished to be treated again	No statistically significant improvement	No statistically significant change
Koller et al[63]	Open trial	?	Bilateral TA	1.0–2.5 U, per side	Significant mean improvement on 0-to-100 scale of function	Not reported	Not reported
Adler et al[66]	Dose-randomized open trial	13	Bilateral TA	1.25 U, 2.5 U or 3.75 U per side	Significant mean improvement on 5-point tremor severity scale	Significant mean improvement on 5-point tremor severity scale	Significant mean improvement in F_0 variation

Abbreviations: U, units of botulinum toxin type A; TA, thyroarytenoid; VAS, 100-mm visual analogue scale; F_0, fundamental frequency.

Botulinum toxin treatment of essential voice tremor yields qualitatively different results than the treatment of spasmodic dysphonia, and personal experience with such treatment has not been entirely consistent with the sanguine reports in the literature. Botulinum toxin does not eliminate the tremor, but rather decreases tremor amplitude. However, this does not always translate reliably into acoustic improvement or greater voice functionality. Not infrequently, treatment of adductor muscles yields prolonged and troublesome breathy dysphonia. Neither injecting abductor muscles nor limiting treatment to one side has yielded reliably better results. Such results are also typical of botulinum treatment of head and hand tremor, in which chemodenervation has not offered consistent and predictable functional benefit.[51,67] Many patients with essential voice tremor do not elect to continue long-term botulinum toxin treatment, in contrast to those with spasmodic dysphonia.

This striking difference may be due to distinctions in the pathophysiology of essential voice tremor and dystonia. There is some evidence to suggest that afferent signal plays some role in dystonia, as discussed earlier, and that botulinum toxin may achieve part of its therapeutic effect by altering feedback to the central nervous system.[68,69] On the other hand, essential tremor is likely the result of abnormalities in cerebellar thalamic outflow pathways without an afferent component, potentially compromising an important part of the effect of botulinum toxin.

Extralaryngeal muscles are commonly involved in essential voice tremor, and extending botulinum toxin treatment to these muscles may offer improved results,[64] although swallowing difficulties are likely to impose limits on such treatment. Because essential voice tremor is a clinically heterogeneous disorder, it may also be possible to select patients who are more likely to benefit from botulinum toxin treatment based on differences in muscle involvement seen in the clinical examination; these studies remain to be performed.

Although benefit is by no means universal, we have occasionally found botulinum toxin to be a useful treatment for essential voice tremor. We offer it as initial treatment in patients whose only complaint is voice tremor, and after failure of pharmacologic treatment in patients with other manifestations of the disease. The effect of combined chemodenervation and medical treatment remains to be determined. As in most voice disorders due to benign pathology, a well-informed and well-advised patient is usually the person best suited to weigh treatment options.

Granuloma

Laryngeal granulomas arise from mucosal injury, usually at the site of the vocal process of the arytenoid, where cartilage lies just under the epithelium. Mechanical trauma and local injury from laryngopharyngeal reflux are the two principal etiologic factors. Granulomas are notorious for recurring after excision, and treatment hinges on treating reflux and modifying harmful laryngeal behaviors such as throat clearing and vocal hyperfunction. In cases that resist these measures, botulinum toxin has been used to weaken adductor muscles to decrease collisional forces at the vocal process. Typically, 10 to 15 U of toxin has been injected into ipsilateral[70,71] or bilateral[72] thyroarytenoid muscles. Reduction in the size of the granuloma is evident as early as 2 weeks following injection,[71] and resolution occurs within 3 months. Repeat treatments appear to be rarely necessary.

Other Laryngeal Disorders

Stuttering blocks, similar to dystonic spasms, are action-induced, task-specific movement abnormalities. When the glottis is affected, botulinum toxin treatment has been shown to increase fluency by both objective and subjective measures.[73] In general, however, stutterers do not choose to undergo long-term botulinum toxin therapy, probably due to the availability of reasonably effective behavioral therapy and different treatment expectations from patients with spasmodic dysphonia.[73]

Among the more intriguing uses of botulinum toxin has been its success in controlling the vocal tics of Gilles de la Tourette syndrome, including coprolalia.[74-76] Its utility in this context again suggests an effect on the central nervous system, possibly mediated through afferent pathways.

In 1998, Rontal and Rontal[77] coined the term *laryngeal rebalancing* to refer to chemodenervation of the interarytenoid muscle and the ipsilateral thyroarytenoid and lateral cricoarytenoid in the treatment of anteromedial cricoarytenoid dislocation. The term can be appropriately applied to an array of uses in which manipulation of neural input to the larynx is used to improve healing or resolution of existing pathology. Various authors have injected botulinum toxin to weaken adductors as an adjunct to treatment of posterior glottic synechiae,[78] dysphonia plica ventricularis and other supraglottic hyperfunction,[79] and vocal process granuloma, as discussed above.

◆ Conclusion

Botulinum toxin is a unique clinical tool for the treatment of certain laryngeal disorders. Skilled application allows selective treatment of individual laryngeal muscles, as well as dose-dependent modulation of effects, offering the clinician an opportunity to modify pathophysiology for symptom control or resolution in these disorders. Because botulinum toxin is nondestructive, its effects are repeatable, apparently indefinitely, in contrast to surgical denervation treatments. At doses required to treat laryngeal disorders, systemic toxicity is extremely unlikely, and most adverse effects are minor and transient. These properties make botulinum toxin a uniquely safe and effective clinical tool whose utility is likely to continue to expand as further insight is gained into neuromotor control of the larynx.

References

1. Sakaguchi G, Kozaki S, Ohishi I. Structure and function of botulinum toxins. In: Alouf JE, ed. Bacterial Protein Toxins. London: Academic Press, 1984;435–443
2. Chen F, Kuziemko GM, Stevens RC. Biophysical characterization of the stability of the 150-kilodalton botulinum toxin, the nontoxic component, and the 900-kilodalton botulinum toxin complex species. Infect Immun 1998;66:2420–2425
3. Sharma SK, Singh BR. Hemagglutinin binding mediated protection of BoNT from proteolysis. J Nat Toxins 1998;7:239–253
4. Aoki KR. A comparison of the safety margins of BoNT serotypes A, B, and F in mice. Toxicon 2001;39:1815–1820
5. Roger-Aoki K. Botulinum neurotoxin serotypes A and B preparations have different safety margins in preclinical models of muscle weakening efficacy and systemic safety. Toxicon 2002;40:923–928
6. Simpson LL. The origin, structure, and pharmacological activity of botulinum toxin. Pharmacol Rev 1981;33:155–188
7. Das Gupta BR, Sugiyama H. Role of a protease in natural activation of Clostridium BoNT. Infect Immun 1972;6:587–590
8. Shone CC, Hambleton P, Melling J. Inactivation of Clostridium botulinum type A neurotoxin by trypsin and purification of two tryptic fragments. Proteolytic action near the COOH-terminus of the heavy subunit destroys toxin-binding activity. Eur J Biochem 1985;151:75–82
9. Mahrhold S, Rummel A, Bigalke H, Davletov B, Binz T. The synaptic vesicle protein 2C mediates the uptake of botulinum neurotoxin into phrenic nerves. FEBS Lett 2006;580:2011–2014
10. Dong M, Yeh F, Tepp WH, et al. SV2 is the protein receptor for BoNT A. Science 2006;312:592–596
11. Dong M, Richards DA, Goodnough MC, et al. Synaptotagmins I and II mediate entry of BoNT B into cells. J Cell Biol 2003;162:1293–1303
12. Nishiki T, Kamata Y, Nemoto Y, et al. Identification of protein receptor for Clostridium botulinum type B neurotoxin in rat brain synaptosomes. J Biol Chem 1994;269:10498–10503
13. Hoch DH, Romero-Mira M, Ehrlich BE, Finkelstein A, DasGupta BR, Simpson LL. Channels formed by botulinum, tetanus, and diphtheria toxins in planar lipid bilayers: relevance to translocation of proteins across membranes. Proc Natl Acad Sci U S A 1985;82:1692–1696
14. Schiavo G, Rossetto O, Benfenati F, Poulain B, Montecucco C. Tetanus and botulinum neurotoxins are zinc proteases specific for components of the neuroexocytosis apparatus. Ann N Y Acad Sci 1994;710:65–75
15. Pellizzari R, Rossetto O, Schiavo G, et al. Tetanus and botulinum neurotoxins: mechanism of action and therapeutic uses. Philos Trans R Soc Lond B Biol Sci 1999;354:259–268
16. Lalli G, Herreros J, Osborne SL, Montecucco C, Rossetto O, Schiavo G. Functional characterisation of tetanus and botulinum neurotoxins binding domains. J Cell Sci 1999;112(Pt 16):2715–2724
17. Blasi J, Chapman ER, Yamasaki S, Binz T, Niemann H, Jahn R. Botulinum neurotoxin C1 blocks neurotransmitter release by means of cleaving HPC-1/syntaxin. EMBO J 1993;12:4821–4828
18. Alderson K, Holds JB, Anderson RL. Botulinum-induced alteration of nerve-muscle interactions in the human orbicularis oculi following treatment for blepharospasm. Neurology 1991;41:1800–1805
19. de Paiva A, Meunier FA, Molgo J, Aoki KR, Dolly JO. Functional repair of motor endplates after botulinum neurotoxin type A poisoning: biphasic switch of synaptic activity between nerve sprouts and their parent terminals. Proc Natl Acad Sci U S A 1999;96:3200–3205
20. Filippi GM, Errico P, Santarelli R, Bagolini B, Manni E. Botulinum A toxin effects on rat jaw muscle spindles. Acta Otolaryngol 1993;113:400–404
21. Rosales RL, Arimura K, Takenaga S, et al. Extrafusal and intrafusal muscle effects in experimental botulinum toxin -A injection. Muscle Nerve 1996;19:488–496
22. Ambache N. A further survey of the action of Clostridium botulinum toxin upon different types of autonomic nerve fibre. J Physiol 1951;113:1–17
23. Bigalke H, Heller I, Bizzini B, Habermann E. Tetanus toxin and botulinum A toxin inhibit release and uptake of various transmitters, as studied with particulate preparations from rat brain and spinal cord. Naunyn Schmiedebergs Arch Pharmacol 1981;316:244–251
24. Lalli G, Bohnert S, Deinhardt K, Verastegui C, Schiavo G. The journey of tetanus and botulinum neurotoxins in neurons. Trends Microbiol 2003;11:431–437
25. Welch MJ, Purkiss JR, Foster KA. Sensitivity of embryonic rat dorsal root ganglia neurons to Clostridium botulinum neurotoxins. Toxicon 2000;38:245–258
26. Durham PL, Cady R, Cady R. Regulation of calcitonin gene-related peptide secretion from trigeminal nerve cells by botulinum toxin type A: implications for migraine therapy. Headache 2004;44:35–42
27. Chuang YC, Yoshimura N, Huang CC, Chiang PH, Chancellor MB. Intravesical botulinum toxin A administration produces analgesia against acetic acid induced bladder pain responses in rats. J Urol 2004;172(4 Pt 1):1529–1532
28. Cui M, Khanijou S, Rubino J, et al. Subcutaneous administration of botulinum toxin A reduces formalin-induced pain. Pain 2004;107:125–133
29. Chitkara A, Meyer TK, Cultrara A, Blitzer A. Dose response of topical anesthetic on laryngeal neuromuscular transmission. Ann Otol Rhinol Laryngol 2005;114:819–821
30. Blitzer A, Brin MF, Stewart CF. Botulinum toxin management of spasmodic dysphonia (laryngeal dystonia): a 12-year experience in more than 900 patients. Laryngoscope 1998;108:1435–1441
31. Mu LC, Yang SL. A new method of needle-electrode placement in the posterior cricoarytenoid muscle for electromyography. Laryngoscope 1990;100:1127–1131
32. Meleca RJ, Hogikyan ND, Bastian RW. A comparison of methods of botulinum toxin injection for abductory spasmodic dysphonia. Otolaryngol Head Neck Surg 1997;117:487–492
33. Green DC, Berke GS, Ward PH, Gerratt BR. Point-touch technique of botulinum toxin injection for the treatment of spasmodic dysphonia. Ann Otol Rhinol Laryngol 1992;101:883–887
34. Ford CN, Bless DM, Lowery JD. Indirect laryngoscopic approach for injection of botulinum toxin in spasmodic dysphonia. Otolaryngol Head Neck Surg 1990;103:752–758
35. Rhew K, Fiedler DA, Ludlow CL. Technique for injection of botulinum toxin through the flexible nasolaryngoscope. Otolaryngol Head Neck Surg 1994;111:787–794
36. Dedo HH. Recurrent laryngeal nerve section for spastic dysphonia. Ann Otol Rhinol Laryngol 1976;85:451–459
37. Byrnes ML, Thickbroom GW, Wilson SA, et al. The corticomotor representation of upper limb muscles in writer's cramp and changes following botulinum toxin injection. Brain 1998;121:977–988
38. Gilio F, Curra A, Lorenzano C, Modugno N, Manfredi M, Berardelli A. Effects of botulinum toxin type A on intracortical inhibition in patients with dystonia. Ann Neurol 2000;48:20–26
39. Bielamowicz S, Ludlow CL. Effects of botulinum toxin on pathophysiology in spasmodic dysphonia. Ann Otol Rhinol Laryngol 2000;109:194–203
40. Hogikyan ND, Wodchis WP, Spak C, Kileny PR. Longitudinal effects of botulinum toxin injections on voice-related quality of life (V-RQOL) for patients with adductory spasmodic dysphonia. J Voice 2001;15:576–586
41. Aronson AE, McCaffrey TV, Litchy WJ, Lipton RJ. Botulinum toxin injection for adductor spastic dysphonia: Patients self-ratings of voice and phonatory effort after three successive injections. Laryngoscope 1993;103:683–692
42. Benninger MS, Gardner G, Grywalski C. Outcomes of botulinum toxin treatment for patients with spasmodic dysphonia. Arch Otolaryngol Head Neck Surg 2001;127:1083–1085
43. Bhattacharyya N, Tarsy D. Impact of quality of life of botulinum toxin treatments for spasmodic dysphonia and oromandibular dystonia. Arch Otolaryngol Head Neck Surg 2001;127:389–392

44. Courey MS, Garrett CG, Billante CR, et al. Outcomes assessment following treatment of spasmodic dysphonia with botulinum toxin. Ann Otol Rhinol Laryngol 2000;109:819–822
45. Bielamowicz S, Stager SV, Badillo A, Godlewski A. Unilateral versus bilateral injections of botulinum toxin in patients with adductor spasmodic dysphonia. J Voice 2002;16:117–123
46. Langeveld TPM, Drost HA, Baatenburg de Jong RJ. Unilateral versus bilateral botulinum toxin injections in adductor spasmodic dysphonia. Ann Otol Rhinol Laryngol 1998;107:280–284
47. Maloney AP, Morrison MD. A comparison of the efficacy of unilateral versus bilateral botulinum toxin injections in the treatment of adductor spasmodic dysphonia. J Otolaryngol 1994;23:160–164
48. Koriwchak MJ, Netterville JL, Snowden T, Courey M, Ossoff RH. Alternating unilateral botulinum toxin type A (BOTOX) injections for spasmodic dysphonia. Laryngoscope 1996;106:1476–1481
49. Adams SG, Hunt EJ, Irish JC, et al. Comparison of botulinum toxin injection procedures in adductor spasmodic dysphonia. J Otolaryngol 1995;24:345–351
50. Elble RJ. Diagnostic criteria for essential tremor and differential diagnosis. Neurology 2000;54(Suppl 4):S2–S6
51. Louis ED. Essential tremor. Lancet Neurol 2005;4:100–110
52. Factor SA, Weiner WJ. Hyperkinetic movement disorders. In: Weiner WJ, Goetz CG, eds. Neurology for the Non-neurologist. Philadelphia: Lippincott Williams & Wilkins; 1999:143–177
53. Louis ED, Ottman R. How familial is familial tremor? The genetic epidemiology of essential tremor. Neurology 1996;46:1200–1204
54. Koller WC, Busenbark K, Miner K. The relationship of essential tremor to other movement disorders: report on 678 patients. Ann Neurol 1994;35:717–723
55. Tomoda H, Shibasaki H, Kuroda Y, Shin T. Voice tremor: dysregulation of voluntary expiratory muscles. Neurology 1987;37:117–122
56. Koda J, Ludlow CL. An evaluation of laryngeal muscle activation in patients with voice tremor. Otolaryngol Head Neck Surg 1992;107:684–696
57. Finnegan EM, Luschei ES, Barkmeier JM, Hoffman HT. Synchrony of laryngeal muscle activity in persons with vocal tremor. Arch Otolaryngol Head Neck Surg 2003;129:313–318
58. Hartman DE, Vishwanat B. Spastic dysphonia and essential (voice) tremor treated with primidone. Arch Otolaryngol 1984;110:394–397
59. Koller W, Graner D, Micoch A. Essential voice tremor: treatment with propranolol. Neurology 1985;35:106–108
60. Busenbark K, Ramig L, Dromey C, Koller WC. Methazolamide for essential voice tremor. Neurology 1996;47:1331–1332
61. Padilla F, Berthier ML, Campus-Arillo VM. Temblor essencial de la voz y tratamiento con gabapentina. Rev Neurol 2000;31:798
62. Warrick P, Dromey C, Irish JC, Durkin L, Pakiam A, Lang A. Botulinum toxin for essential tremor of the voice with multiple anatomical sites of tremor: A crossover design study of unilateral versus bilateral injection. Laryngoscope 2000;110:1366–1374
63. Koller WC, Hristova A, Brin M. Pharmacologic treatment of essential tremor. Neurology 2000;54(Suppl 4):S30–S38
64. Hertegard S, Granqvist S, Lindestad PA. Botulinum toxin injections for essential voice tremor. Ann Otol Rhinol Laryngol 2000;109:204–209
65. Warrick P, Dromey C, Irish JC, Durkin L. The treatment of essential voice tremor with botulinum toxin A: a longitudinal case report. J Voice 2000;14:410–412
66. Adler CH, Bansberg SF, Hentz JG, et al. Botulinum toxin type A for treating voice tremor. Arch Neurol 2004;61:1416–1420
67. Lyons KE, Pahwa R, Comella CL, et al. Benefits and risks of pharmacologic treatment for essential tremor. Drug Saf 2003;26:461–481
68. Hallett M. How does botulinum toxin work? Ann Neurol 2000;48:7–8
69. Sulica L. Contemporary management of spasmodic dysphonia. Curr Opin Otolaryngol Head Neck Surg 2004;12:543–548
70. Nasri S, Sercarz JA, McAlpin T, Berke GS. Treatment of vocal fold granuloma using botulinum toxin type A. Laryngoscope 1995;105:585–588
71. Pham J, Yin S, Morgan M, Stucker F, Nathan CA. Botulinum toxin: helpful adjunct to early resolution of laryngeal granulomas. J Laryngol Otol 2004;118:781–785
72. Orloff LA, Goldman SN. Vocal fold granuloma: successful treatment with botulinum toxin. Otolaryngol Head Neck Surg 1999;121:410–413
73. Brin MF, Stewart C, Blitzer A, Diamond B. Laryngeal botulinum toxin injections for disabling stuttering in adults. Neurology 1994;44:2262–2266
74. Salloway S, Stewart CF, Israeli L, et al. Botulinum toxin for refractory vocal tics. Mov Disord 1996;11:746–748
75. Scott BL, Jankovic J, Donovan DT. Botulinum toxin injection into vocal cord in the treatment of malignant coprolalia associated with Tourette's syndrome. Mov Disord 1996;11:431–433
76. Trimble MR, Whurr R, Brookes G, Robertson MM. Vocal tics in Gilles de la Tourette syndrome treated with botulinum toxin injections. Mov Disord 1998;13:617–619
77. Rontal E, Rontal M. Laryngeal rebalancing for the treatment of arytenoid dislocation. J Voice 1998;12:383–388
78. Nathan CO, Yin S, Stucker FJ. Botulinum toxin: adjunctive treatment for posterior glottic synechiae. Laryngoscope 1999;109:855–857
79. Kendall KA, Leonard RJ. Treatment of ventricular dysphonia with botulinum toxin. Laryngoscope 1997;107:948–953

Chapter 19

Pyramidal Disease

Satish Mistry, Maxine Power, and Shaheen Hamdy

Diseases of the larynx encompass a wide spectrum of problems including inflammation, cysts, benign and malignant tumors, and trauma. This chapter focuses on problems of pharyngolaryngeal function associated with pyramidal disease (i.e., stroke) and consequent dysphagia. It also discusses some new research in assessing the neuroanatomy of the pharyngolarynx and swallowing. Problems with speech (dysphonia) are briefly covered.

♦ Neuroanatomy of the Pyramidal Tracts

As the name suggests, the pyramidal tracts, better known as the corticospinal tracts (CSTs) and corticobulbar tracts (CBTs), are a set of approximately one million nerve fibers that travel down from the motor cortex to the spinal cord and are predominantly involved in the regulation of all voluntary movements, in particular discrete, skilled movements. They are composed of cortical neurons, named pyramidal cells because their cell bodies resemble small pyramids, that collectively give rise to the single most important output tract of the motor cortex. They have an average conduction velocity of 60 m/s, indicating an average fiber diameter of 10 μm; however, fibers arising from the leg area of motor cortex can be up to 20 μm in diameter and account for approximately 3% of the total number of fibers.

Approximately 80% of the tracts extend from upper motor neurons in the primary motor cortex to lower motor neurons in the anterior horn of the spinal cord as shown in **Fig. 19.1**, with the remaining 20% of fibers originating in the premotor cortex and supplementary motor area. Upper motor neurons reside in the precentral gyrus of the frontal lobe, also known as the "motor strip," and are arranged in a somatotopic fashion. Neurons controlling facial movements are located near the sylvian or lateral fissure, whereas neurons controlling limb muscles are located near the medial longitudinal fissure and within the central sulcus. The representations of the various body parts are often depicted graphically by a distorted human figure known as the motor homunculus as shown in **Fig. 19.2**.

Axons extending from upper motor neurons in the motor strip traverse deep brain matter through the corona radiata and coalesce to form the internal capsule of the forebrain and then descend through the midbrain in the cerebral peduncle. Here axons of the CST condense and form the structure known as the pyramids; as in the motor strip, these axons are also arranged somatotopically. Axons innervating facial muscles are located medially and are collectively known as the CBT. These axons exit at their appropriate levels to synapse with their lower motor neurons in the cranial nerve nuclei. Axons innervating limbs are located laterally within the cerebral peduncle and are thus known as the lateral CST (LCST). These axons aggregate to form the pyramids in the medulla oblongata, hence the term *pyramidal tract*. In the distal medulla, approximately 80% of CST axons cross to the contralateral side in a very distinct area (on cross section) known as the pyramidal decussation. The pyramidal decussation separates the medulla, above, from the spinal cord, below. Injuries to upper motor neurons in the cortex or their axons prior to entering the pyramidal decussation result in contralateral spastic paralysis, whereas injuries below the decussation or to the lower motor neurons in the spinal cord usually cause ipsilateral flaccid paralysis. Approximately 10% of axons that do not cross over continue from here to join the lateral CST. The remaining 10% of axons that also do not cross over form the anterior CST (ACST) and supply motor neurons serving deep muscles in the neck.

Beyond the pyramidal decussation, the upper motor neurons synapse on lower motor neurons in the anterior horn of the spinal cord, exiting via the ventral root. Damage to lower motor neurons can also cause flaccid paralysis. The ventral root then joins the dorsal root to form the spinal nerve, which finally innervates skeletal muscles.

♦ Definition of Pyramidal Disease

Pathologic processes that damage the pyramidal tracts (**Table 19.1**) are often associated with disability and suffering and are thus grouped together as pyramidal disease. Stroke is the main pathologic condition affecting the pyramidal tracts that will be discussed in this chapter.

A stroke, or cerebrovascular accident, is the temporary or permanent loss of functioning brain tissue due to an

19 Pyramidal Disease

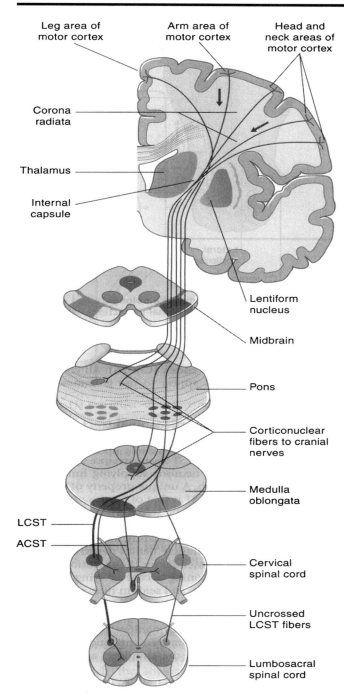

Fig. 19.1 The corticospinal/pyramidal tracts. The pyramidal shape of the axons lead to the term pyramid. The corticobulbar tracts are also referred to as the corticonuclear tracts by some authors. (From FitzGerald MJT, Folan-Curran J. Spinal cord: descending pathways. In: FitzGerald MJT, Folan-Curran J, eds. Clinical Neuroanatomy and Related Neuroscience. 4th ed. Philadelphia: WB Saunders, an imprint of Elsevier Science; 2002:125. Reprinted with permission from Elsevier.)

Regardless of the type, stroke is a devastating affliction resulting in a catastrophic cerebral injury that removes both independence and dignity from many of its survivors. It is also the most common cause of pyramidal tract disease, and is recognized to affect pharyngolaryngeal function, resulting in conditions such as dysphagia,[1] dysphonia,[2] dysphasia,[3] and dysarthria.[4]

◆ Role of Pharyngolarynx in Swallowing

The three functions of the pharyngolarynx are (1) protective, (2) respiratory, and (3) phonatory. This chapter focuses on the protective role of the pharyngolarynx during swallowing.

Normal Swallowing Function

For most people, swallowing or deglutition is a normal and effortless task, but despite its effortlessness, it is a complex and dynamic sensorimotor activity involving 26 pairs of muscles and five cranial nerves. The complexity of the swallowing process is a consequence of the common shared pathway between the respiratory and gastrointestinal tracts that has arisen to avoid the threat of food or liquid entering the airway. Therefore, swallowing enables the safe delivery of ingested food, as a bolus, from the mouth to the stomach while ensuring protection of the airway. It is an integral component of feeding learned during gestation, organized at birth,[5] and essential for the continuation of life.

Traditionally, swallowing is divided into three conventional phases: (1) oral, (2) pharyngeal, and (3) esophageal. Mastication and the oral phase refer to the volitional transfer of ingested material, as a bolus, from the mouth into the oropharynx and is controlled by the motor cortex and premotor areas of the brain.

During the oral phase food is taken into the mouth, manipulated, mixed with saliva, and formed into a bolus. This repetitive cycle of chewing is bolus dependent and regulated via sensory receptors in the tongue, alveolar ridge, and infrahyoid structures, which modify the activity of motor neurons in the trigeminal nucleus.[6] A sophisticated peripheral feedback mechanism prevents injury to the oral structures and gives proprioceptive feedback about bolus position. Once prepared, the bolus is held in a central groove formed by the positioning of the tongue against the hard palate.[7] It is prevented from moving backward by closure of the velum against the pharyngeal aspect of the posterior tongue, which acts as a gateway to the hypopharynx and allows continued respiration.

Once the bolus has been adequately prepared, the oral phase of the swallow commences. The velum elevates, the lips and buccal muscles contract, the posterior aspect of the tongue depresses, and the remainder of the tongue presses against the hard palate to propel the bolus to the hypopharynx.[8] At the point where the bolus passes the anterior faucial arches, the oral stage of swallowing is complete, usually taking less than one second.

interruption in the blood supply. There are two classifications of stroke: (1) those resulting from full or partial blockage of an artery, which is called an infarct; and (2) those caused by hemorrhages or ruptures of intracranial blood vessels.

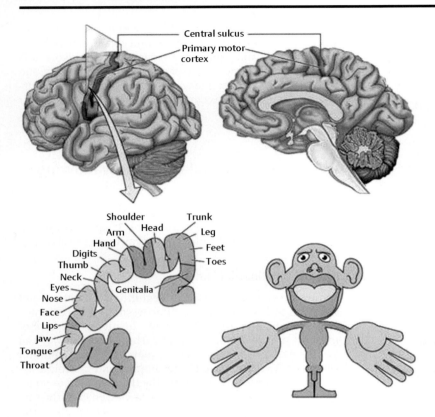

Fig. 19.2 The motor homunculus. The disproportionate anatomy of the homunculus arises from the number of neurons that innervate that area. The larger the body part the greater the number of innervating neurons.(From Purves D, Augustine GJ, Fitzpatrick D, Katz LC, LaMantia AS, McNamara JO. Descending control of spinal cord circuitry. In: Purves D, et al, eds. Neuroscience. Sunderland, MA: Sinauer Associates; 1997:316. Reprinted with permission from Sinauer Associates.)

The pharyngeal phase is the first reflexive component triggered by activation of the central pattern generator in the brainstem, which subsequently controls muscles in the oropharynx to deliver the bolus from the oropharynx to the relaxed cricopharyngeal muscle (upper esophageal sphincter, UES). The oropharyngeal swallow has been described as a single pressure-driven event during which the mouth and pharynx form a continuous tube with four valves: the lips, velopharyngeal port, larynx, and UES.[9]

As the bolus is pushed backward by the tongue, there is a rise in intraoral pressure that marks the beginning of a series of pressure changes that occur during swallowing.[10] A peristaltic-like wave activated by contraction of the constrictor muscles occludes the pharynx by squeezing together the pharyngeal walls behind the bolus.[11]

The nasopharynx is blocked off by the elevation of the soft palate and retraction of the tongue base. The palatopharyngeal folds are pulled together to form a cylindrical passage for the bolus, and the intrinsic muscles of the pharynx shorten, eliminating the pharyngeal recesses. Laryngeal closure is necessary to avoid aspiration and is achieved by a fixed sequence of motor events, which involves cessation of respiration, adduction of the vocal cords, approximation of the arytenoids, laryngeal ascent, and epiglottic descent.[12] The elevation of the larynx also seats the epiglottis over the laryngeal vestibule as a secondary level of airway protection.

Upon closure of the UES, the esophageal phase of swallowing begins. This second reflexive component serves the primary function of transporting food from the UES to the stomach through the lower esophageal sphincter. The sequential contraction of muscles initiated in the pharynx continues down the esophagus and in combination with gravity pushes the bolus down the esophagus. Relaxation of the lower esophageal sphincter allows passage of the bolus into the stomach for digestion.

Sensation

Sensory input to the swallowing tract has three primary functions: (1) to assist in initiating swallowing, (2) to modify the threshold for a pharyngeal swallow, and (3) to alter the level of muscle recruitment during swallowing.

Appropriate preparation of food is reliant upon continuous sensory feedback from receptors in the tongue, soft palate, floor of mouth, and tooth pulp, which detect the size and texture of the bolus, thereby determining the chewing action required from masticatory muscles. The pharyngeal phase of swallowing relies on sensory input from the posterior oral region and pharynx to initiate the response.[13] The intensity of pharyngeal muscle activity and overall duration of this phase are not constant, and in fact vary in

Table 19.1 Some Common Causes of Pyramidal Disease

Multiple sclerosis (MS)
Motor neuron disease (MND)
Space occupying lesions that affect the pyramidal tracts
Stroke

response to sensory information relayed from afferent receptors about the unique characteristics of the bolus.[14] Topical anesthesia of these mucosal regions increases the time to evoke repeated swallows and may disrupt swallowing modulation but does not eliminate swallowing completely.[15]

Sequential Swallowing

Much of what is known about swallowing physiology has been derived from studying single (discrete) swallows. However, the physiology of drinking, a more spontaneous activity composed of multiple swallows (known as sequential swallowing) is a prevalent behavior that warrants our further attention. Recent studies have suggested that two types of sequential swallowing can be observed that vary in their laryngeal closure patterns.[16] In type 1 participants, the larynx rises and lowers for each separate bolus, whereas in type 2, the larynx stays elevated throughout a sequence of bolus ingestions. Both closure patterns are associated with laryngeal penetration, and older participants having significantly higher penetration-aspiration scores,[17] something that has not been found in the study of discrete swallows. Sequential swallows have also been described as being "significantly shorter than discrete swallows in oral transit, pharyngeal response, UES opening, and total swallow durations, but significantly longer in pharyngeal transit and stage transition durations."[18]

Innervation

Motor innervation of the pharynx and larynx is provided through several cranial nerves (CNs) including CN V (trigeminal), XI (glossopharyngeal), and X (vagus) and its branches. A detailed description of laryngeal sensory and motor innervation has been covered earlier in this book and so will not be discussed here.

All the muscles of the pharynx are innervated by the pharyngeal plexus of nerves, which run along its lateral aspect, except the stylopharyngeus, which receives its motor innervation from CN IX. The inferior constrictor is also supplied by additional branches from the external laryngeal and recurrent laryngeal nerves.

The pharyngeal plexus is formed by CNs IX and X and by sympathetic branches from the superior cervical ganglion. Motor fibers are derived from the cranial root of CN XI (the accessory nerve), and are carried by the vagus to all muscles of the pharynx and soft palate, except the stylopharyngeus (supplied by glossopharyngeal) and the tensor veli palatini (supplied by CN V3, the mandibular branch of the trigeminal). Pharyngeal sensory innervation is supplied by the CN IX and the superior laryngeal nerve (SLN) (part of CN X).

Swallowing Dysfunction

Difficulty swallowing, termed dysphagia, is identified as a major clinical problem and can occur during either oropharyngeal or esophageal phases of swallowing. The causes of dysphagia may be neurologic, mechanical, or obstructive in origin, but all have the same outcome: a disruption of bolus flow. This places patients at considerable risk of morbidity and mortality, and particularly at risk for aspiration pneumonia.[19] For the purpose of this chapter, we discuss only oropharyngeal dysphagia, which can be subdivided into structural and neurogenic in origin.

Structural dysphagias (**Table 19.2**) refer to congenital malformations of the lip or palate and usually cause dysphagia from infancy. In adult life, structural resections of the tongue, mandible, pharynx, or neck due to carcinoma are associated with marked swallowing difficulty.

Neurogenic dysphagias (**Table 19.3**) refer to those that have a neurologic basis. Some have a slow onset, associated with progressive neurologic conditions such as Parkinson disease, motor neuron disease, or myasthenia gravis.[20] Others have a sudden onset associated with acute brain injury such as stroke and head trauma.[21] Many diseases of the muscle (e.g., myotonic or oculopharyngeal dystrophy, dermatomyositis, etc.) or cranial nerves (e.g., Guillain-Barré syndrome, facial

Table 19.2 Structural Causes of Dysphagia

Amyloidosis
Cervical spine osteophytes
Congenital anatomic abnormalities, e.g., cleft palate
Iron and B_{12} deficiency
Oral malignancies of the tongue and palate
Pharyngeal malignancy of the epiglottis, tongue base, or larynx
Salivary gland disease
Skull base tumors
Thyroid disease
Thyroid tumors
Zenker's diverticulum

Table 19.3 Neurogenic Causes of Dysphagia

Cerebral palsy
Guillan-Barré and other polyneuropathies
Head trauma*
Huntington disease
Infectious disorders, e.g., meningitis, syphilis, diphtheria, botulism, and encephalitis
Medication side effects
Motor neuron disease (MND)*
Multiple sclerosis (MS)*
Myasthenia gravis
Myopathy, e.g., polymyositis, dermatomyositis, sarcoidosis
Neoplasms, e.g., brain tumor
Parkinson disease and other movement and neurodegenerative disorders
Postpolio syndrome
Progressive supranuclear palsy
Stroke*
Torticollis
Tardive dyskinesia
Wilson disease

*Conditions that specifically cause pyramidal disease. In the United Kingdom, stroke is the most common cause of neurogenic dysphagia.

nerve paralysis, and sarcoidosis) may also affect swallowing.[22] However, the commonest cause of dysphagia is stroke.[23] Dysphagia after stroke is a major cause of morbidity related to respiratory complications and malnutrition.[24] Oropharyngeal dysphagia is also frequently reported as a complication of progressive diseases such as Alzheimer disease and also following long-term use of medication used to control psychogenic conditions.[25]

♦ Dysphagia Post-Stroke

The most common cause of oropharyngeal dysphagia in the United Kingdom is stroke, and it is associated with malnutrition and pulmonary aspiration.[19] Dysphagia and related complications of stroke lead to hospital admissions and greater demands on health service resources, estimated to cost an extra $600 million per year in the United Kingdom.[26] Fortunately, oropharyngeal dysphagia is often transient and is commonly observed to resolve itself in patients who have suffered a unilateral hemispheric stroke.

Characteristics

Hemispheric Stroke

It is well documented that stroke patients aspirate on videofluoroscopy[27]; however, information about the pharyngolaryngeal abnormalities that underpin this aspiration remains limited.

Observational studies suggest that patients who aspirate have a combination of both oral and pharyngeal impairments, which impact on bolus retention in the oral cavity and pharyngolaryngeal function.[19] Release of liquids from the mouth into the hypopharynx, prior to the onset of laryngeal closure, due to poor velopharyngeal closure, termed "premature spillage," has been repeatedly cited as a major contributor.[28] Delayed laryngeal elevation has also been reported and strongly correlated with chest infection at 6 months after the stroke.[29] These observations suggest a breakdown in the synchrony between bolus transport and laryngeal closure, however, without an absence or inability to adequately elevate the larynx.

Post–Brainstem Stroke

Brainstem or infratentorial strokes, as opposed to cortical or supratentorial strokes, affect swallowing in approximately 40% of patients.[30] Brainstem strokes to the middle or lower levels of the medulla are typically associated with more persistent and serious problems with aspiration and pharyngeal dysphagia.[31] Observational studies using videofluoroscopy report adequate oral control associated with an inability or impairment in the initiation of laryngeal closure and pharyngeal contraction.[32] The bolus enters the hypopharynx and travels into the laryngeal recesses; however, repeated attempts to elevate the larynx and relax the cricopharyngeal sphincter fail. Thus liquid is tipped into the larynx during the repeated movements of the tongue base and extrinsic laryngeal muscles.

♦ The Role of the Cerebral Cortex in Swallowing

The importance of the cortex in the initiation and regulation of human swallowing has been recognized for some time now.[1] Unfortunately, much of our understanding of the central brain control of swallowing has come from invasive animal studies, artificially stimulating cortical swallowing areas. In anesthetized animals, electrical microstimulation of the cortex, from either hemisphere, is capable of inducing full swallow responses visible to the investigator, providing evidence that swallowing musculature is bilaterally controlled.[33-36] This may suggest that both hemispheres play an equal role in controlling swallowing[37]; however, pathophysiologic evidence resulting from cerebral injury such as stroke has begun to suggest that one hemisphere may be dominant over the other.[19]

Transcranial Magnetic Stimulation (TMS) Findings

In recent years there has been an increase in the use of neurophysiologic imaging techniques that have improved our understanding of swallowing and its cortical control. One such technique is transcranial magnetic stimulation (TMS), a safe, noninvasive neurophysiologic tool that in combination with electromyography (EMG) has been used to map the cortical representation of swallowing musculature in healthy subjects and in stroke patients recovering from dysphagia.[1] TMS uses rapidly changing magnetic fields to stimulate neural tissue and elicit electromyographic motor responses in the form of motor evoked potentials (MEPs) recorded using an intraluminal catheter (**Fig. 19.3**).

Transcranial magnetic stimulation mapping studies by Hamdy et al[1] have demonstrated that human swallowing musculature is represented on both hemispheres (bilaterally) but that one representation tended to be larger than the other (asymmetric in size), implying the existence of dominant and nondominant swallowing hemispheres. This finding from a large group of subjects was independent from handedness and discordant in a pair of identical twins, suggesting little genetic contribution to its development.

In the field of neurolaryngology, progress in studying the neural control of laryngeal musculature has also been slowed by difficulties in accessing the laryngeal muscles and the inability to noninvasively study the human motor cortex. Recently, however, several investigators[38-41] have used TMS-elicited MEPs, in a similar fashion to studies of the pharynx by Hamdy et al,[1] to record directly from laryngeal musculature either transcutaneously using concentric needle electrodes or transorally using hooked-wire electrodes. Using these methods the investigators have been able to begin studying corticolaryngeal nerve conduction time and cerebral representation. Similar to pharyngeal cortical motor representation, the larynx is also bilaterally

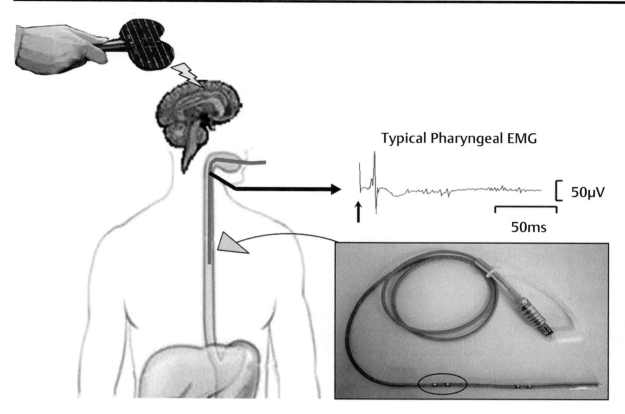

Fig. 19.3 Transcranial magnetic stimulation (TMS) and motor evoked potential (MEP) recording. TMS of the swallowing motor cortex noninvasively elicits an MEP recordable using an intraluminal catheter. Pharyngeal MEP mean onset latency is typically 6 to 10 ms.

represented with MEPs found to be elicitable 2 to 13 cm lateral from the vertex on the interaural line with a mean onset latency of approximately 10 ms, indicating primary motor cortex as the site of excitation. However, it is important to remember that this research is still in its infancy, and to the best of our knowledge the neurophysiologic evidence documenting bilateral cortical innervation of all laryngeal musculature is still scarce.

Although TMS has helped delineate some details of the organization of projections from the motor cortex to swallowing and laryngeal muscles, this approach does not allow an assessment of cerebral activity associated with functional swallowing. The recent technologic advances in functional imaging of human brain have revolutionized our understanding of how the cerebral cortex operates in processing sensory and motor information. In particular, positron emission tomography (PET) and functional magnetic resonance imaging (fMRI) have become established as useful methods for exploring the spatial localization of changes in neuronal activity during tasks, within both cortical and subcortical structures. These techniques have been applied to the study of human swallowing,[42–47] and, broadly speaking, the results have been similar, confirming that this seemingly simple task recruits multiple discrete regions of the brain.

Positron Emission Tomography Findings

Positron emission tomography studies have shown activations in loci **(Fig. 19.4)** including the right orbitofrontal cortex, left mesial premotor cortex and cingulate, right caudolateral sensorimotor cortex, left caudolateral sensorimotor cortex, right anterior insula, left temporopolar cortex merging with left amygdala, right temporopolar cortex, left medial cerebellum merging across the midline with the right medial cerebellum, and dorsal brainstem. The strongest activations were found to be in the sensorimotor cortices, insula, and cerebellum. Therefore, swallowing recruits multiple cerebral regions, often in an asymmetric manner, particularly in the insula, which was predominantly on the right and in the cerebellum, being mainly on the left. These latter observations are in keeping with earlier TMS observations, that motor cortex representation of swallowing musculature displays degrees of asymmetry.

Functional Magnetic Resonance Imaging Findings

Activations seen during fMRI studies[44–46] **(Fig. 19.5)** have been in the primary motor cortex, sensory motor cortex, supplementary motor cortex, anterior cingulated, insular cortex, and parieto-occipital cortex. The cerebellum and brainstem have also been inconsistently implicated in deglutition; however, using current fRMI techniques, subcortical activations are more difficult to identify and have previously been attributed to the different swallowing tasks and functional modalities employed by the researchers.

Using fMRI Kern et al[44] compared cerebral activations during swallowing with activations during jaw clenching, lip pursing, and tongue rolling, and found that similar areas of

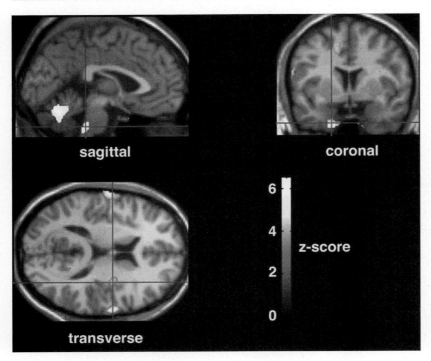

Fig. 19.4 Activations in cerebral loci as identified with positron emission tomography (PET). Activation of swallowing loci observed after a 10-minute swallowing task using radiolabeled H_2O^{15} rendered onto normalized T1-weighted magnetic resonance imaging (MRI) brain slices. The color scale indicates the z-score level for each locus depicted. Cerebellar and dorsal brainstem loci activations are demonstrated in the sagittal section, the right and left sensorimotor cortex and right anterior insula loci are demonstrated in the transverse section, and the left mesial frontal and cingulate cortex and left temporoamygdala loci are demonstrated in the coronal section. (From Hamdy S, Rothwell JC, Brooks DJ, Bailey D, Aziz Q, Thompson DG. Identification of the cerebral loci processing human swallowing with $H_2^{15}O$ PET activation. J Neurophysiol 1999;81:1917–1926. Reprinted with permission from the American Physiological Society.)

activation were seen, suggesting that cerebral regions activated during swallowing may not be specific to deglutition.

Unfortunately, although both PET and fMRI have good spatial resolution (2 mm or less), they have a rather low temporal resolution of several seconds, due to dependency on changes in hemodynamic flow. These technical limitations have prohibited researchers from delineating the functional connectivity between cortical regions and dissociating their specific contributions to the different aspects of swallowing. With the development of magnetoencephalography (MEG), however, researchers are now able to overcome some of these limitations.

Magnetoencephalography Findings

Magnetoencephalography is a newly applied brain imaging approach that is capable of recording the minute electrical signals emanating from the whole brain using ultrasensitive magnetic detection coils. MEG also has the advantage of recording functional information from magnetic fields generated by groups of active neurons, giving a temporal resolution of 1 ms and a spatial resolution equal to PET and fMRI. Essentially, MEG directly records neural activity dynamically with high temporal resolution.

Recently, Furlong et al[48] dynamically imaged human cortical neuronal activity during swallowing using MEG. Utilizing MEG and a new analysis technique known as synthetic aperture manetometry (SAM), they were able to dissociate the spatiotemporal cortical neuronal characteristics of volitional swallowing in healthy subjects **(Fig. 19.6)**. They found infusing water into the oral cavity preferentially activated the caudolateral sensorimotor cortex, whereas during volitional swallowing and tongue movement, the superior sensorimotor cortex was more strongly activated. Temporal analysis indicated that sensory input from the tongue simultaneously activated caudolateral sensorimotor and primary gustatory cortex, which appeared to prime the superior sensory and motor cortical areas involved in volitional swallowing. These data support the existence of a temporal synchrony across the whole cortical swallowing network, with sensory input from the tongue being critical. The importance of sensory input for the production of normal swallowing has previously been reported.[49] To date, all functional imaging studies have assessed swallowing in healthy adults; however, studies comparing dysphagic and nondysphagic stroke patients are eagerly awaited.

Mechanisms of Pharyngolaryngeal Dysfunction and Dysphagia Post-Stroke

Following stroke, swallowing problems are extremely common. What was less clear is why unilateral stroke still produced dysphagia, despite evidence for bilateral swallowing control. Our hypothesis might be that the previously observed asymmetry for swallowing in the cerebral cortex may be important.

Based on this observation that oropharyngeal dysphagia is transient, Hamdy et al[50] studied a large series of pure unilateral stroke patients, half of whom had dysphagia. The authors reasoned that if there were a true asymmetry of swallowing representation in normal subjects, then perhaps dysphagia would occur if the damage had affected the side of the brain with the largest, most dominant projection. The results showed that although stimulation of the damaged hemisphere produced little or no response in either group of patients, stimulation of the undamaged hemisphere

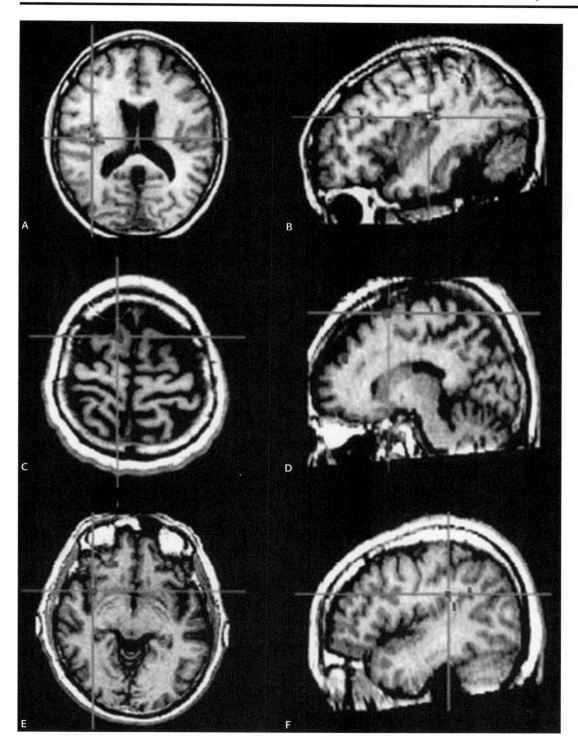

Fig. 19.5 Activations in cerebral loci as identified with functional MRI. MRI orthogonal planes **(A–F)** show cortical activations patterns in an individual after a simple 10-minute swallowing task. Activations shown include right caudolateral pericentral gyri (somatosensory cortex, Brodmann areas 2, 3; **[A]** and **[B]**), bilateral (right > left) middle and superior frontal gyri (premotor cortex, Brodmann areas 6, 8; **[C,D]**), right anterior insula cortex **(E)**, and right caudolateral posterior parietal cortex/precuneus (Brodmann areas 7, 39; (From Hamdy S, Mikulis DJ, Crawley A, et al. Cortical activation during human volitional swallowing: an event-related fMRI study. Am J Physiol 1999;277(1 Pt 1):G219–G225. Reprinted with permission from the American Physiological Society.

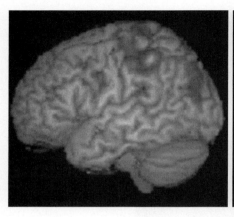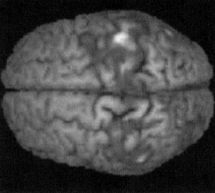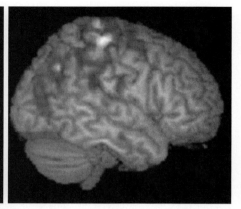

Fig. 19.6 Cerebral loci activations as identified with magnetoencephalography (MEG). MEG activations seen during a simple water-swallowing task. Statistical nonparametric permutation testing maps (SnPM) of group synthetic aperture manetometry results show significant event-related desynchronization effects revealed by the active–passive comparisons in swallowing (5–15 Hz). Blue/pink colors represent ERD (i.e., negative) group scores. (From Furlong PL, Hobson AR, Aziz Q, et al. Dissociating the spatio-temporal characteristics of cortical neuronal activity associated with human volitional swallowing in the healthy adult brain. Neuroimage 2004;22: 1447–1455. Reprinted with permission.)

in the nondysphagia patients evoked a much larger response than in the dysphagia patients. Thus, the size of the hemispheric projection to swallowing muscles may have determined the presence or absence of dysphagia.

Cortical Reorganization and Spontaneous Recovery of Swallowing Post-Stroke

Following the earlier research using TMS,[50] Hamdy et al[51] serially mapped dysphagic and nondysphagic stroke patients over several months while their swallowing ability recovered (**Fig. 19.7**). They found that the area of pharyngeal representation in the undamaged hemisphere increased markedly in patients who recovered, whereas there was no change in patients who had persistent dysphagia or in patients who were nondysphagic. No changes were seen in the damaged hemisphere in any of the groups. These observations implied that over a period of weeks, the recovery of swallowing after stroke was dependent on compensatory reorganization in the undamaged hemisphere. In comparison, TMS studies in recovery of limb function have demonstrated increases in activity within the viable cortex of the damaged hemisphere.[52]

Treatments for Dysphagia Post-Stroke

The current treatments for dysphagia, such as percutaneous endoscopic gastrostomy and speech and language therapy, are controversial with little evidence to suggest that they influence swallowing recovery or the risk of pulmonary aspiration.[53,54] Unfortunately, research into therapeutic areas has suffered from the fact that dysphagia is difficult to categorize and quantify. In addition, there are ethical issues surrounding allocation of patients in control groups. Unfortunately, this and many other factors have led to a lack of good research evidence on which management decisions can be based, and there are still no active therapies with proven efficacy.

♦ Dysphonia

Spasmodic dysphonia (SD) is an idiopathic laryngeal motor control disorder observed after stroke (lateral medullary infarcts involving the nucleus ambiguus and pontine ischemia due to basilar artery occlusive disease).[55] Like stroke, SD can be highly debilitating, resulting in social, financial, and personal hardship.[56] Factors involved in the development of SD are shown in **Table 19.4**.

The two types of SD that have been identified, adductor spasmodic dysponia (ADSD) and abductor spasmodic dysponia (ABSD), affect quiet breathing, swallowing, and voice control during speech.[57–59] ADSD is the most common form and is characterized by a strained or strangled vocal quality or phonatory offset with irregular voice stoppages due to hyperadduction of the vocal folds.[60] ABSD is associated with hypoabduction of the vocal folds and is the less common subtype of the spasmodic dysphonias. ABSD is characterized by a breathy voice or brief vocal loss due to prolongation of voiceless consonants such as /s/, /h/, /f/, /p/, /t/, /k/,

Table 19.4 Factors Involved in Spasmodic Dysphonia Development

- Central nervous system disease
- Emotional trauma (e.g., stress from work or family, interpersonal conflicts, and suppression of aggression)
- Other focal dystonias
- Sore throat
- Stroke
- Traumatic head/neck injury or laryngeal surgery
- Tremor
- Viral infection

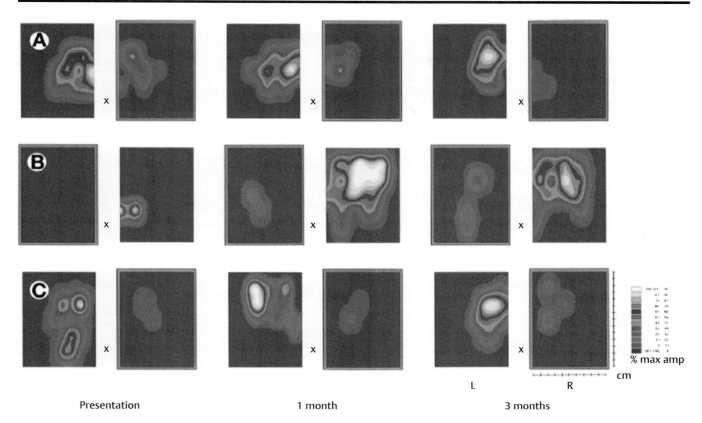

Presentation 1 month 3 months

Fig. 19.7 Transcranial magnetic stimulation (TMS) swallowing musculature representational maps. Topographic TMS maps of the pharynx from three different stroke patients at presentation, 1 month, and 3 months. Patient A was nondysphagic throughout the study, patient B was dysphagic at presentation but had recovered swallowing by month 1, and patient C had persistent dysphagia throughout the study. (From Hamdy S, Aziz Q, Rothwell JC, et al. Recovery of swallowing after dysphagic stroke relates to functional reorganization in the intact motor cortex. Gastroenterology 1998;115:1104–1112. Reprinted with permission.)

and "th."[61] Face and neck grimaces often accompany phonation in SD patients.

◆ Conclusion

The neurologic study of pharyngolaryngeal function after disease such as stroke is an exciting area of research with numerous unanswered questions. In this chapter we have highlighted the current understanding of the neurologic control of the pharyngolarynx and its dysfunction following pyramidal disease. We propose that significant advances in our understanding will emerge with the application of modern imaging techniques such as TMS, PET, fMRI, MEG, and videofluoroscopy to this important research field. A better understanding of the neural control of the pharyngolarynx should ultimately lead to the development of clinically important therapies for the future rehabilitation of patients.

References

1. Hamdy S, Aziz Q, Rothwell JC, et al. The cortical topography of human swallowing musculature in health and disease. Nat Med 1996;2:1217–1224
2. Woo P, Casper J, Colton R, Brewer D. Dysphonia in the aging: physiology versus disease. Laryngoscope 1992;102:139–144
3. Pedersen PM, Vinter K, Olsen TS. Aphasia after stroke: type, severity and prognosis. The Copenhagen aphasia study. Cerebrovasc Dis 2004;17:35–43
4. Sellars C, Hughes T, Langhorne P. Speech and language therapy for dysarthria due to nonprogressive brain damage: a systematic Cochrane review. Clin Rehabil 2002;16:61–68
5. Hooker D. Early human fetal behavior, with a preliminary note on double simultaneous fetal stimulation. Res Publ Assoc Res Nerv Ment Dis 1954;33:98–113
6. Miller AJ. Neurophysiological basis of swallowing. Dysphagia 1986;1:91–100

7. Logemann JA. Swallowing physiology and pathophysiology. Otolaryngol Clin North Am 1988;21:613–623
8. Lowe A. The neural regulation of tongue movements. In: Lowe A, ed. Progress in Neurobiology. New York: Pergamon Press; 1980
9. McConnel FM, Cerenko D, Jackson RT, Guffin TN Jr. Timing of the major events of pharyngeal swallowing. Arch Otolaryngol Head Neck Surg 1988;114:1413–1418
10. Castell JA, Dalton CB, Castell DO. Pharyngeal and upper esophageal sphincter manometry in humans. Am J Physiol 1990;258(2 Pt 1): G173–G178
11. Pouderoux P, Kahrilas PJ. Function of upper esophageal sphincter during swallowing: the grabbing effect. Am J Physiol 1997;272(5 Pt 1): G1057–G1063
12. Shaker R, Dodds WJ, Dantas RO, Hogan WJ, Arndorfer RC. Coordination of deglutitive glottic closure with oropharyngeal swallowing. Gastroenterology 1990;98:1478–1484
13. Shaker R, Ren J, Zamir Z, Sarna A, Liu J, Sui Z. Effect of aging, position, and temperature on the threshold volume triggering pharyngeal swallows. Gastroenterology 1994;107:396–402
14. Dodds WJ, Man KM, Cook IJ, Kahrilas PJ, Stewart ET, Kern MK. Influence of bolus volume on swallow-induced hyoid movement in normal subjects. AJR Am J Roentgenol 1988;150:1307–1309
15. Mansson I, Sandberg N. Effects of surface anaesthesia on deglutition in man. Laryngoscope 1974;84:427–437
16. Daniels SK, Foundas AL. Swallowing physiology of sequential straw drinking. Dysphagia 2001;16:176–182
17. Daniels SK, Corey DM, Hadskey LD, et al. Mechanism of sequential swallowing during straw drinking in healthy young and older adults. J Speech Lang Hear Res 2004;47:33–45
18. Chi-Fishman G, Sonies BC. Motor strategy in rapid sequential swallowing: new insights. J Speech Lang Hear Res 2000;43:1481–1492
19. Robbins J, Levine RL, Maser A, Rosenbek JC, Kempster GB. Swallowing after unilateral stroke of the cerebral cortex. Arch Phys Med Rehabil 1993;74:1295–1300
20. Bucholz D. Neurologic causes of dysphagia. Dysphagia 1987;1:152–156
21. Kirshner HS. Causes of neurogenic dysphagia. Dysphagia 1989;3: 184–188
22. Wiles CM. Neurogenic dysphagia. J Neurol Neurosurg Psychiatry 1991; 54:1037–1039
23. Kuhlemeier KV. Epidemiology and dysphagia. Dysphagia 1994; 9:209–217
24. Veis SL, Logemann JA. Swallowing disorders in persons with cerebrovascular accident. Arch Phys Med Rehabil 1985;66:372–375
25. Deron P. Dysphagia with systemic diseases. Acta Otorhinolaryngol Belg 1994;48:191–200
26. Smithard DG, O'Neill PA, Park C, et al. Complications and outcome after acute stroke: does dysphagia matter? Stroke 1996;27:1200–1204
27. Kidd D, Lawson J, Nesbitt R, MacMahon J. Aspiration in acute stroke: a clinical study with videofluoroscopy. Q J Med 1993;86:825–829
28. Mann G, Hankey GJ. Initial clinical and demographic predictors of swallowing impairment following acute stroke. Dysphagia 2001;16:208–215
29. Mann G, Hankey GJ, Cameron D. Swallowing function after stroke: prognosis and prognostic factors at 6 months. Stroke 1999;30:744–748
30. Teasell R, Foley N, Doherty T, Finestone H. Clinical characteristics of patients with brainstem strokes admitted to a rehabilitation unit. Arch Phys Med Rehabil 2002;83:1013–1016
31. Kim H, Chung CS, Lee KH, Robbins J. Aspiration subsequent to a pure medullary infarction: lesion sites, clinical variables, and outcome. Arch Neurol 2000;57:478–483
32. Martino R, Terrault N, Ezerzer F, Mikulis D, Diamant NE. Dysphagia in a patient with lateral medullary syndrome: insight into the central control of swallowing. Gastroenterology 2001;121:420–426
33. Hamdy S, Xue S, Valdez D, Diamant NE. Induction of cortical swallowing activity by transcranial magnetic stimulation in the anaesthetized cat. Neurogastroenterol Motil 2001;13:65–72
34. Sumi T. Some properties of cortically-evoked swallowing and chewing in rabbits. Brain Res 1969;15:107–120
35. Martin RE, Kemppainen P, Masuda Y, Yao D, Murray GM, Sessle BJ. Features of cortically evoked swallowing in the awake primate (Macaca fascicularis). J Neurophysiol 1999;82:1529–1541
36. Jean A. Brain stem control of swallowing: neuronal network and cellular mechanisms. Physiol Rev 2001;81:929–969
37. Martin RE, Sessle BJ. The role of the cerebral cortex in swallowing. Dysphagia 1993;8:195–202
38. Ludlow CL, Yeh J, Cohen LG, Van Pelt F, Rhew K, Hallett M. Limitations of electromyography and magnetic stimulation for assessing laryngeal muscle control. Ann Otol Rhinol Laryngol 1994;103:16–27
39. Sims HS, Yamashita T, Rhew K, Ludlow CL. Assessing the clinical utility of the magnetic stimulator for measuring response latencies in the laryngeal muscles. Otolaryngol Head Neck Surg 1996;114: 761–767
40. Rodel RM, Olthoff A, Tergau F, et al. Human cortical motor representation of the larynx as assessed by transcranial magnetic stimulation (TMS). Laryngoscope 2004;114:918–922
41. Thumfart WF, Pototschnig C, Zorowka P, Eckel HE. Electrophysiologic investigation of lower cranial nerve diseases by means of magnetically stimulated neuromyography of the larynx. Ann Otol Rhinol Laryngol 1992;101:629–634
42. Hamdy S, Rothwell JC, Brooks DJ, Bailey D, Aziz Q, Thompson DG. Identification of the cerebral loci processing human swallowing with H2(15)O PET activation. J Neurophysiol 1999;81:1917–1926
43. Mosier K, Bereznaya I. Parallel cortical networks for volitional control of swallowing in humans. Exp Brain Res 2001;140:280–289
44. Kern M, Birn R, Jaradeh S, et al. Swallow-related cerebral cortical activity maps are not specific to deglutition. Am J Physiol Gastrointest Liver Physiol 2001;280:G531–G538
45. Kern MK, Jaradeh S, Arndorfer RC, Shaker R. Cerebral cortical representation of reflexive and volitional swallowing in humans. Am J Physiol Gastrointest Liver Physiol 2001;280:G354–G360
46. Hamdy S, Mikulis DJ, Crawley A, et al. Cortical activation during human volitional swallowing: an event-related fMRI study. Am J Physiol 1999; 277(1 Pt 1):G219–G225
47. Zald DH, Pardo JV. The functional neuroanatomy of voluntary swallowing. Ann Neurol 1999;46:281–286
48. Furlong PL, Hobson AR, Aziz Q, et al. Dissociating the spatio-temporal characteristics of cortical neuronal activity associated with human volitional swallowing in the healthy adult brain. Neuroimage 2004;22: 1447–1455
49. Fraser C, Rothwell J, Power M, Hobson A, Thompson D, Hamdy S. Differential changes in human pharyngoesophageal motor excitability induced by swallowing, pharyngeal stimulation, and anesthesia. Am J Physiol Gastrointest Liver Physiol 2003;285:G137–G144
50. Hamdy S, Aziz Q, Rothwell JC, et al. Explaining oropharyngeal dysphagia after unilateral hemispheric stroke. Lancet 1997;350:686–692
51. Hamdy S, Aziz Q, Rothwell JC, et al. Recovery of swallowing after dysphagic stroke relates to functional reorganization in the intact motor cortex. Gastroenterology 1998;115:1104–1112
52. Turton A, Wroe S, Trepte N, Fraser C, Lemon RN. Contralateral and ipsilateral EMG responses to transcranial magnetic stimulation during recovery of arm and hand function after stroke. Electroencephalogr Clin Neurophysiol 1996;101:316–328
53. Dennis MS, Lewis SC, Warlow C. FOOD Trial Collaboration. Effect of timing and method of enteral tube feeding for dysphagic stroke patients (FOOD): a multicentre randomised controlled trial. Lancet 2005;365:764–772
54. Dennis MS, Lewis SC, Warlow C. FOOD Trial Collaboration. Routine oral nutritional supplementation for stroke patients in hospital

55. (FOOD): a multicentre randomised controlled trial. Lancet 2005;365: 755–763

55. Caplan LR. Stroke syndromes. In: Ashbury AK, McKhann GM, McDonald IW, Goadsby PJ, McArthur JC, eds. Diseases of the Nervous System. Cambridge: University Press; 2002:1345–1361

56. Blitzer A, Brin MF, Stewart CF. Botulinum toxin management of spasmodic dysphonia (laryngeal dystonia): a 12-year experience in more than 900 patients. Laryngoscope 1998;108:1435–1441

57. Nash EA, Ludlow CL. Laryngeal muscle activity during speech breaks in adductor spasmodic dysphonia. Laryngoscope 1996;106: 484–489

58. Cyrus CB, Bielamowicz S, Evans FJ, Ludlow CL. Adductor muscle activity abnormalities in abductor spasmodic dysphonia. Otolaryngol Head Neck Surg 2001;124:23–30

59. Edgar JD, Sapienza CM, Bidus K, Ludlow CL. Acoustic measures of symptoms in abductor spasmodic dysphonia. J Voice 2001;15:362–372

60. Parnes SM, Lavorato AS, Myers EN. Study of spastic dysphonia using videofiberoptic laryngoscopy. Ann Otol Rhinol Laryngol 1978;87(3 Pt 1): 322–326

61. Blitzer A, Brin MF, Stewart C, Aviv JE, Fahn S. Abductor laryngeal dystonia: a series treated with botulinum toxin. Laryngoscope 1992;102: 163–167s

Chapter 20

Neuromuscular Disorders of the Larynx

David S. Younger

The cardinal functions of the larynx include phonation and breathing, as well as airway protection. Laryngeal paralysis results when some or all of the intrinsic laryngeal muscles fail to contract, causing decreased or absent motion and abnormal positions of the vocal cords. Neuromuscular diseases that lead to weakness of laryngeal muscles and paralysis of the vocal cords notably include disorders of the neuromuscular junction, peripheral nerve, and motor neuron disease. Myasthenia gravis (MG), botulism, Lambert-Eaton myasthenic syndrome (LEMS), and drugs that block neuromuscular transmission can result in laryngeal paralysis. Laryngeal nerve injury can result from nerve compression, trauma, tumor metastasis, local tumor extension, and connective tissue disorders. Bulbar amyotrophic lateral sclerosis (ALS), poliomyelitis and postpolio syndrome, syringomyelia, and brainstem encephalitis can all result in laryngeal dysfunction. Primary muscle disease rarely affects the larynx. The chapter reviews the anatomy, examination, laboratory evaluation, etiopathogenesis, differential diagnosis, and treatment of neuromuscular disorders of the larynx.

♦ Laryngeal Anatomy

Contraction of the lateral cricoarytenoid and interarytenoid muscles adduct and appose the vocal cords. Contraction of the posterior cricoarytenoid muscle abducts and separates the cords. Contraction of the thyroarytenoid, vocalis, and cricothyroid muscles tighten and change vocal cord shape. Motor innervation of the intrinsic laryngeal muscles originates in the nucleus ambiguus of the brainstem and in corresponding visceral efferent fibers of the vagus nerve, the principal branches of which include the superior and inferior laryngeal or recurrent nerve. The course of the trunk of the vagus nerve in the neck and anterior mediastinum makes it particularly susceptible to surgical and traumatic injury, as well as compression by mass lesions. The nerve descends in the sheath common to the internal carotid artery and internal jugular vein in the neck. The left nerve is displaced ventrally onto the anterior surface of the esophagus. The inferior laryngeal or recurrent nerve ascends in the mediastinum on the right, posteriorly under the right subclavian artery, and, on the left, under the aortic arch. The recurrent nerves ascend in the tracheoesophageal sulcus and divide into anterior and posterior rami that supply all laryngeal muscles except for the cricothyroid. The superior laryngeal nerve innervates the cricothyroid muscle by an external ramus; an internal terminal ramus pierces the thyrohyoid membrane and carries sensory fibers from the larynx.

♦ Laryngeal Function

The larynx normally closes during swallowing, thereby preventing epitracheal aspiration of secretions or food. Aberrant exaggerated reflex activity is observed in laryngospasm, which may be precipitated by endotracheal intubation, presence of a foreign body, or manipulation of the larynx during surgery. During normal breathing, the glottic opening widens by active abduction of the vocal cords during inspiration. Cough and clearing of the airway is produced by tight glottic closure, increasing subglottic pressure, sudden glottic release, and a burst of airflow clearing the airway. Speech results from the combined action of the larynx, tongue, and palate. Sound is generated by isotonic tension and vibration of the vocal cords. The shape and positioning of the vocal cords during normal speech result from the combined action of the cricothyroid and thyroarytenoid muscles, which are involved in fine tuning of the voice, thereby affecting pitch and volume.

♦ Patient Evaluation

Clues to the cause of laryngeal weakness can be ascertained by analysis of a careful history that may include recent neck or mediastinal surgery, local trauma, tracheostomy, recent stroke, or transient ischemic attack. The neurologic examination includes assessment of language, cranial nerve function, muscle strength, cerebellar function, sensation, and tendon reflexes. Direct examination of the larynx should determine if the patient has normal sensation and reflex responses. In particular, the clinician should observe the pattern of breathing, the quality and character of phonation, and the active swallowing of liquids and solids.

Examination of the neck is necessary for detection of masses in the lymphatics or thyroid, and assessing the mobility of the laryngeal framework. Sudden interruption of the sensory supply to the larynx may cause difficulty with swallowing and aspiration. This is usually due to a lesion of the internal ramus of the superior laryngeal nerve. The syndrome may result from surgical trauma, such as radical neck dissection, or operations on the supraglottic portion of the larynx. If the cricothyroid muscle is affected or if signs implicate other cranial nerves or medullary pathways, the lesion is proximal to the bifurcation of the superior laryngeal nerve. When paralysis of the larynx is unilateral, symptoms are minimal and compensation is rapid. Absence of reflex response to palpation of the larynx may be an indication of sensory paralysis, but may also be seen in psychogenic disorders.

Two procedures, laryngeal electromyography (EMG) and direct laryngoscopic examination, are essential in the evaluation of laryngeal paralysis. Laryngeal EMG can assist in the differentiation of mechanical fixation from true weakness and paralysis. Direct laryngoscopic evaluation is essential in the identification of normal anatomy, vocal cord weakness, paralysis, and associated mass lesions such as laryngeal cancer.

Isolated paralysis of the superior laryngeal nerve is less common because it has a short course. Respiration is usually unaffected, but the voice may have a lower pitch and tire easily. Combined paralysis of the superior and recurrent laryngeal nerve may be caused by separate lesions in the respective nerves or an isolated vagal nerve lesion. Combined paralysis can also result from lesions in the upper part of the neck or in the region of the jugular foramen. In bilateral cases, however, the lesion is usually in the medulla and, hence, other cranial nerves are often affected. In unilateral cases, the voice is hoarse, weak, and easily fatigued. Respiration is not affected and the glottic reflex is preserved by the bilateral sensory innervation. In bilateral cases, however, the voice is almost nonexistent, with a monotonous tone and lack of pitch change. Expectoration of secretions is difficult and stridor may be present. Aspiration is common.

Idiopathic vocal cord paralysis is diagnosed by exclusion. Complete evaluation includes indirect laryngoscopy, neurologic examination, and complete serum blood tests for diabetes and thyroid disease. Chest radiograph and chest computed tomography (CT) or magnetic resonance imaging (MRI) should be performed in patients with left-sided paralysis to identify causative lesions before they enlarge enough to be palpable. Skull x-ray, head CT, and MRI evaluate the jugular foramen for mass erosion. Endoscopy should include the nasopharynx as well as the air and food passages.

♦ Differential Diagnosis

Laryngeal or vocal cord paralysis may be classified by either the site of the lesion, whether supranuclear, bulbar, peripheral nerve, or muscle, or by the nature of the disorder, including inflammatory, neoplastic, traumatic, postsurgical, or idiopathic. Although in most instances, the causative lesion lies between the jugular foramen and the port of entry into the larynx, the disorder may also be caused by an intralaryngeal and intramedullary lesion. Lesions of the cerebral cortex and supranuclear corticobulbar pathways, usually evidenced by corticospinal tract signs with bilaterally overactive reflexes, Babinski signs, pseudobulbar palsy, and frontal release signs, can be the cause of spastic vocal cord paralysis, the underlying causes of which include possible cerebral concussion, encephalitis, multiinfarct disease of the hemispheres, and basilar artery insufficiency.

The causative lesions of bilateral vocal cord paralysis are similar to those that cause unilateral lesions. The clinical consequences of bilateral paralysis usually depend on the position of the cords; in general, the prognosis is more serious in cases of sudden onset. Bilateral paralysis after surgical injury may demand urgent relief by tracheostomy, but compression by tumor or aneurysm may cause only exertional dyspnea and stridor. In general, the nearer the cords to the midline, the greater the risk for respiratory insufficiency and more normal the voice. Conversely, the more the cords separate from the midline, the better the laryngeal airway, but the voice is weaker.

♦ Central Nervous System Disorders

Sporadic and Familial Amyotrophic Lateral Sclerosis

Motor neuron disease (MND) comprises a group of disorders characterized by progressive lower motor neuron (LMN) signs including weakness, wasting, and fasciculation, often with superimposed upper motor neuron (UMN) signs, including hyperreflexia, the Hoffman and Babinski signs, and clonus, the combination of which makes the diagnosis of ALS inescapable.[1] About 10% of ALS cases are inherited as an autosomal dominant (AD) trait in adults, the majority of whom have bulbar oropharyngeal and laryngeal involvement. One-fifth of familial ALS (FALS-AD) cases are associated with mutations in the copper/zinc-dependent superoxide dismutase *(SOD1)* gene located on chromosome 21 in ALS1. Bilateral vocal cord paralysis was the presenting manifestation of ALS in one patient with ALS1 due to missense mutation resulting.[2] Paralysis of the abductor muscles of the vocal cords was reported in non-FALS.[3]

X-Linked Spinal Bulbar Atrophy

X-linked spinal bulbar atrophy presents with slowly progressive lower motor neuropathy in men, which, unlike ALS, is confined to the LMN, with a time course slower than in ALS, in association with gynecomastia and testicular atrophy. Affected patients can manifest laryngeal involvement. The molecular defect is an expansion of a CAG repeat in the first exon of the androgen receptor gene, which expands a polyglutamine tract within the receptor. As the length of the tract of CAG increases, the illness becomes more severe; however, it is not clear how the molecular lesion causes MND. One affected patient developed bilateral abductor vocal cord paralysis.[4] Cranial MRI of the brainstem was normal. Direct laryngoscopy showed a complete paralysis of both vocal cords in the paramedian position. Respiratory distress improved after tracheostomy. Most experts agree that it is clinically important to perform a careful assessment of vocal cord function in patients with X-linked spinal bulbar atrophy, as in other similar patients because when found, vocal cord paralysis can shorten life expectancy.

Spinal Muscular Atrophy

Childhood spinal muscular atrophy (SMA) presents with significant bulbar involvement and vocal cord paralysis.[5-8] Children with SMA type 1 or Werdnig-Hoffmann disease, present at birth or in the first few months of life with hypotonia, and LMN signs in the limbs and oropharynx, leading to death by 2 years of age from recurrent aspiration due to laryngeal paralysis and respiratory failure. Those with type 2 SMA achieve normal milestones up to approximately 8 months of age, including sitting, without support in spite of hypotonia, but they fail to walk normally and can display variable oropharyngeal involvement. Many affected children can survive into the third or fourth decade. Individuals with SMA type 3 or Wohlfart-Kugelberg-Welander syndrome, have an onset any time after 18 months, typically in late childhood and adolescence as a proximal neurogenic muscular atrophy that may be confused with limb girdle muscular dystrophy. There may be an elevated serum creatine kinase (CK). Such patients present with a waddling gait, lumbar lordosis, genu recurvatum, and protuberant abdomen, or may appear thin like a stick man. Childhood SMA manifests autosomal recessive (AR) inheritance and linkage to chromosome 5q11.2–13.3, in two genes, one for neuronal apoptosis inhibitory protein (NAIP) accounting for up to 67% of cases, and another, in the survival motor neuron (SMN) gene, which was found to contain greater than 98% of deletions. The protein product of SMN is known to interact with RNA binding proteins and may actually be a spliceosome. Distal hereditary motor neuronopathy type VII is an AD disorder characterized by distal muscular atrophy and vocal cord paralysis, linkage of which was established to chromosome 2q14 in a large Welsh pedigree.[9] The management of the oropharyngeal, laryngeal, and respiratory symptoms in the various syndromes of MND includes airway protection and voice, which may be improved with local therapy of the vocal cords, cricopharyngeal muscle myotomy, tracheostomy, feeding gastrostomy, parasympatholytic drugs, and if necessary, laryngeal diversion, the primary disadvantage of which is the complete loss of phonation.[10]

Poliomyelitis

Acute poliomyelitis, now a rare cause of acute lower motor neuron paralysis in industrialized countries, is due to poliovirus infection of spinal anterior horn cells and other motor neurons. A minor illness occurs 1 to 3 days before onset of paralysis, with gastrointestinal complaints of nausea and vomiting, abdominal cramps, pain, diarrhea, and the systemic manifestations of sore throat, fever, malaise, and headache. The major illness, which includes all forms of central nervous system (CNS) disease caused by the poliovirus, including aseptic meningitis or nonparalytic polio, polioencephalitis, bulbar polio, and paralysis, follows the minor illness by 3 to 4 days. Such patients can present with stiff neck, back pain, photophobia, headache, tremulousness, obtundation, agitation, myalgia, cramps, fasciculation, and radicular pain. Bulbar poliomyelitis, which occurs in 10 to 15% of paralytic patients, involves cranial nerves VII, IX, and X and the medullary reticular formation, resulting in facial weakness, difficulty swallowing, and phonation, as well as variable respiratory difficulty, ataxic breathing, lethargy, obtundation, hypotension, hypertension, and arrhythmias. One reported patient with spinobulbar poliomyelitis had residual dysfunction of cranial nerves IX and X, producing bilateral vocal cord paralysis and recurrent aspiration.[11] Critical glottic stenosis developed 28 years after the initial episode of poliomyelitis, which appeared to be related to fibrosis of the intrinsic laryngeal muscles and ankylosis of the right cricoarytenoid joint. Accordingly, significant upper airway obstruction may develop as a late complication in those with stable neurologic deficits and chronic immobility of the vocal cords.

Postpolio Syndrome

Of the approximately 250,000 survivors of the polio epidemics, up to a quarter experience progressive muscle weakness known as postpolio syndrome. Myopathic symptoms are associated with, in order of decreasing occurrence, fatigue, arthralgia, myalgia, muscle atrophy, cold intolerance, respiratory insufficiency, and dysphagia. Nine patients with postpolio syndrome were evaluated for swallowing complaints with comprehensive history, physical examination, acoustic voice analysis, and laryngeal videostroboscopic endoscopy, including three with laryngeal EMG[12] that revealed some degree of phonatory and laryngeal deficit, and in those with prominent dysphagia, vocal cord paralysis. Bilateral vocal cord paralysis was noted in one affected patient with bulbar and spinal involvement beginning at age 13, resulting in left facial, vocal cord, and hemidiaphragm paralysis that was treated by mechanical ventilation.[13] Thirty-five years later, she noted inspiratory and expiratory stridor, leading to respiratory failure and tracheostomy. Laryngoscopic examination revealed bilateral vocal cord paralysis with near-midline fixation of the cords and pooling of secretions. The syndrome was attributed to progressive bulbar motor neuron weakness. Three patients with prior polio infection who presented with new complaints, including slowly progressive dyspnea, dysphagia, and hoarseness, were evaluated by videostroboscopy and EMG that showed vocal cord abductor and adductor weakness, and recurrent posterior glottic web in one patient, and laryngeal muscle denervation and reinnervation in two others.[14] Treatment was directed at attempting to maintain the airway and optimize vocal quality. One patient benefited from tacheostomy, one from vocal cord medialization, and one from resection of interarytenoid scarring. Three additional patients with laryngeal changes in postpolio syndrome presented with dysphonia, vocal weakness, and fatigue. All three manifested abnormalities on videostroboscopic and laryngeal EMG.

Syringomyelia

Laryngeal weakness with vocal cord paralysis occurs in syringomyelia.[15–17] In one case there was progressive loss of the pharyngeal reflexes with pooling of secretions in the upper esophagus and lower pharynx, requiring endotracheal intubation and feeding jejunostomy.[18] At cervical laminectomy, the cavity was drained and repaired with improvement of pharyngeal reflexes, but there was aspiration 2 days after cervical laminectomy. Presumably, the syrinx had extended into the brainstem to affect neurons of the nucleus ambiguus that normally control pharyngeal, laryngeal, and esophageal muscles. One 35-year-old patient who complained of noisy breathing for 15 years and had been treated for chronic asthma, developed acute breathing difficulty and was found to have stridor and bilateral abductor vocal fold palsy.[19] A syrinx was found with associated type I Chiari malformation. Three other patients with communicating syringomyelia had acute presentations, including one with paraplegia, a second with acute respiratory distress secondary to bilateral vocal cord paralysis, and a third with symptoms of brainstem ischemia.[20] Each had a communicating spinal cord syrinx associated with a posterior fossa and foramen magnum region anomaly, including a large posterior fossa arachnoid cyst in one, and Chiari malformations in the other two. Syringobulbia was found to be the cause of laryngeal stridor in an 11-year-old patient who had chronic symptoms since birth, and suddenly died after development of respiratory obstruction due to vocal cord paralysis.[21] Postmortem examination showed extensive bilateral syringobulbia with the greatest involvement in the nucleus ambiguus. Other brainstem tracts and nuclei were partially affected.

Arnold-Chiari Malformations

The classification of Arnold-Chiari malformations, now termed Chiari complex,[22] is based on the relative position of the cerebellum and brainstem in relation to the foramen magnum and the upper cervical canal.[23] Types I and II are degrees of a similar abnormality in which a conical deformity of the posterior midline cerebellum and the elongated brainstem that lies at or below the foramen magnum. Type I is divided into a classic and myelencephalic form; symptomatic patients are treated with occipitocervical surgical decompression. One MRI classification designated Chiari malformation in association with syringomyelia as type A, and those with evidence of frank herniation of the cerebellar tonsils below the foramen magnum alone as type B.[24] Those with Chiari type II present with progressive hydrocephalus and typically require insertion of a cerebrospinal fluid (CSF) shunt. Chiari type III is associated with an occipitocervical cephalocele and severe CNS malformations. Chiari type IV designates patients with myelomeningocele and severe cerebellar hypoplasia, the most common of which is probably the Dandy-Walker malformation, in which a defect in the inferior vermis is congruent with a ventriculocele of the enlarged fourth ventricle. Adults and infants alike can present symptomatic laryngeal symptoms.

The Arnold-Chiari malformation, in association with myelomeningocele, was considered the cause of progressive choking, apnea, and aspiration of 42 infants.[25] Shunts were already in place and were thought to be functioning normally; however, at posterior fossa craniotomy, all had compression of the upper spinal cord. Mortality was highest (71%) in infants with rapidly progressive, irreversible symptoms. The Arnold-Chiari malformation and shunted myelomeningocele presented with adductor vocal cord paralysis and loss of laryngeal sensation for 10 months.[26] In that infant, consideration was not given to posterior fossa exploration; treatment was supportive, including gastrostomy and close observation for several years. Bilateral abductor vocal cord paralysis due to Arnold-Chiari formation should be suspected in neonates and infants who present with high-pitched inspiratory stridor and airway compromise.[27] Unilateral vocal cord paralysis suspected in an infant or child with hoarse voice, low-pitched cry, and breathy cry or voice should be evaluated with direct laryngoscopy with flexible fiberoptic nasopharyngolaryngoscope and photodocumentation using a videocassette recorders.

Chiari malformation was suspected in a previously healthy 13-year-old boy without myelodysplasia who had mild scoliosis and complaints of nasal congestion, noisy nighttime breathing, and difficulty sleeping.[28] Flattening of the inspiratory loop on the flow-volume curve was found on pulmonary function testing, suggesting a variable extrathoracic obstruction due to a laryngeal lesion. Bilateral abductor vocal cord paralysis and sleep apnea developed precipitously following general anesthesia. Chiari malformations were discerned among six children by T1- and T2-weighted MRI with syndromes of failure to thrive, velopharyngeal incompetence, gastroesophageal reflux, or vagal hypertonia, leading to laryngeal obstruction due to vocal cord paralysis, paradoxical vocal cord motion, or laryngomalacia,[29] and treated symptomatically before decompressive surgery, which led to full functional recovery in five children. Adults likewise present with symptomatic vocal cord paralysis due to type I Chiari malformations.[30] Similarly, stridor and bilateral abductor vocal fold palsy was noted as well in a 35-year-old with complaints of noisy breathing for 15 years previously treated for chronic asthma[19]; subsequent evaluation revealed syringomyelia with a Chiari type I malformation.

Linder and Lindholm[31] evaluated children born with a Chiari II malformation during their first 18 months; four of the 22 children studied by flexible fiberscopes had disturbed breathing, and among those, two suffered from central apneic attacks as well as bilateral vocal fold motion impairment, one from apneic spells only, and one from bilateral vocal fold motion impairment. All four had dysphagia with aspiration and respiratory symptoms within the first 3 to 6 months of life. One infant with severe symptoms expired at age 3 months. The vocal fold paralysis, apneic spells, and swallowing difficulties of another infant resolved following neurosurgical intervention. Choi and coworkers[32] studied airway abnormalities in 16 patients with type I and eight patients with type II Chiari malformation. Vocal cord impairment was noted in three patients with type II Chiari, including one each with unilateral paralysis, bilateral paresis, and paralysis, but in none of those with type I disease. Tracheostomy was necessary in three, all Chiari type II; Central sleep apnea was noted in five of six patients, and tracheostomy was needed in three patients, all with type II malformations, but in none of those with type I disease.

Stroke

Laryngeal dysfunction occurs with infarcts of the brain, especially of the medulla. Venketasubramanian and colleagues[33] noted an overall frequency of 20.4% of vocal cord paresis first-ever acute ischemic stroke among 54 patients, of which 65% were lacunar, 22% cortical or subcortical, 9% lateral medullary, and 4% other brainstem infarcts. Vocal cord paresis was a constant feature of those with brainstem infarcts, but in only 11% of cortical and subcortical infarcts, and in 16% of those with lacunar infarcts. The vocal cord paresis was ipsilateral to the brainstem lesion in 80%, and contralateral to the lesion in all of those with cortical, subcortical, and lacunar infarcts.

Laryngeal hemiplegia caused by infarction of the medulla was recognized by Avillis in 1891, and named in his honor.[34] Properly defined, affected patients manifest ipsilateral palatolaryngeal paresis and contralateral hemiparesis with or without hemihypesthesia. One affected 72-year-old man with left supranuclear hypoglossal nerve palsy and right Avellis syndrome due to medullary infarction, was associated with a small lesion on brain MRI in the reticular formation medial to the nucleus ambiguus.[35] Walther and Alevisopoulos[36] described a 65-year-old man with dysphagia and aspiration, associated with Horner syndrome, paralysis of the soft palate and one vocal cord, meeting the criteria of the Avillis syndrome of palatolaryngeal hemiplegia. Brain MRI demonstrated contrast enhancement in the dorsal upper medulla in the area of the nuclei of cranial nerves IX and X. He was clinically improved without residual neurologic deficits 3 weeks later.

In 1895 Wallenberg[37] described a syndrome of the lateral medulla supplied by the posterior inferior cerebellar artery (PICA), which was later confirmed as postmortem examination and reported 6 years later.[38] As summarized by Pearce,[39] Wallenberg's patient presented with an attack of vertigo without loss of consciousness, and at the same time developed pain and hyperesthesia on the left side of the face and body, hypoesthesia of the right half of the face, and loss of pain and temperature sensitivity in the right limbs and right half of the torso, with retention of touch sensation. There was, in addition, paralysis of the left recurrent laryngeal nerve and paresis of the left hypoglossal muscle, with impaired swallowing, impaired sensation of the mucosa of the mouth, throat, and palate, and disturbed motility of the soft palate, which on the first day was bilateral, and later left sided.

It may be difficult for the examiner to recognize whether laryngeal muscle paresis or paralysis results from an upper or lower motor lesion, especially when the findings of Wallenberg syndrome are incomplete. Palmer and colleagues[40] assessed the utility of laryngeal EMG in patients with UMN and LMN disorders, including patients with Wallenberg syndrome, and noted that EMG abnormalities were significantly associated with LMN disease, whereas motor unit action potential recruitment was the most sensitive indicator of an UMN etiopathogenesis. The etiopathogenesis of the lateral medullary syndrome principally results from atherothrombotic short segment distal vertebral artery, long segment vertebral artery lesions sparing or involving the proximal portion of the vertebral artery with concomitant occlusion of the PICA, followed by arterial dissection, isolated atherothrombotic PICA disease, moyamoya disease, and cardiogenic embolism.[41,42] Sacco and colleagues[43] collected retrospective data from large reported series of Wallenberg's syndrome. Brain MRI abnormalities were evident in more than 90% of patients, and varied in size. The prognosis for the majority of patients was good, with a large measure of functional independence.

The presence of dysphonia and soft palate dysfunction increase the accuracy of detecting aspiration after ischemic stroke in the medulla.[44] Dysfunction of pharyngeal and laryngeal branches of cranial nerves IX and X and ipsilateral vocal cord after brainstem infarct lead to swallowing difficulty and aspiration revealed on a modified barium swallow as sluggish pharyngeal peristalsis and absent swallowing reflex, treatment of which typically includes a multidisciplinary approach that includes percutaneous esophageal gastrostomy tube and intensive dysphagia rehabilitation.[45]

♦ Peripheral Nervous System Disorders

Lesions at or Proximal to the Nodose Ganglion

In general, lesions at or proximal to the nodose ganglion lead to involvement of the ipsilateral half of the larynx, often with the involvement of other cranial nerves, whereas more distal lesions lead to selective neuropathic and muscular branch involvement. Disorders of the posterior cranial fossa, including meningioma, meningitis, or trauma, may affect several cranial nerves. If the lesion is near the jugular foramen, cranial nerves IX, X, and XI are affected. Cranial nerve XII is not involved because it lies above the hypoglossal canal. Symptoms and signs include dysphagia, dysphonia, nasal regurgitation, torticollis, and an inability to raise the ipsilateral arm above shoulder level. This syndrome is most often caused by lymphadenopathy of the jugular foramen; other causes include thrombophlebitis, and basilar skull fractures. Tapia syndrome includes ipsilateral paralysis of the tongue and vocal cord. The soft palate and cricothyroid muscles may be involved. The usual cause is a neoplasm in the lateral pharyngeal space where the hypoglossal nerve crosses the vagus nerve and internal carotid artery. General clues to the presence of laryngeal paralysis in association with paralysis of cranial nerves IX to XII is always an indication for careful investigation of the upper neck, base of the skull, and posterior pharyngeal fossa, as well as examination of the middle ear and nasopharynx with CT and MRI.

Jugular bulb diverticula and tumors can be associated with lower cranial nerve palsies including laryngeal dysfunction. Kobanawa[46] and colleagues described a 54-year-old woman with acute swallowing disturbances and hoarseness. Neuroimaging showed a jugular bulb diverticulum as well as unruptured internal carotid and basilar tip aneurysms on the same side. Corticosteroids for one month led to clinical improvement.

Inherited Conditions

Glomus vagale due to paraganglioma should be considered in the presence of a palpable neck mass, vocal cord paralysis, multiple lesions, and a family history of paragangliomata.[47] An inherited basis for laryngeal dysfunction should be considered when the family pedigree reveals a possible genetic basis for concomitant peripheral and central nervous system disorders. Barbieri and colleagues[48] studied two brothers with AR late-onset cerebellar ataxia and severe dysphonia. Brain MRI showed vermian and hemipheric cerebellar atrophy. Laryngofiberoscopy revealed laryngeal abductor paralysis. Neurophysiologic studies showed a pure motor neuropathy. Abductor vocal fold palsy presented in the Shy-Drager syndrome with snoring and sleep apnea.[49] Blumin and Berke[50] noted a frequency of 7% of patients with the diagnosis of multiple system atrophy (MSA) from among those with systemic neurodegenerative diseases presenting to a laryngologist for workup of dysphonia and later found to have bilateral vocal fold paresis. Isozaki and colleagues[51] found that vocal cord paralysis in hereditary cerebellar ataxia of the spinocerebellar ataxia (SCA) types 1 and 3 contrasted with that of MSA, with a more frequent occurrence of MSA than of SCA 1 and 3, 82% versus 29% and 16%, respectively. In addition, those with SCA generally showed no exacerbation with a sleep needs. All of the intrinsic laryngeal muscles including the cricothyroid, interarytenoid, and posterior cricoarytenoid muscles showed neurogenic atrophy in one autopsied patient with SCA1 and in four others with SCA3. Acute vocal cord paralysis was reported in hereditary neuropathy with liability to pressure palsies,[52] which shares a common inheritance with AD Charcot-Marie-Tooth neuropathy due to a mutation at the 17p chromosome. Laryngeal EMG is essential in the clinical categorization of the diverse forms of hereditary demyelinating and axonal neuropathy of the Charcot-Marie-Tooth (CMT) type before molecular genetic analysis for the causative gene mutation.[53] One reported family with CMT2C manifested AD vocal cord paralysis during the first two decades of life due to recurrent laryngeal nerve palsy, in association with symptomatic chronic axonal polyneuropathy, abducens nerve palsy, and diaphragm weakness, and distinguished from types IIA in which axonal polyneuropathy was restricted to the limbs, and IIB, which is of early onset and associated with foot ulceration. Bilateral adductor vocal cord paralysis presenting with features of laryngeal incompetence is a rare form of congenital bilateral vocal cord paralysis, as an isolated disturbance, or associated with Robinow syndrome and 22q chromosome deletion.[54] Bilateral vocal cord paralysis was the presenting feature of a 9-year-old girl with Williams syndrome, manifested by growth deficiency, learning impairment, and typical facies.[55] Azevedo and colleagues[56] noted the occurrence of dysphonia, laryngeal paralysis, and dysphagia in a review of 21 patients with Portuguese hereditary amyloid neuropathy.

Autoimmune Disorders

Laryngeal paresis may be the presenting feature of diverse acute and chronic autoimmune neuropathies including acute inflammatory polyradiculoneuritis or Guillain-Barré syndrome (GBS)[57] and chronic motor axonal neuropathy,[58] with associated dyspnea, dysphonia, respiratory failure, and bilateral vocal cord paralysis responsive to immunomodulating therapy with intravenous gammaglobulin and plasmapheresis. One patient with idiopathic brachial plexopathy[58] presented with laryngeal paresis.

Systemic Conditions

A systemic cause of presenting laryngeal dysfunction should be sought in those with persistent constitutional complaints, as well as in chronic illness, debilitation, or a preexistent systemic condition. Dysphonia was the first clinical manifestation of Churg-Strauss syndrome of granulomatous vasculitis in a patient with video-laryngostroboscopic evidence of paresis of the right vocal fold and reduction in adduction together with incomplete glottic closure.[60] Other patients with systemic necrotizing arteritis of the polyarteritis nodosa type have been described.[61] Laryngeal paralysis of the cricoarytenoid joint due to gouty arthritis with associated denervation atrophy of the posterior cricoarytenoid and arytenoideus muscles was reported by Gacek and colleagues.[62] Other causes of bilateral vocal cord paralysis include diabetes mellitus,[63] B12 deficiency,[64] sarcoidosis,[65] porphyria,[66] mediastinal light chain (AL) amyloidosis,[67] complete lung collapse and consolidation in cystic fibrosis,[68] relapsing polychondritis,[69] and lupus.[70]

Infectious Agents

Bacteria infections can lead to a paraglottic laryngeal abscess with the result of life-threatening laryngeal dysfunction and vocal cord paralysis.[71] Other reported infectious cases include bilateral vocal cord paralysis associated with multifocal neuropathy and tick-borne relapsing fever[72]; unilateral vocal cord paralysis in Lyme neuroborreliosis 7 days after commencement of ceftriaxone[73]; recurrent laryngeal nerve palsy due to intrathoracic mycobacteriosis[74]; unilateral vocal cord paralysis homolateral to laryngeal mucosal zoster lesions localized to the larynx covering the vestibule, arytenoid, false cord, and true vocal cord, but not extending to the hypopharynx or oropharynx[75]; and bilateral vocal cord paralysis in association with herpes simplex infection[76] and human T-cell leukemia virus-1 (HTLV-1) infection.[77]

Cancer

If a patient with known systemic cancer develops hoarseness, there is usually pressure on the recurrent laryngeal nerve by hilar adenopathy, direct tumor spread, compression, a history of neurotoxic chemotherapy or mediastinal radiation, or infection in association with immunocompetence. Patients with immunosuppression are at high risk for pharyngeal infection, especially of the lateral retropharyngeal space, as occurred in an immunocompromised patient with unilateral vocal cord paralysis in association with lymphoma and *Nocardia farcinica* laryngeal abscess.[78] Carcinoma of bronchogenic origin and mediastinal metastases are the most frequent causes of left recurrent nerve paralysis and are an indication of unresectability. Postoperative recurrent laryngeal nerve paralysis followed transhiatal resection for esophageal carcinoma in one series.[79] Those patients who underwent transhiatal resection with cervical esophagogastrostomy developed recurrent laryngeal nerve palsy more frequently than did those undergoing abdominothoracic resection. One unusual patient with laryngeal mycosis fungoides reported by Kuhn and colleagues[80] presented with vocal cord paresis progressing to paralysis. One other patient presented with vocal cord paralysis in association with prostatic carcinoma resulted from metastasis to the larynx.[81] Nonmalignant thyroid swelling in the correct anatomic site can cause recurrent laryngeal nerve paralysis. The neurologic complications of carcinoid tumor can include recurrent laryngeal nerve paralysis. Vocal cord paralysis occurred in 12 of 150 (8%) of breast cancer patients treated with postoperative therapy after radical mastectomy[82]; 11 of the 12 vocal cord paralyses were left sided, and symptoms did not appear until 2 to 25 years after irradiation. Both mediastinal fibrosis and late radiation injury were proposed as explanations for the observed vocal cord paralysis. Vincristine-induced bilateral recurrent laryngeal nerve paralysis is a rare but potentially life-threatening complication, and should be suspected when stridor is present. Vocal cord paralysis was the cause of stridor and dysphagia in a 5-month-old infant with acute lymphoblastic leukemia after administration of four weekly doses of vincristine during induction therapy.[83] Superior mediastinal syndrome due to a large unresectable cervicomediastinal neuroblastoma had Horner syndrome, phrenic nerve palsy, and ipsilateral recurrent laryngeal nerve palsy.[84] The child required prolonged mechanical ventilation but responded to chemotherapy and was free of tumor and completely recovered. Unilateral vocal cord paralysis occurred in an immunocompromised host with lymphoma resulting from *Nocardia farcinica* laryngeal abscess.[78]

Cardiovascular Disease

Pediatric patients with congenital cardiac disease are predisposed to laryngeal anomalies owing to frequent intubation, prolonged ventilatory support, and recurrent laryngeal nerve injury leading to true vocal cord paralysis after repair surgery of the aortic arch.[85] Nonsurgical vocal cord paralysis occurs in association with thoracic aortic aneurysm, as did an equal number who underwent artificial vessel replacement.[86] Pulmonary arterial stenting with occlusion of the arterial duct led to entrapment of the left recurrent laryngeal nerve between the coil used to close the arterial duct and the stent placed in the left pulmonary artery.[87] Aortic aneurysm and atherosclerotic plaque are a rare cause of left vocal cord paralysis.[88] Syphilitic aortic aneurysm, left auricular hypertrophy, atrial dilatation due to mitral stenosis, and cardiomegaly are all associated with lesions of the recurrent nerve. A 40-year-old man developed right vocal cord paralysis in association with dissection of the extracranial internal carotid artery with paresis of the right side of the soft palate.[89]

Intoxications

Vocal cord paralysis can follow inadvertent injections and indirect exposure to medications and environmental toxins. Peritonsillar bupivacaine was administered preoperatively for an otherwise uneventful tonsillectomy in a 5-year-old girl.[90] She developed stridor and respirator distress following extubation, and bilateral vocal cord paralysis was seen on laryngoscopy. A patient who underwent 131_I therapy for a solitary toxic thyroid nodule experienced vocal cord paralysis and was examined because of hoarseness one week after treatment; indirect laryngoscopy at the time confirmed right vocal cord paralysis.[91] A 76-year-old man developed vocal cord paralysis due to lymph node involvement by silicosis identified by video-mediastinoscopy, which revealed granulomatous and fibrosed recurrent lymph node encasing the left recurrent laryngeal nerve; the nerve was dissected and released from scar tissue, and the patient had total recovery of his voice 15 weeks later.[92] Organophosphate poisoning leading to laryngeal paralysis was reported in a patient leading to a difficult extubation due to bilateral vocal fold palsy, that slowly recovered over time.[93] Although collagen injections of the vocal fold rarely result in complications, Anderson and Sataloff[94] reported two patients in whom injected collagen formed firm submucosal deposits that interrupted the normal mucosal wave and produced significant dysphonia. Other complications included local abscess formation at the injection sites, hypersensitivity reactions, and induction of collagen vascular disease.

Trauma

Unilateral recurrent laryngeal neuropraxia was reported following placement of a laryngeal mask airway in a patient with CREST syndrome (calcinosis cutis, Raynaud's phenomenon, esophageal dysfunction, sclerodactyly, and telangiectasia).[95] Laryngeal examination revealed unilateral vocal cord paralysis. Recurrent bronchial cysts led to recurrent laryngeal nerve palsy in another patient.[96] Of 521 patients undergoing total lobectomy and thyroidectomies, 37 patient (7%) experienced recurrent laryngeal nerve palsies, of whom 35 experienced complete recovery.[97] Operations for thyroid cancer, Graves' disease, and recurrent goiter demonstrated significantly higher recurrent laryngeal nerve palsy. Invasion of the recurrent laryngeal nerve was identified in 19% of patients with thyroid cancer. Total lobectomy with routine recurrent laryngeal nerve identification was recommended as a basic procedure in thyroid operations. Bilateral vocal cord paralysis was reported in a patient admitted with exacerbation of achalasia who developed acute respiratory distress from bilateral immobile vocal cords in whom imaging studies revealed impressive dilation of the cervical esophagus causing compression of both recurrent laryngeal nerves.[98] Recurrent laryngeal nerve injury was reported in association with central venous catherization in a 29-year-old woman with aplastic anemia admitted for bone marrow transplantation[99]; two other reported patients developed right vocal fold paralysis following right venous catheterization.[100]

Tracheal tear, which requires fast and proper treatment, was reported in a 55-year-old man who struck his neck, causing blunt trauma with cervical bruising, neck emphysema, and dyspnea.[101] An end-to-end anastomosis of the trachea as well as tracheostomy were performed, and because of fracture of the larynx, an endolaryngeal stent was employed to stabilize the lumen. Due to injury to both laryngeal nerves, the patient suffered dysphagia, whispered speech, and dyspnea on minimal exertion as long-term sequelae. Tracheal diverticulum may similarly present with recurrent laryngeal nerve paralysis.[102] Delayed onset of vocal cord paralysis occurred 2 weeks after explantation of a left vagus nerve stimulator in a child with intractable complex partial and generalized seizures.[103] Unilateral vocal cord paralysis similarly developed after nasogastic tube insertion.[104] Any process involving the vagus nerve, its recurrent laryngeal branch, or the external branch of the superior laryngeal nerve may cause paralysis of the vocal fold. One reported a patient with degenerative disease of the cervical spine resulting in compression of the recurrent laryngeal nerve, which led to unilateral vocal cord paralysis.[105] Up to 80% of vocal fold paralyses occur after acute cervical diskectomy and fusion, and patients recover within 12 months of the procedure.[106] Vocal cord paralysis secondary to impacted esophageal foreign bodies was reported in two young children with respiratory symptoms, one of whom developed aphonia, and the other with stridor.[107] Among 35 patients with blunt trauma injury from a motor vehicle accident or penetrating injury from stab wound, 86% experienced acute external laryngeal injury leading to unilateral and bilateral vocal cord paralysis.[108] Another reported patient who sustained blunt trauma to the neck suffered a fracture of the thyroid cartilage, and a retropharyngeal hematoma was the explanation for vocal cord paralysis.[109] Self-injection injuries of the neck by intravenous drug users who lose peripheral venous access can lead to vocal cord paralysis and fragment foreign bodies.[110] Pneumothorax is another proximate cause of vocal cord paralysis in patients with chronic obstructive pulmonary disease.[111]

Neuromuscular Junction Disorders

Myasthenia gravis, an autoimmune disorder of the neuromuscular junction, is characterized by fluctuating ocular or oropharyngeal weakness, often with limb weakness. Weakness improves after administration of cholinergic drugs. Abnormal neuromuscular transmission is indicated by a decremental response of evoked motor responses after repetitive 3-per-second nerve stimulation. Circulating antibodies to the acetylcholine receptor are detected in almost 80% of patients. Severe oropharyngeal and laryngeal weakness and ineffective cough predispose the patient to aspiration, and overt aspiration causes myasthenic crisis[112] defined by use of a mechanical ventilator. Respiratory failure with airway obstruction produced by myasthenic weakness of the vocal cord abductors can occur. Drugs may produce a myasthenic syndrome or unmask or exacerbate a preexisting disorder of neuromuscular transmission. Quinidine, a cardiovascular drug, may unmask myasthenia gravis. A drug-induced disorder should be considered in any patient with myasthenic syndrome and concomitant possible adverse drug usage. In general, withdrawal of the offending drug is followed by clinical improvement. Evaluation by injection of edrophonium, repetitive nerve stimulation, and acetylcholine receptor antibody titers should be performed in all cases to confirm the diagnosis of myasthenia gravis and provide basic data for further evaluation and management. Acute botulism and the LEMS are also neuromuscular disorders caused instead by presynaptic blockade. Both may cause severe weakness of cranial muscles with risk of laryngeal weakness and aspiration. In suspected cases of botulism intoxication, laboratory confirmation includes detection of toxin in serum, in stool, and in the contaminated food. Electrophysiologic studies help to establish the diagnosis, particularly if serologic and toxologic confirmation cannot be obtained.

Muscular Disorders

If muscles of the oropharynx and larynx are involved, there is a risk of aspiration. Polymyositis is an acquired myopathy characterized by acute or subacute weakness evolving in weeks or months. There is usually histologic evidence of muscle inflammation. Dermatomyositis is defined by a characteristic rash in addition to proximal limb weakness. In one series of patients with confirmed pathology, oropharyngeal weakness with dysphagia was severe in 13 of 21 who had clinical evidence of overt aspiration and respiratory complications.[113] Nine had rapidly progressive and unremitting symptoms, lasting a few months to 1 year before they died of respiratory complications. Six had histologic and clinical findings of dermatomyositis, two had polymyositis with either lupus or carcinoma of the lung; only one patient had "uncomplicated" polymyositis. Advances in therapy of respiratory failure have improved prognosis for survival. So-called myopathic pharyngoparalysis and layrngoparalysis were reported in three affected patients who presented with dysphagia, phonasthenia, abnormal EMG, and elevated CK; all were treated with corticosteroids with favorable outcome.[114]

The muscular dystrophies are characterized by inherited, progressive weakness with variable age at onset, distribution, and disability. In infantile myotonic muscular dystrophy, severe oropharyngolaryngeal weakness may complicate feeding and lead to aspiration. In adult-onset cases, there is usually evidence of myotonia with facial, oropharyngeal, and limb weakness. Severe oropharyngeal weakness occurs late in the disease. Patients with oculopharyngeal muscular dystrophy can likewise have oropharyngeal and laryngeal weakness with aspiration in advancing age. Myotonic muscular dystrophy type 1 (DM1) presented with laryngeal stridor and vocal cord paralysis in a 47-year-old man with an 8-year course of slowly progressive dyspnea and episodic stridor. Laryngeal paresis was documented with videostroboscopy and laryngeal EMG, and treated with tracheotomy and antimyotonia agents.

The metabolic myopathies, defined by known biochemical defects, can present with severe generalized weakness, infantile hypotonia, and feeding and respiratory difficulties. These include acid maltase deficiency, brancher enzyme deficiency, and cytochrome c-oxidase deficiency. Episodic muscular weakness severe enough on rare occasions to cause complete paralysis can occur in the disorder called periodic paralysis. It is due to primary excessive fluctuations of total body potassium, often precipitated by exogenous factors, including diet, cold, medication, and intercurrent infection.

Acknowledgment This study has been supported by the Neurology Research Foundation, Inc.

References

1. Younger DS, Rowland LP, Latov N, et al. Lymphoma, motor neuron disease, and amyotrophic lateral sclerosis. Ann Neurol 1991;29:78–86
2. Fukae J, Kubo S, Hattori N, et al. Hoarseness due to bilateral vocal cord paralysis as an initial manifestation of famileal amyotrophic lateral sclerosis. Amyotroph Lateral Scler Other Motor Neuron Disord 2005; 6:122–124
3. Raverdy P, Richer-Bigo A. Slowly progressive motor neuron disease associated with paralysis of the abductor muscles of the vocal cords. Rev Neurol 1990;146:445–447
4. Tomiyasu K, Saito T, Nukazawa T, et al. A case of X-linked bulbospinal muscular atrophy with bilateral abductor vocal cord paralysis. Rinsho Shinkeigaku 1996;36:683–686
5. Young ID, Harper PS. Hereditary distal spinal muscular atrophy with vocal cord paralysis. J Neurol Neurosurg Psychiatry 1980;43:413–418
6. Boltshauser E, Lang W, Spillmann T, et al. Hereditary distal muscular atrophy with vocal cord paralysis and sensorineural hearing loss: a dominant form of spinal muscular atrophy? J Med Genet 1989;26:105–108
7. Lapena JF Jr, Berkowitz RG. Neuromuscular disorders presenting as congenital bilateral vocal cord paralysis. Ann Otol Rhinol Laryngol 2001;110:952–955
8. Roulet E, Deonna T. Vocal cord paralysis as a presenting sign of acute spinal muscular atrophy SMA type 1. Arch Dis Child 1992;67:352
9. McEntagart M, Norton N, Williams H, et al. Localization of the gene for distal hereditary motor neuronopathy VII (dHMN-VII) to chromosome 2q14. Am J Hum Genet 2001;68:1270–1276
10. Carter GT, Johnson ER, Bonekat HW, et al. Laryngeal diversion in the treatment of intractable aspiration in motor neuron disease. Arch Phys Med Rehabil 1992;73:680–682
11. Nugent KM. Vocal cord paresis and glottic stenosis: a late complication of poliomyelitis. South Med J 1987;80:1594–1595
12. Driscoll BP, Gracco C, Coelho C, et al. Laryngeal function in postpolio patients. Laryngoscope 1995;105:35–41
13. Cannon S, Ritter FN. Vocal cord paralysis in postpoliomyelitis syndrome. Laryngoscope 1987;97:981–983
14. Robinson LR, Hillel AD, Waugh PF. New laryngeal muscle weakness in post-polio syndrome. Laryngoscope 1998;108:732–734
15. Willis WH, Weaver DF. Syringomyelia with bilateral vocal cord paralysis. Report of a case. Arch Otolaryngol 1968;87:468–470
16. Lopez Gaston JI, Errea JM. Syringomyelobulbia and bilateral paralysis of vocal cords. Neurologia 1990;5:298–299
17. Holinger LD, Holinger PC, Holinger PH. Etiology of bilateral abductor vocal cord paralysis: a review of 389 cases. Ann Otol Rhinol Laryngol 1976;85:428–436
18. Bleck TP, Shannon KM. Disordered swallowing due to syrinx: correction by shunting. Neurology 1984;34:1497–1498
19. Abraham-Igwe C, Ahmad I, O'Connell J, et al. Syringomyelia and bilateral vocal fold palsy. J Laryngol Otol 2002;116:633–636
20. Zager EL, Ojemann RG, Poletti CE. Acute presentations of syringomyelia. Report of three cases. J Neurosurg 1990;72:133–138
21. Alcala H, Dodson WE. Syringobulbia as a cause of laryngeal stridor in childhood. Neurology 1975;25:875–878
22. Cama A, Tortori-Donati P, Piatelli GL, et al. Chiari complex in children-neuroradiological diagnosis, neurosurgical treatment and proposal of a new classification (312 cases). Eur J Pediatr Surg 1995; 5(Suppl 1):35–38
23. Caviness VS. The Chiari malformations of the posterior fossa and their relation to hydrocephalus. Dev Med Child Neurol 1976;18:103–116
24. Amer TA, el-Shman OM. Chiari malformation type 1: a new MRI classification. Magn Reson Imaging 1997;15:397–403
25. Park TS, Hoffman H, Hendrick E, et al. Experience with surgical decompression in young infants with myelomeningocele. Neurosurgery 1983;13:147–152
26. Birns JW. An unusual form of laryngeal paralysis associated with Arnold-Chiari malformation. Ann Otol Rhinol Laryngol 1984;93: 447–451
27. Grundfast KM, Harley E. Vocal cord paralysis. Otolaryngol Clin North Am 1989;22:569–597
28. Ruff ME, Oakes WJ, Fisher SR, et al. Sleep apnea and vocal cord paralysis secondary to type 1 Chiari malformation. Pediatrics 1987;80: 231–234
29. Portier F, Marianowski R, Morisseau-Durand MP, et al. Respiratory obstruction as a sign of brainstem dysfunction in infants with Chiari malformations. Int J Pediatr Otorhinolaryngol 2001;57:195–202
30. Blevins NH, Deschler DG, Kingdom TT, et al. Chiari-I malformation presenting as vocal cord paralysis in the adult. Otolaryngol Head Neck Surg 1997;117:S191–S194
31. Linder A, Lindholm CE. Laryngologic management of infants with Chiari II syndrome. Int J Pediatr Otorhinolaryngol 1997;39:187–197
32. Choi SS, Tran LP, Zalzal GH. Airway abnormalities in patients with Arnold Chiari malformation. Otolaryngol Head Neck Surg 1999; 121:720–724
33. Venketasubramanian N, Seshadri R, Chee N. Vocal cord paresis in acute ischemic stroke. Cerebrovasc Dis 1999;9:157–162
34. Krasnianski M, Neudecker S, Schluter A, et al. Avellis' syndrome in brainstem infarctions. Fortschr Neurol Psychiatr 2003;71:650–653
35. Nakaso K, Awaki E, Isoe K. A case of supranuclear hypoglossal nerve palsy with Avellis' syndrome due to a medullary infarction. Rinsho Shinkeigaku 1996;36:692–695
36. Walther EK, Alevisopoulos G. "Palatolaryngeal hemiplegia" in transient brain ischemia-a contribution to neurogenic dysphagia. Laryngorhinootologie 1992;71:588–591
37. Wallenberg A. Akute bulbaraffektion (Embolie der arteria cerebelli post inf sinistra). Arch Psychiatr 1895;27:504–540
38. Wallenberg A. Anatomischer befund in einen als acute bulbaraffection (Embolie der art. Cerebellar post. Sinister) beshriebenen falle. Arch Psychiatr Nervenkr 1901;34:923–959
39. Pearce JM. Wallenberg's syndrome. J Neurol Neurosurg Psychiatry 2000;68:570

40. Palmer JB, Holloway AM, Tanaka E. Detecting lower motor neuron dysfunction of the pharynx and larynx with electromyography. Arch Phys Med Rehabil 1991;72:214–218
41. Kim JS, Lee HJ, Choi CG. Patterns of lateral medullary infarction: vascular lesion-magnetic resonance imaging correlation of 34 cases. Stroke 1998;29:645–652
42. Wilkins RH, Brody IA. Wallenberg's syndrome. Arch Neurol 1970; 22:379–382
43. Sacco RL, Freddo L, Bello JA, et al. Wallenberg's lateral medullary syndrome: clinical-magnetic resonance imaging correlations. Arch Neurol 1993;50:609–614
44. Kim H, Chung C-S, Lee K-H, et al. Aspiration subsequent to a pure medullary infarction. Arch Neurol 2000;57:478–483
45. Saltzman LS, Rosenberg CH, Wolf RH. Brainstem infarct with pharyngeal dysmotility and paralyzed vocal cord: management with a multidisciplinary approach. Arch Phys Med Rehabil 1993;74:214–216
46. Kobanawa S, Atsuchi M, Tanaka J, et al. Jugular bulb diverticulum associated with lower cranial nerve palsy and multiple aneurysms. Surg Neurol 2000;53:559–562
47. Urquhart AC, Johnson JT, Myers EN, et al. Glomus vagale: paraganglioma of the vagus nerve. Laryngoscope 1994;104:440–445
48. Barbieri F, Pellecchia MT, Esposito E, et al. Adult-onset familial laryngeal abductor paralysis, cerebellar ataxia, and pure motor neuropathy. Neurology 2001;56:1412–1414
49. Brown LK. Abductor vocal fold palsy in the Shy-Drager syndrome presenting with snoring and sleep apnea. J Laryngol Otol 1997; 111:689–690
50. Blumin JH, Berke GS. Bilateral vocal fold paresis and multiple system atrophy. Arch Otolaryngol Head Neck Surg 2002;128:1404–1407
51. Isozaki E, Naito R, Kanda T, et al. Different mechanism of vocal cord paralysis between spinocerebellar ataxia (SCA1 and SCA3) and multiple system atrophy. J Neurol Sci 2002;197:37–43
52. Ohkoshi N, Kohno Y, Hayashi A, et al. Acute vocal cord paralysis in hereditary neuropathy with liability to pressure palsies. Neurology 2001;56:1415
53. Dray TG, Robinson LR, Hillel AD. Laryngeal electromyographic findings in Charcot-Marie-Tooth disease type II. Arch Neurol 1999;56:863–865
54. Berkowitz RG. Congenital bilateral adductor vocal cord paralysis. Ann Otol Rhinol Laryngol 2003;112:764–767
55. Stewart FJ, Dalzell M, McReid M, et al. Bilateral vocal cord paralysis in Williams syndrome. Clin Genet 1993;44:164–165
56. Azevedo EM, Scaff M, Caneias HM, et al. Type 1 primary neuropathic amyloidosis (Andrade, Portuguese). Arq Neuropsiquiatr 1975;33: 105–118
57. Yoskovitch A, Enepekides DJ, Hier MP. Guillain-Barre syndrome presenting as bilateral vocal cord paralysis. Otolaryngol Head Neck Surg 2000;122:269–270
58. Marchant H, Supiot F, Choufani G, et al. Bilateral vocal fold palsy caused by chronic motor axonal neuropathy. J Laryngol Otol 2003; 117:414–416
59. Hyde GP, Postma GN, Caress JB. Laryngeal paresis as a presenting feature of idiopathic brachial plexopathy. Otolaryngol Head Neck Surg 2001;124:575–576
60. Mazzantini M, Fattori B, Matteucci F, et al. Neuro-laryngeal involvement in Churg Strauss syndrome. Eur Arch Otorhinolaryngol 1998; 255:302–306
61. Fujiki N, Nakamura H, Nonomura M, et al. Bilateral vocal fold paralysis caused by polyarteritis nodosa. Am J Otolaryngol 1999;20:412–414
62. Gacek RR, Gacek MR, Montgomery WW. Evidence for laryngeal paralysis in cricoarytenoid joint arthritis. Laryngoscope 1999;109:279–283
63. Sommer DD, Freeman JL. Bilateral vocal cord paralysis associated with diabetes mellitus: case reports. J Otolaryngol 1994;23:169–171
64. Ahn TB, Cho JW, Jeon BS. Unusual neurological presentations of vitamin B(12) deficiency. Eur J Neurol 2004;11:339–341
65. Witt RL. Sarcoidosis presenting as bilateral vocal fold paralysis. J Voice 2003;17:265–268
66. Ratnavalli E, Veerendrakumar M, Christopher R, et al. Vocal cord palsy in porphyric neuropathy. J Assoc Physicians India 1999;47: 344–345
67. Conaghan P, Chung D, Vaughan R. Recurrent laryngeal nerve palsy associated with mediastinal amyloidosis. Thorax 2000;55:436–437
68. Thompson RD, Empey DW, Bailey CM. Left recurrent nerve paralysis associated with complete lung collapse with consolidation in an adult with cystic fibrosis. Respir Med 1996;90:567–569
69. Hussain SS. Relapsing polychondritis presenting with stridor from bilateral vocal cord palsy. J Laryngol Otol 1991;105:961–963
70. Hari CK, Raza SA, Clayton MI. Hydralazine-induced lupus and vocal fold paralysis. J Laryngol Otol 1998;112:875–877
71. Fernández Pérez A, Fernández-Nogueras Jiménez F, Moreno León JA. Paraglottic laryngeal abscesses. Acta Otorrinolaringol Esp 2002; 53:435–438
72. Olchovsky D, Pines A, Sadeh M, et al. Multifocal neuropathy and vocal cord paralysis in relapsing fever. Eur Neurol 1982;21:340–342
73. Neuschaefer-Rube C, Haase G, Angerstein W, et al. Unilateral recurrent nerve paralysis in suspected Lyme borreliosis. HNO 1995;43:188–190
74. Yew WW, Chau CH, Lew J, et al. Hoarseness due to recurrent laryngeal nerve palsy from intrathoracic mycobacteriosis. Int J Tuberc Lung Dis 2001;5:1074–1075
75. Nishizaki K, Onoda K, Akagi H, et al. Laryngeal zoster with unilateral laryngeal paralysis. ORL J Otorhinolaryngol Relat Spec 1997;59: 235–237
76. Pou A, Carrau RL. Bilateral abductor vocal cord paralysis in association with herpes simplex infection: a case report. Am J Otolaryngol 1995;16:216–219
77. Noda K, Isozaki E, Miyamoto K, et al. HTLV-1 associated myelopathy with bilateral abductor vocal cord paralysis-case report. Rinsho Shinkeigaku 1992;32:324–326
78. Cohen E, Blickstein D, Inbar E, et al. Unilateral vocal cord paralysis as a result of a Nocardia farcinica laryngeal abscess. Eur J Clin Microbiol Infect Dis 2000;19:224–227
79. Gockel I, Kneist W, Keilmann A, et al. Recurrent laryngeal nerve paralysis (RLNP) following esophagectomy for carcinoma. Eur J Surg Oncol 2005;31:277–281
80. Kuhn JJ, Wenig BM, Clark DA. Mycosis fungoides of the larynx. Report of two cases and review of the literature. Arch Otolaryngol Head Neck Surg 1992;118:853–858
81. Park YW, Park MH. Vocal cord paralysis from prostatic carcinoma metastasizing to the larynx. Head Neck 1993;15:455–458
82. Johansson S, Lofroth PO, Denekamp J. Left sided vocal cord paralysis: a newly recognized late complication of mediastinal irradiation. Radiother Oncol 2001;58:287–294
83. Anghelescu DL, De Armendi AJ, Thompson JW, et al. Vincristine-induced vocal cord paralysis in an infant. Paediatr Anaesth 2002; 12:168–170
84. Kapoor V, Lodha R, Agarwala S. Superior mediastinal syndrome with Rowland-Payne syndrome: an unusual presentation of cervicomediastinal neuroblastoma. Pediatr Blood Cancer 2005;44:280–282
85. Khariwala SS, Lee WT, Koltai PJ. Laryngotracheal consequences of pediatric cardiac surgery. Arch Otolaryngol Head Neck Surg 2005; 131:336–339
86. Ishii K, Adachi H, Tsubaki K, et al. Evaluation of recurrent nerve paralysis due to thoracic aortic aneurysm and aneurysm repair. Laryngoscope 2004;114:2176–2181
87. Assaqqat M, Siblini G, Fadley FA. Hoarseness after pulmonary arterial stenting and occlusion of the arterial duct. Cardiol Young 2003; 13:302–304
88. Gupta KB, Tendon S, Yadav RK. Left vocal cord paralysis and aortic arch aneurysm: an unusual presentation. Indian J Med Sci 2002; 56:443–444

89. Nusbaum AO, Somo PM, Dubois P, et al. Isolated vagal nerve palsy associated with a dissection of the extracranial internal carotid artery. AJNR Am J Neuroradiol 1998;19:1845–1847
90. Weksler N, Nash M, Rozentsveig V, et al. Vocal cord paralysis as a consequence of peritonsillar infiltration with bupivicaine. Acta Anaesthesiol Scand 2001;45:1042–1044
91. Coover LR. Permanent iatrogenic vocal cord paralysis after I-131 therapy: a case report and literature review. Clin Nucl Med 2000;25:508–510
92. Lardinois D, Gugger M, Balmer MC, Ris HB. Left recurrent laryngeal nerve palsy associated with silicosis. Eur Respir J 1999;14:720–722
93. Indudharan R, Win MN, Noor AR. Laryngeal paralysis in organophosphorous poisoning. J Laryngol Otol 1998;112:81–82
94. Anderson TD, Sataloff RT. Complications of collagen injection of the vocal fold: report of several unusual cases and review of the literature. J Voice 2004;18:392–397
95. Kawauchi Y, Nakazawa K, Ishibashi S, et al. Unilateral recurrent laryngeal nerve neuropraxia following placement of a ProSeal laryngeal mask airway in a patient with CREST syndrome. Acta Anaesthesiol Scand 2005;49:576–578
96. Rice DC, Putnam JB Jr. Recurrent bronchogenic cyst causing recurrent laryngeal nerve palsy. Eur J Cardiothorac Surg 2002;21:561–563
97. Chiang FY, Wang LF, Huang YF, et al. Recurrent laryngeal nerve palsy after thyroidectomy with routine identification of the recurrent laryngeal nerve. Surgery 2005;137:342–347
98. Chegar BE, Emko P. Bilateral vocal cord paralysis secondary to esophageal compression. Am J Otolaryngol 2004;25:361–363
99. Salman M, Potter M, Ethel M, Myint F. Recurrent laryngeal nerve injury: a complication of central venous catheterization-a case report. Angiology 2004;55:345–346
100. Martin-Hirsch DP, Newbegin CJ. Right vocal fold paralysis as a result of central venous catherization. J Laryngol Otol 1995;109:1107–1108
101. Sobiegalla M, von Hintzenstern U, Weidenbecher M Jr, et al. Tracheal rupture—a rare and dramatic emergency. Anaesthesiol Reanim 2003;28:79–81
102. Caversaccio MD, Becker M, Zbaren P. Tracheal diverticulum presenting with recurrent laryngeal nerve paralysis. Ann Otol Rhinol Laryngol 1998;107:362–364
103. Vassilyadi M, Strawsburg RH. Delayed onset of vocal cord paralysis after explantation of a vagus nerve stimulator in a child. Childs Nerv Syst 2003;19:261–263
104. To EW, Tsang WM, Pang PC, et al. Nasogastric-tube-induced unilateral vocal cord palsy. Anaesthesia 2001;56:695–696
105. Yoskovitch A, Kantor S. Cervical osteophytes presenting as unilateral vocal fold paralysis and dysphagia. J Laryngol Otol 2001;115:422–424
106. Morpeth JF, Williams MF. Vocal fold paralysis after anterior cervical diskectomy and fusion. Laryngoscope 2000;110:43–46
107. Virgilis D, Weinberger JM, Fisher D, et al. Vocal cord paralysis secondary to impacted esophageal foreign bodies in young children. Pediatrics 2001;107:E101
108. Sittitrai P, Ponprasert V. Acute external laryngeal injury. J Med Assoc Thai 2000;83:1410–1414
109. Levine RJ, Sanders AB, LaMear WR. Bilateral vocal cord paralysis following blunt trauma to the neck. Ann Emerg Med 1995;25:253–255
110. Kay DJ, Mirza N. Diagnosis and management of complications of self-injection injuries of the neck. Ear Nose Throat J 1996;75:670–676
111. Lazaro MT, Gonzalez-Anglada MI, Uson J, et al. Vocal cord paralysis due to pneumothorax in a patient with COPD. Chest 1994;105:1297–1298
112. Cohen MS, Younger DS. Aspects of the natural history of myasthenia gravis: crisis and death. Ann N Y Acad Sci 1981;377:670–677
113. Walton J, Adams R. Polymyositis. Edinburgh: Livingstone; 1958:38–74
114. Liu Z, Gu C, Hua W. The clinical characters of myopathic pharyngoparalysis and laryngoparalysis with 3 case reports. Lin Chuang Er Bi Yan Hou Ke Za Zhi 1999;13:246–247

Index

Note: Page numbers followed by *f* and *t* indicate figures and tables, respectively.

A

Abdominal breathing, 99–100
Abdominal force, 67
Abscess(es), laryngeal, 221, 222
ABSD. *See* Spasmodic dysphonia, abductor
Acanthocytosis, 184–185
Acetylcholine receptor antibody assay, 55, 114, 223
Acid maltase deficiency, 224
Acoustic assessment
    in laryngeal paralysis/paresis, 115
    of vocal function, 74–84. *See also* Vocal acoustic analysis
ACST. *See* Corticospinal tract(s), anterior
Adam's apple, 3
Adaptive equipment, for patients with dysphagia, 155–156
ADSCAs. *See* Autosomal dominant spinocerebellar ataxias
ADSD. *See* Spasmodic dysphonia, adductor
Aerodigestive tract
    configuration
        for breathing, 149, 149*f*
        for swallowing, 149, 150*f*
    upper, 149
Aerodynamic analysis, in laryngeal paralysis/paresis, 115
Airway(s), conducting, 59
Airway protective capacity, age-related changes in, 89–90
Akinesia, 160
ALS. *See* Amyotrophic lateral sclerosis (ALS)
Alveolar hypoventilation, 62
Alveolar pressure, 62–63
Alveolar ventilation (V_A), 59
    calculation, 59
    decreased, causes, 59
Amyloidosis, 117
    mediastinal light chain, 221
Amyotrophic lateral sclerosis (ALS)
    familial, 217
    and laryngeal dysfunction during sleep, 72
    phonatory instability in, 100
    respiratory dysfunction in, 72
    sialorrhea in, botulinum toxin injection for, 151
    spastic, and vocal fold hyperadduction, 99
    sporadic, 217
    vocal acoustic analysis in, 78
    and vocal fold hypoadduction, 96–98
    and vocal fold paralysis/paresis, 108*t*
    vocal tremor in, 176
    voice modulation analysis in, 80–81, 80*f*–81*f*
Anatomic dead space, 59
Anatomy
    of arytenoid cartilage, 3, 4–5, 4*f*
    of corticobulbar tract, 204, 205*f*
    of corticospinal tract, 204, 205*f*
    of cricoid cartilage, 3, 4, 4*f*
    of cricothyroid muscle, 6*f*, 7
    of epiglottis, 3, 4*f*, 5
    of interarytenoid muscle, 6*f*, 7
    laryngeal, 3–9, 216
    of lateral cricoarytenoid muscle, 6*f*, 7
    of posterior cricoarytenoid muscle, 6*f*, 7
    of pyramidal tract, 204, 205*f*
    of recurrent laryngeal nerve, 32
        and laryngeal reinnervation, 144
    of superior laryngeal nerve, 32
    of thyroarytenoid muscle, 7
    of thyroid cartilage, 3, 4*f*
Ankylosing spondylitis (AS), laryngeal involvement in, 114
Ansa cervicalis–recurrent laryngeal nerve neurorrhaphy, 145–146
Antineutrophil cytoplasmic antibody (ANCA), cytoplasmic, 114
Antinuclear antibody(ies), 114

Aortic aneurysm
  syphilitic, 222
  thoracic, 222
Apraxia, of speech, disordered prosody in, 101
Aprosody, secondary to neurologic disorders, 101
Arnold-Chiari malformation
  type I, 219
  type II, 219-220
    and vocal fold paralysis/paresis, 107, 108t
Arteritis, systemic necrotizing, 221
Articular receptors, 16-17
Artificial larynx, 103
Aryepiglottic fold(s), 4f, 5, 6f, 7
Aryepiglottic muscle, 7
Arytenoid adduction, 128, 152
  Netterville technique, 139-143, 142f-143f
Arytenoid cartilage(s), 6f, 8f
  anatomy, 3, 4-5, 4f
  anterolateral surface, 5
  apex, 5
  base, 5
  medial surface, 5
  movement, intrinsic laryngeal muscle contraction and, 6f
  muscular process, 4f, 5
  posterior surface, 5
  processes, 5
  superior depression, 5
  surfaces, 5
  vocal process, 5
Arytenoid muscle(s). See also Interarytenoid muscle
  oblique, 6f, 7
  transverse, 6f, 7
    action, 6f
Aspiration, 110, 149
  after eating, 149
  chorea and, 182
  during eating, 149
  laryngeal incompetence and, 151-152
  management, general procedures for, 153-154
  in muscular disorders, 223
  myasthenia gravis and, 223
  stroke and, 208, 220
Aspiration pneumonia
  chorea and, 182
  dysphagia and, 89-90
Asterixis, 179
Ataxia
  and disordered prosody, 101
  laryngeal disorders secondary to, 96, 96t
  and vocal tremor, 100
Atmospheric gases, partial pressures of, 60, 60t
  changes during ventilation, 60, 61f
Attention-deficit/hyperactivity disorder, with tic disorder, 182
Augmentative communication, 103
Autoimmune disorders, laryngeal involvement in, 221
Autosomal dominant spinocerebellar ataxias, and laryngeal
    dysfunction in sleep, 71

B

Baclofen, intrathecal, for dystonia, 172
Bacterial infection(s), and vocal fold paralysis/paresis,
    108t, 221
Barium swallow
  in laryngeal paralysis/paresis, 113t, 114
  modified, 90, 181
Basal ganglia
  in dystonia, 171
  sensory function, 169
  in stuttering, 177-178
Belching, recurrent, 181
Biofeedback, in speech therapy
  for phonatory instability, 101
  for vocal fold hypoadduction, 97
Bioimplants, for injection laryngoplasty, 119-120, 120t
Bioplastique, for injection laryngoplasty, 119-120, 120t
Birth trauma, and vocal fold paralysis/paresis, 107-110
Blepharospasm, 165t, 166
Blood supply, laryngeal, 9
Botox®. See Botulinum toxin
Botulinum toxin
  clinical effects, 196-197
  commercial preparations, 196
  injection
    for dystonia, mechanism of action, 168-169
    for essential tremor, 200-201, 200t
    laryngeal, techniques for, 197-198, 197f, 198f
    for laryngeal dystonia, 172
    for laryngeal granulomas, 201
    in multisystem atrophy, 70
    for posterior glottic synechiae, 201
    for sialorrhea, 151
    for spasmodic dysphonia, 197-200, 197f, 198f
      electromyography-guided, 52, 197-198, 199
    for stuttering, 179, 201
    for tics, 182, 201
    for upper esophageal sphincter dysfunction, 151
    for ventricular dysphonia, 201
  pharmacology, 196-197
  type A, 196-197
  type B, 196
Botulism, 223
Boyle's law, 62
Brachial plexopathy, idiopathic, 221
Bradykinesia
  movement disorders with, 160, 160t
  in Parkinson disease, 161
Bradyphrenia, in Parkinson disease, 162
Brancher enzyme deficiency, 224
Breath control, terminology for, 67
Breath patterns, terminology for, 67
Broca's area, 26
  and subcortical pathways, 26-27
Broyles' ligament, 5
Buccinator apparatus, 154
Bupivacaine, for tonsillectomy, and vocal cord paralysis, 222

C

CA. See Cricoarytenoid
Calcitonin gene-related peptide(s) (CGRP)
  in laryngeal sensory nerves, 11
  in taste buds, 11
Cancer
  laryngeal involvement in, 221-222
  and vocal fold paralysis/paresis, 107, 108t
Carbon dioxide (CO_2)
  partial pressure of
    in lungs, blood, and tissues, 60, 61f
    at sea level, 60t
  release rate (VCO_2), 60
Carcinoid tumor, 222
Cardiovascular disease, laryngeal involvement in, 222
Cartilage(s), laryngeal, 3-5

paired, 3
unpaired, 3
Cartilago triticea. *See* Triticeal cartilage
Catechol-*O*-methyltransferase inhibitors, for Parkinson disease, 163
Cavity, of larynx, 6*f*, 7–8
CBT. *See* Corticobulbar tracts
Central nervous system (CNS)
    disorders, 217–220
        affecting swallowing, 150, 150*t*
    injury, laryngeal paresis caused by, 108*t*
        neuropathology, 110–111
Central sleep apnea, in multisystem atrophy, 69–71
Cerebellar ataxia
    laryngeal involvement in, 221
    vocal acoustic analysis in, 78
    vocal tremor in, 176
Cerebellum, and vocal motor coordination, 26–27
Cerebral cortex
    reorganization, post-stroke, and spontaneous recovery of swallowing, 212, 213*f*
    respiratory centers, 24
    role in swallowing, 208–212
    and vocal motor coordination, 25–28
Cerebral palsy, spastic, and vocal fold hyperadduction, 99
Cerebrovascular accident. *See* Stroke
Cervical diskectomy and fusion, laryngeal complications, 223
Charcot-Marie-Tooth disease, 221
    and laryngeal dysfunction during sleep, 72
    and vocal fold paralysis/paresis, 108*t*
Chemoreceptor(s), 11–14
    neurophysiology, 11–13
    and reflexes, 13–14
Chemoreflex(es), laryngeal, 10
Chest pneumographs, 67
Chest x-ray, in laryngeal paralysis/paresis, 113–114, 113*t*
Child(ren), vocal fold paralysis/paresis in
    etiology, 107–110, 109*t*
    management, 115
    prognosis for, 115
    signs and symptoms, 110
Choline acetyltransferase, in laryngeal sensory nerves, 11
Chorea, 182–185
    causes, 182, 182*t*–183*t*
    chemical-induced, 183*t*, 184
    classification, 182, 182*t*–183*t*
    drug-induced, 183*t*, 184
    in endocrine disorders, 183*t*, 184
    of Huntington disease, 182
    infectious, 183*t*, 184
    laboratory evaluation, 185
    laryngeal involvement in, 182
    in metabolic disorders, 183*t*, 184
    primary, 182, 182*t*–183*t*
    secondary, 182, 183*t*
    of Sydenham's chorea, 182
    toxin-induced, 183*t*, 184
    vascular, 184
    and vocal fold hyperadduction, 98–100
Choreic disorders, 182–185
Chronic obstructive pulmonary disease (COPD), and laryngeal injury, 223
Churg-Strauss syndrome, 221
Circular breathing, 67
Clavicular breathing, 67
Clomipramine, for stuttering, 178

Closed phase, of vocal fold vibration, 85–86, 86*f*
Closing phase, of vocal fold vibration, 85–86, 86*f*
CMT. *See* Charcot-Marie-Tooth disease
Collagen injection(s)
    autologous, for injection laryngoplasty, 119–120, 120*t*
    bovine, for injection laryngoplasty, 119–120, 120*t*
    of vocal folds, complications, 222
Computed tomography (CT), in laryngeal paralysis/paresis, 113–114, 113*t*
Continuous positive airway pressure, in multisystem atrophy, 71
Contrast swallow study, in laryngeal paralysis/paresis, 113*t*, 114
Conus elasticus. *See* Triangular membrane (conus elasticus)
Conversion disorder, and spastic dysphonia, 99–100
Corniculate cartilage, 4*f*, 5
Corticobulbar tracts, neuroanatomy, 204, 205*f*
Corticospinal tract(s)
    anterior, 204
    lateral, 204
    neuroanatomy, 204, 205*f*
CPAP. *See* Continuous positive airway pressure
Cranial nerve palsy(ies), laryngeal involvement in, 220–221
CREST syndrome, 222
Cricoarytenoid joint
    fixation, 117
    involuntary motion, 117
Cricoarytenoid muscle(s), 216
    lateral, 5
        action, 6*f*, 7
        anatomy, 6*f*, 7
        disorders, and vocal fold hypoadduction, 97–98
        innervation, 8
        needle electrode placement and verification for, 43, 43*f*
        nerve supply, 7
    posterior, 4, 5, 216
        action, 6*f*, 7
        anatomy, 6*f*, 7
        botulinum toxin injection into, 197–198, 198*f*
        denervated, regeneration, 35
        denervation, 35
        innervation, 8, 33–34, 33*f*
        needle electrode placement and verification for, 43, 43*f*
        nerve supply, 7
Cricoid cartilage, 6*f*, 8*f*, 9*f*
    anatomy, 3, 4, 4*f*
    ossification, 4
    partial resection, 154
Cricopharyngeus muscle, 8
    dilation, 151
    dysfunction, treatment, 152–153
    myotomy, for neurogenic dysphagia, 151, 152–153
    needle electrode placement and verification for, 43
Cricothyroid joint, 3, 4, 4*f*
Cricothyroid ligament, 3, 5
Cricothyroid muscle, 8, 9*f*, 216
    action, 6*f*, 7
    anatomy, 6*f*, 7
    innervation, 33–34, 33*f*
    needle electrode placement and verification for, 42, 43*f*
    nerve supply, 7
CSA. *See* Central sleep apnea
CST. *See* Corticospinal tract(s)
Cuneiform cartilage, 5
Cystic fibrosis, 221
Cytochrome c-oxidase deficiency, 224
Cytomegalovirus (CMV), and vocal fold paralysis/paresis, 108*t*, 110

D

Dalton's law, 60
Deep brain stimulation
 for dystonia, 172
 for Parkinson disease, 164
 for tics, 182
Delphian lymph node, 9
Dementia, in Parkinson disease, 162
Depression, in Parkinson disease, 162
Dermatomyositis, 223
Diabetes mellitus, 221
 laboratory diagnosis, 114
Diaphragmatic breathing, 67
Diaphragmatic flutter, 181
Diet modification, for patients with dysphagia, 156
Diffusing capacity (D_L), 60
 limitation, and hypoxemia, 62
Diffusion
 Fick's law of, 60–61
 of respiratory gases, 60–61
Digastric muscle, 7
Diplophonia, 100–101, 110
 neuropathology, 111
 vocal fold hypoadduction and, 97
Distal hereditary motor neuronopathy type VII, 218
Dopamine agonists, for Parkinson disease, 163
Dopamine releasers, for Parkinson disease, 163
Dopaminergic neurons, transplantation, for Parkinson disease, 164
DRD3 gene, 174
Drive, definition, 17
Drive receptors, 18
Drooling
 botulinum toxin injection for, 151
 in Parkinson disease, 161
Dysarthria(s)
 ataxic, disordered prosody in, 101
 hyperkinetic, disordered prosody in, 101
 vocal tract characteristics in, 96, 97*f*
Dysfluency. *See also* Stuttering
 normal, during speech development, 176
Dyskinesia, and vocal fold hyperadduction, 99–100
Dysphagia, 110, 149, 207–208
 and aspiration pneumonia, 89–90
 chorea and, 182
 combined interventions for, 156
 compensatory interventions for, 154–156
 diagnosis, techniques for, 90–91
 epidemiology, 89
 etiology, 89–90
 in muscular disorders, 223
 neurogenic, 207–208, 207*t*
  diagnosis, 151
  etiology, 150, 150*t*
  signs and symptoms, 151
  treatment
   evaluation, 151
   medical, 150*t*, 151
   surgical, 150*t*, 151–154
 post-stroke, 208
  mechanisms, 210–212
  treatment, 213
 rehabilitative interventions for, 154, 156
 in stroke patients, 89–90
 structural, 207, 207*t*
 treatment
  behavioral, 154–157
  medical, 150*t*
  surgical, 150*t*
Dysphonia, 110, 212–213
 muscle tension, 110, 170
 in Parkinson disease, management, 98
 ventricular, botulinum toxin injection for, 201
Dyspnea, acute, in Parkinson disease, 71
Dysport®. *See* Botulinum toxin
Dystonia, 164–172
 adult onset, 165*t*, 166
 age at onset, 165–166, 165*t*, 166*f*
 biochemistry, 171
 brain pathology in, 171
 cervical, 168
 childhood onset, 165*t*, 166
 classification, 165, 165*t*
 definition, 164
 environmental causes, 165*t*
 epidemiology, 164
 focal, 165*t*, 166, 166*f*, 167*t*
  treatment, 172
 generalized, 165*t*, 166, 166*f*, 167*t*
  treatment, 172
 genetics, 170–171, 171*f*
 hereditary, 165*t*
 hereditary autosomal dominant myoclonus, 170
 with hereditary neurologic syndromes, 165*t*
 idiopathic, childhood-onset, 170
 infantile onset, 165*t*, 166
 laboratory evaluation in, 171
 laryngeal, 165*t*, 166, 166*f*, 167–168, 167*t*. *See also* Spasmodic dysphonia
  abductor, 167–168
  adductor, 167–168
  and essential tremor, differentiation, 167
  respiratory adductor, 168
  treatment, 172
 levodopa-responsive, 171
 lingual, 172
 mandibular, 172
 metabolic findings in, 171
 neuroimaging in, 171
 oropharyngeal, 172
 pharmacotherapy for, 171–172
 pharyngeal, 172
 primary, 165*t*, 166, 166*f*, 167*t*
 psychogenic, 169–170
 secondary, 165*t*, 166
 segmental, 165*t*, 166, 166*f*, 167*t*
  treatment, 172
 segmental-cranial, 167, 167*t*
 sensory system and, 168–169
 sporadic, 165*t*
 surgical treatment, 172
 tardive, 172
 torsion
  idiopathic, 170
  primary generalized, 170
 trauma and, 169
 treatment, 171–172
 viral illness and, 169
 and vocal fold hyperadduction, 98–100
Dystonia musculorum deformans, 170
DYT1 gene mutations, and dystonia, 169, 170–171

E

Eating
  rate of, for patients with dysphagia, 155
  recommended techniques for, for patients with dysphagia, 155
Edrophonium (Tensilon) test, 55, 114, 223
Elderly
  airway protective capacity in, 89–90
  dysphagia in, 89–90
  laryngeal muscle changes in, 157
  superior laryngeal nerve changes in, 89–90
  swallowing changes in, 156–157
  vocal fold changes in, 117, 118, 119f
Electromyography (EMG)
  craniocervical muscles amenable to, 43, 43t
  laryngeal, 41–53, 217
    clinical uses, 41, 41t, 49–52, 55
    electrode placement and verification in, 42–43, 43f
    fibrillation potentials in, 44–45, 44f
    guidance, for laryngeal injections, 52
    historical perspective on, 41
    insertional activity in, 44
    in laryngeal dystonia, 174, 174f
    in laryngeal paralysis/paresis, 114
    motor unit potentials in, 45–47, 45f
      amplitude of, 45–46, 46f
      brief small-amplitude polyphasic, 46
      duration of, 45–46
      interference patterns, 46–47, 47f
      with myopathic process, 45f, 46–47
      with neuropathic process, 45–47, 45f, 46f
      normal, 45, 45f
      number of phases in, 45
      "picket fence" pattern, 45f
      polyphasic, 45–46
      recruitment patterns, 45f, 46–47, 48f
    multiple fine-wire, 49.50f, 51f
    patient positioning for, 42
    patient preparation for, 42
    patterns, 44–47
    positive sharp waves in, 44–45, 44f
    recording, 41–42
    repetitive stimulation in, 47, 48f
    in spasmodic dysphonia with tremor, 175, 175f
    spontaneous activity in, 44–45, 44f
      pathologic, 44–45, 44f
    techniques, 42–43, 42t
    volitional activity in, 45–47
Embryology, laryngeal, 3
EMG. See Electromyography (EMG)
Emphysema, and hypoxemia, 62
Enkephalin, in taste buds, 11
Epiglottic cartilage, 5
Epiglottis, 7
  anatomy, 3, 4f, 5
  taste buds in, 11
Epithelium. See also Specific laryngeal sensory epithelium (SLSE)
  laryngeal, 8
    sensory structures in, 10
Epstein-Barr virus (EBV), and vocal fold paralysis/paresis, 108t, 110
Esophagostomy, cervical, 154
Esophagus, foreign bodies in, laryngeal complications, 223
Essential tremor, 174–176
  botulinum toxin injection for, 200–201, 200t
  and laryngeal dystonia, differentiation, 167
  vocal acoustic analysis in, 78
  and vocal tremor, 100
ETM2 locus, 174
Exercise(s)
  for elderly, 157
  for improving swallowing function, 156, 157
Expiration, active and passive mechanisms during, 63, 63f
Extrapyramidal disorders
  laryngeal disorders secondary to, 96, 96t
  speech/voice therapy in, 100
  and vocal fold hyperadduction, 98–100

F

Falsetto register, and stroboscopic examination, 87
Fat, autologous, for injection laryngoplasty, 119–120, 120t
Fatigue, vocal, 110
Feeding, nonoral, 154
FEES. See Fiberoptic endoscopic examination of swallowing
FEESST. See Flexible endoscopic evaluation of swallowing with sensory testing
FEF. See Forced expiratory flow
Festination, in Parkinson disease, 161
FET1 locus, 174
FEV_1. See Forced expiratory volume in 1 second (FEV_1)
Fiberoptic endoscopic examination of swallowing, 90
Fiberoptic laryngoscopy, 55–57, 57t
  in multisystem atrophy, 70
  during sleep, 69
Fick's law, 60–61
FIF. See Forced inspiratory flow
Fine-wire laryngeal electromyography, 49.50f, 51f
Flexible endoscopic evaluation of swallowing with sensory testing, 89–92
Flexible fiberoptic laryngoscopy, 56, 57f, 57t
Flexible laryngoscope(s), 56–57, 57f, 57t
  tip-chip, 56, 57f
Flow receptors, 17–18
Flow-volume loops, 66–67, 66f
Fluorescent treponemal antibody absorption test (FTA-ABS), 114
Flutter, 180–181
  disorders associated with, 176
fMRI. See Magnetic resonance imaging (MRI), functional
Forced expiratory flow
  at 25% of FVC (FEF_{25}), 66, 66f
  at 50% of FVC (FEF_{50}), 66f, 67
  at 75% of FVC (FEF_{50}), 66f, 67
Forced expiratory volume in 1 second (FEV_1), 66
Forced inspiratory flow
  at 25% of FVC (FIF_{25}), 66f, 67
  at 50% of FVC (FIF_{50}), 66f, 67
  at 75% of FVC (FIF_{75}), 66f, 67
Forced vital capacity (FVC), measurement, 66
FRC. See Functional residual capacity (FRC)
Frontal operculum, and vocal motor coordination, 26
Functional magnetic resonance imaging. See Magnetic resonance imaging (MRI), functional
Functional residual capacity (FRC), 63, 64f
  measurement, 66
Fundamental frequency
  analysis, 74
  in stroboscopic examination of vocal fold vibrations, 86, 87
FVC. See Forced vital capacity (FVC)

G

Gait, in Parkinson disease, 161
Galanin, in taste buds, 11
Gas exchange, respiratory, 59, 60–61

Gastroesophageal reflux, 149
Gastrostomy, feeding, 154
Gelfoam, for injection laryngoplasty, 119–120, 120t
Gestes antagonistes, 168, 169, 178
Gilles de la Tourette syndrome. *See* Tourette syndrome
Globus pallidus, and dystonia, 171, 172
Glomus vagale, 221
Glossoepiglottic fold(s)
   lateral, 5
   median, 5
Glottal fry, 100
Glottal incompetence
   etiology, 117
   treatment, surgical, 152
Glottic closure
   stroboscopic examination, 87
   surgical technique for, 153–154
Glottis, 6f, 8
Gore-Tex implants, use of
   technique for, 135–139, 136f–140f
   Zeitel's rationale for, 135
Granuloma(s), laryngeal, botulinum toxin injection for, 201
Granulomatous vasculitis, 221
Guide plane prosthesis, 154
Guillain-Barré syndrome, 221
   and vocal fold paralysis/paresis, 108t

H

Haloperidol
   for stuttering, 178
   for tics, 182
Head injury, closed, and brainstem contusion, and vocal fold hypoadduction, 96–98
Heimlich maneuver, 156
Herpes simplex virus (HSV), 221
   and vocal fold paralysis/paresis, 108t, 110
Herpes zoster, 221
Hiccup, 179
Human leukocyte antigen (HLA) B27, 114
Human T-cell leukemia virus (HTLV), type 1, 221
huntingtin gene, 183, 185
Huntington disease, 182, 183
   phonatory instability in, 100
   vocal acoustic analysis in, 78
   and vocal fold hyperadduction, 99–100
5-Hydroxytryptamine, in taste buds, 11
Hyoid bone, 3, 4f, 6f
   greater horn, 3, 4f
   lesser horn, 3, 4f
Hyperkinesia, movement disorders with, 160, 160t
Hypertonicity, and vocal fold hyperadduction, 98–100
Hypopharyngeal diverticulum, 153
Hypopharyngoplasty, 152
Hypophonia, in Parkinson disease, management, 98
Hypoxemia, 62
   hypoxic, 62

I

Iatrogenic injury
   to recurrent laryngeal nerve, 222–223
   and vocal fold paralysis/paresis, 107, 108t
Imaging, laryngeal, 55
Immunocompromised patient(s), 222
Infection(s)
   bacterial, and vocal fold paralysis/paresis, 108t, 221
   chorea associated with, 183t, 184
   laryngeal involvement in, 221
   streptococcal, and tics, 182
   viral, and vocal fold paralysis/paresis, 108t, 110, 221
Inferior constrictor muscle, 3, 9f
Inferior laryngeal nerve. *See* Recurrent laryngeal nerve
Inferior thyroid artery, 8, 9
Infraglottic/subglottic cavity (space), 6f, 7, 8
Infrahyoid muscles, 7
Injection(s). *See also* Botulinum toxin, injection
   laryngeal, electromyography-guided, 52
Injection laryngoplasty, for vocal fold incompetence, 118–123
   goals, 118–119
   materials, 119–120, 120t
      selection, 120–121
   outcomes, 123
   techniques, 121–123, 121f, 122f
Injection thyroplasty, 152
Innervation, laryngeal, 8, 9f. *See also* Reinnervation procedure(s); *specific nerve*
Inspiration, 62–63
Interarytenoid muscle, 216. *See also* Arytenoid muscle(s)
   action, 7
   anatomy, 6f, 7
   disorders, and vocal fold hypoadduction, 97–98
   innervation, 8, 33–34, 33f
   needle electrode placement and verification for, 43
   nerve supply, 7
Interarytenoid notch, 7
Intraoral air pressure (P_{io}), measurement, 65
Intravenous (IV) drug abuse, and laryngeal injury, 223
Intubation, and vocal fold paralysis/paresis, 107, 108t, 222
Iodine-131 therapy, for thyroid nodule, and vocal cord paralysis, 222

J

Jaw sling, 154
Jejunostomy, feeding, 154
Jitter
   analysis, practical and theoretical considerations in, 74
   in neurologic disorders, 100
Jugular bulb diverticula, 221
Juvenile rheumatoid arthritis (JRA), laryngeal involvement in, 114

K

KayPENTAX Motor Speech Profile™, 81
KayPENTAX Multi-Dimensional Voice Program™, 76–77
KayPENTAX Real-Time Pitch™ software, 76
Kinesie paradoxale, 169

L

Laboratory study(ies), in laryngeal paralysis/paresis, 114
Lamina propria, and vocal fold incompetence, 117–118
Laryngeal disorders, secondary to neurologic disorders, 96t
   perceptual characteristics, 96, 96t
   speech treatment for, 95–96
   therapy goals and techniques for, 96, 96t
Laryngeal dystonia. *See also* Spasmodic dysphonia
   vocal acoustic analysis in, 78
Laryngeal framework, 3
Laryngeal framework surgery
   anesthesia for, 128–129
   Isshiki classification, 127–128
   preparation for, 128–129, 128f
   principles, 128–129
   procedures, 129–144

sedation for, 128
theory, 128–129
Laryngeal incompetence. *See also* Vocal fold(s), incompetence
   and aspiration, 151–152
   surgical treatment, 151–152
Laryngeal nerve paralysis
   unilateral, phonatory instability in, 100
   and vocal fold hypoadduction, 96, 96*t*, 97–98
Laryngeal obstructive sleep apnea/hypopnea syndrome, 72
Laryngeal prominence, 3, 4*f*
Laryngeal rebalancing, 201
Laryngeal tension-fatigue syndrome, 170
Laryngeal veins, 9
Laryngoparalysis, myopathic, 223
Laryngopharynx, 3, 8
Laryngoscopy, 8. *See also* Videolaryngoscopy
   direct, 217
      in laryngeal paralysis/paresis, 114–115
   fiberoptic, 55–57, 57*t*
      in multisystem atrophy, 70
      during sleep, 69
   flexible fiberoptic, 56, 57*f*, 57*t*
   indirect, in laryngeal paralysis/paresis, 112, 112*f*, 113*f*
   mirror, 55–56
   stroboscopic, 55–57. *See also* Stroboscopic examination
   telescopic, 55–57, 57*f*, 57*t*
Laryngospasm
   adductor, 99
   sleep-related, 72
Laryngostroboscopy, 55–57, 57*t*. *See also* Stroboscopic
      examination
Larynx
   artificial, 103
   function, 216
   motor innervation, 207
   neurological disorders of, 96, 96*t*
Lateral medullary syndrome, 220
Lateral thyroid ligament, 3
LCST. *See* Corticospinal tract(s), lateral
Lee Silverman Voice Treatment®, LOUD program, 95
   for disordered prosody, 102–103
   for vocal fold hypoadduction, 97
LEMG. *See* Electromyography (EMG), laryngeal
Levodopa, for Parkinson disease, 163
Ligament(s), laryngeal, 5
   extrinsic, 5
   intrinsic, 5
Lower lip, of vocal fold vibration, 85–86, 86*f*
Lower motor neuron(s), 204
Lower motor neuron disease, 217
   and vocal fold hypoadduction, 96–98
LSVT. *See* Lee Silverman Voice Treatment®
Lubag, 171
Lung cancer, and vocal fold paralysis/paresis, 107, 108*t*
Lung volume(s), static, measurement, 65–66
Lyme disease, 221
   laboratory diagnosis, 114
Lymphatics, laryngeal drainage, 9
Lymphoma(s), 222

M

Machado-Joseph disease, and laryngeal dysfunction in sleep, 71
Magnetic resonance imaging (MRI)
   functional, of cerebral cortical loci activated in swallowing,
      209–210, 211*f*
   indications for, 55
   in laryngeal paralysis/paresis, 113–114, 113*t*
Magnetoencephalography, of cerebral cortical loci activated in
      swallowing, 210, 212*f*
Magnetometers, 67
Male(s), laryngeal development in, 3
Malignancy. *See* Cancer
Mask area, 99–100
Maximum expiratory pressure, measurement, 64–65
Maximum inspiratory pressure, measurement, 64
MBS. *See* Modified barium swallow
Mechanoreceptor(s), 14–18
Medullary reticular formation, and vocal motor coordination, 24
MEG. *See* Magnetoencephalography
Meige disease, 167
Membrane(s), laryngeal, 4*f*, 5
   extrinsic, 5
   intrinsic, 5
MEP. *See* Maximum expiratory pressure
MEPs. *See* Motor evoked potentials (MEPs)
Metabolic myopathy, laryngeal involvement in, 224
Micrographia, in Parkinson disease, 161
Midbrain centers, and vocal motor coordination, 24–25
Minute ventilation, 59
Minute volume ventilation, 59
MIP. *See* Maximum inspiratory pressure
Mirror laryngoscopy, 55–56
Mitochondrial mutations, and dystonia, 171
Modified barium swallow, 90, 181
Modulation analysis, 80–81, 80*f*–81*f*
   in amyotrophic lateral sclerosis, 80–81, 80*f*–81*f*
Mogigraphia, 167
Mogiphonia, 167
Motor cortex, 204, 206*f*. *See also* Cerebral cortex
   and vocal motor coordination, 27–28, 27*f*
Motor evoked potentials (MEPs), in swallowing motor cortex,
      208–209, 209*f*
Motor homunculus, 204, 206*f*
Motor impersistence, 182
Motor innervation, laryngeal
   central pathways, 21–28
   peripheral, 32–37
   respiratory, 23
   for vocalization and speech, 24–25
Motor neuron disease, 217–218. *See also* Amyotrophic lateral
      sclerosis (ALS)
Motor strip, 204
Movement disorders. *See also specific disorder*
   bradykinetic, 160, 160*t*
   diagnosis, 160
   hyperkinetic, 160, 160*t*
   idiopathic, 160
   laryngeal, 160–195
   psychogenic, 169
   symptomatic, 160
   treatment, 160
MSA. *See* Multisystem atrophy
Mucosa
   laryngeal, 3, 5, 8
      sensory structures in, 10
   laryngopharyngeal, 3
Mucosal wave, stroboscopic examination, 87
Multiple sclerosis (MS)
   vocal acoustic analysis in, 78
   vocal fold hyperadduction in, 99
   and vocal fold paralysis/paresis, 108*t*
   vocal tremor in, 176

Multisystem atrophy
  cerebellar type, 162
  fiberoptic laryngoscopy in, 70
  and laryngeal dysfunction during sleep, 69–71
  laryngeal involvement in, 221
  laryngeal obstruction in, 69–71
    pathophysiology of, 70
  nocturnal stridor in, 69–70
  parkinsonian type, 162
  sleep-disordered breathing in, 69–71
  speech in, 162
  upper airway obstruction in, 69–71
    management, 70–71
  videopolysomnography in, 70
Muscle(s), laryngeal, 5–7
  adductor, disorders, and vocal fold hypoadduction, 97–98
  age-related changes in, 157
  denervated, regeneration, 35
  denervation, 35
  extrinsic, 5–7
  intrinsic, 6f, 7, 216
    denervation, 117
    innervation, 33–34, 33f
  motor innervation, 216
Muscle spindles, 14–15
Muscle tension dysphonia, 110, 170
Muscular disorders
  dysphagia in, 223
  laryngeal involvement in, 223–224
Muscular dystrophy
  laryngeal involvement in, 223–224
  myotonic, 223
    phonatory instability in, 100
  oculopharyngeal, 223
Myasthenia gravis (MG)
  aspiration in, 223
  diagnosis, 223
  laboratory diagnosis, 55, 114, 223
  laryngeal electromyography in, 51–52, 51f
  laryngeal involvement in, 223
  medical management, 98
  pathophysiology, 223
  and vocal fold hypoadduction, 96–98
  and vocal fold paralysis/paresis, 108t
  vocal tremor in, 176
Myasthenic syndrome, drug-induced, 223
Mycobacteriosis, 221
Mycosis fungoides, 222
Mylohyoid muscle, 7
Myobloc®. See Botulinum toxin
Myoclonus, 179–181
  classification, 179, 179t
  definition, 179
  epileptic, 179t
  essential, 179t
  etiology, 179t
  negative, 179
  palatal, 179–181, 180f
  phenomenology, 179t
  physiologic, 179t
  positive, 179
  respiratory, 181
  singulus, 179
  symptomatic, 179t
  and vocal fold hyperadduction, 99

Myopathy
  laryngeal involvement in, 223–224
  and vocal fold paralysis/paresis, 108t

N

Nasogastric tube feeding, 154
  laryngeal complications, 223
National Center for Voice and Speech, standards for vocal acoustic analysis, 76–77
NCVS. See National Center for Voice and Speech
Neonate(s), vocal fold paralysis/paresis in
  etiology, 107–110, 109t
  signs and symptoms, 110
Neoplasm(s), and vocal fold paralysis/paresis, 108t
Nerve(s), laryngeal. See also specific nerve
  injury, 144
  regeneration, 144
  repair, 144
Neuroacanthocytosis, 181, 184–185
Neuroblastoma, 222
Neurolaryngologic evaluation, 54–55
Neurologic disorders. See also specific disorder
  affecting swallowing, 150–151, 150t
  laryngeal disorders secondary to, 96t
    speech treatment for, 95–106
  speech treatment for, 95–106
  and vocal fold paralysis/paresis, 107, 108t
Neuromuscular disorders
  autoimmune, laryngeal involvement in, 221
  infectious, laryngeal involvement in, 221
  inherited, laryngeal involvement in, 221
  of larynx, 216–226
    differential diagnosis, 217
    patient evaluation, 216–217
  systemic, laryngeal involvement in, 221
  and vocal fold paralysis/paresis, 108t
Neuromuscular junction (NMJ), 35, 35f
Neuromuscular junction (NMJ) disorders, laryngeal involvement in, 223
Neuronal apoptosis inhibitory protein (NAIP), 218
Neurotransmitter(s)
  in laryngeal sensory nerves, 11
  in taste buds, 11
Nitric oxide (NO), in laryngeal sensory nerves, 11
Nodose ganglion, lesions at/proximal to, and laryngeal involvement, 220–221
Nucleus ambiguus, laryngeal motoneurons in, functional organization, 21–23
Nucleus retroambiguus, and vocal motor coordination, 24
Nucleus tractus solitarius, 23
Nystagmus, 179

O

Oblique line, 3
Obsessive-compulsive disorder (OCD)
  and stuttering, 178
  with tic disorder, 182
Obstructive sleep apnea/hypopnea
  in amyotrophic lateral sclerosis, 72
  in Charcot-Marie-Tooth disease, 72
  in multisystem atrophy, 69–71
  in syringomyelia and syringobulbia, 71–72
Obstructive sleep apnea/hypopnea syndrome, 72
  secondary, 72
Odynophonia, 110
Omohyoid muscle, 7

Opening phase, of vocal fold vibration, 85–86, 86f
Oppenheim's dystonia, 170
Organophosphates, and vocal cord paralysis, 222
Oromandibular dystonia, 165t, 166
OSAH. See Obstructive sleep apnea/hypopnea
OSAHS. See Obstructive sleep apnea/hypopnea syndrome
Oxygen
  consumption (VO_2), 60
  partial pressure of
    in alveoli (P_AO_2), 60
    arterial (PaO_2), 60
    in inspired air (P_IO_2), 60
    in lungs, blood, and tissues, 60, 61f
    at sea level (PO_2), 60, 60t

P

Palatal lift prosthesis, 154
Palatal myoclonus, 179–181, 180f
Palatal reshaping/augmentation prosthesis, 154
Palatopharyngeus muscle, 7
PANDAS, 182
Paraganglia, 18
Paraganglioma, and glomus vagale, 221
Paraglottic space, 8
Parakinesia, 182
Paralysis
  laryngeal, 107–116
    in adults, etiology, 107, 108t–109t
    in autoimmune disorders, 221
    causes, 217
    classification, 217
    etiology, 107–110, 108t, 111
    evaluation, 111–115, 111f
    familial, 108t, 110
    and fixation, differentiation, laryngeal electromyography for, 50, 55
    historical perspective on, 107
    history-taking in, 111–112
    laboratory diagnosis, 114
    management, 115
    mechanical versus neurogenic causes, differentiation, laryngeal electromyography and, 50, 55
    in neonates and children, etiology, 107, 109t
    neuropathology, 110–111
    physical examination in, 112
    prognosis for, 115
      laryngeal electromyography and, 49–50
    signs and symptoms, 110
    staging, 115
    vincristine-related, 108t, 110
    work-up for, 55
  laryngeal nerve
    unilateral, phonatory instability in, 100
    and vocal fold hypoadduction, 96, 96t, 97–98
  recurrent laryngeal nerve, 217
  superior laryngeal nerve, 117, 217
  vocal fold
    and aspiration, 151–152
    bilateral, 217
    in cardiovascular disease, 222
    classification, 217
    congenital bilateral, 221
    familial, 108t, 110
    in inherited conditions, 221
    toxin-related, 222
    trauma-related, 222–223
    unilateral, etiology, 117
    vocal acoustic analysis in, 78–79
Paratracheal lymph nodes, 9
Parenteral alimentation, 154
Paresis
  laryngeal. See also Paralysis
    in adults, etiology, 107, 108t–109t
    definition, 107
    etiology, 107–110, 108t, 111
    evaluation, 111–115, 111f
    history-taking in, 111–112
    in neonates and children, etiology, 107, 109t
    physical examination in, 112
    signs and symptoms, 110
  vocal fold, familial, 108t, 110
Parkinson disease (PD), 160–164
  aprosody in, 101
  biochemistry, 162
  clinical features, 161–162
  definition, 160–161
  diagnostic criteria for, 161, 161t
  epidemiology, 162
  glottal incompetence in, 117
  laryngeal disorders secondary to, 96, 96t
  and laryngeal dysfunction in sleep, 71
  neurosurgery for, 163–164
    ablative, 163–164
  pathology, 162
  pharmacotherapy for, 163
  phonatory instability in, 100
  sialorrhea in, botulinum toxin injection for, 151
  speech in, 162
  speech treatment for, 95
    combined with medical management, 98
    with LSVT LOUD, 102–103
  treatment, 162–164
  vocal acoustic analysis in, 78
  and vocal fold hypoadduction, 97–98
  vocal tremor in, 100, 174, 176
Parkinsonism
  classification, 160, 161t
  definition, 160–161
  idiopathic (primary), 160, 161t
  postencephalitic, vocal tremor in, 100
  symptomatic (secondary), 160, 161t
Parkinsonism-plus syndrome(s), 160, 161t
Paroxetine, for stuttering, 178
PD. See Parkinson disease (PD)
Peak expiratory flow rate, 66, 66f
Peak inspiratory flow rate, 67
PEFR. See Peak expiratory flow rate
Periaqueductal gray, and vocal motor coordination, 24–25
Peripheral nervous system disorders
  affecting swallowing, 150–151, 150t
  laryngeal involvement in, 220–224
Petiole, 4f, 5, 8
Pharyngeal constrictor(s)
  inferior, 7
  middle, 7
Pharyngeal plexus, 207
Pharyngeal receptors, 17–18
Pharyngolarynx
  post-stroke dysfunction, mechanisms, 210–212
  in swallowing, 205–208

Pharyngoparalysis, myopathic, 223
Pharynx
    motor innervation, 207
    sensory innervation, 207
Phenothiazines
    adverse effects and side effects, 182
    for tics, 182
Phonation
    assessment, 54–55, 100
    exertional, 110
    glottal fry, 100
    hyperfunctional (strained), stroboscopic examination, 87
    hypofunctional (asthenic), stroboscopic examination, 87
    ventricular (false) fold, 100
Phonatory-articulatory incoordination, secondary to neurologic disorders, 96, 96t
Phonatory instability
    long-term, 100
    perceptual characteristics, 96t, 100
    secondary to neurologic disorders, 96, 96t, 100–101
    short-term, 100
    speech therapy for, 101
        combined with medical management, 101
    types, 100
Phonatory stability, and voice production, 100
Phonetogram. See Voice range profile
Physical examination, of larynx, 54–55
Pill-rolling tremor, in Parkinson disease, 161
Piriform sinus (fossa), 6f, 8
Pneumothorax, 223
Poliomyelitis, 218
Polyarteritis nodosa, 221
Polymyositis, 223
Polysomnography, with video recording, 69. See also Videopolysomnography
Pontine vocalization area, ventrolateral, 25
Porphyria, 221
Portuguese hereditary amyloid neuropathy, 221
Positron emission tomography (PET)
    of cerebral cortical loci activated in swallowing, 209, 210f
    in dystonia, 171
Postpolio syndrome
    laryngeal involvement in, 218–219
    and vocal fold paralysis/paresis, 108t, 110
Postural adjustments, for airway protection in swallowing, 155, 155f
Postural support, 97–98, 99
Posture, in Parkinson disease, 161
Pre-epiglottic space, 8
Prelaryngeal lymph node, 9
Premotor areas, medial, and vocal motor coordination, 25–26
Premotor neurons, and vocal motor coordination, 24
Presbylaryngis, 117
Presbyphagia, 156–157
Pressure receptors, 17–18
Pressure-volume curve(s)
    for chest wall, 63, 63f
    for lung, 63, 63f
    for total respiratory system, 63, 63f
Propargylamines, for Parkinson disease, 163
Prosody
    disordered
        neurologic disorders and, 96, 96t, 101–103
        perceptual characteristics, 96t, 101
        speech therapy for, 101–103
    vocal control prerequisites for, 101

Prosthetic devices, for management of dysphagia, 154
Pseudobulbar palsy, and vocal fold hyperadduction, 99
Pseudodystonia, 165t
Psychogenic dystonia, 169–170
Pulmonary edema, and hypoxemia, 62
Pulmonary function testing, 59–68
    devices for, 67
Pyramidal disease, 204–215
    causes, 204–205, 206t
    definition, 204–205
Pyramidal tracts, neuroanatomy, 204, 205f

Q

Q (perfusion), 61–62
Quadrangular membrane, 4f, 5, 6f
Quinidine, and unmasking of myasthenia gravis, 223

R

Radiesse, for injection laryngoplasty, 119–120, 120t
Radiesse Light, for injection laryngoplasty, 119–120, 120t
Radiography, in laryngeal paralysis/paresis, 113–114, 113t
Rasagiline, for Parkinson disease, 163
Recurrent laryngeal nerve, 8, 9f, 10, 216
    anatomy, 32
        and laryngeal reinnervation, 144
    complete transection, and laryngeal paralysis, 107
    iatrogenic injury, 222–223
    immunohistology, 34
    injury
        and aspiration, 110
        laryngeal electromyography with, 47f
        laryngeal paresis caused by, neuropathology, 111
        and vocal fold hypoadduction, 97–98
    malignancy and, 221–222
    muscles supplied by, 7, 33, 33f
    paralysis, 217
    physiology, 34
    reinnervation, evaluation using laryngeal electromyography, 50
    and superior laryngeal nerve, intralaryngeal connections, 33
    topography, 34–35
Reflex(es)
    chemoreceptors and, 13–14
    laryngeal, 10
Reinke's space, 8
Reinnervation procedure(s), 143–147
    anatomical considerations, 144
    historical perspective on, 145
    indications for, 146–147
    options for, 145
    Smith's rationale for, 143–144
    techniques for, 145
Reiter's arthritis, laryngeal involvement in, 114
Relapsing polychondritis, 221
Respiration, laryngeal disorders and, 217
Respiratory centers, cortical, 24
Respiratory dysfunction, management, 97–98
Respiratory function testing, 59–68
Respiratory myoclonus, 181
Respiratory-phonatory incoordination
    management, 98
    secondary to neurologic disorders, 96, 96t
Respiratory pressure(s), maximum, measurement, 63–64, 64f
Respiratory-related pressure(s), measurement, 63–67
Respiratory system, active and passive properties of, 63, 63f
Reticular formation, and vocal motor coordination, 24–25
Rheumatoid arthritis (RA)

laboratory diagnosis, 114
and vocal fold immobility, 114
Rigidity, in Parkinson disease, 161
Rima glottidis, 6f, 7
Rima vestibuli, 6f, 7–8
RLN. *See* Recurrent laryngeal nerve
Robinow syndrome, 221

S

Saccule, 6f, 8
Sarcoidosis, 117, 221
    laboratory diagnosis, 114
Sarcopenia, and senescent swallowing, 157
SB. *See* Syringobulbia
SD. *See* Spasmodic dysphonia
Selegiline, for Parkinson disease, 163
Senescent swallowing, 156–157
Sensory deficits, and dysphagia, 89–90
Sensory receptor(s), laryngeal, 10–20
    morphology, 10–11
Sensory trick(s), for ameliorating dystonia, 168
Sertraline, for stuttering, 178
SGCE gene mutations, and dystonia, 170
Shimmer, in neurologic disorders, 100
Shy-Drager syndrome, 221
Sihler's staining, 33
Silastic implants, Netterville technique for, 129–131, 129f–131f
Silicosis, vocal cord paralysis in, 222
Singing, and dystonia, 168
Singulus myoclonus, 179
Sleep
    laryngeal dysfunction in, 69–73
        amyotrophic lateral sclerosis and, 72
        in autosomal dominant spinocerebellar ataxias, 71
        Charcot-Marie-Tooth disease and, 72
        in multisystem atrophy, 69–71
        neurologic diseases causing, 69
        syringobulbia and, 71–72
        syringomyelia and, 71–72
    laryngeal function during, evaluation, 69
    non–rapid eye movement (NREM), 69
    physiology, 69
    rapid eye movement (REM), 69
Sleep-related laryngospasm, 72
SLN. *See* Superior laryngeal nerve
SM. *See* Syringomyelia
SMA. *See* Spinal muscular atrophy
SOD1 gene, 217
Solitary chemoreceptor cells, in specific laryngeal sensory epithelium, 11
Sound pressure levels
    clinical evaluation, 75–76, 75f
    in stroboscopic examination of vocal fold vibrations, 87
Spasmodic dysphonia, 165t, 166, 167–168, 212–213
    abductor, 167–168, 212
        botulinum toxin injection for, 197–198, 198f, 199
    adductor, 99, 167–168, 175, 175f, 212
        botulinum toxin injection for, 197–198, 197f, 199
        phonatory instability in, 100
    amelioration, sensory tricks for, 168
    botulinum toxin injection for, 198–200
        adverse effects, 199–200
        dosage, 199
        electromyography-guided, 52
        rationale for, 198–199
        strategies for, 199
    as dystonia, 167–168
    glottal incompetence in, 117
    laboratory testing in, 55
    laryngeal electromyography in, 51f, 52
    neurologically based, 167
        management, 99–100
    perceptual characteristics, 167
    psychogenic, management, 99–100
    vocal acoustic analysis in, 78
Spastic dysphonia. *See* Spasmodic dysphonia
Spasticity, and vocal fold hyperadduction, 96, 96t, 98–100
Specific laryngeal sensory epithelium (SLSE), 11
Speech
    laryngeal motor innervation for, 24–25
    in multiple system atrophy, 162
    in Parkinson disease, 162
    production, 216
Speech mechanism
    functional components, 96, 96f
    neuropathology, vocal tract characteristics in, 96, 96f
Speech treatment
    for laryngeal disorders, secondary to neurologic disorders, 95–96
    for neurologic disorders, 95–106
        goals for, 103
        intensive, 103
    for phonatory instability, 101
    for stuttering, 178
    for vocal fold hyperadduction, 99–100
    for vocal fold hypoadduction, 97
Spinal muscular atrophy, 218
    type 1, 218
    type 2, 218
    type 3, 218
    and vocal tremor, 100
Spinocerebellar ataxia, 221
Spirometry, 66–67, 66f
SPL. *See* Sound pressure levels
Stent(s)
    laryngeal, 154
    pulmonary artery, 222
Sternohyoid muscle, 7
Sternothyroid muscle, 3, 7
Strap muscles, 7
Streptococcal infection, and tics, 182
Stridor, 110
    inspiratory, in Parkinson disease, 71
    nocturnal, 69
    in multisystem atrophy, 69–70
Stroboscopic examination, 85–88
    principles, 85, 85f
    results recording, form for, 87f
    video recording, 88
Stroboscopic laryngoscopy, 55–57. *See also* Stroboscopic examination
Stroke
    and aspiration, 208, 220
    bilateral, and vocal fold hyperadduction, 99
    brainstem
        dysphagia caused by, 208
        and vocal fold hypoadduction, 96–98
    definition, 204–205
    dysphagia caused by, 89–90, 150, 150t, 208
    hemispheric, dysphagia caused by, 208
    laryngeal dysfunction after, 220
    pharyngolaryngeal dysfunctions caused by, 205
    types, 205

Stuttering, 176–179
  adult-onset, 176
  clinical presentation, 176
  definition, 176
  and dystonia, association between, 177–178
  epidemiology, 176
  etiology, theories about, 177
  factors affecting, 176–177
  historical perspective on, 176
  as movement disorder, 176
  pharmacotherapy for, 178
  phenomenology of, 176, 177–178
  spontaneous recovery from, 176
  therapy for, 178–179
  and tic-like movements, 178
Stylohyoid ligament, 3
Stylohyoid muscle, 7
Stylopharyngeus muscle, 7
Subclavian artery, 8, 9
Substance P
  in laryngeal sensory nerves, 11
  in taste buds, 11
Sudden infant death syndrome (SIDS), 10
Superior laryngeal aperture, 7
Superior laryngeal artery, 9, 9f
Superior laryngeal nerve, 8, 10, 216
  age-related changes in, 89–90
  anatomy, 32
  complete transection, and laryngeal paralysis, 107
  external branch, 8, 9f, 32
    muscles supplied by, 7
  injury
    and aspiration, 110
    laryngeal paresis caused by, neuropathology, 111
  internal branch, 8, 9, 9f
  muscles supplied by, 33–34, 33f
  paralysis, 117, 217
  physiology, 34
  and recurrent laryngeal nerve, intralaryngeal connections, 33
Superior thyroid artery, 9
Support (breathing), 67
Supraglottic closure technique(s), 153
Surgery. *See also* Laryngeal framework surgery; Reinnervation procedure(s)
  for dystonia, 172
  for glottal incompetence, 152
  for glottic closure, 153–154
  laryngeal, in multisystem atrophy, 70
  for laryngeal incompetence, 151–152
  for neurogenic dysphagia, 150t, 151–154
  for Parkinson disease, 163–164
Survival motor neuron (SMN), 218
Swallowing
  age-related changes in, 156–157
  anatomical considerations, 149, 150f, 205–208
  biomechanics, 149, 150f, 205–208
  cerebral cortex and, 208–212
  dysfunction. *See* Dysphagia
  esophageal function in, 149, 150f
  evaluation, 151
  fiberoptic endoscopic examination, 90–91
  flexible endoscopic evaluation, with sensory testing, 89–92
  improvement, prosthetic devices for, 154
  innervation for, 207
  laryngeal function in, 149, 150f, 205–208
  neurologic disorders affecting, 150–151, 150t

  pharyngolarynx in, 205–208
  phases, 205–206
  senescent, 156–157
  sensory input in, 206–207
  sequential, 207
  spontaneous recovery of, post-stroke, cortical reorganization and, 212, 213f
Sydenham's chorea, 182, 184
Synkinesis, laryngeal, 47, 49f, 144
  evaluation using laryngeal electromyography, 50
Syringobulbia
  and laryngeal dysfunction during sleep, 71–72
  laryngeal involvement in, 219
Syringomyelia
  and laryngeal dysfunction during sleep, 71–72
  laryngeal involvement in, 219
Systemic lupus erythematosus (SLE), 221
  chorea in, 184
  laboratory diagnosis, 114
  and vocal fold immobility, 114

T

Tapia syndrome, 220
Tardive dyskinesia, 182
  and vocal fold hyperadduction, 98–100
Tardive dystonia, 182
Taste buds
  epiglottal, 11
  laryngeal
    anatomic distribution, 11
    cellular distribution, 11
    morphology, 11
    ultrastructure, 11
  reflex actions, 11
Teflon, for injection laryngoplasty, 119–120, 120t
Telescopic laryngoscopy, 55–57, 57f, 57t
Tetrabenazine, for tics, 182
Thyroarytenoid muscle, 5, 6f, 8f, 216
  action, 7
  anatomy, 7
  botulinum toxin injection into, 197–198, 197f
  innervation, 8, 33–34, 33f
  needle electrode placement and verification for, 42–43, 43f
  nerve supply, 7
  neuromuscular junctions in, distribution, 35, 35f
Thyroepiglottic ligament, 5
Thyrohyoid ligament(s)
  lateral, 5
  median, 5
Thyrohyoid membrane, 3, 4f, 5, 9f
Thyrohyoid muscle, 3, 7
Thyroid cancer, recurrent laryngeal nerve involvement in, 222
Thyroid cartilage, 4f, 6f, 8, 8f, 9f
  anatomy, 3, 4f
  inferior horn, 3, 4f
  ossification, 3
  superior horn, 3, 4f
Thyroidectomy, and vocal fold paralysis/paresis, 107, 108t
Thyroid function test(s), 113t, 114
Thyroid-stimulating hormone (TSH), evaluation, in spasmodic dysphonia, 55
Thyroplasty. *See also* VoCoM (nonporous hydroxylapatite ceramic) prosthesis
  injection, 152
  medialization, 152

type I, 127, 127f, 152
type II, 128
type III, 128
type IV, 128
Tic(s)
 classification, 181, 181t
 complex, 181, 181t
 definition, 181
 familial occurrence, 181
 laryngeal, 181
 motor, 181, 181t
 phonic, 181, 181t
 simple, 181, 181t
 vocal, 181, 181t
 and vocal fold hyperadduction, 98–100
Tic disorders, 181–182
 comorbidities, 182
 genetics, 181–182
 pharmacotherapy for, 182
Tick-borne relapsing fever, 221
Tidal volume (TV), 59
Tissue engineering, 123–124
TLC. *See* Total lung capacity
TMS. *See* Transcranial magnetic stimulation (TMS)
Tone focus, 99–100
TorsinA, 170
Torticollis, 165t, 166
Total lung capacity, 63
Touch receptors, 15–16
Tourette syndrome, 181
 and stuttering, 178
 vocal tics in, botulinum toxin injection for, 201
Toxin(s). *See also* Botulinum toxin
 chorea induced by, 183t, 184
 vocal cord paralysis caused by, 222
Tracheal cartilage, first, 4f, 6f
Tracheal motion receptors, 17–18
Tracheal tears, repair, laryngeal complications, 223
Tracheoesophageal diversion, 154
Tracheostomy, 153
 in multisystem atrophy, 70–71
Transcranial magnetic stimulation (TMS), of swallowing motor cortex, 208–209, 209f
 and cortical reorganization post-stroke, 212, 213f
Transplantation therapy, for Parkinson disease, 164
Trauma
 and dystonia, 169
 laryngeal involvement in, 222–223
 and vocal fold paralysis/paresis, 107, 108t
Tremor
 abnormal (pathologic), 173
 action, 173
 classification, 173, 173t
 contraction, 173
 definition, 173
 dystonic, 168
 kinetic (intention), 161, 173
 with laryngeal dystonia, 167–168
 normal physiologic, 173
 in Parkinson disease, 161
 postural, 161, 173
 resting, 161, 173
 terminology for, 173, 173t
 vocal, 80–81, 100, 167
  in amyotrophic lateral sclerosis, 176
  anatomic bases, 173–174
  in cerebellar ataxia, 176
  with essential tremor, 175–176
  in multiple sclerosis, 176
  in myasthenia gravis, 176
  neural bases, 100, 173–174
  in Parkinson disease, 174, 176
  pharmacotherapy for, 175–176
  secondary to neurologic disorders, 100
  voice analysis in, 173–174, 174f
  voice characteristics with, 173–174
Triangular membrane (conus elasticus), 4f, 5, 6f
Triticeal cartilage, 4f, 5

U
Ultrasound, in laryngeal paralysis/paresis, 114
Upper esophageal sphincter, 149, 149f, 150f
Upper lip, of vocal fold vibration, 85–86, 86f
Upper motor neuron(s), 204
Upper motor neuron disease, 217
Upper motor neuron injury
 evaluation using laryngeal electromyography, 51
 and vocal fold hyperadduction, 98–100

V
Vagus nerve, 8, 216
 high lesion, laryngeal paresis caused by, neuropathology, 111
 injury, laryngeal paresis caused by, 223
  neuropathology, 111
  signs and symptoms, 110
 lesions, site of, determination using laryngeal electromyography, 50
 neuropathic lesion, and laryngeal synkinesis, 47, 49f
Vallecula, 5, 8
V_A/Q imbalance, 62
V_A/Q ratio, 61–62
Varepsilon-sarcoglycan, and dystonia, 170
Vascular chorea, 184
Vasculitis, systemic, laboratory diagnosis, 55
Velopharyngeal insufficiency, management, 98
Venereal Disease Research Laboratory (VDRL), 114
Ventilation
 changes of partial pressures of atmospheric gases during, 60, 61f
 evaluation, 59–62
Ventilation/perfusion matching, 61–62
ventilation/perfusion mismatch, 61–62
Ventral respiratory group, 23
Ventricle, 6f, 7, 8, 8f
Ventricular dysphonia, botulinum toxin injection for, 201
Ventricular (false) fold phonation, 100
Vestibular ligament, 4f, 5, 6f, 8
Vestibule, 6f, 7
Videofluoroscopic swallow study (VSS), 151
Videolaryngoscopy, 55–57
 stroboscopic, 55–57, 57t. *See also* Stroboscopic examination
Videopolysomnography, 69
 in multisystem atrophy, 70
Videostroboscopy
 in laryngeal paralysis/paresis, 112–113
 in vocal fold atrophy, 118, 119f
 in vocal fold incompetence, 118, 119f
Vincristine chemotherapy, and vocal fold paralysis/paresis, 108t, 110, 222
Viral infection(s), and vocal fold paralysis/paresis, 108t, 110, 221
Vitamin B_{12} deficiency, 221

Vocal acoustic analysis, 74–84
   acquisition strategies for, 75–76
   advances in (future directions for), 79–82
   analysis strategies for, 76–77
   equipment for, 74
   limitations, 74
   literature review, 77–80, 77t–78t, 82
   practical considerations in, 74–75
   recording configuration for, 75, 75f
   theoretical considerations in, 74–75
Vocal arrest, secondary to neurologic disorders, 99
Vocal cord(s), 8f
   false (vestibular), 7, 8f
   movement, intrinsic laryngeal muscle contraction and, 6f
   true, 8
Vocal fold(s)
   adduction
     problems, secondary to neurologic disorders, 96–100, 96t
     reduced, 117
   age-related changes in, 117, 118, 119f
   atrophy, 118, 119f
   bilateral symmetry of movements, stroboscopic examination, 86–87
   extirpative procedures on, 117–118
   horizontal excursion, amplitude, stroboscopic examination, 87
   hyperadduction, 98–100
     compensatory, 99
     perceptual characteristics, 96t, 99
     secondary to neurologic disorders, 96, 96t, 98–100
     speech therapy for, 99
       combined with medical management, 99–100
     support systems for, 99
   hypoadduction
     case example, 98
     perceptual characteristics, 96t, 97
     secondary to neurologic disorders, 96–98, 96t
     speech therapy for, 96t, 97
       combined with medical therapy, 98
     support systems for, 97–98
   incompetence, 117–118
     clinical presentation, 118
     endoscopic findings in, 118, 119f
     etiology, 117–118
     injection laryngoplasty for, 118–123
     patient findings in, 118
     repair
       advances in (future directions for), 123–124
       research on, 123–124
   nonvibrating portion, stroboscopic examination, 87
   paralysis
     bilateral, systemic disorders and, 221
     in cardiovascular disease, 222
     congenital bilateral, 221
     in inherited conditions, 221
     toxin-related, 222
     trauma-related, 222–223
     unilateral, etiology, 117
     vocal acoustic analysis in, 78–79
   paresis
     bilateral, etiology, 107
     unilateral, etiology, 107
   vibrations
     normal patterns, 85–86, 86f

     normal variations, 87
     regularity (periodicity), stroboscopic examination, 87
   stroboscopic examination
     parameters for, 86–87
     principles, 85, 85f
   vibratory cycle, phases, 85–86, 86f
   viscoelasticity, changes in, 117
   volume, reduced, 117
Vocalis muscle, 5, 6f, 216
   innervation, 8
Vocalization, laryngeal motor innervation for, 24–25
Vocal ligament, 4f, 5, 6f
Vocal motor coordination
   cerebellum and, 26–27
   cortical neurons/pathways and, 25–28
   midbrain centers and, 24–25
   motor cortex and, 27–28, 27f
   periaqueductal gray and, 24–25
   premotor neurons and, 24
   reticular formation and, 24–25
   ventrolateral pontine vocalization area and, 25
VoCoM (nonporous hydroxylapatite ceramic) prosthesis, 132f
   complications, 135
   results, 135
   revision, 135
   use of
     Meyer and Blitzer's rationale for, 131–132
     technique for, 132–135, 133f–135f
Voice
   evaluation, 54–55
   production, phonatory stability and, 100
   strained-strangled, 99
   tremulous, 173–174
Voice disorders
   neurologic
     assessment and differential diagnosis, studies of, 77–78, 77t–78t
     onset and course, studies of, 78, 79t
     treatment outcomes, studies of, 78–79, 79t
   in Parkinson disease, 71
Voice range profile, clinical evaluation, 75–76, 76f
Voice therapy
   for vocal fold hyperadduction, 99–100
   for vocal fold hypoadduction, 97–98
Voice-voiceless contrast, neurologic disorders and, 96, 96t

W

Wegener's granulomatosis
   laboratory diagnosis, 114
   and vocal fold immobility, 114
Werdnig-Hoffmann disease, 218
Williams syndrome, 221
Wilson disease, 172
Wohlfart-Kugelberg-Welander syndrome, 218
Writer's cramp, 165t, 166, 167

X

X-linked dystonia-parkinsonism, 171
X-linked spinal bulbar atrophy, 217–218

Z

Zenker's diverticulum, 153